The Diagnostic Process

The Diagnostic Process

Graphic Approach to Probability and Inference in Clinical Medicine

RUDOLF ZALTER, M.D.

Library of Congress Control Number: 2013910345
ISBN: Hardcover   978-1-4836-5031-9
                  Softcover   978-1-4836-5030-2
                  Ebook   978-1-4836-5032-6

Print information available on the last page.

Rev. date: 08/16/2013

To order additional copies of this book, contact:
Xlibris
1-888-795-4274
www.Xlibris.com
Orders@Xlibris.com
127427

This book addresses the decision making process under uncertainty. The process commonly encountered in all fields of human endeavor is called the diagnostic process in this monograph.

The thrust of this book is to help the struggling student, of all ages, in all fields, to cross the threshold from rote to comprehension, thus bridging an intuitive gap left in many a reader's mind regarding the significance and clinical implication of the accompanying probability data.

The text is, in essence, a verbal and graphic portrait of the basic ideas and symbolic structure of probability and statistical inference with particular stress on the Bayesian version. It aims to expound in words, simile, and diagrams the inherent connections obtained between a given event and its sample space or between a given random sample and a hypothesized population. In this sense, no formula is left naked to be absorbed on its face value without the support of a graphic cover. The final result is a firm grasp of the simple concepts that make the infrastructure (not the superstructure) of the subject.

Nonetheless, this is not another book on statistics. It certainly is not a textbook geared for the classroom, and it contains no problem to solve other than those structured and graphed examples needed to clarify and illustrate the thrust of the point under consideration. The book deals exclusively with the two topics that I tend to believe are the core thesis of statistics, namely, probability and its counterpoint, inference, supported by the necessary exposition of sets. Thus, the book does not include the mandatory and important chapters on analysis of variance, regression, and correlation.

Contents

The Graphic Interpretative Approach of Symbolic Idiom
The Ideal Mode of Comprehending the Subject

Introduction

The diagnostic enterprise is a multifaceted systematic approach to the central issue of clinical medicine. This monograph is an attempt to introduce the interested reader to the use of probabilistic logic as a practical tool in clinical medicine. To this end, I tend to believe that the use and manipulation of mathematical symbols as a pure logical instrument, although scientifically irreplaceable, seem to detract from its wider application as a practical tool in everyday communication.

This is particularly true in dealing with uncertainty, where an intuitive appreciation of probability, perhaps more than the capacity to manipulate its symbolic language, is essential. In this case, more so than in other branches of mathematics, the exclusive use of symbolic notation devoid of its graphic equivalent is a restrictive impediment that tends to curtail the imaginative thrust in visualizing the interrelations the problem presents. The same reservation could be raised at the higher levels of mathematical endeavor, although here again the advent of computer-generated graphic analogs to the complex mathematical functions makes it possible to configure at least in the three-dimensional space the structural anatomy of the function.

Nonetheless, this is not another textbook on statistics. It is, in essence, a verbal and graphic portrait of the basic ideas of statistical inference and Bayesian decision analysis so that once a firm grasp of the simple concepts that make the infrastructure of this subject, indeed of all subjects including this one, has been assimilated, the subject matter, no matter how esoteric, is at once rendered comprehensible, logically obvious, and certainly less formidable.

Bayesian decision theory in its modern context is being increasingly applied in diverse fields ranging from business management to medical diagnosis, where the decision-making process under uncertainty is commonly encountered.

In the medical field, the focal point of the diagnostic process is concerned with the resolution of uncertainty through the ability to zero in on the tentative diagnosis and either confirm or rule it out. It is only with this purpose in mind that a given test is ordered and its results evaluated. With the tentative diagnosis in the background, a given test result confronts the physician with the problem of assessing the test result's credibility in contrast to the prior perception in the given case. At its basic level, the credibility factor may be reduced to one of two possible alternatives, either in support or in denial of what had been formulated up to this moment as a tentative diagnosis or working hypothesis to use the mathematical jargon, which is considered as the best fit to account for the clinical data thus far available.

Yet despite the seemingly complex rules and quaint mathematical script, the core idea underlying the act of decision making is a common tool of everyday experience, which can be summarized as follows.

Given a test result, specifically ordered in connection with a tentative diagnosis previously promulgated on the available evidence, the formal approach, impractical as it may appear, is to determine the predictive accuracy of a positive test result in support of the disease in question or equally the predictive accuracy of the negative result in excluding the disease in question.

Alternatively, the question may be phrased in terms of the predictive error incurred, given a positive result in the absence of disease or a negative result albeit the presence of disease. To answer the two basic accuracy parameters, one needs to appreciate that predictive value or accuracy is a complex function of three independent variables, namely, that of sensitivity, specificity, and prevalence.

What Bayes' theorem offers is a quantitative appraisal of the credibility factor attached to the given test result. The quantification of a yes or no decision is the extra dimension required to fine-tune the diagnostic process, which is, in essence, an iterative and sequential pattern of inductive reasoning leading to a final conclusive diagnosis.

This approach to diagnosis may not be practical at all levels of the diagnostic process. Other modalities of diagnosis, including the intuitive pattern recognition, are powerful tools in the hands of experienced clinicians. It is however in the area of decision making, which requires the integration of diverse and specific information, that a quantitative probabilistic approach to decision assumes its unique function. Under certain conditions, decision making is not an optional exercise in judgment strategy that can be dispensed with; it is in effect the only mode of rational decision applicable under the complex circumstances of therapeutic or diagnostic decisions.

This definitive assertion must be partially retracted or modified in field. The numerical manipulation of the data, other than being not always practical in the clinical setting, is of marginal accuracy in view of the fact that prevalence data in particular for the relevant patient subset is most often lacking and at best subjective.

In the modern medical literature, Bayes' theorem in its esoteric probabilistic form and in its simplified variant of sensitivity, specificity, and predictive value has now been in vogue for several decades. It has by all accounts penetrated the medical literature such that all new therapeutic modalities and diagnostic procedures are routinely bolstered by the basic quota of relevant probabilistic data. Yet despite the ubiquitous routine derivation of the necessary fundamental characteristics of a given procedure or test, an intuitive gap is left in many a reader's mind regarding the significance and clinical implication of the accompanying probabilistic data.

Given the previously mentioned considerations, the road to a graphic interpretation of probability theory including its Bayes' formulation must perforce detour through the domain of set theory as the graphic adjunct necessary to the understanding of probabilistic logic of inductive and deductive inference.

With this in mind, a great deal of effort has been made at the graphic level to unravel among other ideas the delicate concepts of dependence and independence in the context of conditional probability.

The monograph is subdivided into four parts:

Part I is an attempt to translate the key concepts of probability into a structured descriptive language, supported and amplified by its graphic counterpart. This approach presupposes a working knowledge of set theory of which the first chapter is a brief introduction supplemented by the necessary counting and enumeration methods.

Part II is formal approach to Bayes' theorem. It is developed utilizing probability rules and set notations. The clinical correlates of sensitivity, specificity, and predictive value are specified both verbally and graphically. The odds and likelihood alternative to probability is considered in a separate chapter.

A special three-part chapter is interposed before the clinical section as an overview of probability and its corollary of frequency distribution supported by a variety of practical examples that may be familiar to the general reader in order to demonstrate the common bond of probabilistic logic, both medical and otherwise.

Part III presents the practical application of the theorem brought forth in a series of detailed relevant clinical situation in which the decision-making process is formulated to reflect the conditional probabilities extant under a given situation.

An optional side trip to symbolic logic as applied to electronic switching circuits is suggested as an additional perspective or a complement to set theory. To this end, a special chapter (chapter 3) has been added to supplement set theory. This may sound as a superfluous assignment for a simple nonmathematical introduction to probability because the diversity of the three subjects may appear on casual inspection to be lacking a common thread with questionable justification for an artificial although optional side trip. Nevertheless, it may be demonstrated that despite the divergence in the subject matter, the theoretical foundation of all three is analogous. It is this analogy in the axiomatic underpinning and the derived operative laws that unifies and simplifies the understanding and practical application of all three subjects. The common unifying language shared by the three related subjects is Boolean algebra using specialized fonts and notation to accommodate the specific subject matter. The diversity of subject as well as the divergent historical development of the individual subject resulted in the application of different sets of notation (one might call it special script or font) to cover the algebraic operations of sets, symbolic logic, and switching circuits. Indeed, it could be argued that all three subjects are special, and a unique application of Boolean algebra if the historical development of the individual subjects is not taken into consideration.

Part IV presents the classical statistical inference both as an estimation or a hypothesis testing approached via the sampling distribution. Here again, the graphic approach to the concept is paramount.

Given the limitations imposed by this approach, the focus on the graphic elements of the theory may prove rewarding if the core idea of probability theory can be transmitted with a minimum of mathematical luggage. In this somewhat unorthodox attempt to present a complex subject, mathematical rigor is perforce a casualty, and the mathematically oriented reader may object to the unwarranted intrusion into a sanctioned territory through simplistic expositions of well-defined algebraic operations and rules. The only consolation that one can offer is that all modalities of human thought are ultimately defined and shared by one unique reasoning process.

Personal Note

This manuscript was relegated to the dormant shelves until now.

A second look prompted by a friendly reviewer initiated this delayed attempt at self-publishing. This monograph is neither a statistical treatise nor a clinical dissertation on selective medical topics. It is essentially an attempt to demystify the logical symbolic steps involved in the diagnostic process and to place them in their correct category as an exercise in Bayesian decision framework with particular emphasis on their graphic analog as the ideal medium of bridging the comprehension gap. Excerpts from a *New York Times* article on a relevant pulse-quickening topic are reprinted at the end of the introduction, illustrating the extent of the logical gap in the process.

In the present medical setting, the diagnostic process is sometimes intuitive, frequently based on pattern identification by the astute clinician and very often unwittingly invoking a probability paradigm, albeit without the solid backing of the conditional order involved.

Please note that tests, procedures, and clinical data used in this book may not be the current standard in medical practice. This should in no way deflect one's attention from the leitmotif of this treatise, namely, the diagnostic process and its graphic match. This of course is independent of new or old medical tests or procedures because it is not the relevance of outmoded clinical data and/or procedures that is at issue but the context in which the data were used in order to graphically illustrate the probabilistic and or inferential model and thus bring to light what may not be apparent to the general science reader, given the abstract contents of solid mathematical reasoning. Nevertheless, a strong caveat about the mathematical rigor needs to be considered, given the graphic and verbal slant of this presentation.

Finally, I am fully aware the no manuscript can escape the editorial scissors and remain intact given that errors, both inadvertent and heuristic, are unavoidable at first try.

Historical Footnote

The principles of the theory of probability are credited to a series of correspondence between Blaise Pascal (1623-1662) and Pierre Fermat (1602-1665) trying to resolve a question regarding the actual odds encountered in a gambling controversy.

Thomas Bayes' (1702-1761) classic paper, "An Essay toward Solving a Problem in the Doctrine of Chance," which is the main topic of this monograph, was published posthumously in 1763. The work antedates Boole's algebraic formulations. It occupies a central position because it is the first attempt at a precise quantitative definition of inductive inference.

Symbolic logic, however, was a fully developed field of mathematics formulated by Gottfried Wilhelm Von Leibnitz (1646-1716) as a system of mathematical logic.

George Boole's (1815-1864) monumental publication, *An Investigation of the Laws of Thought on Which Are Founded Mathematical Theories of Logic and Probabilities*, laid the foundation for the unique algebra common to both fields.

Set theory in its present form owes its formal inception to George Cantor (1845-1918). The Venn diagrams extensively used in this monograph owes its current perfected version to John Venn (1834-1923).

Symbolic logic transformation from a language technique to an indispensable tool of modern digital electronic may be dated as late as 1938 when Claude Shannon (1916-2001) published his seminal paper "A Symbolic Analysis of Relay and Switching Circuits," which was to become the basis for the logical design of digital computers and switching systems.

The diversity of subject ranging from symbolic logic to switching circuits as well as the divergent historical development of the individual subject may have been a factor in the application of different sets of notation (one might call it special Script or Font) to cover the algebraic operations of the individual subject.

The New York Times: Opinionator
April 25, 2010
Chances Are
by Steven Strogatz

Excerpts from the Article

Perhaps the most pulse-quickening topic of all is "conditional probability." In one study, Gerd Gigerenzer (the author of *Calculated Risk*) asked doctors in Germany and the United States to estimate the probability that women with a positive mammogram actually has breast cancer given the following statistics:

The probability that one of these women has breast cancer is 0.8 percent. If a woman has breast cancer, the probability is 90 percent that she will have a positive mammogram.

If a woman does not have breast cancer, the probability is 7 percent that she will still have a positive mammogram.

Imagine a woman who has a positive mammogram. What is the probability that she actually has breast cancer?

When Gigerenzer asked twenty-four German doctors the question, their estimate whipsawed from 1 percent to 90 percent. Imagine how upsetting it would be as a patient to hear such divergent opinions.

Of one hundred American doctors, ninety-five estimated the woman's probability of having breast cancer to be somewhere around 75 percent.

For a detailed answer, please refer to the end of chapter 5 on conditional probability.

Part I

Sets, Counting, and Probability

Chapter 1

Sets

1.1 Sets in Perspective

In the context of this monograph, the concept of sets and its corollary of counting the elements in a given set need to be fully explored as the necessary background to the all-important subject of probability.

1.2 Definition

In general, a set defines a collection or aggregate of distinct elements (objects and points), real or conceptual. The elements of a set run the gamut from the finite number of the letters of the alphabet to the infinite number of integers.

We call the objects that make up an arbitrary set the *members* of the set of the elements of the set.

Sets are represented by one of two methods:

1. Roster method. In this method, the elements that belong to the set are individually listed and enclosed in braces. The order of listing being immaterial. Thus, each of the symbols {a, b, c}, {a, c, b}, and {b, a, c} stands for the same set, namely, the set consisting of the elements a, b, and c. In general, a set is known once its members are known.

$N = \{1, 2, 3, 4, 5, 6\}$, a set of six elements comprising the integers 1 through 6.
$S = \{a, b, c, d\}$; S is the set of elements a, b, c, and d.

2. Descriptive method. In this method, the elements are not listed individually. Instead, the properties common to all elements are listed as necessary qualification for each and every element of the set in question.

$$A = \{ \underset{\text{Set of all letters}}{L} \ \Big| \underset{\text{Such that}}{} \ L \text{ is a vowel}\}$$

$N = \{n \mid 0 < n < 7\}$, the set of all numbers, such that n is between 0 and 7.

$D = \{d \mid$ male patient members of a pulmonary clinic, with resting $PO_2 < 60$ mm Hg$\}$, the set of all male patients, d, such that d satisfies the previously noted restrictions.

Lowercase letters are usually used for elements and capital letters for sets.

1.3 Sets and Subsets

If A and B are sets, and if every member of A is also a member of B, then set A is said to be a proper subset of the set B (i.e., A is included in, or is contained in, B). Thus, A is a proper subset of B if and only if every element of A is an element of B and there exists at least one member of B that is not a member of A.

For example, the set $\{1, 2\}$ is a subset of the set $\{1, 2, 3\}$, but $\{4\}$ is not a subset of $\{1, 2, 3\}$.

The improper subset of set B is the set itself. Thus, the improper set of $\{1, 2, 3\}$ is identically the set itself.

1.4 The Universal Set and Its Subsets

The universal set U is defined as the set containing all the elements, objects, subjects, or members under consideration. All other sets under current consideration are thus subsets of the universal set.

The null set or empty set, $\{ \ \}$, denoted by $\varnothing$ (to be distinguished from the Greek letter phi φ), is the set whose members are listed inside the braces "$\{ \ \}$." In other words, it has no members.

Thus, it is the flip side or reverse of any given "full" set or subset. Because the null set is an empty set, it is easy to visualize Ø as a legitimate subset of every set.

The empty set (Ø) is unique in set theory in that it is the set that has no elements and is therefore a subset of every set. The empty set must not be confused with zero number of elements despite the apparent similarity in context. Zero by itself as 0 is a decimal digit, not a set, but {0} is the set containing one element, namely, 0. On the other hand, Ø is the empty set { } = Ø, that is, the set with no elements.

Note that a set consisting of a single object is not equivalent to the object itself. In other words, {1} is not the same as 1, in the sense that an object within a box is not the same as the naked object itself.

The relationship between the universal set and its possible subsets is best illustrated by enumerating the subsets of a universal set consisting of three elements only; $U = \{a, b, c\}$ (Table 1.1).

Number of Elements in Subset	Subsets of {a, b, c}	Category
None	{ } = Ø	Null subset
1	{a}, {b}, {c}	Single element proper subsets
2	{a, b}, {a, c}, {b, c}	Multielements proper subsets
3	{a, b, c}	Improper subset

Table 1.1. Subsets of a three-element universal set

Note that besides the six subsets composed of one or two elements, two additional subsets need to be included, the null subset and the set itself, U in this case, for a total of eight possible subsets. This relationship can be generalized to apply to any set containing n elements where the number of all possible subsets is equal to 2^n subsets of U.[1] In the case just cited, the number $2^3 = 8$ subsets, as noted earlier. Note also that the order in which the elements of a

---

[1] This derivation will be fully explored in chapter 2.

set are listed does not affect the basic property of the set because the elements only and not their order characterize the set. Similarly, each subset is unique as to its constituent elements irrespective of their order within the subset.

1.4.1 Combining and Comparing Sets

Two sets are defined to be equal or identical if they contain exactly the same number of identical elements irrespective of order, so that if $A = \{1, 2, 3\}$ and $B = \{2, 3, 1\}$, then $A = B$. That is, a set A is equal to a set B if and only if every member of A is a member of B, and every member of B is a member of A.

In general, two sets are unequal provided at least one of them has a member that is not a member of the other.

The union of any two sets A and B, written $A \cup B$, is the set of all elements that are members of A, B, or both.

Thus, if $A = \{1, 2, 3\}$ and $B = \{4, 5\}$, then $A \cup B = \{1, 2, 3, 4, 5\}$.

The intersection of any two sets A and B, written $A \cap B$, is the set of all elements common to A and B, that is, elements shared by both A and B.

Thus, if $A = \{1, 2, 3, 4\}$ and $B = \{4, 5\}$, then $A \cap B = \{4\}$.

The relationship between a set and its complement may be graphically represented and verbally described as follows:

Set A and its complement $\overline{A}$ are subsets of the universal set U (Figure 1.1). Note that set A and its complement, $\overline{A}$, subdivides the universal set into mutually exclusive, exhaustive, and disjoint sets—mutually exclusive because no element in A is shared by its complement $\overline{A}$, exhaustive because the universal set is fully occupied by set A and its complement $\overline{A}$, and disjoint because set A and its complement $\overline{A}$ do not intersect and thus have no elements in common.

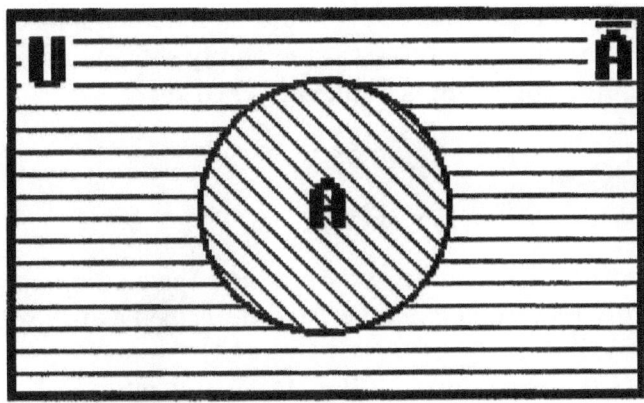

Figure 1.1. Venn diagram of the exhaustive and exclusive partition of the U set by set A and its complement

1.5 Rules Governing Set Operations

1. The union of any set and its complement equals the universal set, and the intersection of any set and its complement equals the null set (Figure 1.7a, panels 2 and 4).

$$A \cup \overline{A} = U \text{ (inversion axiom)} \quad A \cap \overline{A} = \varnothing$$

2. The union of any set with the null set is equal to itself, and the intersection of any set with the null set equals the null set (Figure 1.7a, panels 1 and 3).

$$A \cup \varnothing = A \text{ (identity axiom)} \quad A \cap \varnothing = \varnothing$$

3. The union of any set with the universal set equals the universal set, and the intersection of any set with the universal set equals itself (Figure 1.7a, panels 1 and 3).

$$A \cup U = U \text{ (union and intersection)} \quad A \cap U = A$$

4. The null set and the universal set are complements of each other; all that is not in the universal set is the empty set, and conversely, all that is not in the empty set is in the universal set.

$$\overline{\varnothing} = U \text{ (complements) } \overline{U} = \varnothing$$

The relationship between the two sets and their complements may be graphically represented and verbally described as follows:

1. Sets A and B are disjoint, $A \cap B = \varnothing$, and mutually exclusive, that is, they have no elements in common; they exclude each other, and no two events occur simultaneously among them (Figure 1.2). The universal set is now partitioned into three mutually exclusive and exhaustive sets in which set A could be construed as the intersection of A with the complement of B, and set B could be construed as the intersection of B with the complement of A and the balance of the universal set as the intersection of the complements of A and B. In formal notation,

$$A = A \cap \overline{B}$$

Note the diagonal \\ of A intersecting the vertical $||$ of the B complement.

$$B = B \cap \overline{A}$$

Note the diagonal // of B intersecting the horizontal = of the A complement.

$$\overline{A \cup B} = \overline{A} \cap \overline{B}$$

Note the grid ++ resulting from the intersection of the complements of A and B.

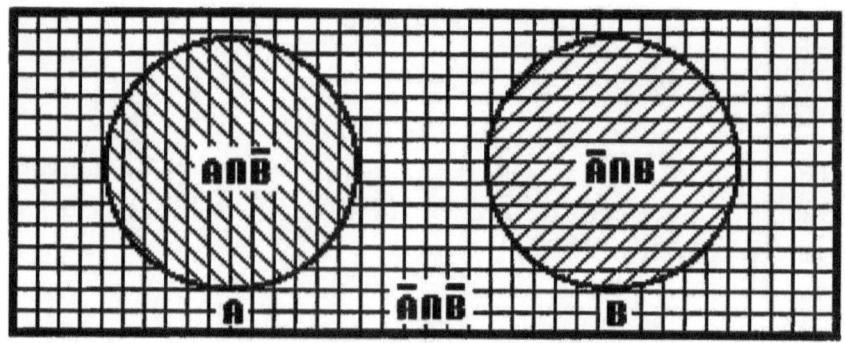

Figure 1.2. Venn diagram of the partition of the U set into three subsets

2. Sets A and B are disjoint, mutually exclusive, and exhaustive, that is, they have no elements in common, and their union comprises the universal set (Figure 1.3). That is, it is impossible that none of them occurred as a result of the experiment.

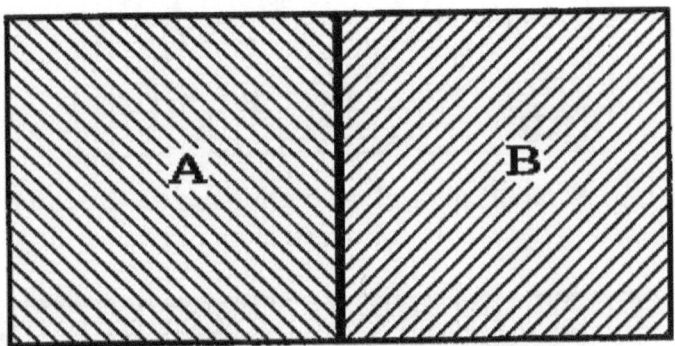

Figure 1.3. Venn diagram of the exhaustive and exclusive partition of the U set by sets A and B

3. Sets A and B are not disjoint, that is, they share a common element(s) at the intersection (Figure 1.4a). Note that A and B and the intersection divide the universal set into four mutually exclusive and exhaustive disjoint subsets, where the intersection area constitute the fourth subset (in contrast to the three subsets of Figure 1.2). The four subsets may thus be categorized as follows (Figures 1.5 and 1.7b):

| $A \cap \bar{B}$ (A but not B) | Panel 6 |

| $\bar{A} \cap B$ (B but not A) | Panel 7 |

| $A \cap B$ (both A and B) | Panel 5 |

| $\bar{A} \cap \bar{B} = \overline{A \cup B}$ (neither A or B) | Panel 7 |

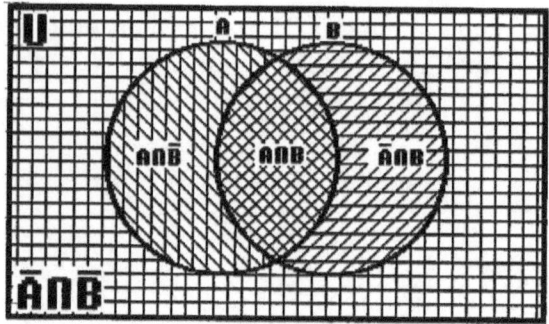

Figure 1.4a. Venn diagram of the partition of the U set into four subsets through the intersection of two sets

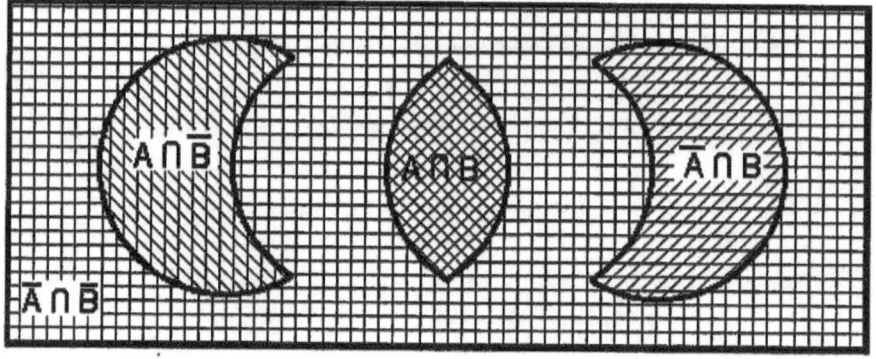

Figure 1.5. Venn diagram of the disjointed subsets of the U set defined by the intersection of the sets and/or their complements

4. Set A is a subset of B, which is a subset of U, which is another way of saying that anything in A is also in B and anything in B is also in U (Figure 1.6). In this case, three disjoint, mutually exhaustive but not mutually exclusive subsets can be recognized.

$$A = A \cap B$$

$$B = \overline{A} \cap B$$

$$\overline{A \cup B} = \overline{A} \cup \overline{B}$$

Note that the intersection of A with the complement of B yields the empty set.

$$A = A \cap \bar{B} = \varnothing$$

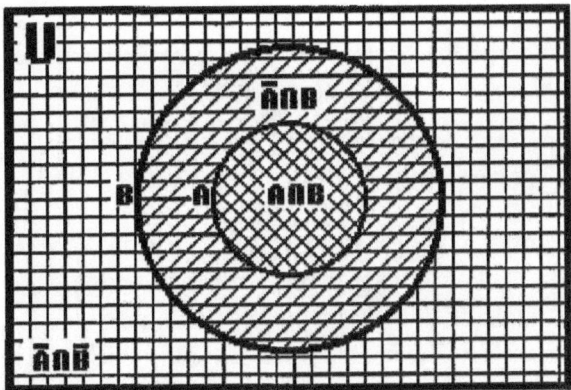

Figure 1.6. Venn diagram of the partition of the U set into three mutually exhaustive, but not mutually exclusive, subsets

1.6 Basic Set Operations

The Venn diagram constitutes the basic graphic element necessary for the intuitive grasp of set interrelations (Figure 1.7b). Traditionally, a rectangle represents the universal set, denoted by U, whereas enclosed circles represent subsets of the universal set. In addition, in order to make full use of the potential of the graphic approach, each given set and its complement will be identified throughout by a distinguishable fill-in pattern, thus allowing instant appraisal of the resultant pattern derived from the interaction of two or more sets.

Four basic operations that may be performed on sets are recognized.

1. Cartesian product. The Cartesian product set of two sets A and B, denoted by $A \times B$, is defined as the set consisting of all possible ordered pairs formed when the first element is taken from the A set and the second element is taken from the B set (Table 1.3).

Thus, if $A = \{a, b\}$ and $B = \{x, y, z\}$, then $A \times B = \{(a, x), (a, y), (a, z), (b, x), (b, y), (b, z)\}$.

Note that $B \times A = \{(x, a), (x, b), (y, a), (y, b), (z, a), (z, b)\}$.

$A \times B$	$\{x, y, z\}$		
$\{a, b\}$	x	Y	z
a	(a, x)	(a, y)	(a, z)
b	(b, x)	(b, y)	(b, z)

Table 1.3. Cartesian product of sets A and B

The elements (ordered pairs) of $B \times A$ are not the same as those of $A \times B$ because the orders are reversed. In other words, (a, x) and (x, a) are distinct elements of their respective sets. Note that the ordered pairs making the elements of the product set $A \times B$ are enclosed in parentheses (not braces) to denote that the order of the individual enclosed elements is important in the differentiation between the resulting ordered pairs.

An ordered pair of elements is not a set because in a set, the order of the elements is completely immaterial: $\{a, b\} = \{b, a\}$. However, in an ordered pair, the additional property of order is essential. The ordered pair (a, b) is to be distinguished from the ordered pair (b, a) if $a \neq b$.

For the sets $B = \{a, b\}$ and $C = \{c, d, e\}$, all possible ordered pairs formed by choosing an element from the set B for the first element and an element from the set C for the second element: $(a, c); (a, d); (a, e); (b, c); (b, d); (b, e)$. This set of ordered pairs is denoted by $B \times C$.

The definition of a Cartesian product set does not specify that the sets used in forming the "product" set need to be the same or different.

For example, if $A = \{1, 2, 3\}$ and $B = \{a, b\}$, then

(a) $A \times B = \{(1,a), (1,b), (2,a), (2,b), (3,a), (3,b)\}$.
(b) $B \times A = \{(a,1), (a,2), (a,3), (b,1), (b,2), (b,3)\}$.
(c) $A \times A = \{(1,1), (1,2), (1,3), (2,1), (2,2), (2,3), (3,1), (3,2), (3,3)\}$.
(d) $B \times B = \{(a,a), (a,b), (b,a), (b,b)\}$.

The ordered pair idea may be generalized to include any ordered arrangements, which may be formed from n objects (ordered n-tuples) constituting the elements of a set. A set may therefore be composed of ordered pairs, ordered triplets, ordered 4-tuples, . . . , ordered n-tuples, but not duplicate elements.

2. Union. The union of two sets, $A + B$, denoted by $A \cup B$, is the set of elements contained within A or B or both, such that an element that belongs to A or B belongs to their union (panel 8).

3. Intersection. The intersection of sets $A \cdot B$, denoted by $A \cap B$, is the set of the elements that belong to both A and B. That is the set of elements shared or common to both A and B.

Note that the shaded area of intersection in panel 5 is actually crosshatched through the intersection the diagonal patterns of set A and set B so as to reflect the shared or common elements of both sets (Figure 1.7b, panel 5).

4. Complement. The complement of a set is the set of elements outside the set but within the universal set U, usually denoted by $\overline{A}$ or A' (Figure 1.7a, panels 2 and 4).

As a concrete example, consider the experiment of rolling a die. The single digit numbers generated are elements of the universal set $S = \{1, 2, 3, 4, 5, 6\}$. Applying the rule defined earlier, the number of subsets that could be derived from the set of six numbers (2^6) equals 64 different subsets ranging in size from no elements of the empty subset to one element per subset up to the total of six elements of the universal set. Within this constraint, we may have 6 one-element subsets, 15 two-element subsets, and so on.

Consider now the subset of even numbers and its complement of odd numbers so that

$$S_{even} \overset{\text{Union}}{\cup} \overline{S}_{odd} = S_{universal} ; \{2, 4, 6\} \cup \{1, 2, 3\} = \{1, 2, 3, 4, 5, 6\}$$

The union of the even subset with the subset made up two elements larger the four is graphically and symbolically denoted as follows:

$$\{2, 4, 6\} \cup \{5, 6\} = \{2, 4, 5, 6\}$$

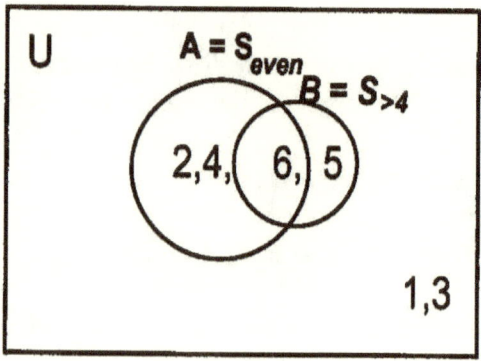

Figure 1.4b

The union of the two subsets is the set that consists of all the elements of S_{even}, $S_{>4}$, or both.

Note that the word *or*, when used in the context of sets interrelationship, carries the exclusive meaning of the equivalent word of union, which is normally symbolized by the set notation $\cup$ or its algebraic counterpart, the plus sign (+).

The intersection of the two subsets, on the other hand, is denoted as follows and graphically as previously mentioned:

$$\{2, 4, 6\} \cap \{5, 6\} = \{6\}$$ diagonal // and diagonal \\ grid ×

The intersection of the two subsets is the set consisting of all the elements common to S_{even} and $S_{>4}$. Note that the word *and*, when used in the context of sets interrelationship, carries the exclusive meaning of the equivalent word of intersection, which is normally symbolized by the set notation $\cap$ or its algebraic counterpart, the dot sign (•).

Comparing Figure 1.4a with Figure 1.4b, it can be readily appreciated that the patterns associated with the subsets of Figure 1.4a correspond to the elements associated with each subset.

$$\overset{A=\text{Seven}}{\{2,4,6\}} \cap \overset{\bar{B}}{\{2,4,1,3\}} = \overset{A\cap\bar{B}}{\{2,4)}$$

diagonal \\ and vertical || pattern

$$\overset{B=S_{>4}}{\{5,6\}} \cap \overset{\bar{A}}{\{5,1,3\}} = \overset{\bar{A}\cap B}{\{5\}}$$

diagonal // and horizontal = pattern

$$\overset{\bar{A}}{\{1,3,5\}} \cap \overset{\bar{B}}{\{2,4,1,3\}} = \overset{\bar{A}\cap\bar{B}}{\{1,3\}}$$

diagonal || and horizontal = grid ++

1.7 Combined Set Operations

1.7.1 Intersection of a Set with the Complement of Another Set

In Figure 1.7b, panel 6, set A is intersecting the complement of set B. The resulting shaded area in this case is crosshatched through the intersection of the diagonal pattern, \\, of set A with the vertical pattern, ||, of the complement of set B.

In Figure 1.7b, panel 7, set B is now intersecting the complement of set A. The resulting shaded area reflects the intersection of the diagonal pattern of set B, //, with the horizontal pattern, =, of the complement of set A.

1.7.2 Union of a Set with the Complement of another Set

In Figure 1.7b, panel 10, the vertical pattern, ||, of the complement of set B is superimposed on the diagonal, \\, pattern of set A. The result of the superimposition (not the intersection) is the complex partitioning the universal set into four distinct patterns.

Panel 11 reverses the union so that the complement of set A, that is, the horizontal pattern, =, is now grafted on the diagonal pattern, //, of set B, resulting in a different partitioning of the universal set into four distinct patterns.

1.7.3 Intersection of the Complements of Two Sets

In Figure 1.7b, panel 12, the complement of set A is intersected with the complement of set B. The intersected area is readily visualized comprising the area outside both set A and set B. In contrast to panel 8, the intersected area excludes the elements in both set A and set B as well as their intersection. The grid pattern of the intersection reflects the super positioning of the horizontal pattern of the complement of set A and the vertical pattern of the complement of set B. Comparing panel 8 with panel 12, it is immediately realized that these two panels are the exact complements of each other.

1.7.4 Union of the Complements of Two Sets

In Figure 1.7b, panel 9, the complement of set A is merged with the complement of set B. The resulting merger, delineated by the superimposition of the horizontal and vertical grids of A and B, includes all the elements that are outside A (horizontal pattern, =) and thus include the part of B that is not in A. The merger also includes all the elements that are outside B (vertical pattern, ||), including the part of A that is not in B. The resulting pattern may be easily visualized by superimposing panel 1a on panel 3a to reflect the common elements, comprising almost the total sample space of the universe, except for the actual area of intersection of set A with set B. What is readily noticeable by comparing panel 9 with panel 5 is that panel 9 may be viewed as the exact complement of panel 5 or, alternatively, panel 5 as the complement of panel 8.

1.7.5 DeMorgan's Laws

The relationship between panels 5 and 8 (Figure 1.7b) is formulated by the first of the two DeMorgan's laws:

1. The complement of the intersection is the union of the complements.

$$1.\ \overline{A \cap B} = \overline{A} \cup \overline{B}$$

The relationship between panels 12 and 8 (Figure 1.7b) is formulated by the second of the two DeMorgan's laws:

2. The complement of the union is the intersection of the complements.

$$2.\ \overline{A \cup B} = \overline{A} \cap \overline{B}$$

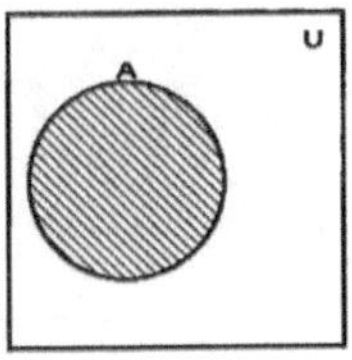	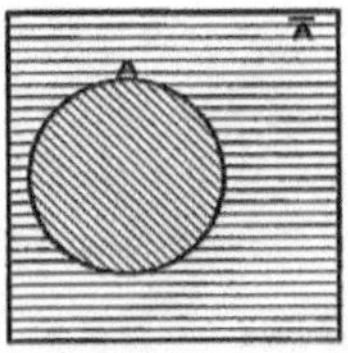	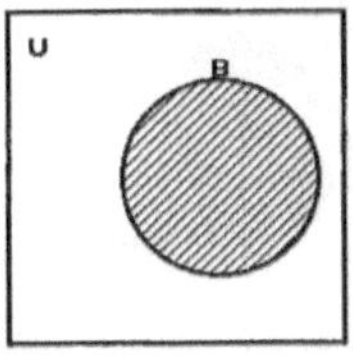	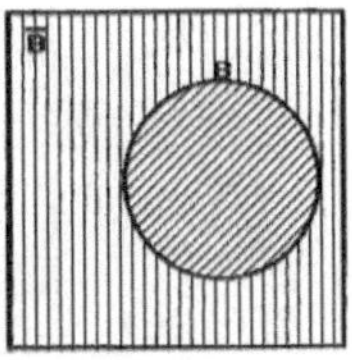
$A \cup \varnothing = A$	$A \cup \overline{A} = U = 1$	$B \cup \varnothing = B$	$B \cup \overline{B} = U = 1$
$A \cap \varnothing = \varnothing$	$A \cap \overline{A} = \varnothing$	$B \cap \varnothing = \varnothing$	$A \cap \overline{B} = \varnothing$
$A \cup U = U$	$A \cup A = A$	$B \cup U = U$	$B \cup B = B$
$A \cap U = A$	$A \cap A = A$	$B \cap U = B$	$B \cap B = A$
Diagonally shaded, \\, set A isolated from the unshaded and excluded universe	Diagonally shaded, \\, set A isolated from its horizontally shaded, =, complement	Diagonally shaded, //, set B isolated from the unshaded and excluded universe	Diagonally shaded, //, set B isolated from its vertically shaded, ‖, complement
Panel 1	Panel 2	Panel 3	Panel 4
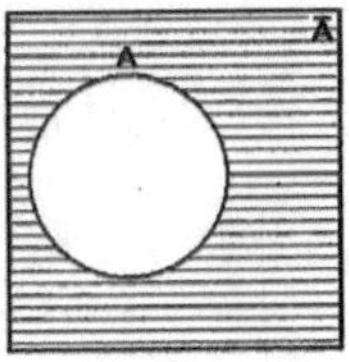		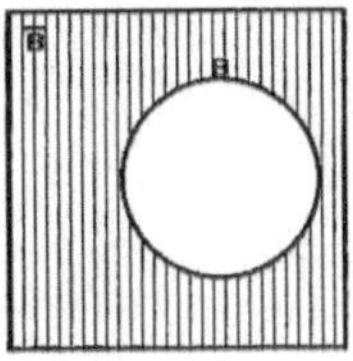	
Horizontally shaded, =, complement of A isolated from the unshaded (deselected, excluded) A		Vertically shaded, ‖, complement of B isolated from the unshaded (deselected, excluded) B	
Panel 1a	Panel 2	Panel 3a	Panel 4

Figure 1.7a. Venn diagram of the basic set operations: complementation

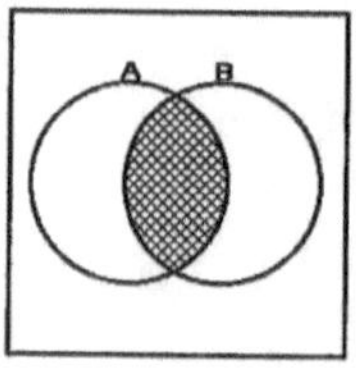	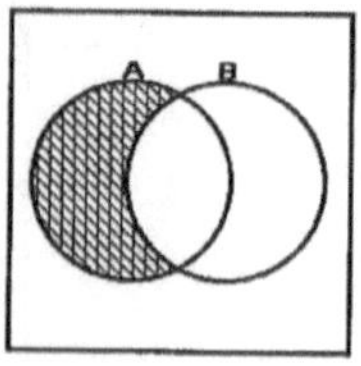	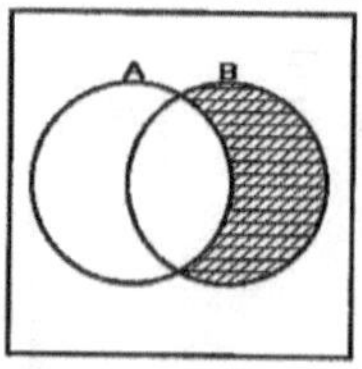	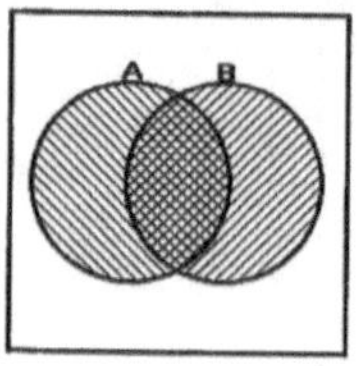
$A \cap B$	$A \cap \overline{B}$	$\overline{A} \cap B$	$A \cup B$
$A \bullet B$	$A \bullet \overline{B}$	$\overline{A} \bullet B$	$A + B$
A and B	A and $\overline{B}$	$\overline{A}$ and B	A or B
Diagonally shaded, \\, A intersecting diagonally shaded, //, B; cross diagonal, ×, intersection	Diagonally shaded, \\, A intersecting vertically shaded B complement	Diagonally shaded, //, B intersecting horizontally shaded A complement	Diagonally shaded, \\, A superimposed on diagonally shaded, //, B
Panel 5	Panel 6	Panel 7	Panel 8
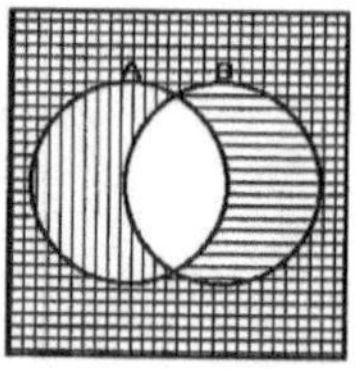	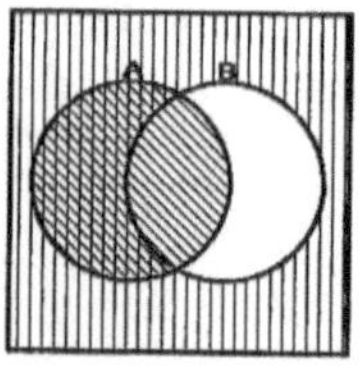	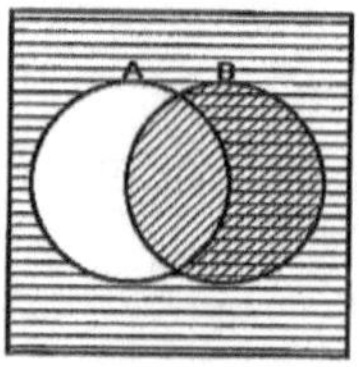	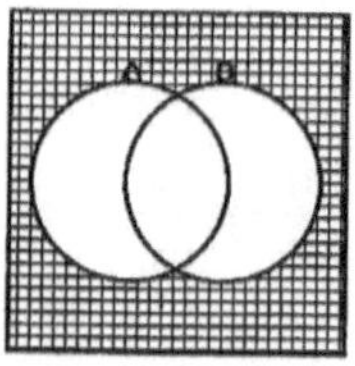
$\overline{A} \cup \overline{B} = \overline{(A \cap B)}$	$A \cup \overline{B}$	$\overline{A} \cup B$	$\overline{A} \cap \overline{B} = \overline{(A \cup B)}$
$\overline{A} + \overline{B} = \overline{A \bullet B}$	$A + \overline{B}$	$\overline{A} + B$	$\overline{A} \bullet \overline{B} = \overline{A + B}$
$\overline{A}$ or $\overline{B} = \overline{A \text{ and } B}$	A or $\overline{B}$	$\overline{A}$ or B	$\overline{A}$ and $\overline{B} = \overline{A \text{ or } B}$
Vertically shaded, ||, complement of B superimposed on the horizontally shaded, =, complement of A	Diagonally shaded, \\, A superimposed on the vertically shaded, ||, complement of B	Diagonally shaded, //, B superimposed on the horizontally shaded, =, complement of A	Vertically shaded, ||, complement of B intersecting the horizontally shaded, =, complement of A; gridlike, +, intersection
Panel 9	Panel 10	Panel 11	Panel 12

Figure 1.7b. Venn diagram of the basic set operations: intersection and union, DeMorgan's laws

1.8 Extended Venn Diagrams

The Venn diagram can be extended to cover the union and intersection of three sets. As noted in Figure 1.8, the union of three distinct sets, A, B, and C, yields eight distinctly patterned subsets resulting from the superposition of three basic patterns. In contrast, the intersection of the three basic patterns yields the composite pattern of the central area whose elements are shared by all three sets. Note that DeMorgan's laws are clearly visualized by comparing each of the middle diagrams with its complement on the bottom as expressed in the following relations:

$$1.\ \overline{A \cap B \cap C} = \overline{A} \cup \overline{B} \cup \overline{C}$$

$$2.\ \overline{A \cup B \cup C} = \overline{A} \cap \overline{B} \cap \overline{C}$$

1.9 Blood Phenotypes

The three-ring Venn diagram provides a lucid graphic depiction of the eight blood phenotypes resulting from the intersection of the three major antigenic sets (Figure 1.9).

A person's ABO blood type depends on the presence or absence of two similar carbohydrate antigens located on the cell membrane of red blood cells. Persons with type A blood possess a network of the A antigen on their red blood cells. Persons with blood type B display antigen B on their red cells surface. Persons with type AB have both antigens on their red blood cells, and finally, persons with type O lack both A and B surface antigens.

The serum of persons with type A antigens on their red blood cells contains antibodies against type B cells (anti-B antibodies). Persons with type B blood have antibodies against type A cells (anti-A antibodies). Type O serum contains antibodies against both A and B cells, and type AB serum contains neither anti-A nor anti-B.

When a transfusion is incompatible, the antigen on the donor cells will react with the recipient's serum antibodies, which in turn activates the complement, resulting in the lysis of the donor's red blood cells.

The Rh factor defines a fourth antigen, Rh^+, normally present on the cell surface in approximately 85 percent of the population. In this case, however, antibodies that react with the Rh antigen do not occur naturally in the serum of Rh^- individuals, although exposure to this antigen can sensitize the exposed Rh^- person to produce anti-Rh antibodies.

All these factors with their numerical counterpart can by succinctly expressed and manipulated through the use of a three-ring Venn diagram as illustrated in Figure 1.9.

The three-ring diagram can be used to solve and illustrate problems with cumbersome data. A maximum of four sets may be graphically handled, although with difficulty.

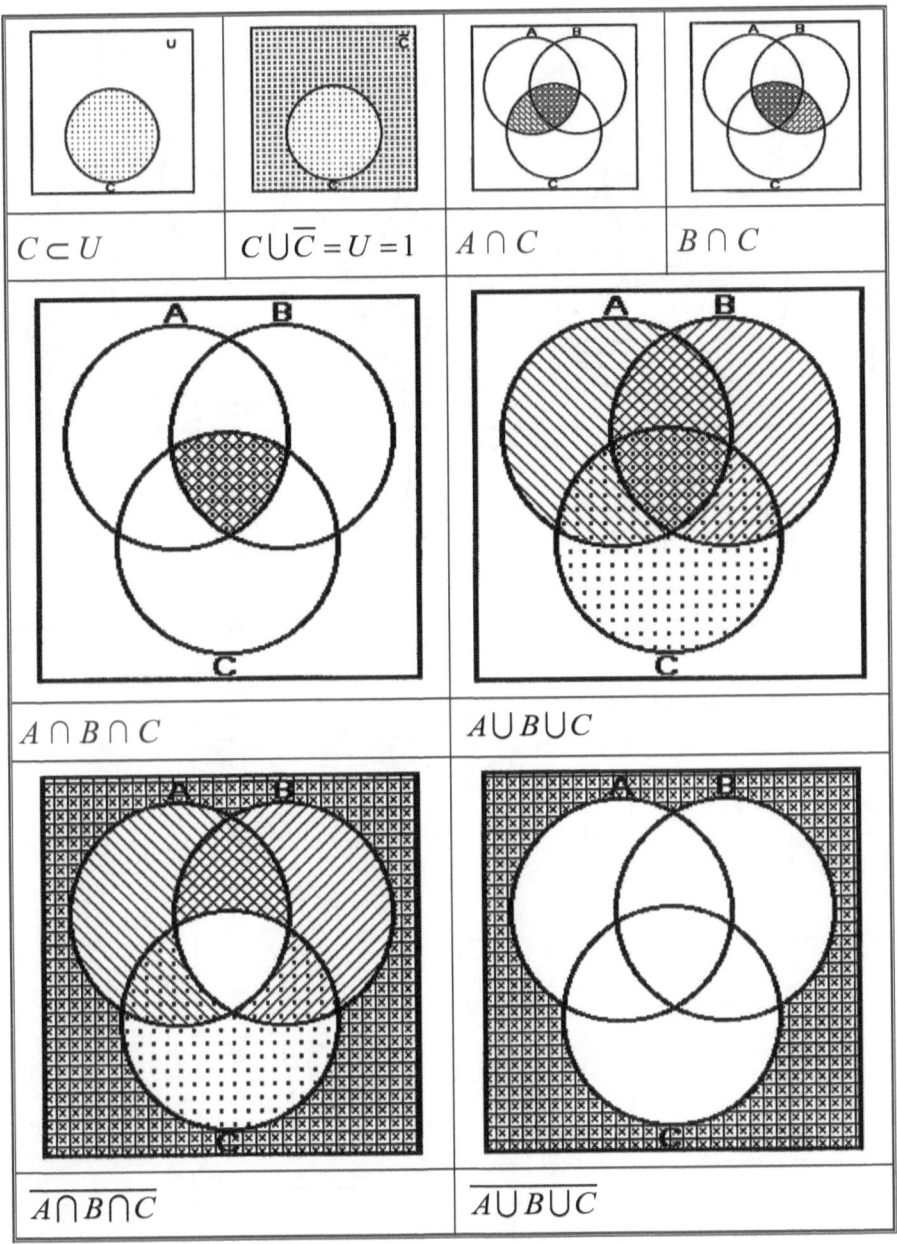

Figure 1.8. Venn diagram of the partition of the universal set into eight mutually exclusive and exhaustive subsets

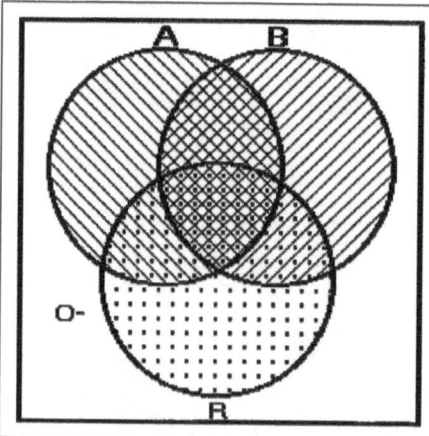

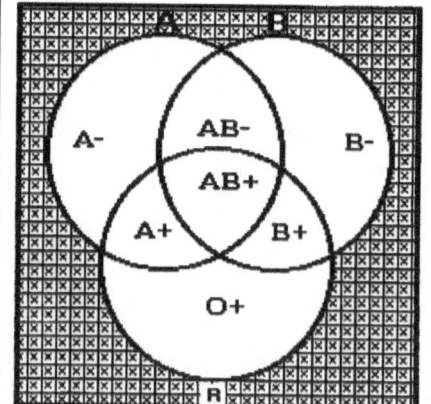

Blood is categorized or typed according to which of the three antigens A, B, and Rh are present. The table lists the eight different blood types

Blood phenotype

Blood phenotype	Antigens		
AB+	A	B	Rh
AB−	A	B	-
A+	A	-	Rh
A−	A	-	-
B+	-	B	Rh
B−	-	B	-
O+	-	-	Rh
O−	-	-	-

$AB+: A \cap B \cap R$

$AB-: A \cap B \cap \overline{R}$

$A+: A \cap \overline{B} \cap R$

$A-: A \cap \overline{B} \cap \overline{R}$

$B+: \overline{A} \cap B \cap R$

$B-: \overline{A} \cap B \cap \overline{R}$

$O+: \overline{A} \cap \overline{B} \cap R$

$O-: \overline{A} \cap \overline{B} \cap \overline{R}$

Figure 1.9. Venn diagram of the graphic and quantitative assignment of the eight blood phenotypes resulting from the intersection of the three major antigenic sets; the corresponding subsets of the universal set

Chapter 2A

Counting Techniques and Enumeration Methods

In chapter 1, a set was defined as a collection or aggregate of distinct elements, real or conceptual, that runs the gamut from finite to infinite numbers. The key question that flows naturally form the stated definition must address the number of elements in any given set. Thus, the number of elements that make up a given set represents a parameter of singular importance, referred to as the cardinality of the set. At the basic level, given a set of primary elements, simple counting is all that is required to answer the question. For the set $S = \{a, b, c, d\}$, composed exclusively of the primary elements, a, b, c, and d, counting the number of elements is a trivial exercise. On the other hand, if it is required to count the number of composite elements or subsets that can be derived from all the possible alignment of the four primary letters, a more elaborate counting technique is required to account for all the possible composite elements that can be derived from the basic set of the four elements.

Because by definition an event is an aggregate of simple or primary elements, the computation of the ways by which the elements of the sample space can be assembled to form a given event requires a thorough familiarity with the counting techniques. In this context, enumeration methods and counting techniques become a prerequisite for set manipulation. Two major principles are involved in the counting process. Together, they provide the framework on which the counting processes are structured.

2A.1 The Multiplication Principle

In the application of the principle, two graphic techniques may prove helpful in configuring all the possible outcomes. The first technique and perhaps the more intuitive method is the use of an array of cells or cubicles to represent each choice separately.

Thus, for the simple question, how many ways can a chairman and a secretary be chosen from a committee of four? the obvious answer is that there are four ways of choosing the chairman; and after he has been chosen, there are three ways of choosing the secretary from the remaining three members. Hence, by the principle, $n \times (n - 1) = 4 \times 3 = 12$ ways of choosing both ($4P_2 = 12$).

Ways of choosing the chairman	Ways of choosing the secretary	Ways of choosing the chairman and the secretary
4	3	$4 \times 3 = 12$

If the four committee members are designated a, b, c, and d, the twelve selections can be shown as follows. In each pair of letters, the first is the chairman and the second is the secretary:

$$\{(a,b);(b,a);(a,c);(c,a);(a,d);(d,a);$$
$$(c,d);(d,c);(b,d);(d,b);(b,c);(c,b)\}.$$

Note that the set of the multiplication result now consists of twelve composite elements, each with equal possibility of being the one chosen.

As a practical application, consider the possible number of the medallion yellow cabs in New York City. For each cab, the medallion number consists of a single digit followed by a single letter of the alphabet followed by two digits (e.g., 4 k 58). Thus, the total number of medallions that could be issued cannot exceed $10 \times 26 \times 10 \times 10 = 26,000$ medallions. In this case, the sample space is made up of 26,000 medallions, each carrying a composite number.

Sample Medallion No.	4	k	5	8
Possible digit-letter-digit-digit sequence	10 (0-9)	26 (letters)	10 (0-9)	10 (0-9)

Note that each numerical cell may be filled by any one of ten digits (0-9) while the letter cell may represent only one of twenty-six letters.

When the number of ways of performing an act remains identical, the multiplication product can be abbreviated. If a coded signal is to be transmitted using a six-digit sequence of 0s and 1s, the possible number of coded words could be simply derived by the so-called pigeon holes technique.

Two ways 0 or 1	Two ways 0 or 1	Two ways 0 or 1	Two ways 0 or 1	Two ways 0 or 1	Two ways 0 or 1
First place	Second place	Third place	Fourth place	Fifth place	Sixth = rth place

$$2 \times 2 \times 2 \times 2 \times 2 \times 2 = n^r = 2^6 = 64$$

Rolling a pair of dice is essentially a compound experiment consisting of two independent trials in which the red die may assume any one of six face values and the white die may likewise turn up in any one of six face values. Hence, by the multiplication principle, the number of ways that a pair of dice may turn up is $6 \times 6 = 6^2 = 36$ (nPn^r; Table 2.17, item 3 of permutations formulae).[2]

The multiplication principle, also called the *fundamental counting principle*, is the basic counting technique or enumeration method that addresses the question, how many ways two or more consecutive acts can be performed? The acts may be independent or dependent and each made up of identical or different elements. The answer needs to consider the number of ways in which each act can be performed as well as the nature of the relation between the consecutive acts.

When consecutive acts are repetitive and independent, that is, the performance of one does not affect the number of ways of doing the other and therefore are not mutually exclusive, the product of such r acts results in a set of composite elements each of which is

---

[2]   Refer to Table 2.17 for a concise listing of relevant formulae.

composed of one defined sequence or permutation of the primary simple elements of the acts performed (Table 6.1, 6b).

The process, both graphic and calculated, utilized in arriving at the number of sequences, stipulates that if an operation consisting of r steps in which the first step assume n_1 possible outcomes, that is, it can be performed in n_1 ways, followed by a second step, similarly assumed to consist of n_2 possible outcomes or performed in n_2 ways (irrespective of the outcome of the first step), and the same of the third and rth steps, then $n_1 \times n_2 \times \ldots n_r =$ the number of all possible outcomes resulting from the performance of the entire sequence, which is also the number of possible ways of performing the entire operation sequence. The derived sequences may now be considered as the elements of a new set made of all the possible sequences.

In formal language, the multiplication principle may be formulated, as noted in Table 2A.1.

	Dependent Events	Independent Events
Mutually exclusive, disjoint, asynchronous	Mutually exclusive events are automatically dependent because they cannot occur simultaneously	Independent events cannot be mutually exclusive; impossible event
	Summation principle: If act I can be performed in n_1 different ways and act II can be performed in n_2 different ways, then either act I or act II can be performed in $n_1 + n_2$ different ways	

Mutually, nonexclusive, conjoint, synchronous	Both general rules of union and intersection are required	The multiplication principle: If act I act can be performed in just n_1 different ways, and if after it has been done in one of those ways, act II can be done in just n_2 different ways, then both acts can be performed in the order stated in just $n_1 \times n_2$ different ways

Table 2A.1. Summation and multiplication principles in relation to timing and dependence

The principle may be extended to include any number of consecutive acts, resulting in a set of ordered r-tuples, which defines all the possible sequence (permutations) of the acts in performing the complete operation,

$$n_1 \times n_2 \times n_3 \times \ldots n_r \text{ set of all possible permutation of the elements in } n_1, n_2, \ldots n_r.$$

On the other hand, when, in addition, the acts are identical with outcome, all the possible sequences now become the product of n identical number of ways of doing each act. The multiplication process can thus be abbreviated to raising the specified number of ways for each act, n, by the exponent, r, the equivalent of the number by which the experiment was repeated [3. nPn^r],

$n \times n \times n \times n = n^r$ set of all possible permutation of the elements in $n \times n \times$.

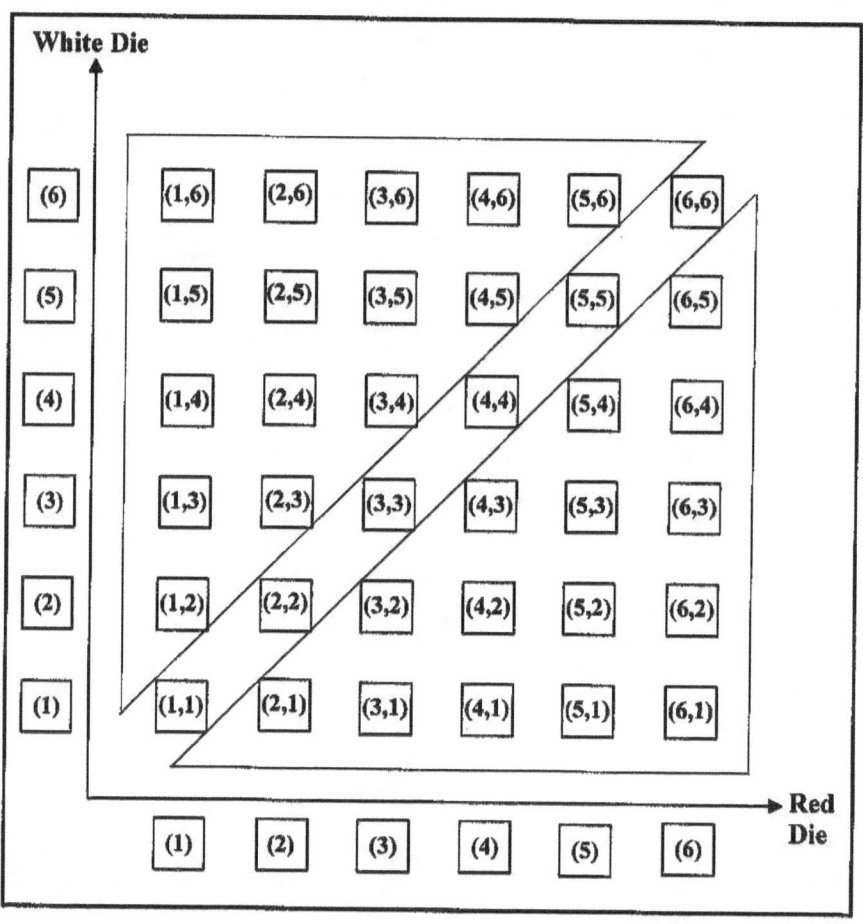

Table 2A.2. Set of all possible ordered pairs (composite elements) obtained on rolling a pair of dice

Table 2A.2 shows the sample space that lists the possible ordered pairs for this experiment. Note that the red die is always recorded first. For example, the sample point (1,6) is obtained when the red die turns up 1 and the white die 6. In other words, each face value on a red die may be coupled to any one of six values on the white, resulting in 36 ordered pairs.

The ordered pairs of the compound experiment constitute the sample points in a sample space in which every point is equally likely to occur as a result of any one roll of the dice (Table 2A.3).

a_1	a_2	a_3	a_4	a_5	a_6
a_7	a_8	a_9	a_{10}	a_{11}	a_{12}
a_{13}	a_{14}	a_{15}	a_{16}	a_{17}	a_{18}
a_{19}	a_{20}	a_{21}	a_{22}	a_{23}	a_{24}
a_{25}	a_{26}	a_{27}	a_{28}	a_{29}	a_{30}
a_{31}	a_{32}	a_{33}	a_{34}	a_{35}	a_{36}

Table 2A.3. Mutually exclusive, exhaustive, and equally likely simple events

In a similar way, tossing a number of coins is actually a compound experiment consisting of independent trials in which the outcome of each tossed coin may turn up head or tail, which is independent of the outcome of any other coin in the experiment. Thus, the sample space for a given experiment of tossing two coins is equal to the Cartesian product: $P \times N = \{H, T\} \times \{H, T\} = 2 \times 2 = 2^2 = 4$ ordered pairs (Table 2A.4).

$P \times N$	Penny	
Nickel	Head	Tail
Head	HH	TH
Tail	HT	TT

Table 2A.4. Set of four ordered pairs

A more practical technique of addressing the same question albeit in different format is to ask, "In how many ways can the outcome of tossing three different coins be arranged?" taking into consideration the fact that simultaneous or successive trials are assumed to yield identical results because the results of flipping one coin at a time is not different from the simultaneous tossing of all three, given that the outcome of each coin is independent from the others. In other words, there are two ways in which the first coin may turn.

Irrespective of the way the first coin turns out, the second coin assumes similarly one of two options. The same applies to the third coin. The classical approach is to deploy an array of empty contiguous cells (pigeon holes) to be consecutively filled out with the number of ways resulting from performing the act. In the case under consideration, consider a series of three cells ready to receive either of the two elements of the three sets.

The first cell may be filled out in two ways: H or T, and the second and third cells may be similarly filled out. Each step consists of either the inclusion or the exclusion of a particular element.

2	2	2

The number of composite elements thus derived is $2 \times 2 \times 2 = 2^3 = 8$. The resultant sample space now consists of eight composite elements corresponding to the eight possible outcomes of the tossing experiment,

$$\{HHH, HHT, HTH, HTT, THH, THT, TTH, TTT\}.$$

The eight outcomes in the above set are the secondary and composite elements of the sample space of the experiment resulting from the performance of a multiple of the basic tossing experiment of a single coin. The eight elements listed above were empirically enumerated because it was practical to cover all the possible sequence in the triads involved with minimal effort. It is, however, the principle underlying the enumeration and counting process of the composite elements in the derivative sample space that is of paramount importance because it allows its application to be universal.

In the previously mentioned experiment, the number of permuted outcomes resulting from tossing three coins is then equal to the product of the numbers in the cells, so that

$$2 \times 2 \times 2 = [\text{No. of outcomes of tossing a coin}]^{\text{No. coins}} = 2^{\text{No. coins}} = 2^3$$
$$= 8 \text{ distinct outcomes.}$$

In a similar vein, for the experiment of rolling a die, the sample space of a single trial, SS = {1, 2, 3, 4, 5, 6}, includes the six possible elemental outcomes of the roll.

The same line of reasoning applies to the SS of rolling two dice, whose Cartesian product sample space, SS = { (1,1); (1,2); . . . ; (6,6)}, is now configured to be composed of thirty-six composite elements (Table 2A.1).

Again, note that the product consists of thirty-six ordered (permuted) pairs such that $(1,6) \neq (6,1)$,

$$SS_{Red} \times SS_{White} = SS_{Product} = \{(\overset{Red}{1}, \overset{White}{6});(\overset{Red}{2}, \overset{White}{6});...;(\overset{Red}{6}, \overset{White}{1})\}$$

$$6 \times 6 = 6^2 = 36$$

For three identical dice rolled simultaneously or consecutively, the sample space now consists of 216 ordered triples. Stated differently, how many three-digit numbers can be made from the six digits {1, 2, 3, 4, 5, 6}? [3. Pn^r]

$$6 \times 6 \times 6 = 6^{No.\ dice} = 6^3 = 216$$

By the same process, tossing four coins results in a sample space made up of $2 \times 2 \times 2 \times 2 = 2^4 = 16$ composite elements (not subsets) represented by the set {HHHH, HHHT, . . . , TTTT}.

The multiplication principle as applied so far to identical repetitive trials may be extended to include the product of two or more sample spaces that characterize the possible outcome of different trials.

Rolling two dice (a cube and a twelve-sided dodecahedron) gives rise to a Cartesian product of $6 \times 12 = 72$ ordered pairs instead of the thirty-six ordered pairs encountered in rolling the pair of standard dice.

In response to the question, "In how many ways can a specific sequence or order of elements chosen from a given sample space be arranged?" the multiplication principle resulted in the enumeration of all possible sequential arrangements in the form of ordered pairs, triplets, or *n*-tuples. This is in effect the concept of permutation, which specifically addressed the question of sequential alignment of the elements of the sample space.

The second graphic technique is the classic tree diagram in which the number of branches corresponds to the actual count of possibilities.

The tree diagram, frequently used to configure all possible outcomes, illustrates a practical technique for the derivation and computation of all possible permutations of a reasonable number of elements.

From a starting point, a line is drawn for each element of the first set (quarter). From the free end of each of the first two lines, attach the two lines corresponding to the two elements of the second set (penny). Repeat the process for the third set (dime). The path crossed from the initial point to the final end point at the end of the terminal line, crossing in the process three serial branches, spells out each of the eight outcomes or elements of the SS of the experiment (Figure 2A.1).

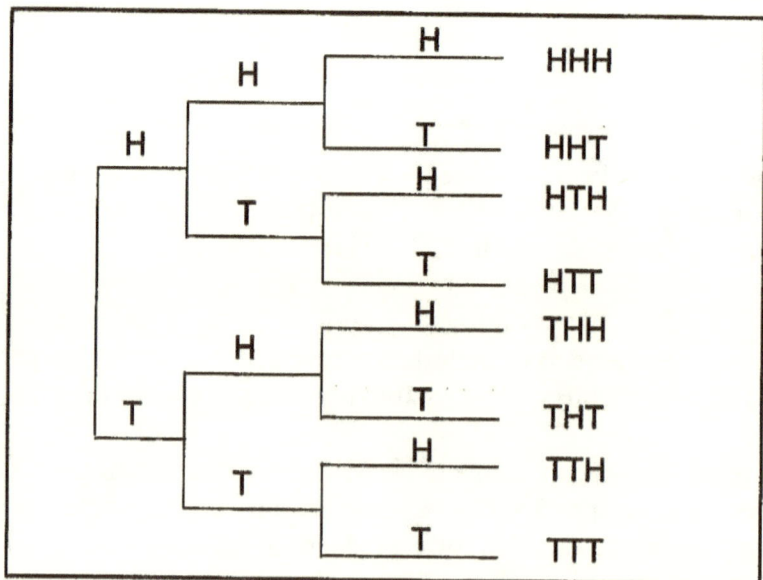

Figure 2A.1. Tree diagram of the graphic technique for the listing of all possible permutations

For the set of SS = {a, b, c, d}, the permutation concept may similarly be visualized as paths of a tree (Figure 2A.2), where each path defines a possible permutation. The twenty-four paths exhaust all possible permutations of the four letters set, taken four at a time [3. Pn^r].

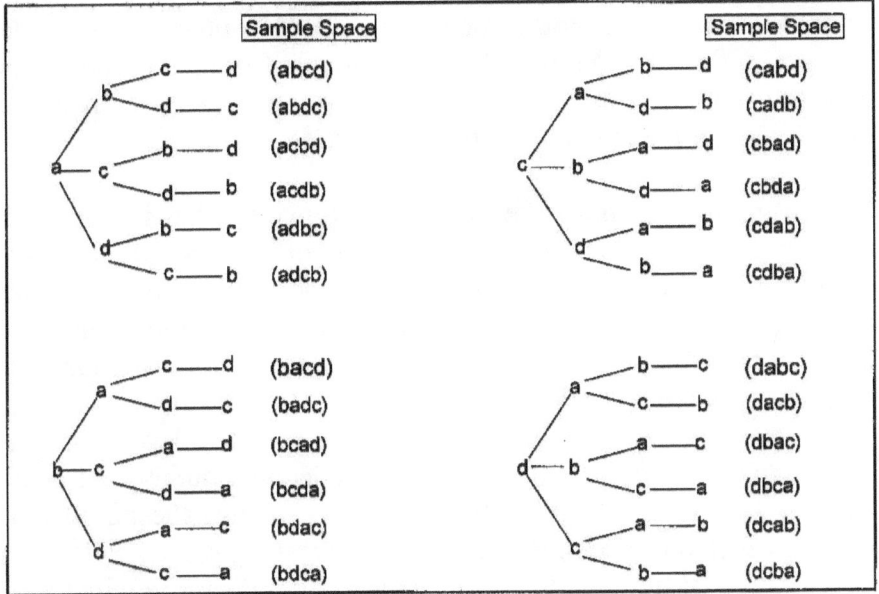

Figure 2A.2. Tree diagram of the sample space structural elements: all possible permutations of four distinct objects taken four at a time

Alternatively, using a series of adjacent cells (pigeon holes) designed to be filled out in a given order, the total number of possible permutations of the same SS elements may also be readily calculated.

Given SS = {a, b, c, d}, the first cell may be filled in one of four ways, that is, by placing a or b or c or d in the first cell. The second cell reduces the choice of filling it to the remaining three letters. The third cell is left with only two options, while the remaining fourth cell may only be filled with the remaining letter (no option). Thus, a total of twenty-four permutations (4 × 3 × 2 × 1 = 24) or sequential arrangement of the letters is possible (Pn, Table 2.17, item 2 of the permutations formulae).

| 4 | 3 | 2 | 1 |

The Summation Principle

Consider a travel plan for which either a bus or a subway is available. If three bus routes and two subway routes are available for the trip, then the number of ways available for making the trip is the sum of the bus routes and the subway routes, $3 + 2 = 5$, because travel by either mode excludes the other mode.

Because both acts cannot be performed together, that is, they are mutually exclusive such that both acts cannot occur simultaneously and therefore they are automatically dependent, in the sense that the occurrence of one preclude the occurrence of the other, then the number of ways in which one or the other may be performed is sum of the ways in which both can occur.

The principle may be extended to include any number of acts, resulting in a sample space whose elements include the number of ways in which any one of the Acts can occur; thus, $n_1 + n_2 + n_3 + \ldots$ n_r = elements of the sample space, the sum of the ways in which one and only one of the acts can occur.

In formal language, the addition principle may be formulated as noted in Table 2A.1.

2A.2 Permutation

2A.2.1 Counting Ordered Arrangements with No Repetition or Replacement

Permutation is any arrangement of the elements of a set in a definite order (Table 2.17, items 1 and 2 of the permutations formulae). Given a set of n objects, arranging r of them in a definite order is referred to as permutation of n objects taken r at a time. Thus, for a given a set of nine objects, arranging five of them in definite order is referred to as the permutation of nine objects taken five at a time. Symbolically, the process can be configured as the number of ways of consecutively placing five different items given nine contiguous cells.

Thus, the first place can be filled in n ways because there are n different objects to place. The second place can be filled in $n - 1$ ways; hence, the first two places are filled in $n \times (n - 1)$ ways. When the two places are filled, the third place can be filled in $(n - 2)$ ways; hence, the first three places are filled in $n \times (n - 1) \times (n - 2)$ ways. The last place can be filled in $(n - 4)$ ways or five ways. This is another way of saying that by the time the last object, the fifth, is to be placed, the distributor has in fact five remaining items at hand, one of which is to be placed in the fifth cell, thus implying that the fifth cell can be filled out in five possible ways. In the generic terms of n and r, the fifth or rth cell can be filled out in $n - r + 1 = 9 - 5 + 1 = 5$ possible ways

$n = 9$	$(n - 1)$ $= 8$	$(n - 2)$ $= 7$	$(n - 3)$ $= 6$	$(n - 4) =$ $5 = n - r$ $+ 1 = 5$	$(n - 5)$ $= 4$	$(n - 6)$ $= 3$	$(n - 7)$ $= 2$	$(n - 8)$ $= 1$
$r = 5$	$r - 1$ $= 4$	$r - 2$ $= 3$	$r - 3$ $= 2$	$r - 4 = 1$				
First place	Second place	Third place	Fourth place	Fifth = rth place	Sixth place	Seventh place	Eighth place	Ninth place

Table 2A.5. Permutation of nine (n) objects taken five (r) at a time

Although most problems involving permutation can be solved by direct application of the multiplication principle, permutation formulae allow the practical application of the principle by noting the number of permutations of n different objects taken r at a time.

Note the formula stipulates r factors or r cells to fill in all, leaving $n - r$ cells empty. Accordingly, the last factor is actually the rth cell (fifth) to be filled in ($n - r + 1 = 5$) ways,

$$nPr = n(n - 1)(n - 2) \ldots (n - r + 1)$$

$9P5 = 9 \times 8 \times 7 \times 6 \times 5 = 15,120$, the number of ways the five items can be permutated.

The formula may be generalized to include the permutation of n different objects taken all at a time, that is, when $r = n$ or the number of cells is equal to the number objects to be placed.

Thus, there are n places in line to be filled and n different objects to fill with. The first place can be filled with any one of the n objects and thus in n ways. The choice for the second place is restricted to the remaining $n - 1$ objects. Similarly, the third place is restricted to the remaining $n - 3$ objects. When the last nth place is reached, we are left with the remaining single object, limiting the choice to one way.

$$nPn = n(n - 1)(n - 2)\ldots 3 \times 2 \times 1 = n! = n \text{ factorial}$$

$$9P9 = 9! = 362{,}880$$

$n = 9$	$(n-1)$ $= 8$	$(n-2)$ $= 7$	$(n-3)$ $= 6$	$(n-4)$ $= 5$	$(n-5)$ $= 4$	$(n-6)$ $= 3$	$(n-7)$ $= 2$	$(n-8)$ $= 1$
First place	Second place	Third place	Fourth place	Fifth place	Sixth place	Seventh place	Eighth place	Ninth = nth place

Table 2A.6. Permutation of nine (n) objects taken all (n) at a time

Note that when r cells are to be filled as in the first formula, $(n - r)$ cells are left vacant only to be filled if all objects, n, are taken at time. Therefore, dividing $n!$ by $(n - r)!$ will restrict the places to be filled to r by canceling the $(n - r)!$ component of $n!$. The permutation formula may thus be simplified and reformatted as follows:

$$nPr = \frac{nPn}{(n-r)!} = \frac{n!}{(n-r)!}$$

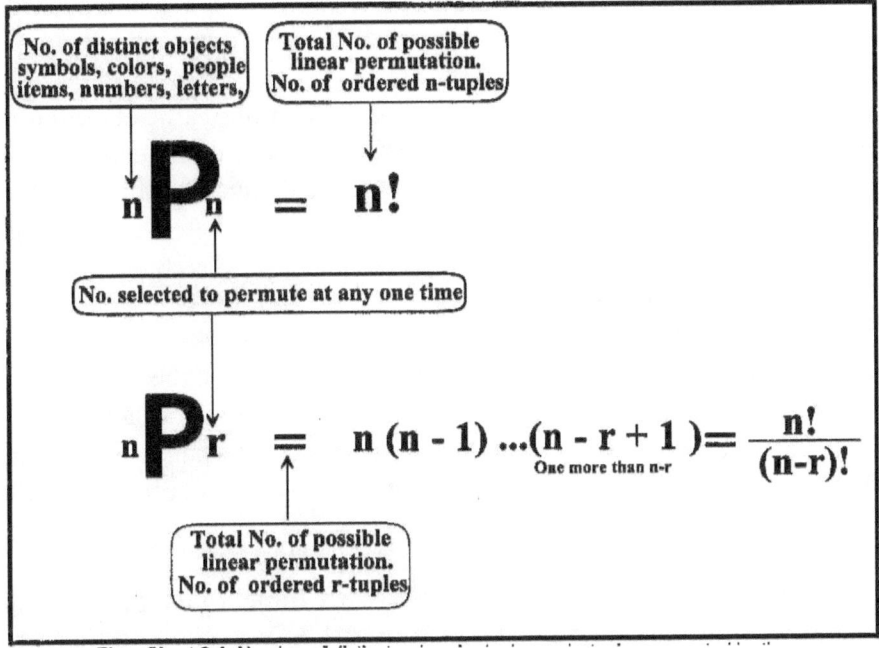

Figure 2A.3. Flow chart of the number of distinct ordered *n*-tuples and *r*-tuples generated by the permutation of *n* objects taken *n* and *r* at a time, respectively, without replacement

2A.2.2 Counting Ordered Arrangements with Repetition or Replacement

In contrast to the process of permutation without repetition or replacement, the process in this method allows for the replacement of the element drawn back into the original set of *n* elements (nPn^r, Table 2.17, item 3 of the permutations formulae). Thus, in choosing the first element in the ordered arrangement, we have at our disposal the whole intact set of *n* elements. On choosing the second element, we have again at our disposal the whole intact set of *n* elements because the element drawn on the first draw has been replaced. Because each of the elements can be chosen in *n* ways, the number of possible arrangements with replacement or repetition is as follows:

$n \times n \times n \ldots \times n = n^r$ permutations of size r of n element with replacement.

In general, if the number of ways of performing an act remains identical, the above relation is obtained. Thus, if a coded signal is to be transmitted using a six-digit sequence of 0s and 1s, the possible number of coded words as noted earlier

$$2 \times 2 \times 2 \times 2 \times 2 \times 2 = n^r = 2^6 = 64$$

Rolling two dice (a cube and a twelve-sided dodecahedron) gives rise to a Cartesian product of $6 \times 12 = 72$ ordered pairs instead of the thirty-six ordered pairs encountered in rolling the pair of standard dice. Note that in this case, the outcome of each die roll is specific and different.

The same logic could be applied to the three dials of the slot machines with numbers of 1-12, 1-8, and 1-6, which could turn out $12 \times 8 \times 6 = 576$ different numbers. The total number of permuted outcomes that can be derived from the simultaneous rotation of the three dials $= n_r$.

2A.2.3 Counting Ordered Arrangements with Fixed Repetition or Replacement

In chapter 2A.2.2 and this chapter, the permutation was exclusively applied to the ordering of one set of n distinct objects taken all or in part with or without replacement (nPn_1n_2, Table 2.17, item 5 of the permutations formulae). In this chapter, the idea is partially generalized to include more than one set of n objects, with the proviso the each set is exclusively made of identical elements. Consider the permutation of an eight-letter word (aaa bbb cc) made up of three, three, and two identical letters.

Taken individually, if the a's were distinguishable, they could have been permuted in 3! ways, the b's similarly in 3! ways, and the c's in 2! ways. Finally, if all the eight letters were distinguishable, they could be similarly permuted in 8! ways, which if actual would result in 40,320 words. The real number of permutation must then account for the permutation of the individual letters. The ratio of 8!/3!3!2! = 560 is now the number of words permutated from the hypothetical eight-letter word.

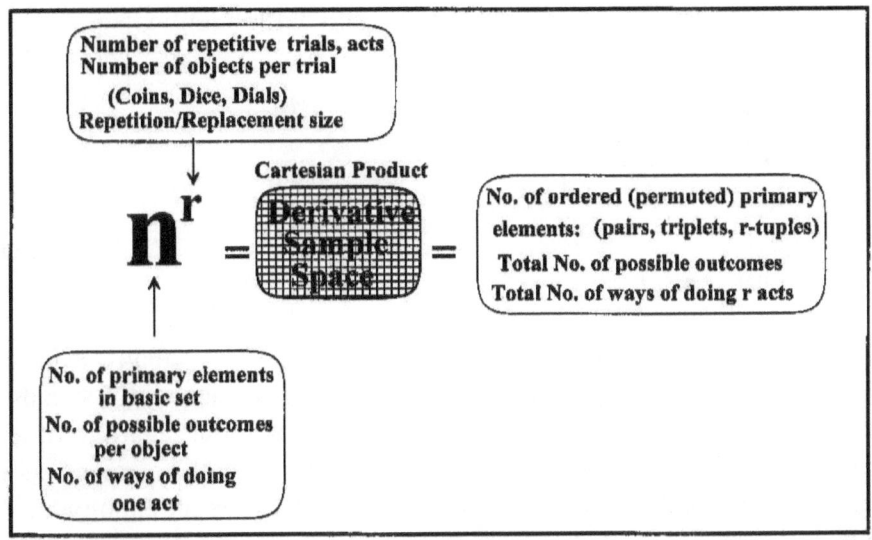

Figure 2A.4. Flow chart of the permutation of identical sets of elements with repetition or replacement

Accordingly, a set of n objects made up of r types of fixed size with each type composed of identical elements that differ from other types such that type 1 is made up of n_1 identical elements, type 2 of n_2 identical elements, and similarly type r of n_r identical elements, so that

$$n = n_1 + n_2 + \ldots + n_r$$

Hence, the number of distinguishable permutation taking all the types of elements in n at a time is given by the following relation

$$nP\,n_1, n_2, \ldots, n_r = \frac{n!}{n_1!n_2!\ldots n_r!}$$

The permutation of n objects consisting of two types of fixed size and distinct identical elements represents a special case of the multiple identical types noted earlier. In this instance, the two types of partition in effect set into an r type and its complement type ($n - r$). The permutation of two types each with identical elements assumes then the following format:

$$nP\,r,(n-r) = \frac{n!}{r!(n-r)!}.$$

2A.3 Combination

The combination concept pauses the question "How many subsets (bunches, groups, clusters, and composite elements) each with a specific number of different elements (e.g., 2 elements), without regard to order within the subset, can the total number of elements in the sample space be separated into?" In the case of the four letters, as an example, six different subsets of two distinct letters each are possible,

ab	cd
ac	bd
ad	bc

Alternatively, only four subsets of three distinct letter can be made out of the same sample space,

abc	acd
abd	bcd

The concept of combination as a collection of different objects in which the order of arrangement is unimportant appears at first sight to be self-evident. In selecting a committee, the order of selection or arrangement of the members (in contrast to a hierarchical election) does not change the composition of the committee. In a similar vein, the arrangement of five cards in a hand does not change the rank of the hand.

Specifically, combination addresses the question "How many different subsets (groups, clusters, bunches, and composite elements) of size r can be made from the n elements of the SS?"

Implicit in this selection is the fact that for each subset made of r elements out of the total n available elements, a complementary subset made up of the balance left after the selection of r elements is automatically produced. We have thus managed through the selection of a subset of specified magnitude to subdivide the SS into a series of paired subsets. One series in the foreground, in which each subset contains exactly the r element, and another series in the background, in which each subset contains exactly the complementary balance of $n - r$ elements, were not included in the r elements chosen for the required subsets.

2A.3.1 Counting Unordered Combinations with No Repetition or Replacement

Combination in contrast to permutation is any unordered selection of different elements from the elements of a set (nCr, Table 2.17, item 1 of the combination formulae). Given a set of n objects selecting r of them without regard to their order, a combination of the n objects taken r at a time is as follows:

r	$n-r$	$nCr = \dfrac{n!}{r!(n-r)!}$
a	bcd	
b	acd	$nC_1 = \dfrac{4!}{1!(4-1)!} = \dfrac{4!}{1!3!} = 4$
c	abd	$nC_3 = \dfrac{4!}{3!(4-3)!} = \dfrac{4!}{3!1!} = 4$
d	abc	
ab	cd	

ac	bd	$nC_2 = \dfrac{4!}{2!(4-2)!} = \dfrac{4!}{2!2!} = 6$
ad	bc	
∅	abcd	$nC_0 = \dfrac{4!}{0!(4-0)!} = \dfrac{4!}{0!4!} = 1$
		$nC_4 = \dfrac{4!}{4!(4-4)!} = \dfrac{4!}{4!0!} = 1$

Table 2A.7. Ordered pattern of partition into two subsets for all possible values of r

As noted in Table 2A.7, the total number of possible subsets correspond to the sum derived from adding the number of subsets calculated by changing the value of r from 0 to 4 so that

$$nC_0 + nC_1 + nC_2 + nC_3 + nC_4 + 2^4 = 16$$

Total number of possible subsets $= 1 + 4 + 6 + 4 + 1 = 16$

Because each combination consists of a subset of r different elements, and because each subset can be arranged in $r! = rPr$ ways, the total number of permutations of r objects taken at a time from a set of n objects can be equally derived from the product of the combinations and the permutation of r elements taken r at a time, so that

$nCr \times rPr = nPr$ or

$$nCr = \frac{nPr}{rPr} = \frac{nPr}{r!} = \frac{n!}{r!(n-r)!}$$

Note that despite the similarity in the format of the special case of "permutation with fixed repetition or replacement consisting of two types" to that of combination with no repetition or replacement, the results are distinctly different, although numerically equivalent. In the combination case, the set is comprised on n distinct objects. In the permutation case, the set is made up of two distinct elements of r and $(n - r)$ types, each with identical elements.

The combination formula addresses the question of how many combinations consisting of r different elements can be derived from a set of n elements. Implicit in the question is that each combination of r objects selected from the set of n objects partitions the set into an equal number of r and $(n - r)$ combinations. The combination formula is thus equally valid when written in terms of the r objects selected or their complement of $(n - r)$ so that

$$nCr = nC(n - r)$$

The permutation formula, on the other hand, addresses the question of the number of distinguishable permutations resulting from the permutation of a set of n objects made up of two distinct elements.

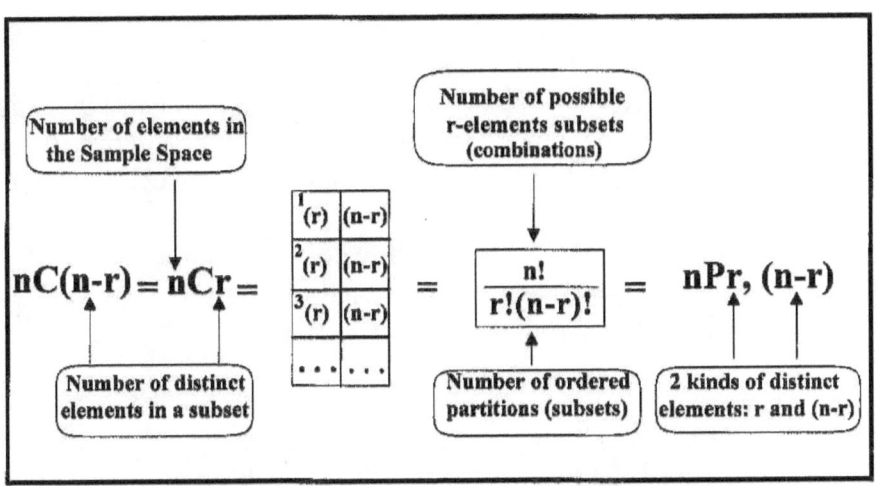

Figure 2A.5. Flow chart of the confluence
between combination and permutation

2A.3.2 Counting Subsets with Repetition or Replacement

The technique of counting the resultant subsets when repetition or replacement is permitted in the combinatory process may now be introduced $[3. (n-1) + rCr]$. This is best illustrated through a practical example.

Consider a set of three elements, {a, b, c}. Recall that the total number of possible combinations with no repetition or replacement that can be made out of the three elements set including the empty set is given by the following:

$$\text{Subsets of the set } S = \{a, b, c\} = 3C0 + 3C1 + 3C2 + 3C3 = 2^3 = 8$$
$$\varnothing, \{a\}, \{b\}, \{c\}, \{a, b\}, \{a, c\}, \{b, c\}, \{a, b, c\}$$

a	b	
b	ac	$3C1\|3C2$
c	bc	
$\varnothing$	abc	$3C0\|3C3$

Table 2A.8. Ordered pattern of partition into two subsets

Implicit in the combination with no replacement is the allocation of all the possible subsets to two contiguous cells separated by a single divider. As can be readily noted, each of the possible subsets is made of distinct elements without repetition. A combination of size 2, for example, yields the three subset, {a, b}, {a, c}, and {b, c}.

For the same set, if repetition is allowed, combination of size 3 yields the following ten different combinations (subsets): {a a a}, {a a, b}, {a a, c}, {b b b}, {b,b, a}, {b b, c}, {c c c}, {c c, a}, {c c, b}, and {a, b, c}.

In other words, how many different arrangements can be made of the three basic characters, {a, b, c}, taken three at a time with replacement? Assume that each letter is represented by a floating ball in a lotto machine.

Number of combinations with replacement $(n-1)+rCr =$ $2+3C3 = 5C3$ $= 10$			Number of permutations coupled to each combination	Number of permutations with replacement $n^r = 3^3 = 27$		
aaa			$1 \times 1 = 1$	**a**	**a**	**a**
aa	b		$1 \times 3 = 3$	a	a	b
				a	b	a
				b	a	a
aa		c	$1 \times 3 = 3$	a	a	c
				a	c	a
				c	a	a
	bbb		$1 \times 1 = 1$	**b**	**b**	**b**
a	bb		$1 \times 3 = 3$	b	b	a
				b	a	b
				a	b	b
	bb	c	$1 \times 3 = 3$	b	b	c
				b	c	b
				c	b	b
		ccc	$1 \times 1 = 1$	**c**	**c**	**c**
a		cc	$1 \times 3 = 3$	c	c	a
				c	a	c
				a	c	c
	b	cc	$1 \times 3 = 3$	c	c	b
				c	b	c

				b	c	c
a	**b**	**c**	$1 \times 6 = 6$	**a**	**b**	**c**
				a	c	b
				b	a	c
				b	c	a
				c	b	a
				c	a	b

Table 2A.9. Parallel and comparative development of counting technique and enumeration methods derived for the combination, permutation, and partition principles (pp. 26-28). Page 44 details the resultant permutation and combination of a set of four letters.

The possible sequence that may result on drawing the first ball, then replacing it; drawing the second ball, then replacing it; and finally, drawing the third ball for a total of three draws with replacement is the equivalent of filling each of three contiguous cells with one of the three basic characters, as noted in Table 2A.9. In this analogy, the first cell may be filled with any one of the three characters and so is the second and third cell.

In order to accommodate the added replacement, it becomes necessary to add an extra contiguous cell, or equivalently to replace the single divider by 2.

A moment's thought might convince the reader that what is being partitioned is not the standard combination whereby the set of the three distinct elements is partitioned into the two complementary subsets, which produced the eight possible subsets, but the controlled allocation of the same elements with the added proviso of replacement into three contiguous cells.

In effect, the distribution includes, in addition to the three basic elements, the two dividers that made it possible to partition the sample space into ten subsets. Stated differently, the distribution of three elements into three cells is equivalent to the possible combination of five objects (two dividers and three elements) taken three at a time,

Dividers   Elements
2 +   3 $C3 = 5C3 = 10$ = number of combination of size 3 with replacement from a set of three elements.

On the other hand, if the permutations of the three elements with replacement is considered, the result is given as $3 \times 3 \times 3 = 3^3 = 27$ possible sequences or permutations of three elements with replacement.

The coupling of the combination of the three elements taken three at time with the permutation of the same elements becomes evident.

Note that the single combination of {a, b, c} is coupled to six permuted subsets of the same cardinality and having the same elements. When the order or alignments of the elements in the subsets is left out of consideration, the subsets are considered essentially equal so that

$$\{a, b, c\} = \{a, c, b\}.$$

If, on the other hand, the order is important in differentiating between the subsets, then

$$(a, b, c) \neq (a, c, b).$$

Note the use of parentheses to indicate order, in contrast to the braces enclosing sets and subsets. When each of the possible combinations with replacements is then multiplied by the number of its associated permutations, the final tally is the same as the number originally derived by the direct computation of the total number of permutations possible.

In the case at hand where repetition is allowed, changing the provision so that the resultant combination cannot exceed the limit of four elements of which at least two may be identical, the number of possible combinations, as noted in Table 2A.10, now becomes fifteen, accounting for all possible repetition of three elements to the limit imposed by the size of the combination prescribed.

a a a a		
a a a	b	
a a a		c
a a	b b	
a a		c c
a a	b	c
	b b b b	
a	b b b	
	b b b	c
	b b	c c
a	b b	c
		c c c c
a		c c c
	b	c c c
a	b	cc

Table 2A.10. Combination with replacement of size 4 from the set
$S = \{a, b, c\}$

The perusal of Table 2A.10 is instructive as to the allocation of the elements to the three cells of the table. Note that the division into three cells was achieved by the insertion of two vertical dividers without the usual initial and terminal dividers customarily included in tabular forms.

Thus, the problem could be considered as the combination of six items taken four at a time, which amounts to filling six positions with four letters and two bars, with no regard to the order of placement; accordingly,

$$(n-1)+rC\,r = 4+2C4 = 6C4 = \frac{n!}{(n-1)!\,r!} = \frac{6!}{2!4!} = 15$$

= number of combination of size 4 with replacement from a set of three elements.

Applying the same technique to a set of four letters, {a, b, c, d), the problem of deriving the combination of five letters becomes inordinately unwieldy, as evidenced from Table 2A.11, enumerating the initial seventeen combination out of the possible total of fifty-six.

a a a a a			
a a a a	b		
a a a a		c	
a a a a			d
a a a	b b		
a a a		c c	
a a a			d d
a a a	b	c	
a a a	b		d
a a a		c	d
a a	b b	c	
a a	b b		d
a a	b	c c	
a a		c c	d
a a		c	d d
a a	b		d d
a a	b	c	d

Table 2A.11. Combination with replacement of size 5 from the set $S = \{a, b, c, d\}$

Note, however, that the number of the dividers in each case is one less than the number of cells in the set under consideration. Thus, the number of combinations could be derived from the combination formula, where n is now the sum of the elements and the dividers, so that

Composite number of dividers and size $(n-1)+r$	=	(No. of elements in the set -1) = number of dividers $n-1$	+	r = combination size required r

The formula for combination with repetition or replacement may now be rewritten in terms of the components of n, so that

Dividers = Set -1 $(n-1)$	Combinations size $+r$	=C	Combinations size r	$= (n-1+r)Cr = \dfrac{(n+r-1)!}{r!(n-1)!}$

Thus, the number of combinations with replacement of size 5 from the set $S = \{a, b, c, d\}$ may now be easily computed using the above relation

Dividers = Set -1 $(4-1)$	Combinations size $+r$	=C	Combinations size r	$= 8C5 = 56$ different combinations

2A.4 Practical Application

A pharmacy shelf displays five kinds of toothpastes. In how many ways can three tubes be chosen? A pictorial representation is to configure the shelf space into a series of five cells corresponding to the five possible varieties separated by four vertical dividers, thus making the number of dividing bars equivalent to one less than the number of cells, or equivalently the number of varieties, that is, ($n - 1$). The choice of three tubes may be made out of the five cells by choosing one, two, or three of the available varieties. In other words, a combination of three tubes is to be made out of the set of five varieties.

A	B	C	D	E
	♦♦		♦	

As noted in the diagram, a choice of two tubes of the B variety and one tube of the D variety was made. This of course is only one of the possible choices available.

The choice in this case may range from one extreme, whereby the three tubes are chosen from one single variety, to the other extreme, where one tube is chosen from each variety.

In order to configure the solution in terms of combination where the subsets may contain more than one element of the same item, the problem needs to be recast in terms of partition into two subsets, which can be formed out of n objects numbering seven, composed of four dividers and three tubes taken r or $(n - r)$ at a time as stipulated in the first case. We are now dealing with seven slots into which the chosen tubes (diamonds) and the vertical dividers (varieties) are to be placed. Three of these slots are reserved for the placement of the diamonds without regard to the order in which they are placed. The balance of the slots is to be filled by the dividers. Accordingly,

$$nCr = nC(n-r) = \frac{n!}{r!(n-r)!} = 7C3 = \frac{7!}{3!4!} = 35.$$

In general, using the diamonds and bars analogy, the combination problem becomes a choice between $(n - 1)$ bars to account for the number of cells (varieties) and r to account for the number of diamonds (tubes of choice). Thus, the number of combination with repetition assumes the following format:

$$\underset{\text{dividers}}{(n-1)}+\underset{\text{diamonds}}{r})Cr = (4+3)Cr = 7C3 = \frac{(n+r-1)!}{r!(n-1)!}$$

Note that the combination format is equally valid when the combination is taken r at a time or $(n - r)$ at a time. This, of course, is derived from the complementary nature of the combination format as noted elsewhere in this chapter.

Table 2A.12 shows a summary of the choice involved in choosing a sample of r elements from a set of n elements by invoking the process of permutation and combination with and without replacement.

The sampling process for deriving all possible combinations or permutations within the imposed constraints	Repetitions	Order: r-tuple	No. of ways of choosing all possible combinations or permutations (samples) derived from the sampling process
Permutation of r distinct objects from a set of n distinct objects	No repetition	Ordered	$nPr = \dfrac{n!}{(n-r)!}$
Permutation of r distinct object from a set of n distinct objects with replacement	With repetition	Ordered	$n \times n \times n \ldots \times n = n^r$
Combination of r distinct objects from a set of n distinct objects	No repetition	Unordered	$nCr = \dfrac{n!}{r!(n-r)!}$
Combination of r distinct objects from a set of n distinct objects with replacement	With repetition	Unordered	$(n+r-1)Cr = \dfrac{(n+r-1)!}{r!(n-1)!}$

Table 2A.12. Combinations and permutations of r elements from a set of n elements with imposed constraints

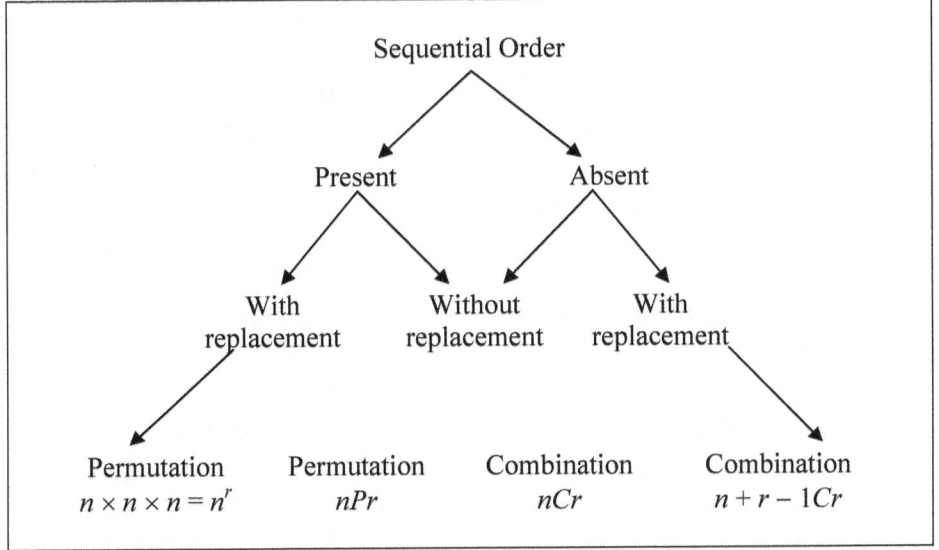

Flow Chart version of Table 2A.12

Sampling without replacement

Items with distinguishable characteristic P (r)	Combinations with distinguishable characteristic kCr	$\times$	Combinations with distinguishable characteristic $(N-k)C\,(n-r)$
$=$	NCn Sample space of combinations from N population		

2A.5 Questionnaire and Review

To further emphasize the central role of the multiplication principle in conjunction with the four sampling techniques that can be used in deriving all possible combinations or permutations of a given set, consider for the final episode the ubiquitous die and the six numbers that make up its six faces, namely, {1, 2, 3, 4, 5, 6}. To this end, four pointed questions will be addressed in order to elicit the extent of the sample space and the makeup of its constituent elements.

Question 1: "How many different two-digit numbers may be formed from the set = {1, 2, 3, 4, 5, 6} if repetitions of digits are allowed?"

Answer: Using the cellular array, the first cell may be filled with any one of the six digits. The second cell may similarly be filled (because with replacement or repetition, six digits are still available after filling the first cell). The Cartesian product is similarly $6 \times 6 = 36$, the same number of ordered pairs encountered in rolling two standard dice. Alternatively, this of course is a problem of permutating six different objects ($n = 6$) with repetition or replacement, taken twice ($r = 2$), relating two trials with identical outcome (rolling the two dice concurrently or sequentially is of course identical). Thus, $n^r = 6^2 = 36$ distinct permutation with repetition (3-Pn^r).

Note that the same question results in a different answer through a simple change of the parameter involved, so that for the question "How many six-digit numbers can be formed from the six numbers if repetitions or replacements of a digit are allowed?" The answer is the number of 6-tuples, where each digit is made of 1, 2, 3, 4, 5, or 6 only. the answer is (i.e., different numbers)

$$n^r = 6 \times 6 \times 6 \times 6 \times 6 \times 6 = 6^6 = 46,656 \text{ ordered 6-tuples.}$$

Question 2: "How many numbers of two different digits can be formed from the same set of six numbers?"

This of course is the same question as previously mentioned, only this time without repetitions or replacement, such that no digit may be used more than once. With the new imposed restriction, the first cell may be filled with any of the six digits, that is, in six different ways. The second cell may now be filled with any of the remaining five digits, resulting in a Cartesian product of $6 \times 5 = 30$ ordered pairs. The SS has now been reduced from the original 36 to 30, composed of the two triangle enclosed areas of Table 2A.1.

Answer: This is a problem of simple permutation of six objects taken two at a time, such that (Pr, Table 2.17, item 1 of the permutations formulae).

$$6P2 = \frac{6!}{(6-2)!} = 30 \text{ different numbers (no doubles or repetitions).}$$

Again, note that the same question results in a different answer through a simple change of the parameter involved, so that for the question "How many six-digit numbers can be formed from the six numbers if no repetitions or replacements of a digit are allowed?" The answer is the number of 6-tuples, only this time, no digit is to be repeated in any one 6-tuple (6P6 = 720; Pn, see Table 2.17, item 2 of the permutations formulae).

The answer is $6 \times 5 \times 4 \times 3 \times 2 \times 1 = 6! = 720$ ordered 6-tuples.

Question 3: "How many two-digit without reference to order can be formed from the set of the 6 numbers?"

Answer: We are dealing here with a straightforward problem of combination, where each subset is made of different number, disregarding order. Thus [=1(Cr)],

$$6C2 = \frac{6!}{2!(6-2)!} = 15 \text{ two-digit combination}$$

The pattern is restricted to the single triangle enclosed area of Table 2A.1, where it is apparent that (1, 2) and (2, 1) are considered identical combinations [1. Cr].

Question 4: "How many different combinations are possible if repetition or replacement is allowed?"

Recall that in this case we are dealing with six different items (numbers, varieties, and types) separated by dividers, to be chosen two at a time.

A	B	C	D	E	F
1	2	3	4	5	6

Answer: Invoking the combination formula with replacement, the following equation is derived ($C(n - 1) + r$; see Table 2.17, item 3 of the combination formulae):

$\underset{\text{dividers}}{(n-1+} \ \underset{\text{choice}}{r})Cr = (6-1) + 2C2 = 7C2 = 21$	different combination with repetition

Note that the number includes, besides the standard fifteen combinations derived in question 3, an additional six combinations of the repeating numbers for a total of 21 combinations ($C(n - 1) + 1$; see Table 2.17, item 3 of the combination formulae).

Question 5 (the final question concerning the random experiment of rolling a die): "How many different subsets can be generated from the SS = {1, 2, 3, 4, 5, 6}?"

Answer: $2^6 = 64$ possible subsets. For each of the six elements, a binary decision needs to be made whether to include the element in the given subset or to exclude it. A two-way answer regarding each element results in $2 \times 2 \times 2 \times 2 \times 2 \times 2 = 2^6 = 64$ possible subsets that may be derived from the experiment. The same number is of course available by toting the number of all possible combinations taken 0, 1, 2, 3, 4, 5, and 6 at a time; thus ($2^6 = 64$; C2^r, see Table 2.17, item 3 of the combination formulae),

$6C0 + 6C1 + 6C2 + 6C3 + 6C4 + 6C5 + 6C6 = 1 + 6 + 15 + 20 + 15 + 6 + 1 = 64$ subsets.

Permutation (Counting Orders)	Combination (Counting Subsets)
1. nPr: number of ordered arrangements (permutations) that can be made using r objects chosen from a set of n distinct objects	1. nCr: number of unordered subsets that can be made using r distinct objects from a set of n distinct objects
Number of permutations of n distinct objects taken r at a time (ordered r-tuples) (without repetition/replacement)	Number of combinations that can be formed out of n distinct objects taken r at a time (unordered r-tuples, subsets) (without repetition/replacement)
$$nPr = n(n-1)\ldots(n-r+1)$$	$$nCr = \frac{n(n-1)\ldots(n-r+1)}{r!}$$
$$nPr = \frac{nPn}{(n-r)!} = \frac{n!}{(n-r)!}$$	$$nCr = \frac{nPr}{rPr} = \frac{nPr}{r!} = \frac{n!}{r!(n-r)!}$$
	Note that because each of these unordered subsets may be permuted in $r!$ ways, it becomes necessary to eliminate the permutation factor from the corresponding permutation formula by dividing nPr by $rPr = r!$ in order to arrive at the unordered combination
	Note that the elements of a set are not repeated, so that the order in which the elements are listed is not pertinent
2. nPn: number permutations of n distinct objects taken n at a time (ordered n-tuples) (without repetition/replacement)	2. 2^n: number of all combinations (unordered r-tuples, subsets) out of n distinct objects taken 0, 1, 2, 3, . . . , n at a time (without repetition/replacement)
$$nPn = n(n-1)(n-2)\ldots 3.2.1 = n!$$	$$nC_0 + nC_1 + nC_2 + \ldots + nC_n = 2^n$$

Table 2A.13. Counting orders versus subsets without replacement

4. $nP_{r,(n-r)}$ **Distinguishable Permutation**	5. nPn_1, n_2 **Distinguishable Permutation**
Permutation of two types with fixed repetition (not all distinct objects)	Permutation of several types with fixed repetition (not all distinct objects)
Number of permutation of n objects, r of which are alike and of one kind and the balance, $(n - r)$, of which are similarly alike and of another kind.	Number of permutations (ordered n-tuples) out of n objects of more than two subsets of the same kind two kinds.
$$nPr = nP(n - r)$$	Number of permutations (distinguishable arrangements) of n objects not all distinct, taken all at a time, of which n_1 is alike and of one kind, n_2 is alike and of another kind, and finally, n_r objects are alike and yet of another kind, such that
$$nP r,(n-r) = \frac{nP r}{rP r} = \frac{nP r}{r!} = \frac{n!}{r!(n-r)!}$$	$$n_1 + n_2 + \ldots + n_r = n$$
Permutation of an eight-letter word made up of three and five identical letters (aaa bbbbb), i.e., permutation of $n = 8$ of which three and five objects are identical results in 8! / 3!(8 − 3)! = 56 different eight-letter words; 56 different sequences of a and b compared with 8! = 40,320 words possible if the eight letters were distinct (abc def gh).	The number of distinguishable permutation (ordered partition) is then given as
	$$nP n_1, n_2, \ldots, n_r = \frac{n!}{n_1! n_2! \ldots n_r!}$$
Note that the number of permutations or orders of n objects, r of which is alike and of one kind and $(n - r)$ of which is alike and of another kind, is equal to the number of combinations of n different objects taken r or equally $(n - r)$ at a time.	Permutation of an eight-letter word (aaa bbb cc) made up of three, three, and two identical letters, i.e., permutation of $n = 8$ of which three, three, and two letters are identical results in 8!/3!3!2! = 560 different eight-letter words; 560 different sequences of a, b, and c compared with 8! = 40,320 words possible if the eight letters were distinct (abc def gh).

Table 2A.14. Distinguishable permutation of
two or more types with fixed repetition

5. $nPr,(n-r)$	1. nCr
Distinguishable Permutation Permutation of size r with fixed repetition (not all distinct objects)	**Paired Combination** (Partition into 2 subsets without repetition)

5. $nPr,(n-r)$

Distinguishable Permutation

Permutation of size r with fixed repetition (not all distinct objects)

SS = number of ordered r-tuples (permutations) out of n objects of (r) and $(n-r)$ kinds (two kinds only).

= number of permutation of n objects, r of which are alike and of one kind and the balance, $(n-r)$, of which are similarly alike and of another kind.

$$nPr,(n-r) = \frac{nPr}{rPr} = \frac{nPr}{r!} = \frac{n!}{r!(n-r)!}$$

Example: Permutation of an eight-letter word made up of three and five identical letters (aaa bbbbb), i.e., permutation of $n = 8$, of which three and five objects are identical, results in $8!\,/\,3!(8-3)! = 56$ different eight-letter words; 56 different sequences of a and b compared with $8! = 40,320$ words possible if the eight letters were distinct (abc def gh).

Note that the number of permutations or orders of n objects, r of which is alike and of one kind and $(n-r)$ of which is alike and of another kind, is equal to the number of combinations of n different objects taken r or equally $(n-r)$ at a time.

1. nCr

Paired Combination

(Partition into 2 subsets without repetition)

SS = number of unordered r-tuples (combinations and subsets) (without repetition), which can be formed out of n distinct objects taken r or $(n-r)$ at a time.

= number of paired subsets of n objects taken r at a time or $(n-r)$ at a time. Resulting in r or $(n-r)$ subsets out of n distinct objects.

$$nCr = nC(n-r)$$

$$nCr = \frac{nPr}{rPr} = \frac{nPr}{r!} = \frac{n!}{r!(n9r)!}$$

Example: Combination of an eight-letter word made up of eight distinct letters, (abc def gh) taken three at a time results in $8!/\,3!(8-3)! = 56$ subsets of three distinct letters and a corresponding balance of 56 subsets of five letters each. Alternatively, when five letters were taken at a time, the result was similarly $8!/\,5!(8-5)! = 56$ subsets of five distinct letters and a corresponding 56 subsets of three letters each.

Table 2A.15. Confluence of notation regarding permutation of two types with fixed repetition and combination with no replacement of subsets r and $n-r$

Given four objects labeled a, b, c, and d, the following ordered arrangements may be realized by different permutations

Number of permutations of four objects taken two at a time (letters cannot be used more than once)

$$nPr = 4P2 = \frac{n!}{(n-r)!} = \frac{4!}{2!} = 12$$

$S = $ {(a,b);(b,a);(a,c);(c,a);(a,d);(d,a); (c,d);(d,c);(b,d);(d,b);(b,c);(c,b)}.

No. of **Permutations** of 4 objects taken 3 at a time

$$nPr = 4P3 = \frac{n!}{(n-r)!} = \frac{4!}{1!} = 24$$

$S = $ {(a,b,c);(a,c,b);(b,c,a);(b,a,c);(c,a,b); (c,b,a);(a,b,d);(a,d,b);(b,d,a);(b,a,d); (d,a,b);(d,b,a);(a,d,c);(a,c,d);(d,c,a); (d,a,c);(c,a,d);(c,d,a);(b,c,d);(b,d,c); (c,d,b);(c,b,d);(d,b,c);(d,c,b)}

Number of permutations of four objects taken one at a time

$$4P_1 = 4$$
$$S = \{a\}; \{b\}; \{c\}; \{d\}$$

Number of permutations of four objects taken zero at a time

$$4P_0 = 1$$

Number of permutations of four objects taken four at a time

$$nPn = 4P4 = n! = 4! = 24$$

$S = $ {(a,b,c,d);(b,a,c,d);(b,c,a,d);(b,c,d,a); (a,b,d,c);(b,a,d,c);(b,d,a,c);(b,d,c,a); (a,c,b,d);(c,a,b,d);(c,b,a,d);(c,b,d,a); (a,c,d,b);(c,a,d,b);(c,d,a,b);(c,d,b,a); (a,d,b,c);(d,a,b,c);(d,b,a,c);(d,b,c,a); (a,d,c,b);(d,a,c,b);(d,c,a,b);(d,c,b,a)}

Given four objects labeled a, b, c, and d, the following unordered subsets may be realized by different combinations

Number of unordered subsets (combinations) of four objects taken two at a time

$$nCr = 4C_2 = \frac{n!}{r!(n-r)!} = \frac{4!}{2!2!} = 6$$

$S = $ {ab};{ac};{ad};{bc};{bd};{cd}

Number of unordered subsets (combinations) of four objects taken three at a time

$$nCr = 4C_3 = \frac{n!}{r!(n-r)!} = \frac{4!}{3!1!} = 4$$

$S = $ {abc};{abd};{adc};{bcd}

Number of unordered subsets (combinations) of four objects taken one at a time

$$4C_1 = 4$$
$$S = \{a\}; \{b\}; \{c\}; \{d\}$$

Number of unordered subsets (combinations) of four objects taken four at a time

$$4C_4 = 1$$
$$S = \{abcd\}$$

Number of unordered subsets (combinations) of four objects taken zero at a time

$$4C_0 = 1$$
$$S = \varnothing = \{ \} = 1$$

Number of all unordered subsets (combinations) of four objects taken 0, 1, 2, 3, and 4 at a time

$$nC_0 + nC_1 + nC_2 + nC_3 + nC_4 = 2^4 = 16$$

Power set $= 1 + 4 + 6 + 4 + 1 = 16$

Table 2A.16. Comparison of permutation and combination elements

Permutations Formulae

1. nPr: permutations of r distinct elements with no repetitions or replacements

$$nPr = n(n-1)(n-2)...(n-r+1) = \frac{nPn}{(n-r)!} = \frac{n!}{(n-r)!}$$

2. nPn: permutations of n distinct elements with no repetitions or replacements

$$nPn = n(n-1)(n-2) \ldots 3 \times 2 \times 1 = n!$$

3. nPn^r: permutations of identical sets of elements with repetitions or replacements of size r

$$n \times n \times n \ldots \times = n^r$$

4. $nPr, (n-r)$: permutations of two types of elements/sets with fixed repetition or replacement

$$nPr,(n-r) = \frac{n!}{r!(n-r)!}$$

5. nPn_1, n_2: permutations of several types of elements/sets with fixed repetition or replacement

$$nPn_1, n_2, \ldots, n_r = \frac{n!}{n_1! n_2! \ldots n_r!}$$

Combination formulae

1. nCr: combination with no replacement of subsets of size r
   Partition into two complementary subsets of r and $(n-r)$

$$nCr = nC(n-r) = \frac{nPr}{rPr} = \frac{nPr}{r!} = \frac{n!}{r!(n-r)!}$$

2. 2^n: total number of possible subsets derived from a given set (n elements) with no replacement

$$2^n = 2^{\text{No. elements}} = \text{No. possible subsets}$$

3. $C(n-1) + rCr$: combination of size r with replacement
   Partition into number of contiguous cells/subsets

$$(n-1)+rCr = \frac{(n+r-1)!}{r!(n-1)!}$$

4. n^r: number of permuted subsets of size r derived from the combination of n elements with replacement

Table 2A.17. Permutations and combinations formulae

Chapter 2B
Partition and Occupancy

In the first part of this chapter, the concept of permutation and combination, with and without replacement or repetition, were fully addressed. In the first case, the stress was on the number of ways distinct (distinguishable) items arrange themselves in defined sequences; in the second case, the subdivisions or partition of distinct items into defined subsets was considered.

This part addressed the corollary of the process of combination or permutation by taking into consideration the distinctiveness or identity of the items being combined or permuted as well as the distinctiveness or identity and of the spatial enclosure into which the elements are being compartmentalized. The problem addressed finds application in fields as diverse as quantum mechanics to genetics. In the classical language of combinatorics, the analogy of balls and cells, either of which may be distinguishable or indistinguishable, is often employed to clarify the issues involved in partition and occupancy.

2B.1 The Distribution of Balls into Cells

In the traditional presentation of probability, the problems revolving around the drawing of colored balls from the urn has been a standard staple from which a multitude of real-life physical analogies can be simulated.

With this in mind, in order to put the problem in perspective, it may be instructive to configure the ordered arrangement of permutation and resultant subsets of combination in terms of colored ball and cells.

Because the balls (a) and (b) can be made distinguishable or indistinguishable through either numbering or coloring and the cells may similarly be made distinguishable or indistinguishable by numbering |1|, |2|, |3|, it follows that we are dealing with a matrix of four possibilities, as can be noted from Table 2B.1. Thus, four possible couplings or placement of items (distinguishable or indistinguishable) into cells (distinguishable or indistinguishable) may be envisaged.

	Distinguishable Cell	Indistinguishable Cell
Distinguishable Balls	(a), (b) → | 1 | 2 | 3 |	(a), (b) → | 1 | 1 | 1 |
Indistinguishable Balls	(a), (a) → | 1 | 2 | 3 |	(a), (a) → | 1 | 1 | 1 |

Table 2B.1. Matrix of the four possibilities

1. Consider the distribution of two distinguishable items, diamond and heart, into three distinguishable numbered cells, 1, 2, and 3. As noted in Figure 2B.1, nine distinct allocation patterns of placement are possible. The experiment may be thought of as a two-step process, whereby the diamond may be placed in any one of the three cells to be followed by the placement of the heart in any one of the three cells. Thus, by the multiplication principle, there are $3 \times 3 = 9$ ways of placing the two distinct object. A moment's thought might convince the reader that the placement of the two distinct objects into the three distinct cells is in effect the permutation of size 2 of the three distinct cells (with replacement),

$$(n_{\text{distinguishable cells}})^{r \text{ distinguishable suits}} = n^r = 3^2 = 9 \text{ possible outcomes.}$$

2. Consider instead the distribution of two indistinguishable diamonds into the same distinguishable numbered cells. As noted in Figure 2B.2, only six distinct allocation patterns are now possible. The second and third rows of the previous distribution are made impossible to differentiate.

Again, a moment's thought might convince the reader that the distribution process is in effect the selection of six different subsets of cells resulting from the combination with replacement of size 2, from a set of three cells, so that,

$$\underset{n}{\text{Distinguishable cells}} + \underset{r}{\text{Indistinguishable diamonds}} - 1 = 3 + 2 - 1 C r = 4C 2 = 6 \text{ possible outcomes}$$

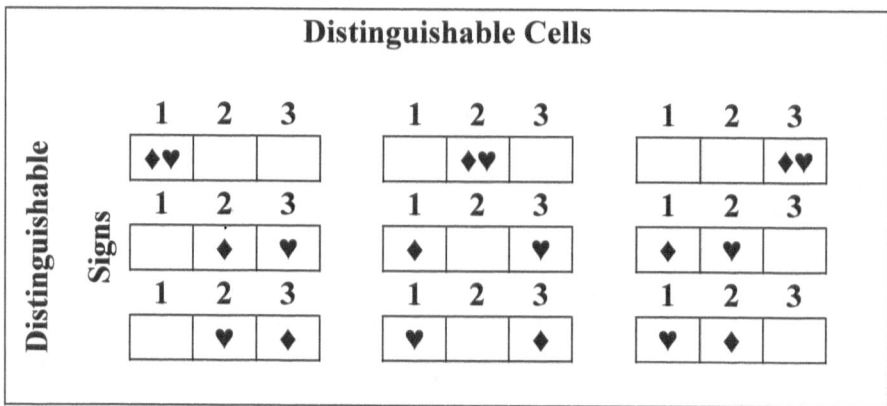

Figure 2B.1. Chart of the possible placements (outcomes) of two distinct elements into three distinct cells

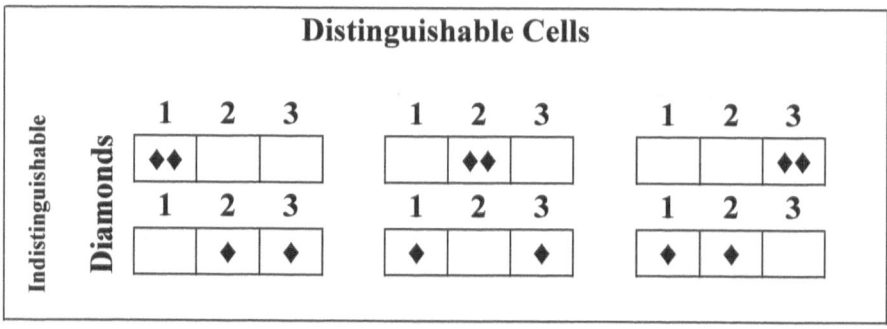

Figure 2B.2. Chart of the possible placements (outcomes) of two indistinguishable elements into three distinct cells

3. Consider the third alternative of distinguishable items to be placed into indistinguishable cells. The cells have the same number and are thus indistinguishable. The perusal of Figure 2B.3 should convince the reader that only two outcomes are possible. The two items may be placed together in one of the three cell, accounting for one outcome; all three distributions in the first row are identical, or alternatively each item may be placed in a separate cell, accounting for the second possible outcome; and the second and third row are similarly indistinguishable.

4. Finally, consider the placement of indistinguishable items into indistinguishable cells. Here again, the perusal of Figure 2B.4 will convince the reader that the three distribution of the first row are indistinguishable and so are the distributions of the second row, resulting in just two possible outcomes.

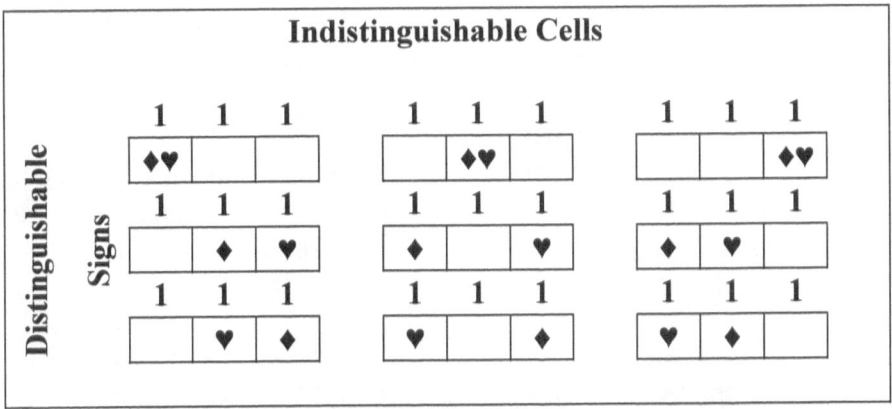

Figure 2B.3. Chart of the possible placements (outcomes) of two distinct elements into three indistinguishable cells

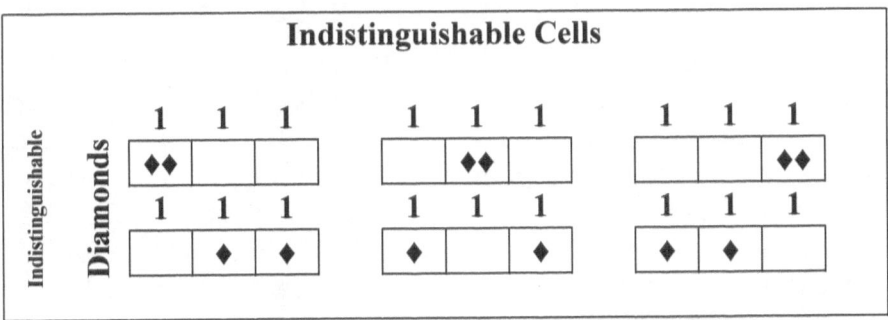

Figure 2B.4. Chart of the possible placements (outcomes) of two indistinguishable elements into three indistinguishable cells

The process of distribution of a number of elements, distinguishable or otherwise, into a series of contiguous cells, distinguishable or otherwise, necessitates, in the light of the new format associated with the set and its elements, a reinterpretation of the symbols so far used in standard permutations and combinations (Table 2B.2).

Permutation and Combination	Partition and Occupancy
n = set of distinct objects	n = set of contiguous cells, distinguishable/undistinguishable
r = size of permutation or combination of an n-set	r = no. of glass balls, letters, distinguishable/undistinguishable

Table 2B.2. Partition and Occupancy: Reinterpretation of the Permutation/Combination symbols

Thus, in the context of partition and occupancy, the old symbols need to be viewed in terms of the new process and its associated format. Nevertheless, despite the change in the format of the variables involved, the underlying principle remains unchanged.

2B.2 Ordered Partition

Recall that the basic combination formula, nCr, partitions the set of n distinct elements into two complementary subsets of distinct elements for any value of r ranging from 0 to n.

For the set {a, b, c, d}, setting $r = 1$, four possible combinations of the set into four subsets of one element each {a}; {b}; {c}; {d} are obtained, and implicitly, an equal number of complementary subsets of $(n - r)$ distinct elements {bcd};{acd};{abd};{abc} are retained. For $r = 2$, three possible combinations of the set into three subsets of two elements each {ab}; {ac}; {ad} are obtained, and implicitly, an equal number of complementary subsets of $(n - r)$ distinct elements {cd}; {bd}; {bc} are retained. For $r = 4$ or $r = 0$, the subset {abcd} or its complement {∅} is obtained.

|1|	|3|	$4C1 = \dfrac{4!}{1!(4-1)!} = 4$	$4C3 = \dfrac{4!}{3!(4-3)!} = 4$
a	bcd		
b	acd		
c	abd		
d	abc		

|2|	|2|	$4C2 = \dfrac{4!}{2!(4-2)!} = 6$	
ab	cd		
ac	bd		
ad	bc		
|0|	|4|	$4C0 = \dfrac{4!}{0!(4-0)!} = 1$	$4C4 = \dfrac{4!}{4!(4-4)!} = 1$
∅	abcd		

Table 2B.3. Partition of the set of n distinct elements into complementary subsets

Table 2B.3 provides the necessary insight into the nature of partition, which may be categorized as follows:

1. For any value of r, a complementary value of $(n - r)$ is automatically chosen.
2. The formula stipulates partition into two cells, with the first cell occupied by the r subsets and the second occupied by the $(n - r)$ subsets.
3. The total number of all possible subsets, derived from the SS = {a, b, c, d}, accounts for all the possible allocation numbers of the SS elements into two contiguous cells.

Viewed in this light, the concept of partition further extends the concept of combination by the controlled division of the elements of the sample space into a specific number of subsets, whereby, in this case, each subset is to contain a distinct and different number of elements.

In effect, the concept of partition may be visualized as the virtual allocation of the resultant subdivision of the sample space to a specific number of contiguous cells in a given order.

For the sample space under consideration, SS = {a, b, c, d}, partition into two subsets with allocation numbers of 1 and 3 results in the four ordered partitions, occupying the top four rows of the table.

When all possible subdivisions of the sample space into two cells are considered, only three allocation ratios are possible, 1:3, 2:2, and 0:4, accounting for a total of sixteen ordered partitions.

The concept is best illustrated by reference to Table 2B.3, where the partition of the four elements with a set of four letters, SS = {a, b, c, d}, into all possible values of r, (0, 1, 2, 3, and 4) is tabled.

The previously mentioned conclusions allow us to consider combination as a special case of partition restricted to two complementary subsets. Thus, the process of combination leads into the more generic concept of partition because, in effect, every simple combination is a partition into two complementary subsets.

As noted in Table 2B.3, the total number of subsets corresponds to the sum derived from adding the number of subsets calculated by changing the value of r from 0 to 4, so that

$$nC_0 + nC_1 + nC_2 + nC_3 + nC_4 = 2^4 = 16$$

$$\text{Power set} = 1 + 4 + 6 + 4 + 1 = 16$$

Note that the denominator in each of the combination relationship partitions the basic set of the four distinct objects into complementary subsets of ordered pairs with occupancy numbers of {1:3}, {2:2}, and {∅:4}, distributed over eight pairs of cells accounting for all the paired subsets.

This pattern of ordered partition may be extended and generalized to include the ordered partition of a given set into r cells, each containing a specific number of elements out of the total set of n elements. The total number of elements of the set, n, are distributed into the given number of cells such that each cell is to contain a prescribed number of distinct elements while retaining its ordered place in the sequence of cells. Thus, for any given distribution, the sum of the subsets distributed over r cells must add up to the number of elements in the original set, so that

$$n = n_1 + n_2 + \ldots n_r.$$

Consequently, for any given pattern of ordered distribution that allows for the occupancy number in each cell and the order of the cells to be defined, the number of distribution possibilities that defines the different possible combination within each cell is given by the following expression:

$$nCn_1, n_2, \ldots, n_r = \frac{n!}{n_1! n_2! \ldots n_r!} \qquad \text{(Table 2B.5)}.$$

Table 2.4 presents in a concise format the correspondence of the combination and permutation formulae and their relationship to the type or distinctness of the items representing the sample space in each case.

Note again the correspondence between the expression for permutation involving identical subsets and that for combination of distinct and ordered subsets.

n = no. of distinct objects r = no. of distinct objects in a subset nCr = no. of subsets of size r	n = no. of distinct objects r = no. of distinct objects out of r nPr = no. of permutations of r objects
$$nCr = \frac{n!}{r!(n-r)!}$$	$$nPr = \frac{n!}{(n-r)!}$$
n = no. of distinct objects r = no. of distinct objects in a subset $(n-r)$ = no. of distinct objects in the complementary subset (two subsets) $nCr = nC(n-r)$ = no. of subsets of size r or their complement size $(n-r)$	n = no. of objects; two kinds only r = no. of objects; one kind $(n-r)$ = no of objects; another kind $nPr, (n-r)$ = no. of permutations of two kinds of objects

$nC(n-r) = nCr = \dfrac{n!}{r!(n-r)!}$	$nPr,(n-r) = \dfrac{n!}{r!(n-r)!}$
n = no. of distinct objects r_1 = no. of distinct objects in the first subset r_2 = no. of distinct objects in the second subset r_k = no. of distinct objects in the last subset $nCr_1, r_2, \ldots, r_k$ = no. of possible ordered partitions (subsets) derived from n distinct objects with $r_1, r_2, \ldots,$ or r_k objects per cell	n = no. of objects; several kinds r_1 = no. of objects; one kind r_2 = no. of objects; another kind r_k = no. of objects; last kind $nPr_1, r_2, \ldots, r_k$ = no. of distinguishable permutations of n objects composed of $r_1 + r_2 + \ldots + r_k$ kinds of objects
$nC\, r_1, r_2, \ldots, r_k = \dfrac{n!}{r_1!, r_2!, \ldots, r_k!}$	$nP\, r_1, r_2, \ldots, r_k = \dfrac{n!}{r_1!, r_2!, \ldots, r_k!}$

Table 2B.4. Correspondence of the combination and permutation formulae and their relationship to the distinctness of the items representing the sample space in each case

The obvious correspondence in the expressions may, however, obfuscate a basic qualitative divergence in the r value when applied to the permutation of indistinguishable objects compared with its value in the combinations requiring ordered partition of distinct objects into a given sequence of subsets, each containing a determined number of elements.

Ordered Partition	$nCr_1, r_2, \ldots, r_k$ $= \dfrac{n!}{r_1, r_2, \ldots, r_k}$	$rP\, r_1, r_2, \ldots, r_k$ $= \dfrac{r!}{r_1, r_2, \ldots, r_k}$	Ordered and Permuted Partitions
	No. of Ordered Partitions for Each Allocation Pattern	No. of Distinguishable Permutations for Each Allocation Pattern	No. of Ordered and Permuted Allocations Patterns

		Allocation patterns of four objects into two cells (3:1, 2:2, 0:4) = 4 + 6 + 1 = 11	Combinations with replacement $n-1+rCr = 1 + $ 4C4 5C4 = 5	Permutations with replacement of size 4 $8 + 6 + 2 = 16$ $2^4 = 16$
$\lvert 1 \rvert$	$\lvert 3 \rvert$	$\dfrac{4!}{1!3!} = 4$	$\dfrac{2!}{1!1!} = 2$	$4 \times 2 = 8$
a	bcd			
b	acd			
c	abd			
the	abc			
$\lvert 2 \rvert$	$\lvert 2 \rvert$	$\dfrac{4!}{2!2!} = 6$	$\dfrac{2!}{2!} = 1$	$6 \times 1 = 6$
ab	cd			
ac	bd			
ad	bc			
$\lvert 0 \rvert$	$\lvert 4 \rvert$	$\dfrac{4!}{0!4!} = 1$	$\dfrac{2!}{1!1!} = 2$	$1 \times 2 = 2$
$\varnothing$	$\lvert 4 \rvert$			
Possible allocation patterns				

Table 2B.5. Partition of a four-element set into two subsets for all possible allocations

Consider now a different allocation pattern for the same SS = {a, b, c, d}. The letters could be distributed instead to a series of three cells as an alternative. By imposing a 1:1:2 allocation scheme, for example, twelve different ordered partitions may be filled out, in which the contents of each cell are different from its adjacent cell for this particular allocation order.

	1			1			2	
c	d	ab
d	c	ab
b	d	ac
d	b	ac
b	c	ad
c	b	ad
a	d	bc
d	a	bc
a	c	bd
c	a	bd
a	b	cd
b	a	cd

Note that the allocation order of 1:1:2 may be similarly achieved by changing the order of the cells, that is, permutating the cells into the three possible sequence of the allocation order: 1:1:2; 1:2:1; 2:1:1.

a	b	cd
a	cd	b
cd	b	a

Alternatively, the SS could be partitioned into an allocation pattern of 3:1:0 or 2:2:0. In each instance, the contents of each cell are different from its neighbor.

Similarly, the allocation ratio pattern may be rearranged or permuted while keeping the contents of the individual cells intact so that for the partition 3:1:0, six different arrangements or sequences are possible. For the occupancy pattern of 2:2:0, the six possible subsets of the basic set of four elements {a, b, c, d}, namely, {ab};{ac};{ad};{bc};{bd}:{cd}, may alternate in filling the cells as follows:

ab	ac	0
ad	bc	0
bd	cd	0

This distribution satisfies the ordered partition into subsets of predefined number of elements; that is, this particular pattern is obtained simply through changing the combination of the elements in the individual cells while keeping the number of elements in the individual cell as well as their sequence unchanged.

Thus, the distribution of four elements into three cells may be accomplished in four different occupancy patterns, namely, {(1), (1), (2)}, {(2), (2), (0)}; {(3), (1), (0)}; {(4), (0), (0)}, with each pattern resulting in a given number of fixed subsets (Table 2B.6).

Ordered Partition			$[nCr_1, r_2, \ldots, r_k]$	$[rP\, r_1, r_2, \ldots, r_k]$	Ordered and Permuted Partitions
			No. of Ordered Partitions for Each Allocation Pattern	No. of Distinguishable Permutations for Each Allocation Pattern	No. of Ordered and Permuted Allocation Patterns
1	1	2	$\dfrac{4!}{1!1!2!} = 12$	$\dfrac{3!}{2!1!} = 3$	$3 \times 12 = 36$
a	b	cd			
2	2	0	$\dfrac{4!}{2!2!0!} = 6$	$\dfrac{3!}{2!1!} = 3$	$6 \times 3 = 18$
ab	cd	$\varnothing$			
3	1	0	$\dfrac{4!}{3!1!0!} = 4$	$\dfrac{3!}{1!1!1!} = 6$	• $4 \times 6 = 24$
• abc	• d	• $\varnothing$			

4	0	0	$\dfrac{4!}{4!0!0!} = 1$	$\dfrac{3!}{1!2!} = 3$	$1 \times 3 = 3$
abcd	∅	∅			
Possible allocation patterns			Allocation patterns of four objects into three cells, 1:1:1, 2:2:0, 3:1:0, 4:0:0 = 12 + 6 + 4 + 1 = 23	No. of combinations with replacement $n - 1 + rCr =$ $6C4 = 15$	No. of permutations with replacement = $36 + 18 + 24 + 3 = 81 = 3^4$ $= 81$

Table 2B.6. Ordered pattern of partition
of four elements into three cells

When this pattern is permuted over the available three cells, the sequence of the partition, but not the contents of the cells, results in three sets of permuted sequence, $\{(2), (2), (0)\}$; $\{(0), (2), (2)\}$; and $\{(2), (0), (2)\}$. The compounded sequence of ordered and permuted subsets results in all the possible allocation of the four elements into eighteen different sequences of subsets in conformity with the given partition. As noted in the table, each ordered partition may be accomplished with a fixed number of subsets, which in turn may be permuted to produce the possible number of ordered and permuted sequences while retaining the partition format but not its order. The sum of all possible partition and permutation is then given by the power formula, which is the equivalent to the sum of the ordered and permuted possible partitions. In other words, the total number of unordered subsets of all sizes that can be selected from a set of n elements when partitioned into r cells is expressed as in the first case involving the allocation of distinct objects to numbered cells by the multiplication principle involving the permutation with the replacement of three cells of size 4, that is, 3^4 distinct allocation patterns. The four objects may thus be assigned to three cells in $3^4 = 81$ different ways. The resulting sample space now contains eighty-one cells of equal probability such that each cell has a probability of $1/81$.

2B.3 Allocation in Practice

Consider the set of six different letters, SS = {a, b, c, d, e, f}, and its possible distribution into three cells. To put the question into a practical format, assume that six patients are to be assigned to three rooms, each room with a two-bed capacity. The perusal of Table 2B.7 shows that the six patients may be allocated to the double rooms, R1, R2, and R3, in ninety different ways depending on the order of their admission. If only two rooms are available, each capable of accommodating in case of an emergency, a maximum of four patients, while the third room is to remain vacant for back up option, the six patients may be accommodated in the available two rooms, two in the first and four in the second or alternatively three to each room.

Finally, if two rooms are to remain vacant, the six patients may be accommodated in the one available room. This situation is identical to the one posed earlier for the six letters, namely, the number of possible ordered partition that can be formed from a set of n objects allocated to r cells having a prescribed occupancy number, that is, the number of elements in each cell.

The ordered partition made to rooms R1, R2, and R3 may be altered if for some reason the patients in room R1 are transferred to R2 while those in R2 are transferred to R1. The patients assigned to a particular room remain unchanged, except for the order of the assigned room, that is, the order or sequence of the occupancy number.

To recapitulate, a set or sample space made up of distinct elements could be partitioned into two or more cells in a given allocation ratio or pattern, where the contents of each cell are distinct and different from its next neighbor.

When the cells, but not their contents, are now permuted, all possible allocation sequence for the given allocation ratio or pattern is obtained.

Finally, when this operation is carried over all the possible allocation patterns, distributed over the given number of cells, the partition of the given SS into all possible ordered allocation ratios is accomplished. Furthermore, when all the possible sequencing or permutation of the allocated cells is considered, the complete ordered partition of the SS into distinct and permuted subsets is derived. This number is equal to the number of cells to which the allocation is made, raised to a power equal to the number of elements in the SS.

Ordered Partitions			$[nCr_1, r_2, \ldots, r_k]$	$[nPr_1, r_2, \ldots, r_k]$	Ordered and Permuted Partitions
			No. of Ordered Partitions for Each Allocation Pattern	No. of Distinguishable Permutations for Each Allocation Pattern	No. of Ordered and Permuted Allocation Patterns
$|1|$	$|1|$	$|4|$	$\dfrac{6!}{1!1!4!} = 30$	$\dfrac{3!}{2!1!} = 3$	$30 \times 3 = 90$
a	b	cdef			
$|1|$	$|2|$	$|3|$	$\dfrac{6!}{1!2!3!} = 60$	$\dfrac{3!}{1!1!1!} = 6$	$60 \times 6 = 360$
a	bc	def			
$|1|$	$|5|$	$|0|$	$\dfrac{6!}{1!5!0!} = 6$	$\dfrac{3!}{1!1!1!} = 6$	$6 \times 6 = 36$
a	bcdef	∅			
2	2	2	$\dfrac{6!}{2!2!2!} = 90$	$\dfrac{3!}{3!} = 1$	$90 \times 1 = 90$
ab	cd	ef			
$|2|$	$|4|$	$|0|$	$\dfrac{6!}{2!4!0!} = 15$	$\dfrac{3!}{1!1!1!} = 6$	$15 \times 6 = 90$
ab	cdef	∅			

|3|	|3|	|0|	$\dfrac{6!}{3!3!0!} = 20$	$\dfrac{3!}{2!1!} = 3$	$20 \times 3 = 60$
abc	def	∅			
|6|	|0|	|0|	$\dfrac{6!}{6!0!0!} = 1$	$\dfrac{3!}{1!2!} = 3$	$1 \times 3 = 3$
abcdef	∅	∅			
Possible allocation patterns			Allocation patterns of six objects into three cells 1:1:4, 1:2:3, 1:5:0 2:2:0, 2:4:0, 3:3:0 6:0:0	No. of combinations with replacement $n - 1 + rCr = 8C6 = 28$	No. of permutations with replacement = $90 + 360 + 36 + 90 + 90 + 60 + 3 = 3^6 = 729$

Table 2B.7. Partition of six distinct objects into three cells

To round up the subject, consider the allocation of four indistinguishable objects to three distinguishable cells.

As noted in Table 2B.8, placing four identical objects into three cells can be made in fifteen different ways, taking into account the allocation number to each cell and the order of the cells.

Stated differently, the possible combination of objects and dividers is in effect a count of the possible ways of placing n identical objects into r cells.

Ordered Partition			
|1|	**|1|**	**|2|**	Permutation of three cells, two which are of one kind
◆	◆	◆◆	$\dfrac{3!}{2!1!} = 3$
◆	◆◆	◆	
◆◆	◆	◆	

|2|	|2|	|0|	Permutation of three cells, two of which are of one kind
♦♦	♦♦	∅	$\dfrac{3!}{2!1!} = 3$
♦♦	∅	♦♦	
∅	♦♦	♦♦	
|3|	|1|	|0|	Permutation of three different cells
♦♦♦	♦	∅	$\dfrac{3!}{1!1!1!} = 6$
♦♦♦	∅	♦	
♦	♦♦♦	∅	
♦	∅	♦♦♦	
∅	♦♦♦	♦	
∅	♦	♦♦♦	
|4|	|0|	|0|	Permutation of three cells, two of which are of one kind
♦♦♦♦	∅	∅	$\dfrac{3!}{1!2!} = 3$
∅	♦♦♦♦	∅	
∅	∅	♦♦♦♦	
			Total number of possible distribution of four identical diamonds into three cells $$3 + 3 + 6 + 3 = 15$$ $$n - 1 + rCr = 2 + 4C4 = 6C4 = 15$$

Table 2B.8. Partition of four identical objects into three cells

The concept of partition in the case of identical objects (Table 2B.8) includes two subsidiary concepts that need to be separately explored. As the name implies, partition is literally the placement of one line divider to affect the separation into two spaces or cells. Two dividers are needed to create three cells so that the number of cells exceeds the number of dividers by one. For n spaces, $(n - 1)$ dividers are needed.

The distribution of r objects into n spaces is equivalent to the number of all possible combinations of r objects and n dividers taken r at time. Thus, distributing five identical objects into three cells may be thought of as the possible combination of seven objects (five real objects and two dividers) taken five at a time. The parallel to the actual combination of seven different objects taken five at a time is noted the following two relations. The first relation gives the number of ways in which five different objects may be placed into three cells. The second relation gives the number of different subsets that may be derived from seven different objects taken five at a time.

No. objects		No. dividers		No. objects			
5	+	2		5	$= \dfrac{(r+(n-1))!}{r![(r+(n-1))-r]} = \dfrac{7!}{5!(7-5)!} = 21$ ways		
r		$(n-1)$	C	r			

$$nCr = \frac{n!}{r!(n-r)!} = 7C5 = \frac{7!}{5!2!} = 21 \text{ ways}$$

Stated differently, the possible combination of objects and dividers is in effect a count of the possible ways of placing n identical objects into r cells.

The perusal of Tables 2B.5, 2B.6, and 2B.7 confirms that the total number of distinguishable permutations (but not the total ordered and permuted) for the distribution of r distinguishable objects into n distinguishable cells may be similarly derived using the sum of the dividers and objects in the combination formula for n elements taken r at a time with replacement.

2B.4 Partition and Occupancy

Instead of the random assignment on arrival of patients to rooms, consider the situation where nine emergent car accident cases arrived simultaneously to the ER and were to be assigned simultaneously to three surgical intensive care units of four-, three-, and two-bed capacity. The question in this case is how many ways can the nine patients be assigned to the three rooms?

Four patients out of the nine could be assigned to room 1 in $9C4$ ways. Of the remaining five patients, three could be assigned to room 2 in $5C3$ ways. The remaining two patients are then assigned to room 3 in $2C2$ ways.

By the multiplication principle, the total number of possible assignments is then the product of the three possible combinations, so that

$$9C4 \times 5C3 \times 2C2 = \frac{9!}{4!5!} \times \frac{5!}{3!2!} \times \frac{2!}{2!0!} = \frac{9!}{4!3!2!} = 126 \times 10 \times 1 = 1260.$$

The problem, however, is essentially one of an ordered partition out of a set of n distinct objects and placed into a sequence of numbered cells, so that

$$nCn_1, n_2, \ldots, n_r = \frac{n!}{n_1!n_2!\cdots n_r!} = 9C4,3,2 = \frac{9!}{4!3!2!} = 1260$$

On the other hand, a strictly random distribution of the nine patients to the three rooms can occur in $3^9 = 19{,}683$ possible assignments because for each patient, a choice of one of the three rooms is possible. Under the circumstances of random distribution, we are dealing with the permutation of three rooms taken nine times with replacement. Stated differently, there are 19,683 possible ways of distributing nine patients to three rooms taking into consideration all possible allocation from all to one room to equal distribution of three to a room. The allocation of four, five, and two to the three rooms resulted in 1,260 possible assignments only. The probability of such an assignment is rather small considering the possible assignments choice available, so that

$$\frac{9C\,4,3,2}{3^9} = \frac{1,260}{19,683} = 0.064.$$

The partition property of the combination process underlies its inherent connection to the binomial theorem, which shall be alluded to later in the discussion.

As a prelude, it is instructive to refocus on the simple events or outcomes derived from the sample space associated with the experiment of tossing n coins. The coin is a representative of a generic object that can assume one of two mutually exclusive states. The sample space associated with the tossing of three coins was noted earlier to equal $2^3 = 8$ possible outcomes.

As can be seen from Figure 2B.3, the value assigned to r in the combination formula nCr addresses the number of elements in a subset chosen from the set of n elements. Where n equals the number of coins, three in this case. The assigned r value in effect addresses the question in one of two formats: "How many heads in a subset of r elements?" or "How many tails in a subset of $(n - r)$ elements?" If the first format is chosen, then the conditions are as follows:

For $r = r$, the query is about the subsets with all heads.
For $r = 1$, the query is about subsets with one head only.
For $r = 0$, the question may be rephrased to ask "How many subsets with zero heads in a set of n elements, that is, tails only?"
Because $nCr = nC(n - r)$, two possibilities are assumed. If r is assigned to the number of heads, then $(n - r)$ is the number of tails.

Putting the question in numerical format and asking "How many subsets with two heads may be obtained from tossing three coins?" the following equation provides the obvious answer:

$$nCr = 3C2 = \frac{3!}{2!1!} = 3 \text{ subsets with two heads each}$$

This, obviously, may be obtained directly from inspection of the sample space of the three coins. What is not apparent is that the number of subsets with 3, 2, 1, or 0 heads may be obtained directly from the combination formula as follows:

$$\underset{\text{quarter penny dime}}{SS \times SS \times SS} = = \{ \quad \underset{3C3}{H \quad H \quad H} \underset{\text{Washington Lincoln Roosevelt}}{}, \underset{+3C2}{HHT, HTH, THH}, \underset{+3C1}{HTT, THT, TTH}, \underset{+3C0}{TTT} \}$$

Possible Outcomes of Tossing Three Coins			Frequency of Occurrence of Each of the Possible Outcomes
H	H	H	$3C3 = 1$
H	H	T	
H	T	H	$3C2 = 3P2,1 = \dfrac{3!}{2!(3-2)!} = 3$
T	H	H	
H	T	T	
T	H	T	$3C1 = 3P1,2 = \dfrac{3!}{1!(3-1)!} = 3$
T	T	H	
T	T	T	$3C0 = 1$

Table 2B.9. Frequency of occurrence of each of the possible outcomes of tossing three coins

When the number of heads or tails in a subset is now transcribed into the standard numerical format, the sample space now assumes the familiar superscripted pattern, indicating the frequency of each element in the subset, whereas the coefficient pertains to the number of subsets of this category.

$$SS_{quarter} \times SS_{penny} \times SS_{dime} = SS = \{ \underset{3C3=1}{1H^3}, \ \underset{3C2=3}{3H^2T^1}, \ \underset{3C1=3}{3H^1T^2}, \ \underset{3C0=1}{1T^3} \}$$

As noted in Table 2B.6, for $r = 2$, $3C2 = 3$, indicating the number of combinations (subsets) with two heads each. Strictly speaking, the three subsets are essentially one combination since

$$\{H, H, T\} = \{H, T, H\}.$$

But

$$(H, H, T) \neq (H, T, H).$$

In this sense, the three subsets are actually permutations of the three elements. This confluence in the formula describing two different processes is unfortunate because it tends to obfuscate rather than enlighten. The practice, however, is standard, sanctified by usage. As noted in Flow Chart 2-3, the permutation formula for two kinds of objects is identical to the combination formula of r objects taken of n distinct objects.

The combination formula for a given n and a variable r may be individually calculated as required. The Pascal triangle in its modified format offers a handy substitute for the hand held calculator when dealing with limited range of numbers, as seen in Table 2B.10. The intimate relationship of Pascal's triangle to the binomial theorem is a subject of major significance that will be alluded to later in this discussion.

	nCr	$r = 0$	$r = 1$	$r = 2$	$r = 3$	$r = 4$	$r = 5$	$r = 6$
$(H + T)^0$	$n = 0$	1						
$(H + T)^1$	$n = 1$	$1H$	$1T$					
$(H + T)^2$	$n = 2$	$1H^2$	$2HT$	$1T^2$				
$(H + T)^3$	$n = 3$	$1H^3$	$3H^2T$	$3HT^2$	$1T^3$			
$(H + T)^4$	$n = 4$	$1H^4$	$4H^3T$	$6H^2T^2$	$4HT^3$	$1T^4$		
$(H + T)^5$	$n = 5$	$1H^5$	$5H^4T$	$10H^3T^2$	$10H^2T^3$	$5HT^4$	$1T^5$	
$(H + T)^6$	$n = 6$	$1H^6$	$6H^5T$	$15H^4T^2$	$20H^3T^3$	$15H^2T^4$	$6HT^5$	$1T^6$

Table 2B.10. Pascal triangle: limited format

Chapter 3

Switching Circuits and Gates: The Alternative to Sets

Set theory plays a central role in bridging the gap between the mathematical deductive logic that applies to statements that are either absolutely true or absolutely false and inductive logic (probability) dealing with statements that range over the whole spectrum of reality from total falsehood to absolute truth.

In 1847, George Boole (1815-1864) published an introductory book titled *The Mathematical Analysis of Logic*, in which he was able to demonstrate the innate analogy between the perceived laws of human reasoning and the symbolic language, adapted to a binary system that can only assume two values, 1 if true and 0 if false. This abstract mathematical structure, devoid of any reference to magnitude or numbers, is based exclusively on symbols and rules of operations without any specific meaning.

Symbolic logic, referred to as Boolean algebra, is essentially a restatement of classical deductive logic. Letter symbols are used to represent variables that are in effect substituting for declarative statements that can be judged true or false, excluding interrogative, imperative, or exclamatory statements. Compound statements can then be constructed from simple ones through logical connectives linking two or more statements.

By assigning the truth value of 1 to a true statement and the truth value of 0 to a false statement, all logical statements are transformed into a binary format. Thus, logical analysis translates the premises into symbols that can be operated on by the rules of logic, leading to the deduction of valid conclusion. The system is not concerned with the truth or credibility of the premises involved, but rather with the validity of the deductive process.

The subsequent reincarnation of Boolean algebra into two additional forms attests to its impact on modern communication: an algebra of sets now commonly used in introductory texts, which gives a graphic interpretations of deductive logic using the ubiquitous Venn diagrams, and a switching algebra, which forms the basis of modern electronic computers.

3.1 Sets and Switching Circuits Operations

The laws of Boolean algebra covering set and switching circuits operations are listed in Table 3.1 and graphically depicted in Tables 3.2A and 3.2B for the basic set operation and Table 3 for the switching circuits operations.

The empty set ($\emptyset$) is unique in set theory in that it is the set that has no elements and is therefore a subset of every set. The empty set must not be confused with 0 number of elements despite the apparent similarity in context. Zero by itself as 0 is not a set, but {0} is the set containing one element, namely, 0. On the other hand, $\emptyset$ is the empty set { }, that is, the set with no elements.

The digital logic for switching circuits is generally concerned with the operation of multiplication (conjunction symbol •), addition (disjunction symbol +), and negation (negation symbol bar or apostrophe, e.g., $\overline{A}$ or A'). Because the binary variable can assume two and only two values, it can be represented by the position of a toggle switch where the on and off positions are representative of 1 and 0, respectively. State 1 is the code for the transmission of current or pulses, and state 0 is the code for the cutoff of transmission.

In this analogy, the off position is the negation of the on position so that if $A = 1$, $\overline{A} = 0$; and if $A = 0$, $\overline{A} = 1$. This definition of complementation is another way of saying that an open circuit is the negation of a closed circuit, $0 = \overline{1}$, and a closed circuit is the negation of an open one, $1 = \overline{0}$. Thus, an open contact is associated with the symbol 0, and a closed contact is associated with the symbol 1. A switching device representing a circuit variable denoted by a letter symbol takes on the values of 0 or 1, depending on its position when open or closed, respectively.

The operation of addition or union when applied to two circuit variables may be represented physically by the parallel connection of the switches corresponding to these variables. Thus, in Table 3.3, panels 7 and 8, the two parallel switches are physical realization of the union noted in panels 2 and 9 of Table 3.2. The parallel connection provides a closed circuit if and only if the *A* switch, the *B* switch ($\overline{A}$), or both are closed.

The operation of multiplication or intersection may be represented physically by the series connection of the two switches, as noted in panels 5 and 6 of Table 3.3. The series connection provides a closed circuit only when both switches are in the closed position.

In the case of the parallel connection, transmission fails, resulting in an open circuit or 0, under one condition only, namely, when both switches are in the open position, all the other positions lead to a closed circuit. This relationship may be symbolized by the following binary outcome:

$$0 + 0 = 0; \; 1 + 0 = 0 + 1 = 1 + 1 = 1.$$

In the case of the series connection, transmission failure, that is, open circuit or 0, results from the open position of one or both of the two switches. This relationship may be symbolized by the following binary outcome:

$$1 \bullet 1 = 1; \; 0 \bullet 0 = 0 \bullet 1 = 1 \bullet 0 = 0.$$

3.2 Logic and Set Operations

This chapter was introduced by comparing sets and circuits because of the intuitive feel for the graphic representation of the variables involved. Boole's original contribution was in fact exclusively related to its application in symbolic logic where in this case simple statements represented by letters stand for the logical variables, which by convention assume the value of 1 if true and 0 if false. Two or more simple statements are then tied together into a compound statement by the appropriate connective.

When two simple statements are tied together by the connective AND, the truth value of the compound statements may be defined by the truth table of the conjunction of p∧q (*p* and *q*) or its equivalent

$A \cdot B$, as shown under the AND connective in Table 3.5. As noted, the compound statement A and B is true if, and only if, A is true and B is true. There are no other possibilities. The second connective is OR, which is the disjunction of p∨q (p or q) or its equivalent $A + B$ shown under the inclusive OR of Table 3.5. The inclusive disjunction in this case is true when A, B, or both are true.

The third basic connective is the negation, which reverses the truth or falsehood of the given statement. Two additional connectives are required to complete the operational system of symbolic logic.

The conditional or implication symbolized by an arrow between two logical variables corresponds to the "If p, then q" compound statement encountered in routine communication. Its truth table is presented under the conditional column in Table 3.5.

The biconditional or equivalence denoted by a double-headed arrow between two logical variables corresponds to the compound statement of "p if and only if q," often abbreviated into an acronym (Iff), often confused as a typographical error. It can be shown, however, that conjunction, disjunction, and negation are sufficient to cover all logical operations.

Table 3.4 presents the equivalent set operations of the corresponding logical operations. Table 3.6. combines the corresponding graphic elements of sets, truth tables, and symbolic gating circuits together with their respective Boolean equations for Conjunction, disjunction, and negation in order to delineate the essential unity of their logical substrate.

The three symbolic logical systems described so far apply to propositions or situations that are bivalent in nature, being either absolutely true or false with no intermediate third possibility in between. Probability theory occupies the range left vacant by symbolic logic where the propositions that describe chance events are analyzed in terms of probability.

The range includes the limiting cases of absolute truth, where the probability of 1 means absolute certainty, and the limiting case of absolute falsehood, where the probability of 0 means absolute impossibility.

3.3 Probability and Set Operations

From this perspective, probability theory may be construed as the complement of deductive logic. The inductive inference involved in probability leads to probabilistic or indirect conclusions in contrast to deductive inference of drawing direct conclusions.

Set theory in this case, as in the case of symbolic logic, provides the necessary theoretical and graphic elements for the elucidation of the laws governing the probabilistic process. The set containing all possible outcomes of a random event constitutes the sample space of the given experiment. A particular outcome, on the other hand, may be considered as a sample point or element of the sample space while an event is a subset of the same space.

Set theory and its graphic counterpart, the Venn diagram, offer the theoretical and graphic tool for the analysis of complex problem. Thus, given the sample space of an experiment, the laws governing set operations may be applied to describe events and to derive their probabilities. On the other hand, any given event may be translated into the language of sets because it is actually a subset of the sample space.

As such, the event E and its complement $\overline{E}$ make up the full sample space, while their intersection consists of the impossible event $E \cap \overline{E} = \varnothing$.

No.	Laws of Boolean Algebra				
	Set Operations			**Switching Circuits Operations**	
No.	Identity	Tables 3.2A-3.2B	Identity		Table 3.3
1	$A \cup \emptyset = A$	Panel 1	$A + 0 = A$		Panel 4
2	$A \cap \emptyset = \emptyset$	Panel 1	$A \bullet 0 = 0$		Panel 2
3	$A \cup U = U$	Panel 1	$A + 1 = 1$		Panel 3
4	$A \cap U = A$	Panel 1	$A \bullet 1 = A$		Panel 1
	Complementarity		**Complementarity**		
5	$A \cup \overline{A} = U$	Panel 2	$A + \overline{A} = 1$		Panel 8
6	$A \cap \overline{A} = \emptyset$	Panel 2	$A \bullet \overline{A} = 0$		Panel 6
	Idempotence		**Idempotence**		
7	$A \cup A = A$	Panel 2	$A + A = A$		Panel 7
8	$A \cap A = A$	Panel 2	$A \bullet A = A$		Panel 5
9	$\overline{\emptyset} = U$		$\overline{0} = 1$		
10	$\overline{U} = \emptyset$		$\overline{1} = 0$		
	Commutative		**Commutative**		
11	$A \cup B = B \cup A$	Panel 8	$A + B = B + A$		Panel 7
12	$A \cap B = B \cap A$	Panel 5	$A \bullet B = B \bullet A$		Panel 5
	Associative		**Associative**		
13	$(A \cup B) \cup C = A \cup (B \cup C)$		$(A + B) + C = A + (B + C)$		
14	$(A \cap B) \cap C = A \cap (B \cap C)$		$(A \bullet B) \bullet C = A \bullet (B + C)$		
	Distributive		**Distributive**		
15	$A \cup (B \cap C) = (A \cup B) \cap (A \cup C)$		$A \bullet (B + C) = A \bullet B + A \bullet C$		
16	$A \cap (B \cup C) = (A \cap B) \cup (A \cap C)$	Panel 8	$A + (B \bullet C) = (B + C) \bullet (A + C)$		
	Absorption		**Absorption**		
17	$A \cap (A \cup B) = A$		$A \bullet (A + B) = A$		
18	$A \cup (A \cap B) = A$		$A + (A \bullet B) = A$		
	DeMorgan's		**DeMorgan's**		
19	$\overline{(A \cup B)} = \overline{A} \cap \overline{B}$	Panel 12	$\overline{A + B} = \overline{A} \bullet \overline{B}$		
20	$\overline{(A \cap B)} = \overline{A} \cup \overline{B}$	Panel 9	$\overline{A \bullet B} = \overline{A} + \overline{B}$		

Table 3.1. Generic format of the basic laws of Boolean algebra as applied to sets and circuits operations

$A \cup \varnothing = A$	$A \cup \overline{A} = U = 1$	$B \cup \varnothing = B$	$B \cup \overline{B} = U = 1$
$A \cap \varnothing = \varnothing$	$A \cap \overline{A} = \varnothing$	$B \cap \varnothing = \varnothing$	$B \cap \overline{B} = \varnothing$
$A \cup U = U$	$A \cup A = A$	$B \cup U = U$	$B \cup B = B$
$A \cap U = A$	$A \cap A = A$	$B \cap U = B$	$B \cap B = B$
Panel 1	Panel 2	Panel 3	Panel 4

Table 3.2A. Basic laws of Boolean algebra as applied to set operations

$A \cap B$	$A \cap \overline{B} = A - (A \cap B)$	$B \cap \overline{B} = B - (B \cap A)$	$A \cup B$
$A \cdot B$	$A \cdot \overline{B}$	$B \cdot \overline{A}$	$A + B$
A and B	A and $\overline{B}$	B and $\overline{A}$	A or B
Panel 5	Panel 6	Panel 7	Panel 8
$A' \cup B' = (A \cap B)'$	$A' \cup B = (A \cap \overline{B})'$	$B' \cup A = (B \cap \overline{A})'$	$A' \cap B' = (A \cap B)'$
$\overline{A} + \overline{B} = \overline{A \cdot B}$	$\overline{A} + B$	$\overline{B} + A$	$\overline{A} \cdot \overline{B} = \overline{A + B}$
$\overline{A}$ or $\overline{B} = \overline{A}$ and $\overline{B}$	$\overline{A}$ or B	$\overline{B}$ or A	$\overline{A}$ and $\overline{B} = \overline{A}$ and $\overline{B}$
Panel 9	Panel 10	Panel 11	Panel 12

Table 3.2B. Basic laws of Boolean algebra as applied to set operations

Boolean algebraic laws

Identity	Identity	Identity	Identity
$A \cdot 1 = A$	$A \cdot 0 = 0$	$A + 1 = 1$	$A + 0 = A$
Multiplication rules	Multiplication rules	Multiplication rules	Multiplication rules
$1 \cdot 0 = 0$ $1 \cdot 1 = 1$ Panel 1	$0 \cdot 0 = 0$ $0 \cdot 1 = 0$ Panel 2	$1 + 1 = 1$ $1 + 0 = 1$ Panel 3	$0 + 1 = 1$ $0 + 0 = 0$ Panel 4
Idempotence	Complementarity	Idempotence	Complementarity
$A \cdot A = A$	$A \cdot \overline{A} = 0$	$A + A = A$	$A + \overline{A} = 1$
$1 \cdot 1 = 1$ $0 \cdot 0 = 0$ Panel 5	$1 \cdot 0 = 0$ $0 \cdot 1 = 0$ Panel 6	$1 + 1 = 1$ $0 + 0 = 0$ Panel 7	$1 + 0 = 1$ $0 + 1 = 1$ Panel 8

Table 3.3. of Boolean algebraic laws as applied
to switching circuits operations

Logic: Operations	Statements	Sets: Operations
p (proposition)		P
q (proposition)		Q
Conjunction $p \wedge q$	**And**	**Intersection** $P \cap Q$
Inclusive Disjunction $p \vee q$	**Or** $p, q,$ or both One or the other or both Legal usage: and/or	**Union** $P \cup Q$
Exclusive Disjunction $p \veebar q$ $(p \vee q) \wedge \sim (p \wedge q)$	**Or** Either p or q, not both False when both are T Legal usage: either/or	
Negation $\sim$ $\sim(p \wedge q) = \sim p \vee \sim q$ $\sim(p \vee q) = \sim p \wedge \sim q$	**Not** It is not the case Not both p and q; not p or not q Neither p nor q Not p or q; not p and not q	**Complement** P' $(P \cap Q)' = P' \cup Q'$ $(P \cup Q)' = P' \cap Q'$
Conditional: **Implication**	p implies q	$P \subset Q$
Conditional $p \rightarrow q = \sim p \vee q$ Premise $\rightarrow$ conclusion Antecedent $\rightarrow$ consequent	If p, then q p is a sufficient condition for q p only if q q is a necessary condition for p q, if p	$(P' \cup Q)$ or $(P' \cup Q')'$
Converse = Inverse $q \rightarrow p = \sim p \rightarrow \sim q$	If q, then p q is a necessary condition for p q, only if p	
Contrapositive = Conditional $\sim q \rightarrow \sim p = p \rightarrow q$	If not q, then not p	
Inverse = Converse $\sim p \rightarrow \sim q = q \rightarrow p$	If not p, then not q p is a necessary condition for q	
Biconditional: **Equivalence** $p \leftrightarrow q$ $(p \equiv q)$ Double conditional $(p \rightarrow q) \wedge (q \rightarrow p)$	p implies q and q implies p p if and only if (Iff) q If p then q, if q then p p is necessary and sufficient for $q \equiv$ $(p \rightarrow q)$ and $(q \rightarrow p)$	$P = Q$ $(P' \cup Q) \cap (Q' \cup P)$ or $(P \cap Q) \cup (P \cup Q)'$

Table 3.4. Generic format of the basic laws of Boolean algebra as applied to symbolic logic and set operations

		Truth Tables and Electronic Gates			
		AND	**NAND**		
A	B	$A \cdot B$	$\overline{A \cdot B} = \overline{A} + \overline{B}$	$A \cdot \overline{B}$	$\overline{A} \cdot B$
1	1	1	0	0	0
1	0	0	1	1	0
0	1	0	1	0	1
0	0	0	1	0	0
		Inclusive OR	**Inclusive NOR**		
A	B	$A + B$	$\overline{A + B} = \overline{A} + \overline{B}$	$A + \overline{B}$	$\overline{A} + B$
1	1	1	0	1	1
1	0	1	0	1	0
0	1	1	0	0	1
0	0	0	1	1	1
		Conditional	Converse	Contrapositive	Inverse
A	B	$A \to B$	$B \to A$	$\sim B \to \sim A$	$\sim A \to \sim B$
1	0	0	1	0	1
0	1	1	0	1	0
0	0	1	1	1	1

		Biconditional			
A	B	$A \leftrightarrow B$			
1	1	1			
1	0	0			
0	1	0			
0	0	1			

Table 3.5. Basic truth tables of symbolic logic:
electronic gates for AND and OR

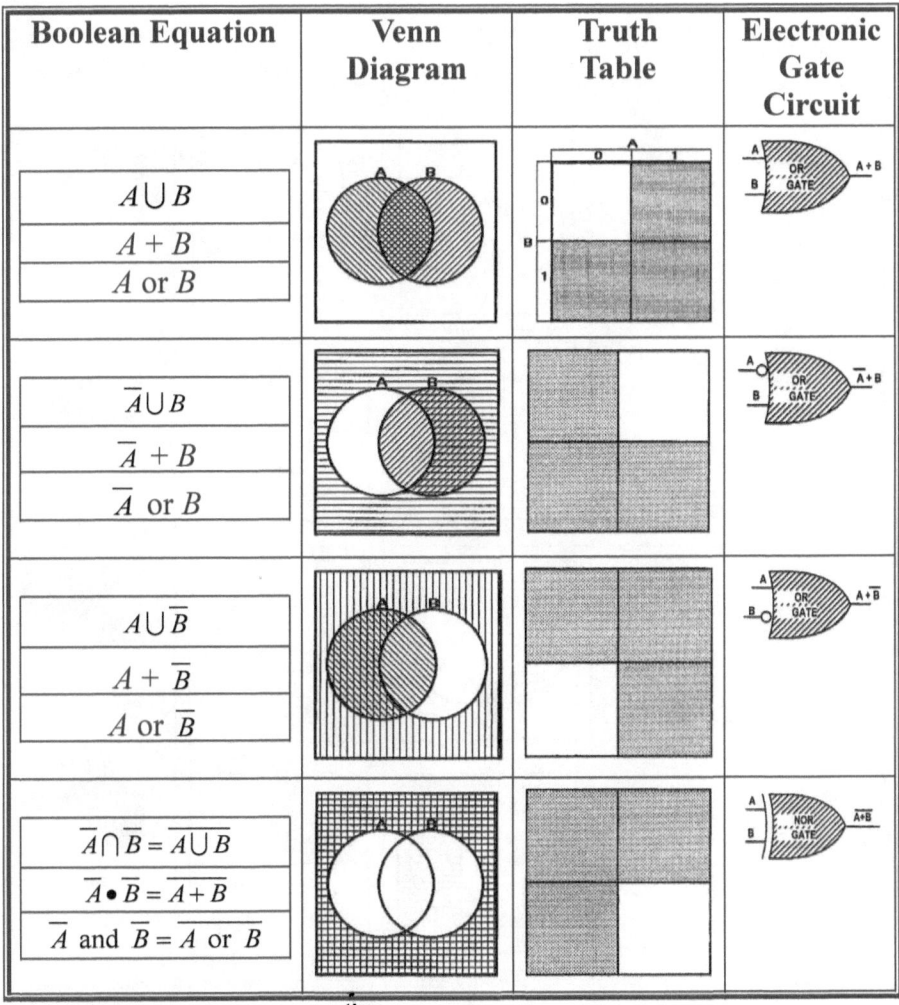

Boolean Equation	Venn Diagram	Truth Table	Electronic Gate Circuit
$A \cup B$ $A + B$ A or B			
$\overline{A} \cup B$ $\overline{A} + B$ $\overline{A}$ or B			
$A \cup \overline{B}$ $A + \overline{B}$ A or $\overline{B}$			
$\overline{A} \cap \overline{B} = \overline{A \cup B}$ $\overline{A} \bullet \overline{B} = \overline{A + B}$ $\overline{A}$ and $\overline{B} = \overline{A}$ or $\overline{B}$			

Table 3.6A. Boolean generic equations and their corresponding graphic equivalents

Boolean Equation	Venn Diagram	Truth Table	Electronic Gate Circuit
$A \cap B$ $A \cdot B$ A and B			
$\overline{A} \cap B$ $\overline{A} \cdot B$ $\overline{A}$ and B			
$A \cap \overline{B}$ $A \cdot \overline{B}$ A and $\overline{B}$			
$\overline{A \cup B} = \overline{A} \cap B$ $\overline{A} + \overline{B} = \overline{(A \cdot B)}$ $\overline{A}$ or $\overline{B} = \overline{A \text{ and } B}$			

Table 3.6B. Boolean generic equations and their corresponding
graphic equivalents

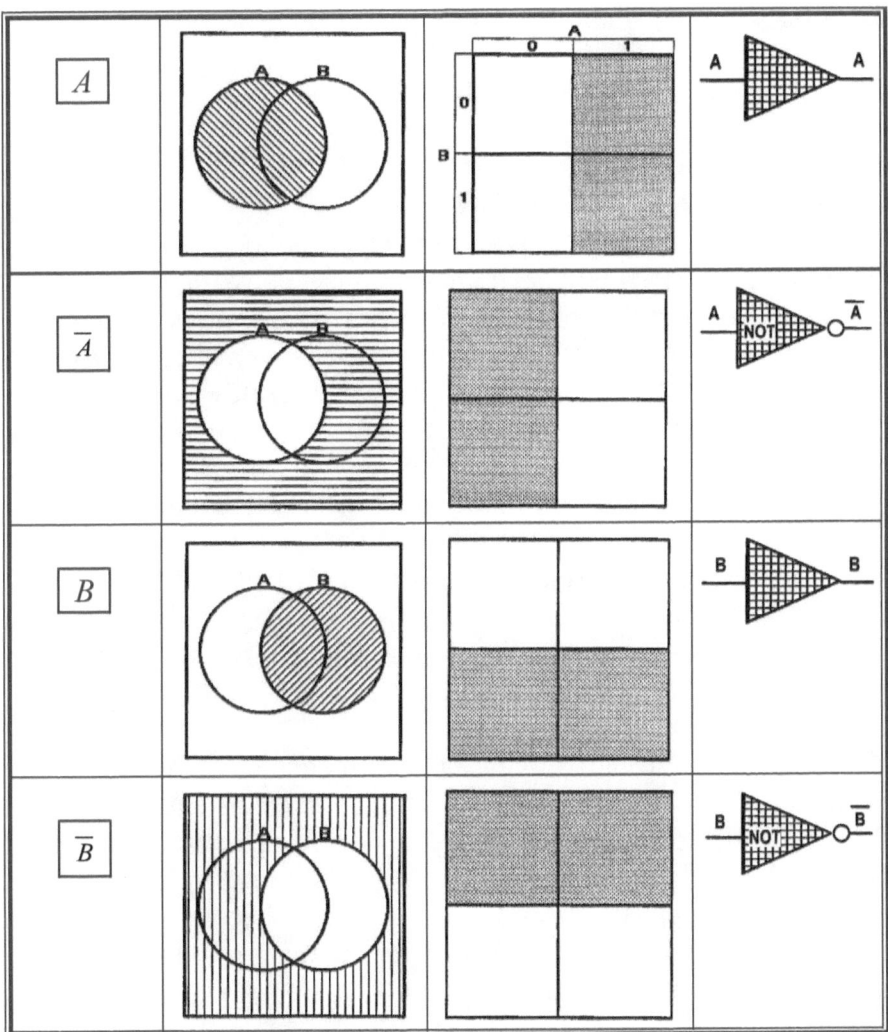

Table 3.6C. Boolean generic equations and their corresponding
graphic equivalents

Chapter 4

Probability

4.1 An Overview

The subject of probability is intriguing in its concepts and logical substrate. Despite its universal application in daily intercourse from weather forecasting to the trend analysis of the stock market, the human mind is not adept at manipulating complex situations where probability is a basic premise, unless specifically trained in the field. To observe a bridge player calculating effortlessly, the odds is to realize that a different category of logical endeavor is at work, equivalent but different from the common deductive logic.

The road to an intuitive approach to probabilistic logic must perforce pass through three stations beginning with the simple artificially structured model to the final station where probability is just a function of a random variable assigned to a particular outcome.

This transition through three stages, which almost replicates the historical development of the subject, may seem as an unwarranted detour with little bearing on the practical side of the reality. It is my belief that this probabilistic mode of thought cannot be acquired and manipulated unless its special rules and terms become a functional tool equivalent to the capacity at manipulating number or the deductive logic of Euclidean geometry.

One may argue that this facility belongs to the province of childhood and youth, a notion that is being gradually instituted with the stated objective.

In the final analysis, however, the subject matter of probability revolves around the idea of chance occurrence of an event or happening, to which the name random event has been affixed, implying the lack of a defined plan in the making process. An element of uncertainty thus underlies all random events. Such being the case, one might be tempted to surmise that by definition, no specific set of rules could possibly apply. This might explain the late entry of probabilistic mode of thought into the main stream of elementary mathematics.

With this in mind, the aim of probability is to investigate whether a discernible pattern or order, hidden in the repetitive scheme of randomness, may be detected. The subject of probability is the elucidation of the rules that might dictate the given occurrence, which in turn may be the very tool of prediction that may be used to constrain the boundaries of randomness.

4.2 A Simple Experiment

Begin with the most ubiquitous gambling tool the tossing of a balance die. This trivial play dignified by the word experiment offers, nonetheless, the basic axioms of classical probability:

1. The outcome of the experiment yields one and only one outcome at a time.
2. Each of the final six outcomes of the experiment is called a *simple event*.
3. If the number of occurrences of each of the six numbers {1, 2, 3, 4, 5, 6} is tallied, it will be found that the frequency and by extension the probability of outcome of each is identically the same; thus, the occurrence of each outcome is equally likely.
4. The individual outcomes correspond to a conceptual sample space, which might be construed as a depot of all the possible outcomes.
5. The elements of the sample space (all the possible outcomes) may be considered as members of a defined set {1, 2, 3, 4, 5, 6}.

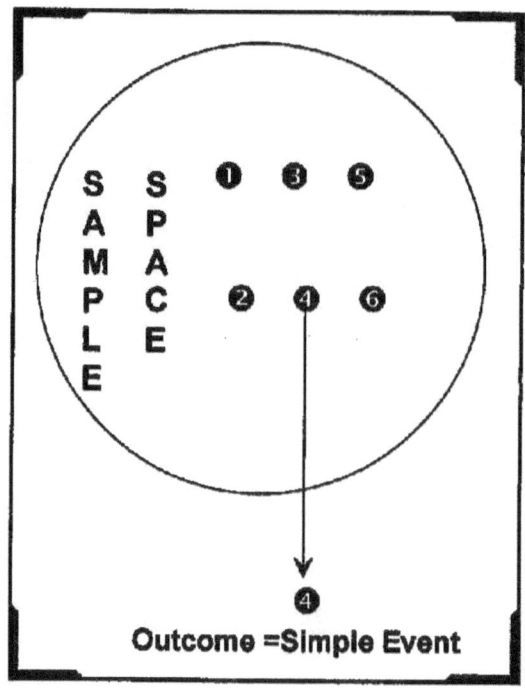

Figure 4.1. Outcome of the Experiment yielding a simple event

If the experiment is identically repeated, then instead of tallying the outcome of the simple events as noted earlier, the outcome of specifically even number is being tallied.

1. With this injunction, the equally likely outcome is no longer in effect. The new tally is that of a compound event that consists of three outcomes.
2. The sample space is now divided into two subsets, each corresponding to the even and odd outcomes.
3. If the outcomes being tallied are stipulated as (a) perfect square, (b) prime numbers, and (c) even numbers, the sample space is now divided into three subsets, two of which are intersecting, which correspond to three compound events, each made up of more than one element.
4. The probability of occurrence deviates sharply from the original equally likely outcome because now the outcome is a function of the frequency of the even subset of 3, the prime subset of 2, and the even/perfect square of 1.

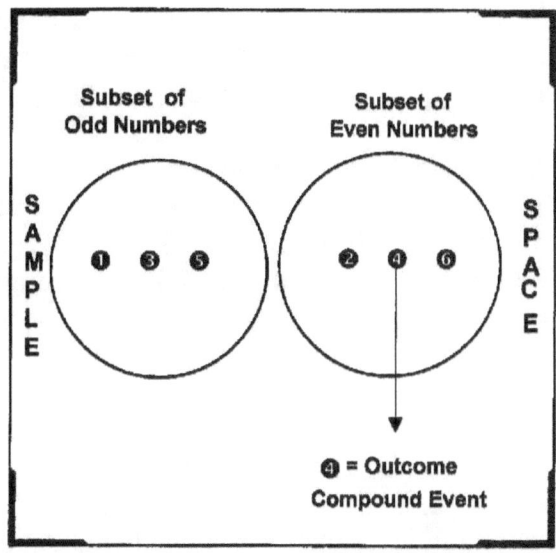

Figure 4.2. Venn diagram of the partition of
the sample space into two subsets

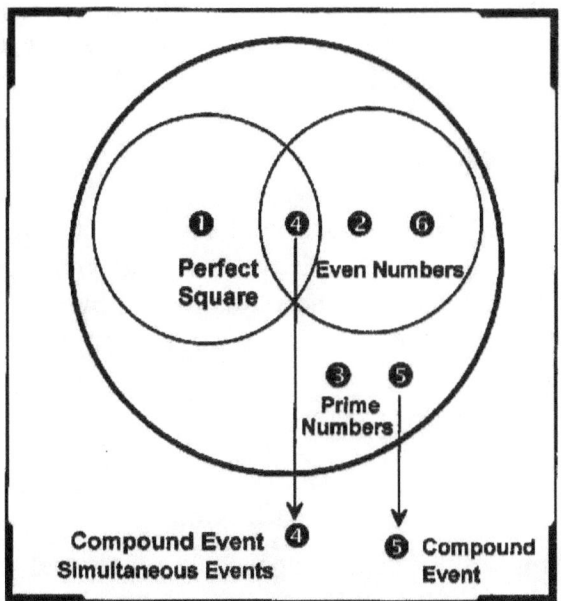

Figure 4.3. Venn diagram of the partition of
the sample space into three subsets

Assigning odd/even outcome to the resulting event of rolling a die implies the partition of the universal set of the six possible singular and indivisible outcomes into two mutually exclusive and exhaustive subsets of even and odd sample point or elements (Figure 4.2).

Assigning perfect square/even/prime outcome to the resulting events of rolling a die implies the partition of the universal set into three subsets not all mutually exclusive (Figure 4.3). No. 4 belongs to both the even and the square subsets. The outcome 4 confirms the simultaneous occurrence of the two events as well as being a compound outcome.

4.2.1 The Experiment

An experiment or trial is defined as a process, physical or conceptual, resulting in more than one possible outcome.

A random experiment (flipping a coin, rolling a die, or drawing a ball from an urn filled with colored balls) is by definition one in which the result is unpredictable. A random experiment may consist of one or several identical trials. Thus, a single toss of a coin is a single trial, whereas an experiment is an organized repetition of the same trial either sequentially or simultaneously.

4.2.2 The Outcome

The result of the random experiment is called the *outcome* of the experiment. An experiment yields one and only one outcome at a time. For a single coin, the outcome is obviously one of two possibilities. Because the outcome of an experiment is any one of possible outcomes, and thus unpredictable, it follows that such an outcome is a random occurrence.

4.3 The Sample Space

As the name implies, the sample space is a conceptual structure from which all possible outcomes are drawn and out of which all possible outcomes are bound to occur. At the basic level, every experiment is associated with its own sample space defined by the conditions and constraints of the experiment. Thus, every random experiment is associated with a sample space composed of the complete list of all the possible outcomes.

Viewed in this light, the single outcome of the experiment makes up the smallest unit of the sample space of the experiment. Alternatively, viewed from the point of view of set theory, the sample space is the set of all possible outcomes (i.e., the actual number of possible outcomes) of the experiment, where each possible outcome is a simple element of the set.

We begin the process of elucidating the structure of the sample space by considering one made exclusively of two distinct element, {0, 1}, which may alternatively be labeled as head or tail {H, T}, success or failure {S, F}, up or down {U, D}, left or right {L, R}, defective or perfect {D, P}, and boy or girl {B, G}. In terms of the set theory, the sample space consists of two mutually exclusive and complementary elements, that is, the number 0 and its complement 1. Three experiments will serve as generic models from which countless analogous variation may be constructed or encountered in reality.

For the trivial experiment of tossing a coin, the outcome of a single trial is the simple event of head or tails, {H, T}, which includes all the possible outcomes of the toss.

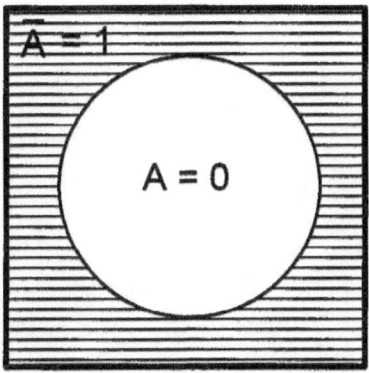

Figure 4.4. Venn diagram of the sample space of the binomial set: two mutually exclusive and complementary elements

For two coins tossed simultaneously or consecutively, the outcome of a single trial is the simple event that includes one and only one of the outcomes of the experiment, configured as follows:

{HH, HT, TH, TT}

The resulting possible outcomes derived from the permutation with repetition of size 2 ($n^r = 2^2 = 4$) of the set {H, T} now becomes the sample space composed of four ordered pairs. The term ordered refers to the definite sequence of binary elements, which differentiates one ordered subset from another subset with the same elements but with different order.

For three coins tossed simultaneously or consecutively, the outcome of a single trial is the simple event that includes one and only one of the outcomes of the experiment, configured as follows:

{HHH, HHT, HTH, THH, HTT, THT, TTH, TTT}

Again, the resulting outcome derived from the permutation with repetition of size 3 ($n^r = 2^3 = 8$) of the binary set {H, T} now becomes the sample space composed of eight ordered triples. As noted in Table 4.1 and depicted in Figure 4.5, the sample space is made up of eight distinctly ordered elements. Thus, for any one toss, the outcome of the experiment can only result in one of the eight possible ordered triples. In other words, each of the ordered triples is a potential outcome and thus may turn up as a simple outcome on any given toss.

As can be surmised from the previous statement, the sample space, physical or conceptual, is not a haphazard collection of elements. Essentially, it is a set whose basic components are simple indivisible elements corresponding to the set of all possible outcomes, such that every element corresponds exactly to one sample point in the set designated as the sample space of the experiment in question.

When the primary simple elements combine to form subsets, the sample space now becomes the subject of structural complexity. Thus, the analysis and formulation of the components of the SS form the substrate on which and from which the complementary concept of probability is based. Such being the case, the structural elements of the sample space need to be specifically counted and numbered if the probability of their distribution is to be considered.

As will be shown, the sample space together with its correlates, the process of sampling and the resultant random samples, constitute the framework within which inferential logic is organized to bear on the chance occurrence of events.

This definition underlines the intimate connection between sets and probability. Linked to the concept of sets representing the sample space of a given experiment is the subject dealing with the enumeration methods necessary to count the possible outcomes in a complex experiment. Familiarity with the subject of permutation and combination is prerequisite if the number of possible outcomes exceeds the trivial example of rolling a pair of dice or cutting a deck of cards.

4.4 The Event: Simple and Compound

Central to the concept of probability is the concept of the event associated with the trial or experiment for which probability is the measure. The physical occurrence of any one element derived from the sample space thus represents the outcome of a selection process dictated by chance. The outcome represented by any one of the eight elements generated on tossing three coins is designated as a *simple event*, representing one element of the sample space. In contrast, when the primary elements combine in an organized pattern to form subsets of the sample space, the outcome of any one of the elements of the subset of 1H triplets, {HTT, THT, TTH}, marks the occurrence of a *compound event*. The compound event thus represents a collection of possible outcomes that make up a subset of the sample space.

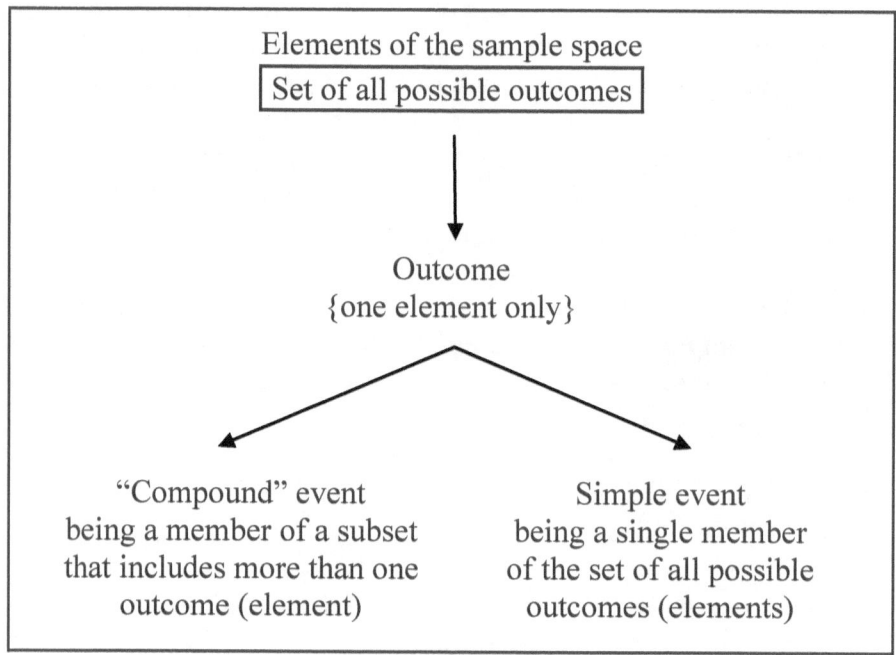

Figure 4.5. Flow chart of the compound and simple
events defined by the nature of the outcome

Note that tossing three coins simultaneously can result in one and
only one outcome composed of one of the elements of the SS. The
"compound" event that qualified for the answer is, however, made
up of three elements (Figure 4.5).

Obviously, one needs to conclude that performance of the trial or
experiment resulting in an event represented by the occurrence
of one and only one outcome, that is, one element, may denote
concurrently the occurrence of a "compound" event, embracing
several elements of the sample space, depending on the constraints
(boundaries and rules) dictated by the requirement of the experiment
and the question demanded from the experimental result.

In other words, depending on the definition of the constraints or
rules that tie up the primary elements, a finite number of questions
may be posed that would require the inclusion of more than one
element of the SS.

In this context, a "compound" event is said to occur when one outcome representative of a primary or simple element of the defined subset being considered (i.e., {H T T, THT, TTH}) occurs. In other words, the occurrence of a one particular primary element which share with other elements a given constraint, is sufficient ground to conclude that the compound event made up of several similarly categorized primary elements also occurred conceptually. Hence, the outcome of a random toss that turn up any one of the three elements previously mentioned is consistent with the occurrence of the compound event (Figure 4.6).

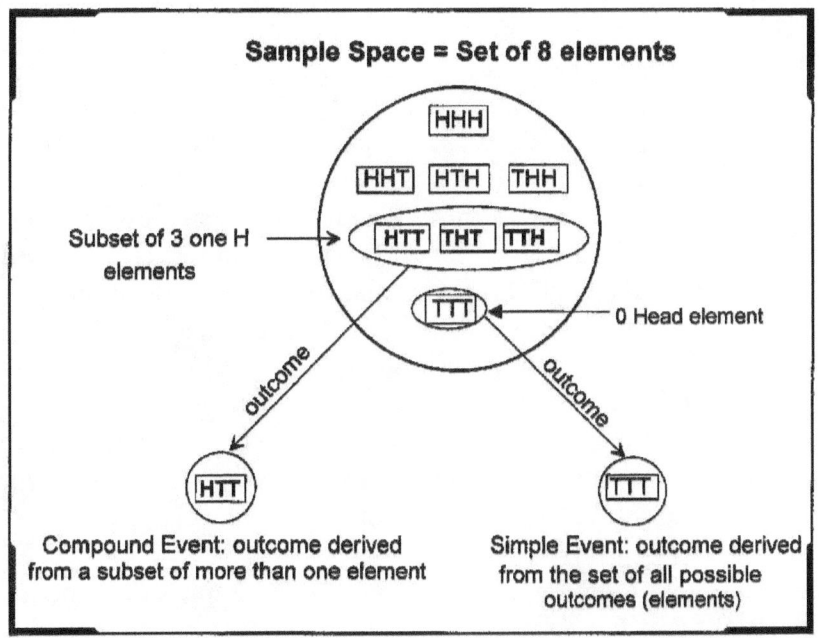

Figure 4.6. Venn diagram of the graphic equivalent of the sample space and its potential outcomes

Furthermore, every conceivable event that may include more than one element of the set corresponds to a subset of the sample space.

In defining the compound event as a specific combination and/or arrangement of the primary elements of the SS begs the question of how many ways can the elements of the SS be partitioned or arranged to form a "compound" event. Stated differently, given a set of primary elements, how many compound events can be expected from the set of the primary elements.

Before addressing this question, it becomes necessary to define the boundary of the sample space of the experiment as to the number and composition of the sample points. Consider the sample space associated with the rolling of six dice (three pairs). As noted in Table 4.2, the experiment may be translated into the permutation of a set of six numbers with replacement resulting in 46,656 distinct arrangements of the six numbers, that is, 46,656 different numbers corresponding to the elements of the sample space. Simultaneously, 462 subsets or combination with repetition can be derived from the permuted results of the six dice experiment. For the ubiquitous two dice, the result of permutation of size 2 with unrestricted repetition of the set {1, 2, 3, 4, 5, 6} is reduced to thirty-six distinct and ordered numbers that fill the sample space. If repetition is excluded, the numbers are reduced to thirty ordered elements confined to the two triangles in Figure 4.6. If, on the other hand, the order within the elements is disregarded, the number of subsets (combination) of size 2 that can be generated with repetition equals 21, whereas the number generated without repetition equals 15, confined to a single triangle in Table 4.1. What needs to be appreciated is that the sample space in each of the above situations is distinctly different given the initial conditions, the size of the set, and the constraints imposed on the elements of the set (permutation or combination).

From the point of view of set theory an event, simple or compound is representative of the particular subset, one of several, that partitions the universal set, which is another way of saying that every possible event, which is in fact the answer to a possible specific question, corresponds to a subset of the sample space. The notion of the compound event may therefore be generalized to include subsets generated by the union and/or intersection of two or more subsets, as well as the complement of a given event as will be demonstrated shortly.

Once the elements of the experiment are defined and the counting process is concluded, the SS of the given experiment may be considered a universal set subject to partition into distinct subsets in response to questions concerning the nature and frequency of a particular compound event. The subsets thus defined may be further combined through union, intersection, and complementation in response to more complex questions related to possible outcomes as will be demonstrate shortly.

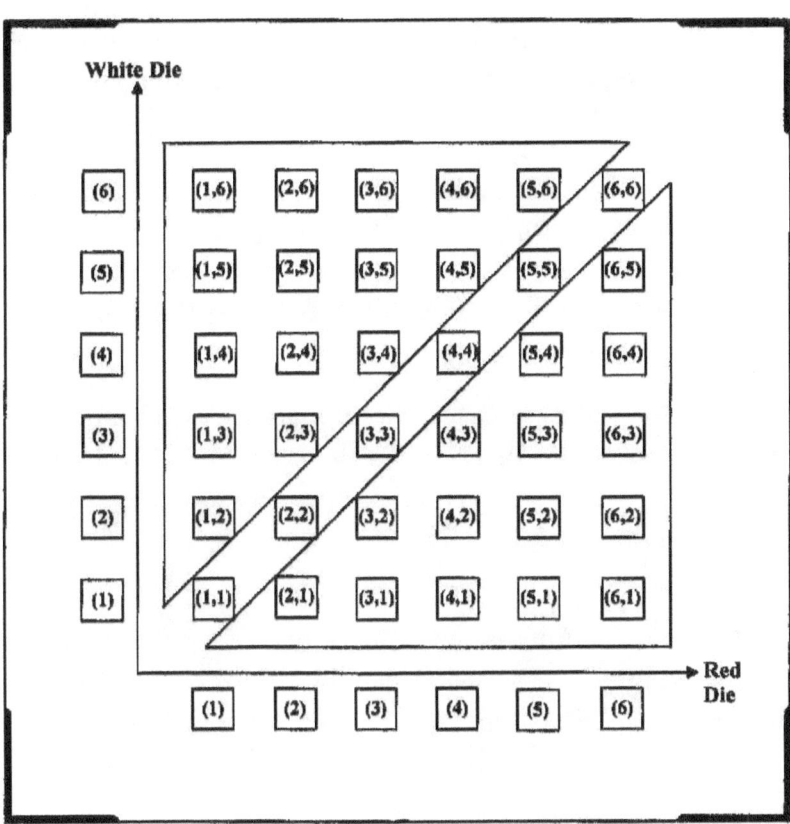

Table 4.1 Sample spaces generated through variation of the experimental constraints

4.5 Probability and Randomness

A random event defines an unpredictable outcome of a given experiment. The event in such an experiment or trial may occur or fail to occur; thus, in tossing a coin, the event "head" may or may not occur. Probability theory is a rational attempt to determine the degree of likelihood or probability of random events. The aim is to predict the outcome of a random phenomenon on the basis of probabilistic estimates. Stated differently, probability theory attempts to quantify the randomness of the event. The quantitative measure of this estimate of probability is at once a basic property and a tool of the theory.

In this scale of measurement, the probability of a sure event is assumed to be equal to one, whereas zero probability is assigned to an impossible event. Thus, in the limit $P(\text{event } A) = 1$ means absolute certainty, whereas $P(\text{event } A) = 0$ means an impossible event. A card selected at random from a bridge deck will certainly turn out to belong to one of the four suits and one of the thirteen denominations. No other possibility exists. At the other end, the drawing of a card bearing a denomination of twenty is an impossible event.

Given these two extreme cases, the probability of a random event, $P(\text{Event A})$, will obviously be in the interval between zero and one, so that

$$\boxed{0 \leq P(A) \leq 1.}$$

The above proposition assumes a more serious tone when the question is rephrased as to the probability of drawing a ten of clubs for instance. The implication of the question is the ability to predict, within the limitation previously noted, the outcome of this simple experiment.

In practice, the rigorous definition of certainty and impossibility needs to be modified so that events are practically sure or practically impossible as they approach one or zero in the limit. The appearance of heads on all one hundred coins tossed is practically impossible but not theoretically impossible.[3]

---

[3]   Law of large numbers: the relative frequency after repeated trials approached the theoretical probability.

Permutation with Unrestricted Repetition of Set {1, 2, 3, 4, 5, 6}	Combination with Unrestricted Repetition of Set {1, 2, 3, 4,5, 6}
One die rolled six times or six dice rolled once Permutations of size 6 with unrestricted repetitions, taken most from set {1, 2, 3, 4, 5,6} $n^r = \{1, 2, 3, 4, 5, 6\}^6 = 6^6 = 46{,}656$ distinct arrangement of the six numbers with repetition	Combinations of size 6 with unrestricted repetitions, taken from set {1, 2, 3, 4, 5, 6} $(n-1) + rCr = (6-1) + 6C6 = 11C6 = 462$ subsets of the six numbers with repetition
One die rolled two times or two dice rolled once Permutations of size 2 with unrestricted repetitions, taken from set {1, 2, 3, 4, 5,6} $n^r = \{1, 2, 3, 4, 5, 6\}^2 = 6^2 = 36$ distinct arrangement of the six numbers with repetition	Combinations of size 2 with unrestricted repetitions, taken from set {1, 2, 3, 4, 5,6} $(n-1) + rCr = (6-1) + 2C2 = 7C2 = 21$ subsets with repetitions
Permutation with No Repetition of Set {1, 2, 3, 4, 5, 6}	**Combination with No Repetition of Set {1, 2, 3, 4, 5,6}**
Permutations of size 6 with no repetitions, taken from set {1, 2, 3, 4, 5, 6} $6P6 = n! = 6! = 720$ distinct arrangement of the six numbers with no repetitions	Subsets of the set {1, 2, 3, 4, 5,6} $= 2^r = 2^6 = 64$ subset = power set = set of all sets $6C0 + 6C1 + 6C2 + 6C3 + 6C4 + 6C5 + 6C6 + 1 + 6 + 15 + 20 + 15 + 6 + 1$
Permutation size 2 with no repetition taken from set {1, 2, 3, 4, 5,6} $6P2 = 720/24 = 30$ distinct arrangement of any two numbers with no repetitions	Combinations of size 2 with no repetitions, taken from set {1, 2, 3, 4, 5,6} $6C2 = 15$ distinct subsets with nor repetition

Table 4.2. Subsets generated through different permutation and combination of a six elements set {1, 2, 3, 4, 5, 6}

Permutation with Unrestricted Repetition of Binary Sets {0, 1} and {H, T}	Combination with Unrestricted Repetition of Binary Sets {0, 1} and {H, T}
Permutations of size 2 from set {0, 1} $\{0, 1\}^2 = 2^2 = 4$ (0, 0) (0, 1) (1, 0) (1, 1)	Combinations of size 2 from set {0, 1} $(2-1) + 2C2 = 3C2 = 3$ {0 0} {0 1} {1 1}

Permutations of size 2 from set {H, T}	Combinations of size 2 from set {H, T}
{H, T}$^{2=2}$2 = 4	(2 − 1) + 2C2 = 3C2 = 3
(H, H) (H, T) (T, H) (T, T)	{H H} {H T} {T T}
Permutations of size 3 from set {0, 1}	Combinations of size 3 from set {0, 1}
{0, 1}^{3} = 2^3 = 8	(2 − 1) + 3C2 = 4C3 = 4
(0, 0, 0) (0, 0, 1) (0, 1, 0) (0, 1, 1)	{0 0 0} {0 01} {0 1 1} (1 1 1}
(1, 0, 0) (1, 0, 1) (1, 1, 0) (1, 1, 1)	
Permutations of size 3 from set {H, T}	Combinations of size 3 from set {H, T}
{H, T}^{3} = 2^3 = 8	(2 − 1) + 3C2 = 4C3 = 4
(H, H, H) (H, H, T) (H, T, H) (H, T, T)	{H H H} {H H T} {H T T} {T T T}
(T, H, H) (T, H, T) (T, T, H) (T, T, T)	
Permutations of size 4 from set {0, 1}	Combinations of size 4 from set {0, 1}
{0, 1}^{4} = 2^4 = 16	(2 − 1) + 4C4 = 5C4 = 5
(0,0,0,0) (0,0,0,1) (0,0,1,0) (0,0,1,1)	{0 0 0 0} {0 0 01 } {0 0 1 1} {0 1 1 1}
(0,1,0,0) (0,1,0,1) (0,1,1,0) (0,1,1,1)	{1 1 1 1}
(1,0,0,0) (1,0,0,1) (1,0,1,0) (1,0,1,1)	
(1,1,0,0) (1,1,0,1) (1,1,1,0) (1,1,1,1)	
Permutations of size 4 from set {H, T}	Combinations of size 4 from set {H, T}
{0, 1}^{4} = 2^4 = 16	(2 − 1) + 4C4 = 5C4 = 5
(H,H,H,H) (H,H,H,T) (H,H,T,H)	{HHHH} {HHHT} {HHTT} {HTTT}
(H,H,T,T)	{TTTT}
(H,T,H,H) (H,T,H,T) (H,T,T,H)	
(H,T,T,T)	
(T,H,H,H) (T,H,H,T) (T,H,T,H)	
(T,H,T,T)	
(T,T,H,H) (T,T,H,T) (T,T,T,H) (T,T,T,T)	
Permutation with No Repetition of Binary Sets {0, 1} and {H, T}	**Combination with No Repetition of Binary Sets {0, 1} and {H, T}**
Permutations of size 2 with no repetitions, taken from set {0, 1}	Subsets of the set {0, 1} = 2^r = 2^2 = power set = set of all sets = 4 subsets
2P2 = n! = 2! = 2 (0, 1) (1, 0)	Ø {0} {1} {0, 1}
Permutations of size 2 with no repetitions, taken from set {H, T}	Subsets of the set {H, T} = 2^r = 2^2 = power set = set of all sets = 4 subsets
2P2 = n! = 2! = 2 (H, T) (T, H)	Ø {H} {T} {H, T}

Table 4.3. Subsets generated through the permutation and combination of binary sets {0, 1} and {H,T}

1. What is the probability of turning up a sum of 7 or 11 on the first roll (Table 4.6)? We are dealing with the probabilities of two events that are mutually exclusive (i.e., cannot occur simultaneously). In this case, the probability of either one or the other occurring may be found by adding the probability of the two events. Thus, if events A and B are mutually exclusive, that is, they share no outcomes in common, then $P(A$ or $B) = P(A \cup B) = P(A) + P(B)$.

Event (sum 7) is represented by the slanted rectangle, whereas event (sum 11) is represented by the slanted rectangle enclosing the elements of (5, 6) and (6, 5). However, because either outcome, 7 or 11, will satisfy the conditions of the compound event, the probabilities of the two subsets are added, the result being the probability of either one or the other (Table 4.9, 3a).

$$P(\text{event sum 7} \overset{\text{Union}}{\text{ or }} \text{event sum 11}) = P(\text{event sum 7}) + P(\text{event sum 11}) = \frac{6}{36} + \frac{2}{36} = \frac{8}{36}.$$

2. What is the probability of the event in which the sum is 7 and the red die (the first number) turns out red 6. In contrast to the first question, the event is this case stipulates the simultaneous concurrence of both events, ruling out mutual exclusiveness. As shown in Table 4.4, it is apparent that only (6, 1) of the six elements, in either the slanted rectangle or the vertical rectangle, qualifies as being a sum of 7 and simultaneously exhibiting red 6 on the first die. In the language of sets, the event so described results from the intersection of subset (sum 7) with that of subset (first red 6) (Table 4.9, 6a).

$$P(\text{sum 7} \overset{\text{Intersection}}{\text{ and }} \text{first red 6}) = P(\text{sum 7}) \times P(\text{red 6}) = \frac{6}{36} \times \frac{6}{36} = \frac{1}{36}.$$

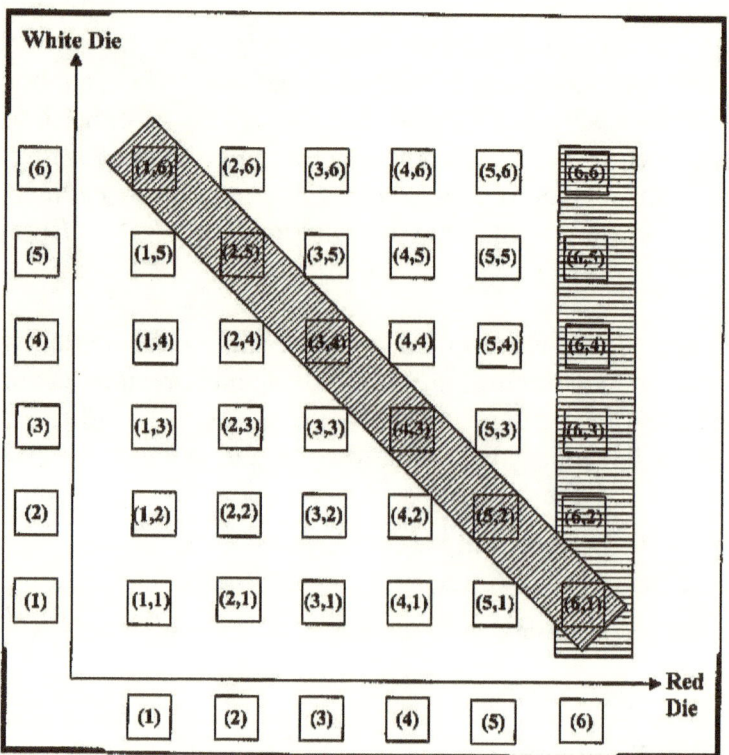

Table 4.4. Probability of the sum, given the
replication of shared element

3. What is the probability of either event (sum 7) or event (first red 6)? In contrast to the first question, the two events in this case share one common element. In other words, they are not mutually exclusive; thus, the sum of their probabilities must consider the replication of the shared element in the sum. Thus (Table 4.9, 4a),

$$P(\text{sum 7} \overset{\text{Union}}{\text{or}} \text{red 6}) = P(\text{sum 7}) \overset{+}{\cup} P(\text{red 6}) - P[(\text{sum 7}) \overset{\times}{\cap} (\text{red 6})] = \frac{1}{6} + \frac{1}{6} - \frac{1}{36} = \frac{11}{36}.$$

As shown in Table 4.4, it is clear that that number of elements in the two rectangles is indeed 11 and not 12, having eliminated the duplicate count of the shared element from the total.

4. What is the probability of the complement to the four heavy bordered elements (Table 4.6)? What is required is the probability of the compound event that excludes the four heavy bordered elements. The probability of the four elements is readily calculated at 4/36 because we are dealing with mutually exclusive and equally likely events. The complement is simply the balance of the total sample space so that the compound event in question includes all the elements of the sample space, excluding the four heavy border elements.

$$1 - P(\text{heavy borders}) = 1 - \frac{4}{36} = \frac{32}{36} = \frac{8}{9}.$$

4.6 Classical Probability: Probability of Simple Events

At the basic discrete level, all the elements are to be considered equally distributed, which carries the implication that the probability of a random selection or chance occurrence is equally weighted, resulting in an equally likely outcome of any one element, out of the total number of elements known to be the constituents of the SS, representing either simple or a compound event.

Dice, coins, and similar implements of the game of chance represent a unique class of objects that exhibit a symmetry of possible outcomes usually referred to as the classical models of probability.

To return to the number of elements in the SS of the tossed three fair coins, that is, the eight ordered triples, it is obvious that each of the elements is equally likely to occur on a given toss (Table 4.3). Equivalently stated, the probability of being randomly selected is equally partitioned among the eight elements, so that the probability of randomly selecting a given element is 1/8. Thus, the probability of tossing three fair coins and having all of them land head on (which is the equivalent of tossing one coin consecutively three times and obtaining three heads in a row) is 1/8 or 0.125. This outcome defines the probability of the simple event. The question need not always be that simple. A more indirect question may take the following form: "What is the probability of getting exactly one head on tossing three coins?" In more relevant terms, the question may be rephrased as follows: "What is the probability of the compound event detailed earlier?"

Consider the permutation of size 2 with unrestricted repetitions of the set {1, 2, 3, 4, 5, 6}, which is the technical expression for the mundane experiment of rolling a pair of dice (Tables 4.2 and 4.4).

The required features of such a model stipulates that all possible outcomes of a trial (rolling a die, tossing a coin, or drawing a ball from an urn) are in compliance with the following restrictions (Table 4.5):

1. Mutually exclusive: the individual outcomes are mutually exclusive in that they exclude each other such that no two events can occur simultaneously. (The unique outcome of rolling a single die excludes the remaining five possible outcomes.)
2. Exhaustive: the complete set of simple events or, alternatively, the elements of the set of sample space is exhaustive if they cover all possible outcomes of the experiment.
3. Equally likely outcome: the condition of the experiment is such as to provide equal possibility for each elementary outcome such that $P(a_1) = P(a_2) = P(a_3) = P(a_n)$.
4. An important corollary of the equally likely outcome is the fact that the sum of the probabilities of all the simple events that ensued from and experiment adds up to 1.

$$P(a_1) + P(a_2) + P(a_3) + \ldots P(a_n) = 1$$

5. Because the total number of the equally probable outcomes of the experiment is n, the probability of any outcome or simple event is

$$\frac{1}{\text{Total number of outcomes for the given experiment}} = \frac{1}{n} = P(a).$$

White Die	Red Die					
	1	2		4	53	6
6	(1,6)	(2,6)	(3,6)	(4,6)	(5,6)	(6,6)
5	(1,5)	(2,5)	(3,5)	(4,5)	(5,5)	(6,5)
4	(1,4)	(2,4)	(3,4)	(4,4)	(5,4)	(6,4)
3	(1,3)	(2,3)	(3,3)	(4,3)	(5,3)	(6,3)
2	(1,2)	(2,2)	(3,2)	(4,2)	(5,2)	(6,2)
1	(1,1)	(2,1)	(3,1)	(4,1)	(5,1)	(6,1)

Sample space
= set of all possible ordered pairs
=$\{(1,6), (2,6), \ldots, (6,1\}$

= 36 simple events

Mutually exclusive: no two events can occur simultaneously

Exhaustive: include all possible outcomes

Equally likely: $P(a_1) = P(a_2) = \ldots = P(a_{36})$

Probability of simple event $a_1 = P(a_1) = 1/36$

Table 4.5 Probability of a simple event

The above-mentioned definition covers all games of chance when all possible tampering with the free flow of pure chance has been eliminated.

The urn model (lottery drum) filled with identical balls of different color fits the requirements of the classical model such that the drawing of any one ball is equally likely and mutually exclusive.

In the game of lotto as played in New York, a sample of six winning numbers (and as additional supplementary number) are drawn on the given day from a rotating drum containing fifty-four balls, numbered and labeled 1 to 54. To figure out the chances of correctly scoring six numbers, not necessarily in sequence out of the fifty-four numbers, one needs to have an idea of the number of subsets made of six numbers each that can be formed from the available fifty-four numbers, out of which only one such subset is the winner. This number (easily obtained using a hand calculator) is 25,827,165 subsets of six different number made from the roster of the fifty-four numbers.

The computation of this number without the ancillary formulae is a formidable if not impossible task. Both the coin tossing and the lotto experiments illustrate the need for basic methods of categorizing and enumerating the sample space given the constraints of the experiment.

4.7 Probability of Compound Events

What needs to be reiterated is that all events are made of single outcomes, that is, one element of the SS or of any subset of the SS.

When the event is an element of a predefined subset, a compound event is presumed to have occurred because, on repeated performances, the elements of the subset occurring individually define the nature and boundary of the compound event. Accordingly, because the compound event is by definition associated with the elements of a subset, its probability of occurrence is the sum of the individual probabilities associated with the outcome of each of the elements of the designated subset.

Having defined the extent of the sample space as well as the composition and the probabilities associated with the individual elements, all questions related to the composition and frequency of any given compound event may now be addressed. To the question regarding the probability of the sum of the dots on the two dice on a given roll being equal to 7, the perusal of Table 4.6 demonstrates that the elements enclosed in the slanted rectangle make up the subset of the compound event consistent with the required answer. Because the probabilities associated with the individual elements are all equally likely and because the elements are mutually exclusive, the probability of the event (i.e., the sum of seven) is the sum of the individual probabilities of the elements in the subset,

$$P(\text{compound event}) = \frac{1}{36} + \frac{1}{36} + \frac{1}{36} + \frac{1}{36} + \frac{1}{36} + \frac{1}{36} = \frac{6}{36} = \frac{1}{6}.$$

Alternatively, because the compound event is represented by any one of the six elements and because the probability of turning up is equally likely for all elements of the set, the probability of the compound event could be considered as the ratio of the number of elements in the rectangular subset to the total number of elements in the sample space,

$$P(\text{compound event}) = \frac{\text{No. of elements in subset (rectangle)}}{\text{No. of elements in sample space}} = \frac{6}{36} = \frac{1}{6}.$$

A sample of the pertinent questions regarding the probability of compound events that may be addressed is shown in Table 4.6.

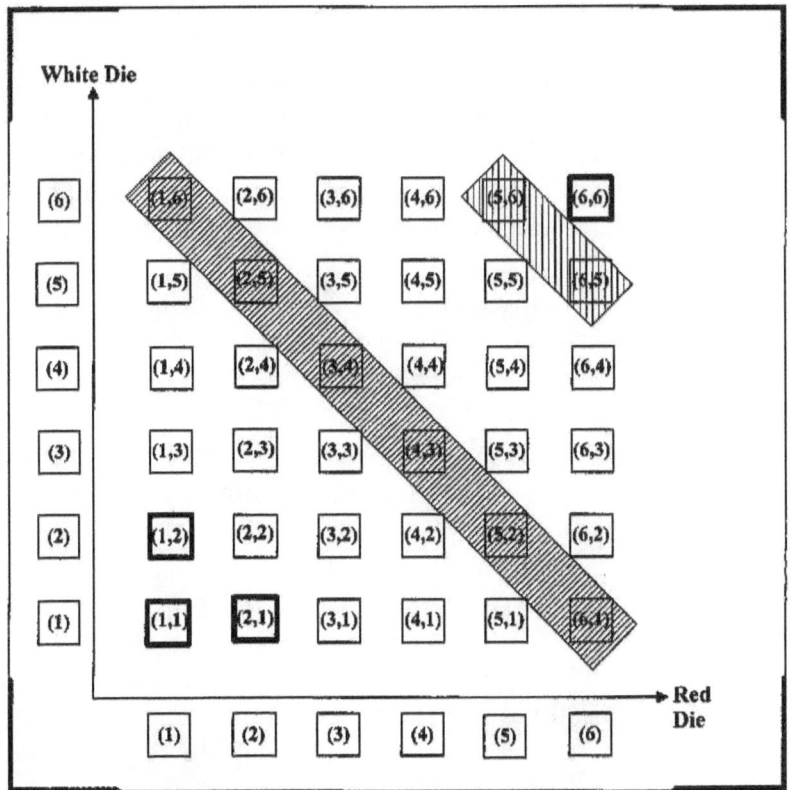

Table 4.6 Probability a compound event

The probability of a compound event A, $P(A)$, may thus be defined as follows:

$$P(A) = \frac{\text{Number of possible outcomes which characterize the compound event}}{\text{Total number of possible outcomes in the sample space}},$$

which may be abbreviated to a simpler format as follows:

$$P(A) = \frac{\text{Number of outcomes favorable to A}}{\text{Number of all possible outcomes}} = \frac{\text{Number of elements in a predefined subset}}{\text{Total number of elements in the sample space}}.$$

When the number of outcomes favorable to the compound event in question is identically associated with success, the definition may assume the following format:

$$P(\overset{\text{success}}{E}) = \frac{\text{No. of successful outcomes}}{\text{No. of possible outcomes}} = \frac{\text{No. of successes}}{\text{No. of successess} + \text{No. of failures}} = \frac{s}{s+f}.$$

Under field conditions, given the above-mentioned definition of random events, the probability of a given simple event may be calculated as the ratio of the number of actual outcomes for a given experiment to the number of possible outcomes encountered in repeated trials of an experiment.

The probability of a compound event, on the other hand, is the ratio of number of occurrence of the event to the number of times the experiment is performed, in repeated trials of the same experiment.

We are faced here with a ratio that involves the relationship between two numbers that need to be counted if the probability of the event is to be determined: a denominator representing the number of elements in the SS and a numerator representing the number of elements in the subset corresponding to the outcomes in the case of a compound event.

The task therefore involves a counting process or enumeration technique that may be used in the calculation of the required ratio.

In a sample space made up of individually equally likely elements, it is still possible to devise a set of outcomes whose probabilities are not equally likely.

In rolling a pair of dice, eleven possible point outcomes comprising the sum of the face values are obtained. The probabilities associated with each pair, however, are not equally likely. Thus, the probability of obtaining any one point outcome (i.e., sum of the two face values), as noted in Table 4.7, varies between 1/36 for the sum of 2 (snake eyes) to 6/36 for the sum of 7 and back again to 1/36 for the sum of 12 (box cars).

Two Dice					
Point Number; Outcome	Combinations Which Make Up the Number	Ways of Rolling the Number	Probability	Odds for	Odds against
2	1-1	1	1/36	1:35 = 1:35	35:1
3	2-1; 1-2	2	2/36 = 1/18	2:34 = 1:17	17:1
4	3-1; 2-2; 1-3	3	3/36 =1/11	3:33 = 1:11	11:1
5	4-1; 3-2; 2-3; 1-4	4	4/36 = 1/9	4:32 = 1:8	8:1
6	5-1; 4-2; 3-3; 2-4; 1-5	5	5/36 ≈ 1/7	5:31 ≈ 1:6	6:1
7	6-1; 5-2; 4-3; 3-4; 2-5;1-6	6	6/36 = 1/6	6:30 = 1:5	5:1
8	6-2; 5-3; 4-4; 3-5; 2-6	5	5/36 ≈ 1/7	5:31 ≈ 1:6	6:1
9	6-3; 5-4; 4-5;3-6	4	4/36 = 1/9	4:32 = 1:8	8:1
10	6-4; 5-5; 4-6	3	3/36 = 1/11	3:33 = 1:11	11:1
11	6-5; 5-6	2	2/36 = 1/18	2:34 = 1:17	17:1
12	6-6	1	1/36	1:35 = 1:35	35:1

Sample space = set of all possible points (sums of the face values)
= {2, 3, . . . , 12}

= 11 compound events

Mutually exclusive: no two events can occur simultaneously

Exhaustive: include all possible outcomes

Not equally likely: $P(7) \neq P(3)$

Probability of compound event 7 = P(7) =

$$\frac{\text{Number of elements (simple events) in event 7}}{\text{Total number of elements in sample space}}$$

$$= \frac{6}{36} = \frac{1}{6}$$

Table 4.7. Probability of compound event 7

4.8 Probability of Not Equally Likely Outcome: Relative Frequency Model

The constraints placed on the above-noted definition of probability is restrictive because most of the experiments with random results cannot be described by the classical model. The artificially designed symmetry of outcome, noted in gambling mechanisms, is not naturally encountered. In actual practice, most of the experiments with random results cannot be described by the classical model. (In such an experiment, where the elementary outcomes are not equally likely, the probability of event A in the same space is the sum of the individual probabilities assigned individually to each elements of the SS.)

The slot machine, on the other hand, offers a system in which the basic elements (sequence of three symbols) are not equally likely. Thus, by varying the number of symbols on the dials, it is possible to assign varying degrees of frequency to specific patterns (Table 4.8).

Thus, any tampering with the symmetry of the model (e.g., artificially loading a die so as to shift its center of gravity) constitutes the first point of departure from the classical model. Such being the case, the probability of a six turning up in a loaded die cannot be predicted on the basis of the theoretical assumption of equally likely outcome assumed to be 1/6. The probability of such an event can only be inferred from the actual frequency of turning up a six in a series of repeated trials of rolling the die. In this case, the statistical probability is actually the ratio of turning a six to the total number of trials.

$$\text{Statistical probability} = \text{frequency} = \frac{\text{Number of repetitions in which the simple event occurred}}{\text{Total number of repetitions}}.$$

In a similar fashion, the probability of a head on tossing a weighted coin cannot be assumed to equal 0.5. The contrast in the corresponding probability between a balanced and a weighted coin is illustrated in the following parallel probabilities of the outcomes on tossing two regular and two weighted coins. The probability of a head, $P(\text{H}) = 1/2$, in the balanced coin can be theoretically assigned, whereas the probability of a head in the weighted coin, $P(\text{H}) = 3/4$, is solely experimentally derived for the particular coin. The probability of a tail is then $P(\text{T}) = 1 - 3/4 = 1/4$.

Balance coin: HH, HT, TH, TT

$$\frac{1}{2} \times \frac{1}{2} = \frac{1}{4}, \quad \frac{1}{2} \times \frac{1}{2} = \frac{1}{4}, \quad \frac{1}{2} \times \frac{1}{2} = \frac{1}{4}, \quad \frac{1}{2} \times \frac{1}{2} = \frac{1}{4}$$

Note that the probability of the ordered pairs is now radically different from those encountered in the balanced coin.

Weighted coin: HH, HT, TH, TT

$$\frac{3}{4} \times \frac{3}{4} = \frac{9}{16}, \quad \frac{3}{4} \times \frac{1}{4} = \frac{3}{16}, \quad \frac{1}{4} \times \frac{3}{4} = \frac{3}{16}, \quad \frac{1}{4} \times \frac{1}{4} = \frac{1}{16}$$

The concept of probability and frequency are nevertheless not identical. It becomes apparent, however, as the total number of repetitions increases, random variation in the manner of conducting each trial as well as the conditions prevailing at the time of each trial cancel out, so that in the long run, the frequency (i.e., the statistical probability) levels out and approaches a particular value unique to the given experiment, which for practical purposes may be considered as the "real probability" of the particular event. Implicit in this statement are two conditions that preclude the derivation of the real probability with absolute certainty, namely, the length of the run, that is, the number of trials undertaken to establish the frequency of the event and the degree of confidence with which we can assert that the obtained frequency and its probability are indeed a valid approximation of the real probability. The words probability and random events are intertwined in a circuitous definition.

In order to focus on the discrepancy between the theoretical probability and the frequency as determined by repeated performance of identical trials, consider the tossing of six coins and the expected number of heads for any given toss.

The event under consideration in this experiment is the resultant number of heads when the six coins are tossed. This is to be differentiated from the one outcome on any given toss, where the sequence or order of the heads and tails for the particular toss is considered. Clearly, $2^6 = 64$; such simple events or outcomes resulting from the permutation of size 6 of the binary element are possible, whereas only seven compound events ranging from 0 head to 6 heads may be realized, which may be restated to imply that out of the sixty-four simple events, only seven such events are possible. Although different in the frequency of their occurrence, the sum of their frequencies adds up to sixty-four.

Therefore, for any given sequence of heads and tails, the number of possible events displaying the same number of heads is the number of possible permutations of n objects (six coins), r of which are alike and of one kind (no. of heads) and the balance $(n - r)$ of which are similarly alike and of another kind (no. of tails).

Calculating individually, the possible number of combinations associated with each event reveal the following distribution of the number of heads theoretically expected in tossing six coins $64^{\times 2}$ times. The combination associated with each event ranging from 0 to 20 to 1 can be seen as the number of possible combinations[4] in each event, which simultaneously doubles up as the binomial coefficient, which is the shorthand way of indicating the expected frequency of the number of heads in each of the seven events,

No. events with x heads frequency	$f=1$	$f=6$	$f=15$	$f=20$	$f=15$	$f=6$	$f=1$
Sample space=	$\{1T^6,$	$6T^5,$	$15H^2T^4,$	$20H^3T^3,$	$15H^4T^2,$	$6H^5T^1,$	$1H^6\}.$
Combination=$6Cx$	$6C0=1$	$6C1=6$	$6C2=15$	$6C3=20$	$6C4=15$	$6C5=6$	$6C6=1$

When the frequency is converted to probability by dividing the frequency of a particular event by the total number of possible outcomes ($2^6=64$), the distribution is now configured as follows:

No. events with x heads frequency	$f=1$	$f=6$	$f=15$	$f=20$	$f=15$	$f=6$	$f=1$
Sample space=	$\{\ 1T^6,$	$6T^5,$	$15H^2T^4,$	$20H^3T^3,$	$15H^4T^2,$	$6H^5T^1,$	$1H^6\ \}.$
Probability	$\frac{1}{64}=0.0156$	$\frac{6}{64}=0.0938$	$\frac{15}{64}=0.2344$	$\frac{20}{64}=0.3125$	$\frac{15}{64}=0.2344$	$\frac{6}{64}=0.0938$	$\frac{1}{64}=0.0156$

Thus, the probability of obtaining exactly twenty heads = 20/64 = 0.3125.

---

[4]   As previously mentioned, the word combination has been traditionally used in this context instead of the correct term of permutation.

Now should the trials be actually conducted under identical conditions, the probability of the seven different events (i.e., seven different frequencies of the number of heads) calculated on the basis of the observed frequencies if actually tossing the six coins repeatedly may deviate from the theoretical values in either direction by a certain percentage depending on the number of trials conducted for the experiment. Nevertheless, it is possible to state with almost (but not quite perfect) certainty that the probability of getting twenty heads, for example, will hover around the theoretical value of 0.3125 within a limited range of slightly less than 10 percent in either direction (0.2198-0.4052), as determined by the following relation:

$$0.3125 \pm 2\sqrt{\frac{0.3125(1-0.3125)}{100}} = 0.3125 \pm 0.0927(0.2198 - 0.4052)$$

If the experiment could be extended to 1,000 trials, the range becomes restricted to 0.3125 ± 0.00927 (0.3032-0.3218), a much narrower latitude than before. In other words, we are now able to predict again with less than 100 percent certainty (95 percent in fact) that the statistical or experimental probability cannot vary from the theoretical probability by more than 0.00927 (i.e., less than 1 percent) in either direction.

To be able to predict with such a degree of confidence, such a tight range of probabilities is impressive enough as a quasi-conclusive evidence. The fact that the results may disprove our predictions must remain in the background as a constant reminder of the fickleness of the situation.

The analogy to the periodic classification of elements is apt. As you may remember, by 1968, 103 simple elements have been identified in nature. Of the millions of compounds both organic and nonorganic known to exist, all are essentially complex combinations of the basic elements. If all the elements in nature were equally distributed (which most emphatically they are not), the probability of randomly selecting one element out of the total would be 1 out of 103 equally distributed elements. If now the question is rephrased as to the probability of randomly selecting a compound substance containing at least one carbon atom, the answer would be a subset of all the existing compounds containing a very large number of compounds with multiple carbon atoms.

If the question is rephrased as to restrict the subset to compounds containing exactly one carbon atom, the size of the subset will be significantly smaller. If now the restriction extends to a single carbon atom in combination with the unrestricted number of oxygen atoms, the subset will shrink to two compounds. Finally, if the single carbon atom is restricted to its elemental state, then we will be left with one of the roster of the 103 elements in existence.

Using the analogy, it can be postulated that every sample space is made up of either primary simple elements or complex elements made up of simple elements fused into indivisible units, now considered to be the new elements of the sample space. In both cases, their number is finite and countable at the discrete level.

What is not discernible from the above-mentioned statements regarding the nature of elements of the sample space is that the elements themselves may also be simple or compound.

The outcome of an experiment is sometimes referred to as a simple event, to be differentiated form a compound event, usually referred to simply as an event when several outcomes are considered together as a group.

The individual element of the sample space, however, may be further considered as being capable of potential transformation into a definite "outcome," which identifies one specific result of an experiment.

Dials on a Typical Slot Machine			
	Dial I	Dial II	Dial III	Probability
Cherries	7	7	0	
Oranges	3	6	7	3×6×7=126/8,000
Lemons	3	0	4	
Plums	5	1	5	5×1×5=25/8,000
Bells	1	3	3	1×3×3=9/8,000
Bars	1	3	1	1×3×1=3/8,000
	20	20	20	

Sample space = set of all possible permutations
(sequence of three symbols)

= 8,000 permutation (not all distinguishable)

Sample space: set of all possible paying permutations
(sequence of three specific symbols)

= 1,169 paying permutations
(not all distinguishable)

Mutually exclusive: no two events can occur simultaneously

Exhaustive: include all possible outcomes

Not equally likely: P(bar, bar, bar) ≠ P(bell, bell, bell)

Probability of a paying permutation

$$= \frac{\text{Number of paying permutations}}{\text{Total number of possible permutations}}$$

Probability of a paying permutation on any one play
$$= \frac{1169}{8000} = 0.146$$

Probability of two paying permutations in a row
$$= 0.146 \times 0.146 = 0.02$$

Table 4.8. Not equally likely event

4.9 Probability Mode: Simple versus Conditional

4.9.1 Simple Probability

Consider an urn containing one hundred balls, a mixture of plastic and glass balls, seventy of which are known to be red and the balance of thirty. Thus, the probability of retrieving a red ball is simply the probability of the red in the urn, so that $P(\text{red}) = 0.7$. The simple probability is thus defined as the probability of a simple event. The key question in this context, however, is to query the probability of drawing a glass ball given that it is red.

4.9.2 Conditional Probability

As the name implies, it is a probability with strings attached, distinctively coded and read as $P(G|R)$, "the probability of G given R," implying that the probability of the event G, referring to the probability of drawing a glass ball in this trial, is conditional, given that another event has already occurred, in this case the ball turned out to be red. Stated more forcefully, the probability of event G is conditional on the knowledge of the probability provided by event R.

4.9.3. The Timing and Interdependence of Events

1. Two events are said to be mutually exclusive if the occurrence of one event precludes the simultaneous occurrence of the other event, thus making the probability of the occurrence of the other event impossible or zero. Alternatively, the chance occurrence of the other event precludes the first event from occurring at the same time. In both cases, the probability of the simultaneous occurrence in both events, that is, the occurrence of one and the other, is impossible; that is,

$P(\text{one and the other}) = P(\text{one}) \times P(\text{other}) = 0$.

On the other hand, the probability of one or the other is the sum of their respective probabilities; thus,

$P(\text{one or the other}) = P(\text{one}) + P(\text{other}) -$ sum of the respective probabilities of one and the other.

	Dependent Events	Independent Events
Mutually exclusive disjoint (or) asynchronous	Events A and B cannot occur simultaneously. Therefore, disjoint events are automatically dependent.	In fact, if A and B are two independent events, then they cannot be mutually exclusive
	3a. Union (Addition)	
	$P(A \cup B) = P(A) + P(B)$	Independent events are never mutually exclusive
Mutually nonexclusive conjoint (and) synchronous	Dependent events: occurrence of one event alters the probability of the occurrence of the other	Independent events: occurrence of one does not alter the probability of the other: $P(A\|B) = P(A)$. The probability of A is not affected by (not conditional upon) the occurrence of the second event B
	4a. Union (Addition)	**4b. Union (Addition)**
	$P(A \cup B) = P(A) + P(B) - P(A \cap B) \Rightarrow\Rightarrow\Rightarrow$	$P(A \cup B) = P(A) + P(B) - P(A) \times P(B)$
	5a. Conditional	**5b. Conditional**
	$P(A\|B) = \dfrac{P(A \cap B)}{P(B)} \Rightarrow\Rightarrow\Rightarrow$	$P(A\|B) = \dfrac{P(A) \times P(B)}{P(B)} = P(A)$
	6a. Intersection (Multiplication)	**6b. Intersection (Multiplication)**
	$P(A \cap B) = P(B) \times P(A\|B) \Rightarrow\Rightarrow\Rightarrow$	$P(A \cap B) = P(B) \times P(A)$

Table 4.9. Dependence Vs. Exclusivity

2. The other implication of mutual exclusiveness is that the two events cannot share a common a single element, which if it does occur as it may, implies the occurrence of both events simultaneously, which rules out mutual exclusiveness as a precondition. In other words, the events are not mutually exclusive. Thus, two events are said to occur simultaneously if one of the elementary events shared by both (i.e., common to both subsets) occurs. Under the circumstances, the occurrence of one and the other is the product of their respective probabilities (given independence); that is,

P(one and the other) = P(one) × P(other) = product of the respective probabilities of one and the other.

3. On the other hand, two events that have an elementary event in common and are thus not mutually exclusive are said to occur simultaneously if one of the elementary events of one or the other or both occurs. Under the circumstances, the occurrence of one or the other event is the sum of their respective probabilities minus the shared replicated elements in the intersection of the subsets (given independence); that is,

P(one or the other) = P(one) + P(other) − P[(one) × P(other)] = sum of the respective probabilities of one plus the other, minus the product of the respective probabilities of one and the other.

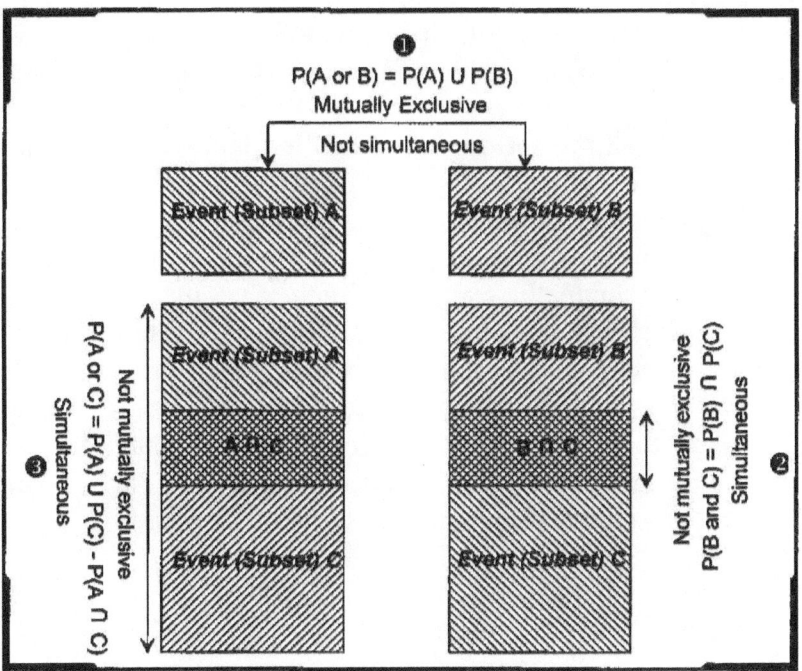

Figure 4.7. For Flow Chart 4-2: Exclusivity Vs Simultaneity

4. Two events are independent if the occurrence of one has no influence the probability the occurrence of the other event. Stated differently, the probability of A is not conditional on the occurrence of the other event B,

$P(A|B) = P(A)$ and $\underline{P}(B|A) = P(B)$.

Two events are dependent if the occurrence of one influences the probability of the occurrence of the other event. Stated differently, the probability of A is conditional on the occurrence of the other event B,

$P(A|B) \neq P(A)$ and $P(B|A) \neq P(B)$.

Given the above-mentioned conditional probability, events A and B are independent if and only if $P(A \cap B) = P(A) \times P(B)$. And if $P(A$ and $B) = P(A) \times P(B)$, then A and B are independent.

4.10 Probability Interaction: The Addition Rule of Probability

The probability of the occurrence of mutually exclusive, asynchronous events is equal to the sum of their respective probabilities. Alternative events that are mutually exclusive imply that they cannot occur simultaneously; that is, they are "either-or" events. Thus, the probability of getting either one or six in a single throw of a die is the sum of the probabilities associated with each throw, so that the chance of getting one or the other is one in three. Stated differently, the probability of alternative results occurring in a single trial will be the sum of their individual probabilities (Table 4.9, 3a).

$$P(1) \text{ or } P(6) = \frac{1}{6} + \frac{1}{6} = \frac{2}{6} = \frac{1}{3}.$$

The rule applies equally to the outcome of sampling from a given set. Thus, the chance of drawing an ace of clubs or an ace of diamonds from a standard pack of cards is one in twenty-six.

$$P(\text{ace} \clubsuit) \text{ or } P(\text{ace} \lozenge) = \frac{1}{52} + \frac{1}{52} = \frac{2}{52} = \frac{1}{26}.$$

Consider the event that the two dice show the same number as given by the following subset:

$$E = \{(1, 1), (2, 2), (3, 3), (4, 4), (5, 5), (6, 6)\}.$$

Therefore, by the addition principle, the probability of the event is the sum of the probabilities of the respective ordered pairs in the subset as given by the following relation:

$$P(E) = P(1,1) + P(2,2) + P(3,3) + P(4,4) + P(5,5) + P(6,6) = \frac{1}{36} + \frac{1}{36} + \cdots + \frac{1}{36} = \frac{6}{36} = \frac{1}{6}.$$

Alternatively, consider the event that the sum of the numbers of the two dice is six, as given by

$$E_6 = \{(1, 5), (2, 4), (3, 3), (4, 2), (5, 1)\}.$$

Therefore, the probability that the sum of the numbers on the two dice is six is the sum of the individual probabilities of the members of the subset as given by following relation:

$$P(E_6) = \{P(1,5) + P(2,4) + P(3,3) + P(4,2) + P(5,1)\} = \frac{1}{36} + \frac{1}{36} + \cdots + \frac{1}{36} = \frac{1}{36}.$$

Because the probability of any single ordered pair is 1/36, the probability of subset S_7 with six ordered pairs may be simply computed as follows:

$$P(E_7) = \frac{1}{36} + \frac{1}{36} + \frac{1}{36} + \frac{1}{36} + \frac{1}{36} + \frac{1}{36} = 6 \times \left(\frac{1}{36}\right) = \frac{6}{36}.$$

Finally, the probability of the occurrence of several mutually exclusive, alternative subsets is equal to the sum of their respective probabilities:

$$P(\text{Sum 7 or Sum 6}) = P(\text{Sum 7}) + P(\text{Sum 6}) = \frac{6}{36} + \frac{5}{36} = \frac{11}{36}.$$

4.11 The Multiplication Rule of Probability

The probability of the joint occurrence of two or more independent events is equal to the product of their respective probabilities. Stated differently, the probability of getting any particular combination of results in two or more independent trials (whether consecutively or simultaneously) will be the product of their individual probabilities.

The rationale underlying the multiplication rule is of course the obvious notion that one-half of one-half equals one-quarter ($\frac{1}{2} \times \frac{1}{2} = \frac{1}{4}$). If the two events are independent (as will be discussed later), then their simultaneous membership in the intersection (a fraction of a fraction of the sample space area) can similarly be interpreted and translated as the product of a (fraction × fraction).

In contrast to the addition rule, the probabilities associated with joint events are independent of their timing (consecutive or simultaneous); that is, they are "and" events. However, the events need to be independent as to their outcome, that is, the result of each event exerts no influence on the outcome of the others.

Thus, the probability of the same face number appearing twice in succession on throwing a single die is the same as the probability getting the same face number on both dice on throwing the pair simultaneously. As noted in the following relation, the probability associated with successive throws or simultaneous throw turns out to be the same, namely, one chance in thirty-six (Table 4.9, 6b).

$$P(6) \text{ and } P(6) = \frac{1}{6} \times \frac{1}{6} = \frac{1}{36}$$

By the same token, the probability of casting two identical ordered pairs in succession is the product of their respective probabilities. Thus, a pair of 6s followed by the same face numbers results in the following diminished probability (Table 4.9, 6b):

$$P(6,6) \text{ and } P(6,6) = \frac{1}{36} \times \frac{1}{36} = \frac{1}{1,296}$$

The multiplication law can be similarly applied to sampling form given sets of elements. Thus, the probability of drawing a specified card from two separate and identical decks will be the product of their respective probabilities of 1 chance in 2,704, as noted in the following relation:

$$P(Ace\clubsuit) \text{ and } P(Ace\diamondsuit) = \frac{1}{52} \times \frac{1}{52} = \frac{1}{2704}.$$

From the foregoing, it is seen that both the addition theorem and the product theorem underlie the determination of the p values for the various combinations of results in the casting of dice. By generalizing, it will be seen that these two theorems are essential to mathematical (a priori) probability theory.

4.12 Contingency Tables, Venn Diagrams, and Tree Diagrams

The contingency table and its graphic equivalents, the Venn diagram or the tree diagrams, are central to the practical application of probability to a variety of scientific, social, and administrative issues.

At the basic level, the contingency table serves as the framework into which the acquired data detailing the frequency for two distinguishing traits are tabulated. The distribution based on the two variables ranges from the classic urn example filled with marbles (plastic or glass) and color (black or white) to the health issues where the test (positive or negative) and well-being (disease or its absence, health) are distributed.

4.12.1 Case 1

Consider the random experiment of drawing a ball from urn filled with ten balls of different colors and makes. The table shows the distribution based on the two variables that characterize the balls: make (glass or plastic) and color (red or white). Note that each ball has two distinguishing characteristics: its color and its make. Accordingly, there are 2 × 2 different kinds of balls; thus, each of the four cells gives the frequency for the distinguishing traits.

	Glass	Plastic	Marginal Total
Red	3	3	6
White	2	2	4
Marginal Total	5	5	Grand total 10

Translating the contingency table into a Venn diagram, the same information assumes a more graphic presence. Note that the R circle encloses all the red balls. Accordingly, all the white balls fall outside the red circle. The same logic applies to the glass circle. The area shared between R and G contains the balls that are red and glass. Finally, the rectangle encloses the grand total, namely, all the marbles in the urn.

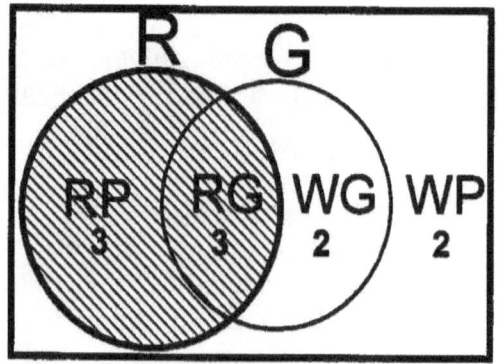

Once tabled and/or translated, the outlay of the data becomes amenable to answer all the probability questions that may arise.

For the simple probability of picking a red ball from the urn, ignoring for the moment the intuitive answer, the answer takes the following format:

$$P(R) = \frac{\text{Marginal total}}{\text{Grand total}} = \frac{6}{10} = 0.6.$$

For the conditional probability of picking a red ball knowing/given that its make is glass,

$$P(R\mid G) = \frac{\text{Cell no.}}{\text{Marginal total}} = \frac{3}{6} = 0.5.$$

For the joint probability of picking glass red ball,

$$P(R\cap G) = \frac{\text{Marginal total}}{\text{Grand total}} \times \frac{\text{Cell no.}}{\text{Grand total}} = \frac{6}{10} \times \frac{3}{6} = \frac{3}{10}.$$

Finally, the check for independence is confirmed,

$$P(G\mid R) = \frac{3}{6} = \frac{1}{2} = P(G) = \frac{5}{10} = \frac{1}{2} \quad P(R\mid G) = \frac{3}{5} = P(R) = \frac{6}{10} = \frac{3}{5}.$$

$$P(G\cap R) = \frac{3}{10} = P(G) \times P(R) = \frac{5}{10} \times \frac{6}{10} = \frac{3}{10}.$$

4.12.2 Case 2

A box contains twenty tablets, four of which are outdate (Od). If two tablets are selected at random (without replacement), what is the probability that both are outdated or both are dated (**D**)?

	D1 = 16	Od1 = 4	20
D2	D2|D1	D2|Od1	
Od2	Od2|D1	Od2|Od1	

Because the first tablet turned out to be outdated, that is, Od1 has already occurred, and because no replacement is possible, we are left with nineteen tablets, three of which are outdated.

$$P(\text{Od1} \cap \text{Od2}) = P(\text{Od1}) \times P(\text{Od2} \mid \text{Od1}) = \frac{4}{20} \times \frac{3}{18} = \frac{3}{95} = 0.0315$$

$$P(\text{D1} \cap \text{D2}) = P(\text{D1}) \times P(\text{D2} \mid \text{D1}) = \frac{16}{20} \times \frac{15}{19} = \frac{12}{19} = 0.6315.$$

4.12.3 Case 3

The following table gives the gender and job classification of an industrial company. If one person is selected at random from the 250 employees, what is probability of being a male or a white-collar worker?

	White Collar	Blue Collar	
Male	80	120	200
Female	40	10	50
	120	130	250

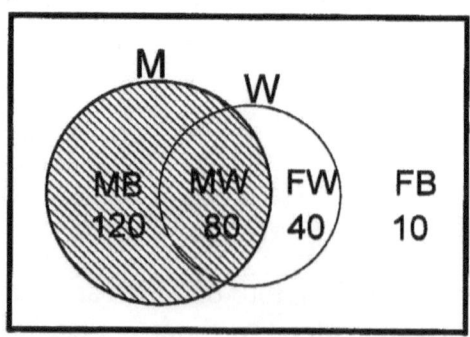

$$P(M) = \frac{200}{250} = \frac{4}{5}$$

$$P(W) = \frac{120}{250} = \frac{12}{25}$$

The joint probability of being a male and white-collar worker is computed as follows:

$$P(M \cap W) = P(M) \times P(W \mid M) = \frac{200}{250} \times \frac{80}{200} = \frac{80}{250} = \frac{2}{5} = 0.4.$$

The probability of the union of two events, a male or white-collar worker, is computed as follows:

$$P(M \cup W) = \frac{200}{250} + \frac{120}{250} - \frac{80}{250} = \frac{2}{5} = \frac{24}{25} = 0.96.$$

Check for independence: denied

$$P(M \mid W) = \frac{80}{120} = \frac{2}{3} \neq P(M) = \frac{200}{250} = \frac{4}{5}.$$

4.12.4 Case 4

The probability that a credit card holder is in debt is 0.6. What is the probability that three randomly selected card holders are all in debt? $(0.6)^3 = 0.216$ $(0.7)^3 = 0.343$.

Concise Overview

Experiment: set of repeated trials (repetitions)

Outcome: chance occurrence of an event that could be counted, measured, or otherwise defined on performing a physical experiment (rolling a die, tossing a coin, spinning a wheel, placing a bet, etc.).

Given the value/type of the experiment, the outcome is the natural expression and chance realization of any one member of the set that constitute possible outcomes of the experiment.

Event: the event in turn defines the actual outcome as a simple event corresponding to a single element subset or as a compound event corresponding to a member element of a multielement subset. The event may thus be viewed as the expression of a particular element in a subset derived from the partition of the sample space into defined subsets dictated by the design of the experiment.

Sample space: the subdivision of the universal set into subsets/cells (that correspond to the design specification of the outcome under consideration) constitutes the sample space of the experiment.

The sample space is thus a specifically partitioned universal set, configured to address the defined or measured outcome. In this sense, the category, value, or property of the outcome defines and determines the unique sample space of the experiment.

Universal set: the set of all possible sample points or elements corresponding to all possible outcomes of the experiment.

Note that every element of the universal set must be in one of subsets/cells that make up the sample space. Furthermore, every possible outcome of the experiment corresponds to exactly one element of the sample space associated with the experiment.

4.13. The Odds Alternative to Probability

The odds approach, essentially a variant of probability, may be easier to comprehend, being the favored mode of predicting the outcome in sporting and gaming events. The concept is intuitive in its evaluation of success versus failure, as applied in the gambling jargon. The relationship between the essential two approaches to probability is not always firmly connected. One usually tends to think in terms of odds or probability depending on habit, training, or experience.

In simple terms, the odds may be defined as the ratio of two mutually exclusive and exhaustive subsets of a given sample universe (e.g., ratio of number of successful outcomes to all possible outcomes in a given defined sample universe). Thus, by splitting all possible outcomes of the sample universe into two distinct and complementary categories that are mutually exclusive and exhaustive, comprising as the situation warrants success (*s*) versus failure (*f*), gain versus loss, for versus against, health versus disease, and so on, the concept of odds pits one subset against its complement in the form of a simple ratio or fraction. By contrast, probability is the ratio of a given subset to the total sample universe of which it is only one subset (Figure 4.8).

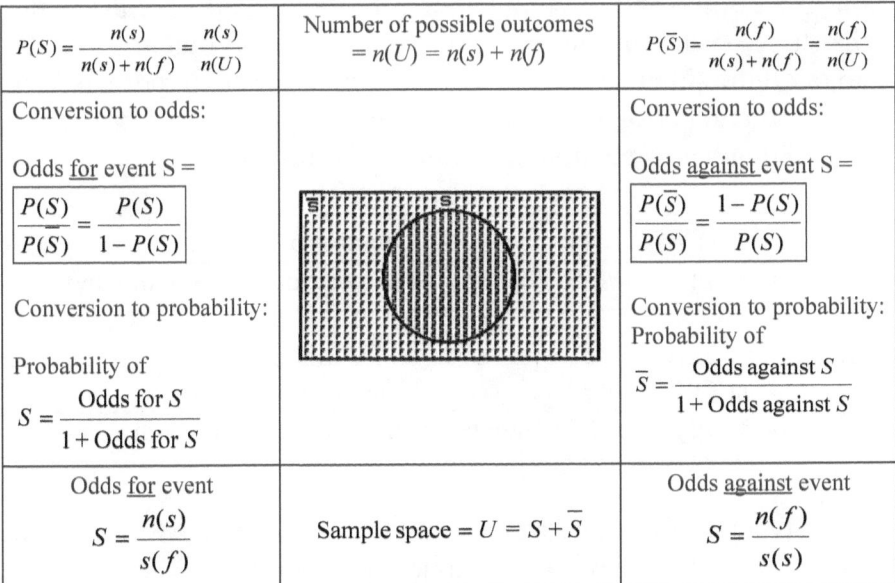

Figure 4.8. Flow chart of the concept of probability versus odds: a two-way reverse conversion

Using success or failure as the defining outcome of a given event (craps, thoroughbred racing, or clinical trials), the odds for (in favor of) an event and against an event (usually given as a ratio rather than a fraction, which is normally used in probabilistic estimates) are stated as follows:

$$\text{Odds } \underline{\text{for}} \text{ event } S = \frac{n(s)}{n(f)} = \frac{\text{number of successes}}{\text{number of failures}} = \frac{\text{Event } S}{\text{Complement } \overline{S}}.$$

Event S is to be differentiated from the simple event s for success, which contains exactly one element in the subset S. Similarly, the complement of event S, $\overline{S}$, is to be differentiated from its constituent elements designated as f for failure. The sum of all the simple elements, both S and F, constitutes the sample space under consideration.

$$\text{Odds } \underline{\text{against}} \text{ event } S = \frac{n(f)}{n(s)} = \frac{\text{number of failures}}{\text{number of successes}} = \frac{\text{Complement } \overline{S}}{\text{Event } S}.$$

Note that event S and its complement, $\overline{S}$, are mutually exclusive and exhaustive, such that the total number of possible outcomes is the sum of all the simple events within the sample space. In probabilistic terms, the number of successes or failures is related as a fraction to the total number of possible outcomes of both s and f.

$$P(S) = \frac{n(s)}{n(s)+n(f)} = \frac{n(s)}{n(U)} = \frac{\text{number of successes}}{\text{number of possible outcomes both } s \text{ and } f)}$$

$$P(\overline{S}) = \frac{n(f)}{n(s)+n(f)} = \frac{n(f)}{n(U)} = \frac{\text{number of failures}}{\text{number of possible outcomes both } s \text{ and } f)}$$

The conversion from one format into another is entered in the side panels for an overview of the inherent relationship (Figure 4.8). As a memory aid, the transition from odds to probability and vice versa may be envisaged as noted in the Venn diagram in terms of the elements and subsets comprising the sample space. Thus, odds are the ratio of the elements within the subset (circle), which are favorable for a particular event to those outside the circle against the event in question. By contrast, the probability is the ratio of a given subset for or against to the total sample space. The conversion from one approach to another is simply a matter of adjusting by subtracting or adding the components of the sample space to fit the mode adopted.

The relationship between probability and odds is perhaps best appreciated using the classical throw of a fair die such that the probability if an ace (a successful event in the old literature) is the event in question. The relationship between the probability of an ace and the odds in favor of an ace is illustrated by the following example of forward and reverse conversion:

Converting to odds using the elaborate conversion format: read left to right

$$P(S) = P(\text{Ace}) = \frac{1}{6} = \frac{s}{s+f} \rightarrow \left[\frac{P(S)}{1-P(S)} \right] \rightarrow \frac{1/6}{1-1/6} = \frac{1/6}{5/6} = \frac{1}{5} = \text{Odds in favor of } S.$$

Again converting to probability using the elaborate conversion formula: read right to left

$$P(S) = P(\text{Ace}) = \frac{1}{6} = \frac{1/5}{6/5} = \frac{1/5}{1+1/5} \leftarrow \left[\frac{\text{Odds}}{1+\text{Odds}} \right] \leftarrow \frac{s}{f} = \frac{1}{5} = \text{Odds in favor of } S \text{ (Ace)}.$$

Similarly, the relationship between the probability of no ace and the odds against an ace is illustrated by the following example of forward and reverse conversion:

$$P(\overline{S}) = P(\text{no ace}) = \frac{5}{6} = \frac{f}{s+f} \rightarrow \left[\frac{1-P(S)}{P(S)} \right] \rightarrow \frac{5/6}{1-5/6} = \frac{5}{1} = \text{Odds against an ace}.$$

$$P(\overline{S}) = P(\text{no ace}) = \frac{5}{6} = \frac{5/1}{1+5/1} \leftarrow \left[\frac{\text{Odds against}}{1+\text{Odds against}} \right] \leftarrow \frac{f}{s} = \frac{5}{1} = \text{Odds against an ace}.$$

At the practical level, a better appreciation of the odds alternative to probability is best illustrated by adopting the parlance of the bookmaker. Consider the odds of 5:2 against Speedy in the second race as made by your trusted bookmaker. The odds in this case are purely subjective based on one's assessment of the variable involved.

The odds that Speedy will lose as quoted are as follows:

$$\text{Odds against Speedy} = \frac{f}{s} = \frac{\overset{\text{bet+win (return) 5+2=\$7}}{5}}{\underset{\text{against}(f)}{}} : \underset{\text{for}(s)}{\overset{\text{risk \$2}}{2}} = \frac{5}{2},$$

which can be translated into probability of winning as follows:

$$\frac{s}{s+f} = \frac{\text{bet(risk)}}{\text{bet+win(return)}} = \frac{2}{2+5} = \frac{2}{7} = 0.28 = P(\text{win}).$$

A bet or $2.0 will net $7.0 contingent on "beating the odds," which in essence negates the given probability of losing calculated at 0.28, or slightly more the one chance in four. Note the ease with which the conversion to probability is made as a simple ratio.

Alternatively, the odds that Speedy will win may be equivalently formulated as follows:

$$\text{Odds for Speedy} = \underset{\text{for}}{\overset{\text{risk \$2}}{2}} : \underset{\text{against}}{\overset{\text{Return (5+2=\$7)}}{5}} = \frac{2}{5},$$

which can similarly be translated into probability of winning as follows:

$$\frac{s}{s+f} = \frac{\text{bet(risk)}}{\text{bet+win(return)}} = \frac{2}{2+5} = \frac{2}{7} = 0.28 = P(\text{win}).$$

Note that the simple reversal of the *for* and *against* position in the odds pattern did not affect the probability of winning $P(W)$, which in both of the above examples is the equivalent of the probability of success $P(S)$, not $P(\overline{S})$.

Note that the odds of 1:1 ordinarily referred to as *even money odds* is the equivalent of 0.5 probability, the probability associated with the tossing of a coin or any bet involving a dichotomous outcome. In the formulation of "odds against," the numerator of the ratio is always the larger integer when the associated probability is less than 0.5

Odds for $n/n - m \Rightarrow s/f = \text{odds}(F)$ $Pr \Rightarrow \text{odds}(F)$	Odds against $n - m/n \Rightarrow f/s = \text{odds}(A)$ $Pr \Rightarrow \text{odds}(A)$	Probability of $s/f + s = n/m = P(S)$ $Odds \Rightarrow P(S)$
9:1	1:9	9/10 = 0.9
4:1	1:4	4/5 = 0.8
3:1	1:3	3/4 = 0.75
2:1	1:2*	2/3 = 0.66
1:1	1:1	1/2 = 0.5
2:3	3:2	2/5 = 0.4
3:5	5:3	3/8 = 0.38
1:2	2:1	1/3 = 0.33
2:5	5:2	2/7 = 0.28
1:3	3:1	1/4 = 0.25
1:4	4:1*	1/5 = 0.2
1:9	9:1	1/10 = 0.11

Table 4.4 A sample of odds *for* and *against* and their corresponding probabilities

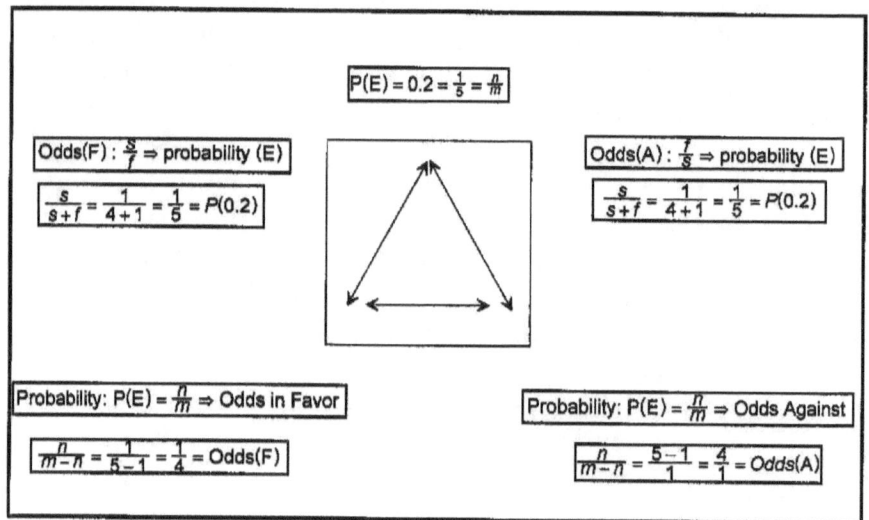

Figure 4.9. Flow chart of the triple two-way conversion between $P(0.2)$, odds in favor and odds against

A detailed triple two-way conversion for the probability of 0.2 associated with the odds in favor of 1:4 and odds against 4:1* is detailed in Figure 4.9. Using the simplified conversion format of n/m and s/f, the chart details the practical two-way conversions between equivalent expressions.

However, as noted in Figure 4.10, where the probability is simply stated as the ratio of n/m, the conversion to odds assumes a simplified and practical format.

Given the probability of (Ace),

$$P(\text{Ace}) = \frac{1}{6} = \frac{n}{m},$$

then the odds against an ace

$$\frac{m-n}{n} = \frac{\text{denominator - numerator}}{\text{numerator}} = \frac{6-1}{1} = \frac{5}{1} = \text{Odds against an ace.}$$

In converting from probability to odds, the numerator is subtracted from the denominator so as to reduce the denominator to the exact complement of the numerator. The reverse process of converting odds to probability involves restoring the denominator to include both subsets of the sample universe. In this case, the numerator is added to the denominator in order to restore the odds ratio to its original probability ratio. Thus, if the odds against an ace is 5/1,

$$\text{Odds against an ace} = 5:1 = \frac{5}{1} = \frac{f}{s},$$

then the probability of an ace is

$$\frac{s}{s+f} = \frac{\text{numerator}}{\text{numerator} + \text{denominator}} = \frac{1}{1+5} = \frac{1}{6} = P(\text{Ace}).$$

In general, the denominator of the ratio is adjusted by adding or subtracting the necessary factor, f or s, to accommodate the desired conversion.

For the ace in question, the arithmetic involved is the addition or subtraction of 1 for the event under consideration and 5 for its complement,

$$P(S) = \frac{s}{s+f} = \frac{1}{6} = \frac{\left[\dfrac{s}{(s+f)-s}\right]}{\underset{\leftarrow}{\overset{\rightarrow}{}} } = \frac{1}{6-1} = \frac{1}{5} = \frac{s}{f} = \text{Odds for } S$$

$$\left[\frac{1}{5+1} = \frac{s}{s+f}\right]$$

$$P(\bar{S}) = \frac{s}{s+f} = \frac{5}{6} = \frac{\left[\dfrac{s}{(s+f)-f}\right]}{\underset{\leftarrow}{\overset{\rightarrow}{}} } = \frac{5}{6-5} = \frac{5}{1} = \frac{f}{s} = \text{Odds against } S$$

$$\left[\frac{5}{5+1} = \frac{f}{s+f}\right]$$

The above-mentioned equations somewhat elaborate attempt to detail that the innate equivalence between the two classical formats of portraying chance events is made in order to facilitate its application as the alternative format in the evaluation of "posterior probability."

Figure 4.10 is essentially a detailed restatement of the triple two-way conversion relation using both the classical and the revised conversion ratios.

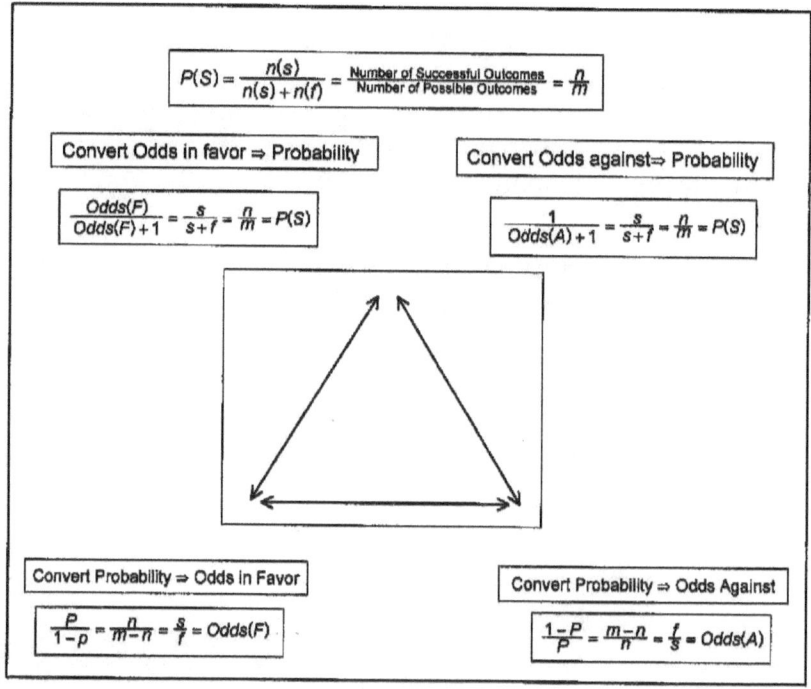

Figure 4.10. Flow chart of the triple two-way conversion between probability, odds in favor and odds against

4.14 The Random Variable

The random variable is a numerical quantity, real number, whose value is defined for each outcome of the experiment and thus indirectly with each element of the sample space corresponding to the resulting outcome. The random variable may thus be represented by a table that lists the elements of a finite sample space and the corresponding number the random variable assumes with each outcome. Because the outcome of any one experiment is unpredictable beforehand, it must, however, correspond to the particular numerical value associated with the particular outcome and ultimately with the corresponding element of the sample space. For the event of two heads outcome, the random variable $X(\text{HHT}) = 2$.

Outcome	HHH	HHT	HTH	THH	HTT	THT	TTH	TTT
No. of Heads	3	2	2	2	1	1	1	0

In the classical case where each outcome is equally likely (i.e., the probability of rolling a one is the same as that of rolling a six), an event as noted previously is defined as a subset of the sample space, that is, any combination from the list of simple events.

Thus, if the sample space of rolling a fair die is given, SS = {1, 2, 3, 4, 5, 6}, the probability of the event of rolling an even outcome,

$$P(\text{even no.}) = P(2 \text{ or } 4 \text{ or } 6) = P(2) + P(2) + P(4) + P(6) = \frac{1}{6} + \frac{1}{6} + \frac{1}{6} = \frac{3}{6} = \frac{1}{2}.$$

Thus, the probability of the compound event is the sum of the individual simple probabilities of the outcomes that comprised the event.

The probability of the simultaneous or consecutive occurrence of two events is equal to the probability of one of them multiplied by the probability of the other provided the first event has occurred (Table 4.3).

Chapter 5

Conditional Probability

Consider an urn containing one hundred balls, a mixture of plastic and glass balls, 70 of which are known to be red and the balance of 30 white. In this case, the reds and the whites are the complementary events so that $P(\text{red}) = 0.7$ and the $P(\text{white}) = 1 - P(\text{red}) = 1 - 0.17 = 0.3$.

Thus, the probability of retrieving a red ball is simply the probability of the red in the urn. The key question in this context, however, is to query the probability of drawing a glass ball given that it is red.

	Glass Balls	Plastic Balls	
Red Balls	Red glass balls	Red plastic balls	$R = 70$
White Balls	White glass balls	White plastic balls	$W = 30$
			100

Table 5.1. The classic Urn mixed contents

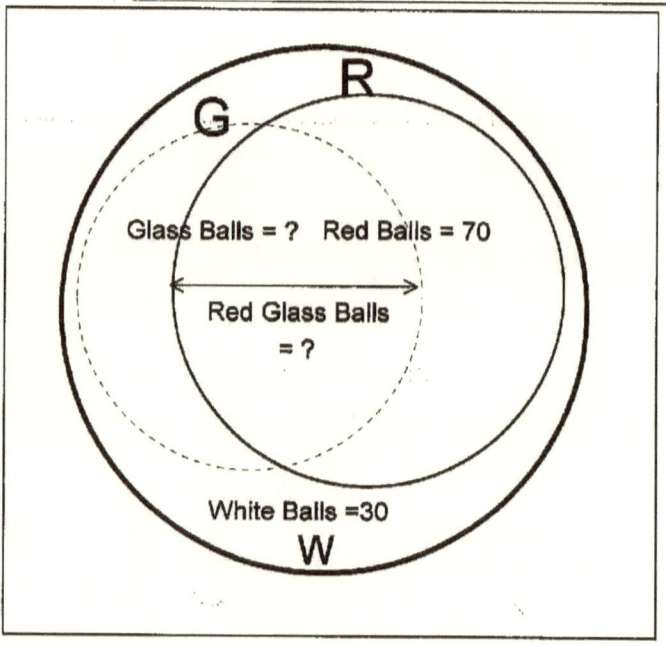

Figure 5.1.

5.1 Conditional Probability

As the name implies, conditional probability is a probability with strings attached, distinctively coded and read as $P(G|R)$ "the probability of G given R," implying that the probability of the event G, in this trial referring to the probability of drawing a glass ball is conditional, given that another event has already occurred, in this case the ball turned out to be red. Stated more forcefully, the probability of event G is conditional on the knowledge of the probability provided by event R.

Having translated the question into the conditional probability, $P(G|R)$, the answer implicitly begs the question as to how many glass balls are red.

From Figure 5.1, the missing link is the area delineated by the tentative intersection of the glass event, G, with the red event, R, namely, $(R \cap G)$, which essentially defines how much of the G event is shared by or is in the R event, which is equal to the ratio of the intersection subset to the whole of the R event.

	Glass Balls	Plastic Balls	
Red Balls	$GR = 50$	$PR = 20$	$50 + 20 = 70$ $R = $ total red
White Balls	$GW = 10$	$PW = 20$	$10 + 20 = 30$ $W = $ total white
	$G = 50 + 10 = 60 =$ =total glass	$P = 20 + 20 = 40 =$ =total plastic	100 =total balls

Table 5.2. The classic Urn defined

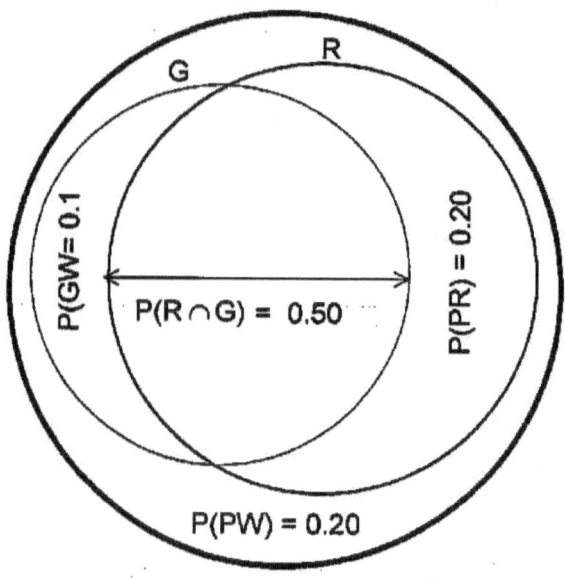

Figure 5.2.

The probability of a drawing a glass ball given that it is red thus depends on the evaluation of the critical ratio in the conditional probability equation.

$$P(G\,|\,R) = \frac{\overset{\text{Unknown}}{P(R\cap G)}}{\underset{=0.7}{P(R)}}$$

Thus, without the missing link $(R \cap G)$, $P(G|R)$ is not amenable to probabilistic solution. However, if any one of the cells associated with the table is determined, Table 5.2 and Figure 5.2 are now completed, subdividing the sample space into four exhaustive and mutually exclusive subsets. Note that the outcome of any given draw results in the simultaneous occurrence of the two events associated with each sample point, its color, and material.

With the information supplied through other means, the conditional probability of having a glass red ball selected may be easily visualized from the Figure 5.2 as being the ratio of the intersection $(R \cap G)$ to the total area R occupied by the red color subset, alternatively the ratio of the GR cell to the total red computed from the table. In both cases, the numerical ratio is 50/70.

From the conditional formula noted previously, the desired conditional probability is derived as follows:

$$P(G \mid R) = \frac{P(G \cap R)}{P(R)} = \frac{0.5}{0.7} = 0.71.$$

Similarly, the conditional probability picking red ball given it is made of glass follows the same derivation process; thus,

$$P(R \mid G) = \frac{P(R \cap G)}{P(G)} = \frac{0.5}{0.6} = 0.83.$$

Note that $P(G|R)$ is not equal to $P(R|G)$.

From the previously mentioned conditional formulae, the formulae for the conjunctive event can be obtained by simple transformation, Thus, the joint probability, that is, the probability of the intersection of the two events, is a measure of the extent to which R and G happen together such that a randomly selected ball is red and glass.

$$P(G \cap R) = P(R) \times P(G \mid R) = 0.7 \times \frac{0.5}{0.7} = 0.5$$

and

$$P(R \cap G) = P(G) \times P(R \mid G) = 0.6 \times \frac{0.5}{0.6} = 0.5.$$

Thus, the probability of drawing a ball that is red and glass ($R \cap G$) is equal to the probability of drawing a ball that is Glass and Red ($G \cap R$).

$$P(R \cap G) = R\,(G \cap R).$$

Finally, in this case, the probability that a randomly selected ball is either red or glass is simply the sum of both probabilities minus the duplicated intersection, as noted by the formula for the union of two disjunctive events,

$$P(R \cup G) = P(R) + P(G) - P(R \cap G)$$

$$= \frac{70}{100} + \frac{60}{100} - \frac{50}{100} = \frac{80}{100} = 0.8 \,.$$

5.2 Graphic Overview

Conditional probability is a central concept in probability theory. It is, in essence, an order to tie together two events, A and B, and to derive the absolute proportion of one with respect to the other. In formal notation, it is expressed as $P(A \mid B)$, read as A given B. In simple terms, the expression is in effect a question to be addressed, namely, what is the new probability of A given that B has occurred already? Or phrased differently, How much of A is in B?

In the context of probability, given two overlapping or intersecting events (Figure 5.3), the question, in fact the order, is to compute the probability of being in A, knowing that we must be in B. In other words, we are now asking, given a new SS, namely, B, what is the proportion of A in it? In graphic terms, we are to compute the fraction of area A that is actually in B. In probabilistic terms, the order is to compute $P(A)$ with respect to the reduced sample space B and not the original sample space, SS.

We have now restricted the universal set to B, one-half the original in this case. The obvious graphic answer is the area of intersection $(A \cap B)$ as a fraction of the B area, both calculated in terms of the universal set. Note that the probability of intersection and that of A or B are usually stated as a fraction of the universal set. This is generally accepted and implicit in the notation of probability such that $P(B)$ is understood to imply $P(B|SS)$, that is, as a fraction of the universal set under consideration. The implicit understanding becomes an exception when it is explicitly specified otherwise, whereby the sample space now put forth is to replace or substitute for the original sample space. This is a key statement that needs to be fully appreciated. $P(A \cap B)$ refers to the area the intersection occupies, as a fraction of the universal set. Similarly, the probability of B, $P(B)$, refers to the area occupied by B as a fraction of the total area of SS. Therefore, the ratio of the intersection area to that of B area now becomes the absolute area shared by A and B as a fraction, this time of the absolute B area and not the universal area.

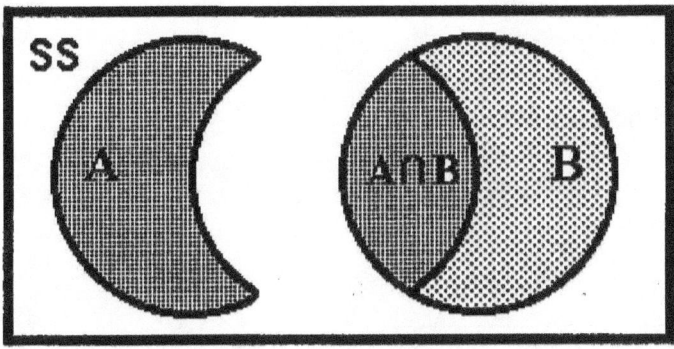

Figure 5.3. Venn diagram of $P(A|B)$: probability of A given B

Because the relationship of A to B is the key element in conditional probability, it is essential to analyze the possible juxtapositions such a relationship may assume.

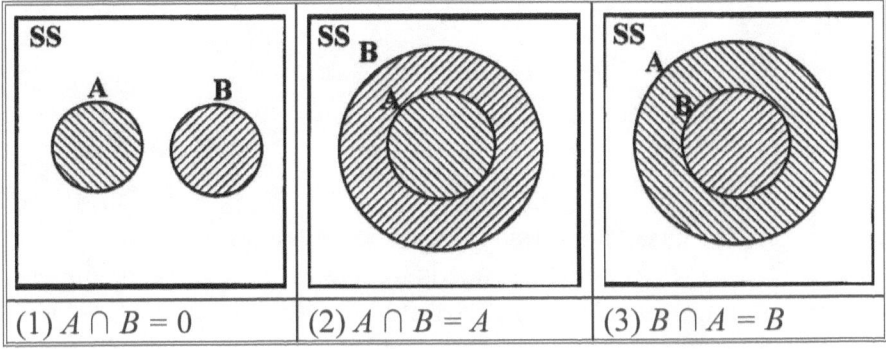

| (1) $A \cap B = 0$ | (2) $A \cap B = A$ | (3) $B \cap A = B$ |

Figure 5.4. Venn diagram of $P(A|B)$: three other possibilities

Thus, in addition to intersection as noted in Figure 5.3, A and B may be mutually exclusive as in equation 1, A may be a subset of B as in equation 2, or B may be a subset of A as in equation 3 (Figure 5.4).

The relative magnitude of $P(A|B)$ and $P(B)$ may accordingly assume one of three possibilities corresponding to the relative positions noted earlier.

In the first instance,

$P(A|B) = 0$ Because A and B are mutually exclusive, the given occurrence of B automatically exclude the occurrence of A.

In the second instance,

$$P(A\,|\,B) = \frac{P(A \cap B)}{P(B)}$$ However, $P\,(A \cap B) = P(A)$, so that

$$P(A\,|\,B) = \frac{P(A \cap B)}{P(B)} = \frac{P(A)}{P(B)}$$

In the third instance,

$$P(A\,|\,B) = \frac{P(A \cap B)}{P(B)}$$ In this case, however, $P\,(A \cap B) = P(B)$, so that

$$P(A\,|\,B) = \frac{P(A \cap B)}{P(B)} = \frac{P(B)}{P(B)} = 1.$$

In the general case of partial intersection of A and B, the relative magnitude of $P(A|B)$ and $P(B)$ needs to be determined by the general formula of conditional probability noted previously,

$$P(A\,|\,B) = \frac{P(A \cap B)}{P(B)}$$,where $P(A \cap B)$ and $P(B)$ are computed with respect to the original SS.

Similarly, the relative magnitude of $P(B|A)$ and $P(A)$ needs to be determined by the general formula of conditional probability,

$$P(B\,|\,A) = \frac{P(B \cap A)}{P(A)},$$ where $P(B \cap A)$ and $P(A)$ are computed with respect to the original SS.

The key factor in the relationship is of course the magnitude of the intersection $(A \cap B)$, which, if known, renders the relationship soluble because B is by definition given.

The previously mentioned definition of conditional probability may be reformulated as follows:

$$\boxed{P(B \cap A) = P(B|A) \bullet P(A),}$$

or equivalently,

$$\boxed{P(A \cap B) = P(A|B) \bullet P(B).}$$

This is known as the multiplication theorem of probability to which we shall return in conjunction with the rules covering probability theory.

5.3 Illustrative Examples

The following examples illustrate in a practical way all the important concepts of conditional probability.

In a survey of 1,000 employees, which included 520 males, 70 were found to be hypertensive, including 40 males and 30 females.

	Hypertensive	Normotensive	Row Total
Male	40	480	M = 520
Female	30	450	F = 480
Column total	H = 70	N = 930	1,000

Table 5.3

The probability that a person chosen at random from this population is hypertensive in probability notation is

$P(H) = 70/1,000 = 0.07.$

And the probability that a person chosen at random is a male is

$P(M) = 520/1,000 = 0.52.$

These data pertain to the total population comprising the sample space. A relevant question in the previously mentioned survey is to address the probability that a male chosen at random is hypertensive. The answer is readily available from the survey data as 40/520.

In probability notation, the probability of being hypertensive given that the person chosen at random is a male is

$$P(H \mid M) = \frac{P(H \cap M)}{P(M)}.$$

The solution requires the evaluation of both the numerator and the denominator. $P(M)$ was already given as 520/1,000. $P(H|M) = $ the number of males found to be hypertensive out of the total population (not just the male population) $= 40/1,000$. Plugging these data into the conditional probability equation yields the required result noted previously:

$$P(H \mid M) = \frac{P(H \cap M)}{P(M)} = \frac{\dfrac{40}{1000}}{\dfrac{520}{1000}} = \frac{40}{520} = \frac{1}{13}.$$

Figure 5.5 is now drawn to represent the partition of the sample space into four disjoint areas: normal males = 480, normal females = 450, hypertensive males = 40, and hypertensive females = 30.

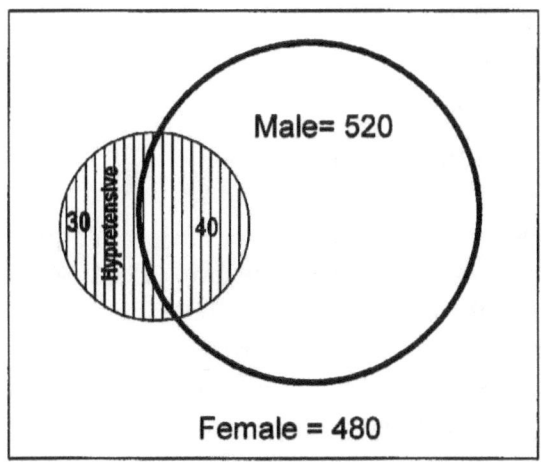

Figure 5.5. Venn diagram of the partition of SS into four disjoint areas.

Note that both $P(H \cap M)$ and $P(M)$ are expressed as a ratio of the sample space of 1,000. The process of division eliminates the common denominator, leaving the conditional probability $P(H|M)$ as a fraction of the reduced sample space now made exclusively of the male circle of 520. Similarly,

$$P(H \mid F) = \frac{P(H \cap F)}{P(F)} = \frac{30}{480}.$$

From Table 5.3 and Figure 5.5, the following relations are easily deduced:

$$P(H \mid M) = \frac{40}{520} = 0.0679$$

$$P(H \mid F) = \frac{30}{480} = 0.0625$$

$$P(N \mid M) = \frac{480}{520} = 0.923$$

$$P(N \,|\, F) = \frac{450}{480} = 0.9375$$

5.4 Basic Rules of Probability Theory

The basic rules of probability theory are concerned with indirect methods which makes it possible to calculate the probability of complex events, given those of the elementary events which combine to make them. All the formulae are based on two main principles or rules: The summation and the multiplication, just as ordinary arithmetic is based on addition and multiplication

5.4.1 Summation Rule

If an experiment results in one and only one of two mutually exclusive events, such that the occurrence of one excludes the possibility of other, then the probability that either one or the other occurs is equal to the sum of the probabilities of both. Note that the probability refers to the possible occurrence of one of two events. In this sense, the probability of occurrence of one is equal to the sum of their individual probabilities,

$$P(A \text{ or } B) = P(A+B) = P(A \cup B) = P(A) + P(B).$$

The probability of getting either one or six on rolling a single die is clearly the sum of their probabilities because the two events are mutually exclusive: $1/6 + 1/6 = 1/3$. The summation rule can be readily extended to cover any number of events, such that the probability that one and only one of several mutually exclusive events occurs is equal to the sum of the respective probabilities of these events.

If A and B are not mutually exclusive, the summation rule needs to be modified to accommodate the synchronous occurrence of the two events. Accordingly, a correction is added in case events A and B are overlapping, so that

$$P(A \cup B) = P(A) + P(B) - P(A \cap B).$$

The need to subtract $P(A \cap B)$ is made obvious by Figure 5.6, where the probability of $P(A \cap B)$ being at once a part of A and part of B is added twice, hence the need for the correction.

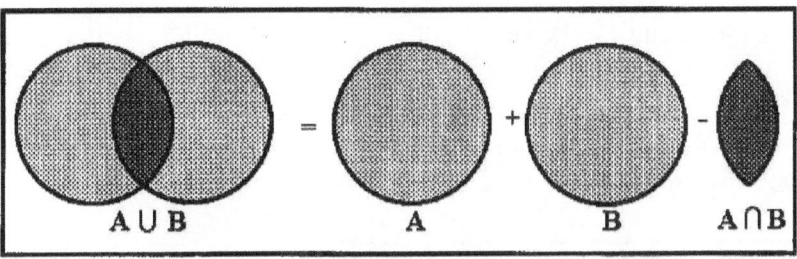

Figure 5.6. Venn diagram of the graphic equivalent
of the summation rule.

The summation rule has two important corollaries:

1. If events (simple or compound) are mutually exclusive and exhaustive, then the sum of their probabilities is equal to one.
2. If A is an event and $\overline{A}$ is the opposite event (i.e., the event of nonoccurrence of A), then the sum of the probabilities of opposite events is equal to one.

$$P(A) + P(\overline{A}) = 1$$

5.4.2 Multiplication Rule

The multiplication rule was fully detailed in chapter 2 as the fundamental counting principle. The rule conceives the process of determining the number of ways a certain procedure may be performed in sequential stages. Thus, if the first stage of the process can occur or be performed in n_1 ways and the second stage can occur or be performed in n_2 ways, then the complete process can occur or be performed in $n_1 \times n_2$ ways.

Recall that in rolling a pair of dice, the experiment may be considered as a two-trial sequence in which the first trial consists of rolling a single die resulting in one of six face values followed by a second identical trial resulting in one of six values. The result of the compound experiment, that is, the number of ways in which the face value of the first die may be followed by the face value of the second die, is thus the equivalent of the result of the first trial, n_1 multiplied by the result of the second, n_2. In this case, $6 \times 6 = 36$ ways of sequencing the two trials of the compound experiment.

The simultaneous or consecutive occurrence of two events is equal to the probability of one of them multiplied by the conditional probability of the other provided the first event has occurred,

$$P(B \text{ and } A) = P(B \bullet A) = P(B \cap A) = P(A) \bullet P(B \mid A).$$

where $P(B|A)$ is the conditional probability of the event B calculated on the assumption that event A has occurred. Note that it is immaterial which of the events is considered the first and which is the second. The rule can thus be rewritten in the following form:

$$P(A \text{ and } B) = P(A \bullet B) = P(A \cap B) = P(B) \bullet P(A \mid B).$$

However, in case events A and B are independent of each other, the intersection formula reverts to the simple multiplication of their respective probabilities,

$$P(B \cap A) = P(B) \times P(A)$$

and

$$P(A \cap B) = P(A) \times P(B).$$

The multiplication rule is simply a restatement of the conditional probability formula elaborated in the previous chapter.

5.5 Probability in Words, Symbols, and Venn Diagrams

The problems encountered in probability are often made unnecessarily complicated by the use of codified or symbolic language that may not be readily understood and appropriately translated into its corresponding Boolean algebraic format. It is with this in mind that a series of problems that address the coded language format will be presented to underscore the inherent simplicity of the mathematical transformation involved.

5.6 Uniform Distribution: The Classical Model

The so-called classical model being the oldest probability model proposed for the practical implementation of probability remains to date despite its limited application, an essential prerequisite in the appreciation of probabilistic logic. To this end, the physical urn filled with identical numbered glass balls is an apt analogy to a sample space made of indivisible primary elements that confirm to the requirements of the classical model and the demand for uniform distribution.

In using the urn model, the probability of outcome following the experiment of drawing a numbered ball fulfills the criteria associated with the classical model, namely, (1) the outcomes are mutually exclusive (not two balls of the same number can be drawn simultaneously), (2) the outcomes are exhaustive (because the experiment covers all possible outcomes), and (3) the outcome is equally likely to result in any one of the numbered balls on performing the "experiment" of drawing any one of the balls at random.

For an urn filled with eight identical numbered balls, the probability of outcome following the experiment of drawing one numbered ball is obviously 1/8.

Consider now the same urn filled with three numbered white balls and five numbered red balls. The random drawing of any one ball does not fundamentally change the initial conditions of the experiment. We are still dealing with the blind choice of one of eight equally likely outcomes, irrespective of the color, that are similarly mutually exclusive and exhaustive.

If color is now specified, the probability of drawing a white ball is 3/8 and the probability of drawing a red ball is 5/8. In this sense, the sample space may now be considered to be made of two elements (instead of eight) whose respective probabilities are 3/8 and 5/8.

Consider instead the drawing of two balls simultaneously (i.e., without replacement). The first thing to notice is that the initial conditions of the experiment have now changed. The new elements of the sample space are now made of "pairs" of balls rather than single balls. Hence, the first step is to consider the size of the configured sample space, that is, counting the number of its newly formed elements as well as the makeup of the individual elements.

This new sample space provides the framework from which the diverse questions encountered in the application of probability may be addressed. As will be demonstrated, the approach to problems of probability must consider the extent (enumeration) of the sample space and the composition of its elements as a prelude or in conjunction with the application of standard formulae. In all such cases, the structure of the sample space constitutes the background for the applications required or the answers sought.

5.6.1 Permutation Approach without Replacement

Using the same urn of three white balls and five red balls, two balls are drawn without replacement. What is the probability that **both** balls turn out to be red?

At the basic level, suppose that the balls are numbered. The basic sample space is made up of eight elements corresponding to eight possible outcomes that are mutually exclusive and equally likely.

White$_1$, W$_2$, W$_3$,	Red$_1$, R$_2$, R$_3$, R$_4$, R$_5$.

The first ball may thus be selected in eight ways. The second ball following the removal of the first may now be selected in seven ways. By the multiplication rule, a total of $8 \times 7 = 56$ ways of selecting two numbered balls is possible, although not visually perceived as different.

This is another way of stating that the SS is composed of fifty-six ordered pairs derived from the permutation of eight "numbered" simple elements taken two at a time ($8P2 = 56$). The fifty-six ordered pairs include $3P2 = 6$ white pairs, the result of permuting the set of three white balls $\{W_1, W_2, W_3\}$; $5P2 = 20$ red pairs, the result of permuting the set of five red balls $\{R_1, R_2, R_3, R_4, R_5,\}$; fifteen white and red pairs as a result of permuting three white and five red; and another fifteen pairs, the result of permuting five red and three white balls as noted in Table 5.4.

Sample space = $\{W_1, W_2, W_3, R_1, R_2, R_3, R_4, R_5\}$				
	(W, W)	(W, R)	(R, W)	(R, R)
$8P2 = 56$ ordered pairs	$3P2 = 6$	$3 \times 5 = 15$	$5 \times 3 = 15$	$5P2 = 20$	$P(R, R) = 20/56 = 10/28$
$8C2 = 28$ unordered pairs	$3C2 = 3$	15		$5C2 = 10$	$P(R, R) = 10/28$
$P(R_A) = 5/8$ $P(R_B \mid R_A) = 4/7$	$P(R_A$ and $R_B) = P(R_A) \cdot$ $P(R_B \mid R_A)$		$P(R_A \cap R_B) = \dfrac{5}{8} \times \dfrac{4}{7} = \dfrac{20}{56} = \dfrac{10}{28}$	

Table 5.4

Because each of the outcomes, that is, the drawing of any one pair, is equally likely, the probability of drawing a given pair corresponds to one of the fifty-six possible outcomes or 1/56.

The probability of drawing two red balls is simply the ratio of the number of red pairs to the total number of possible pairs in the sample space,

$$P(R, R) = \frac{20}{56} = \frac{10}{28}.$$

Because the total number of red ordered pairs may simply be obtained from the permutation of five red balls taken two at a time, which essentially defines the possible choices of red pairs out of the five numbered balls shown as follows:

$$P(R_1R_2 \text{ or } R_1R_3 \text{ or } R_1R_4 \text{ or } \ldots \text{ or } R_4R_5) = 5P2 = 20.$$

The probability of drawing a red pair is then

$$P(R,R) = \frac{5P2}{8P2} = \frac{20}{56} = \frac{10}{28}.$$

Finally, note that the probability associated with any one pair, red or otherwise, is identically equal to 1/56. Thus, the probability of the 20 red pairs is simply the sum of their individual probabilities, i.e., $1/56 + 1/56$, etc.

$$P(R_1R_2 \text{ or } R_1R_3 \text{ or } \ldots \text{ or } R_4R_5) = P(R_1R_2 + R_1R_3 \ldots + R_4R_5) = \frac{20}{56} = \frac{10}{28}.$$

5.6.2 Permutation Approach with Replacement

Using the same urn of three white balls and five red balls, two balls are drawn sequentially with replacement. What is the probability that **both** balls turn out to be red?

Sample space = $\{W_1, W_2, W_3, R_1, R_2, R_3, R_4, R_5\}$					
	(W, W)	(W, R)	(R, W)	(R, R)	
$n^r = 8^2 = 64$ ordered pairs	$W^2 = 9$	3×5 $= 15$	5×3 $= 15$	$R^2 = 25$	$P(R, R) = 25/64$
$P(R_A) = 5/8$ $P(R_B \mid R_A) = 5/6$	$P(R_A \text{ and } R_B) = P(R_A) \cdot$ $P(R_B \mid R_A)$			$P(R_A \cap R_B) = \frac{5}{8} \times \frac{5}{8} = \frac{25}{64}$	

Table 5.5. The classic Urn Probability model

The number of ordered pairs possible with replacement is now $8^2 = 64$ ordered pairs, whereas the number ordered red pairs is $5^2 = 25$. The probability of sequentially picking two red balls is 25/64 as noted in Table 5.5. The same result is obtained by noting that the conditional probability following the replacement of the first red ball remains the same as obtained with the first ball. Thus, the conditional probability is the product of the probability of the first red ball × the probability of the second red ball.

5.6.3 Combination Approach

A simpler approach is to consider combination rather than permutation because order is irrelevant in the case of both balls being red. The sample space of unordered pairs may be derived from the combination formula, $8C2 = 28$ unordered pairs (Table 5.4). Similarly, a total of ten combinations may be made from the five numbered red balls taken two at a time, $5C2 = 10$. The probability of drawing two red balls in succession assumes the simple ratio between the two combinations:

$$P(R,R) = \frac{5C2}{8C2} = \frac{10}{28}$$

5.6.4 Conditional Probability Approach

This approach is carried out through the application of the multiplication rule for dependent events (conditional probability) because the drawing of the second red ball is dependent on the first ball being red. When the above statement is translated into its conjunctive counterpart, the following analogous formulation of the probability multiplication rule results:

$$P(A \cap B) = P(A) \bullet P(B \mid A)$$

$$P(R_A \cap R_B) = P(R_A) \bullet P(R_B \mid R_A) = \frac{5}{8} \times \frac{4}{7} = \frac{20}{56} = \frac{10}{28}.$$

Note that the conjunctive event of "R_A and R_B" stipulates that the drawing of the second red ball, R_B, is conditional on the drawing of the first red ball, R_A, because no replacement is assumed. This being the case the probability of drawing R_B, given that R_A has been drawn, implies a reduction in the sample space from 8 to 7 and equal reduction in the subset of the red balls from 5 to 4.

5.6.5 Complement Approach

Using the same urn of three white balls and five red balls, two balls are drawn without replacement. What is the probability that at least one ball turns out to be red?

Note that at least one is red implies that either A or B is red. The statement is indefinite as to the number of red in the pair, which may vary from a minimum of one to the maximum possible of two. The statement, however, is definite in excluding the white pairs by subtracting $P(WW)$ from the total probability pool of one, such that [1 − neither (W_1 or W_2)] includes all the RR pairs as well as the RW pairs.

$$1 - P(\overset{\text{and}}{W \cap W}) = 1 - P\left(\overset{\text{and}}{\overline{R} \cap \overline{R}}\right) = 1 - \frac{3}{28} = \frac{25}{28}.$$

Alternatively, using direct approach the $P(A \text{ or } B)$ may be translated into either $P(RR \text{ or } RW)$ because this combination includes all possibilities excluding WW. Accordingly,

$$P(RR \overset{\text{or}}{\cup} RW) = \frac{20}{56} + \frac{30}{56} = \frac{50}{56} = \frac{25}{28}$$

5.6.6 Double Combination Approach

At a slightly more complex level, the question may be reconfigured to inquire as to the probability of two red balls and one white ball if three balls are drawn instead of two. The combination approach offers the most direct method.

Note that the sample space in this case is the set of all possible unordered triples, readily derived from a set of eight elements taken three at a time, $8C3 = 56$ subsets of three elements each.

The two red balls, on the other hand, may be chosen out of the five red balls in $5C2 = 10$ ways. In a similar mode, out of the three white balls, one white ball may be chosen in $3C1 = 3$ ways. The number of possible combinations of two red balls and one white ball is the product of the ways two red balls and one white ball can be chosen, or

$5C2 \cdot 3C1 = 10 \times 3 = 30$ ways of choosing two red balls and one white ball.

The sample space, however, is made up of fifty-six distinct triples; therefore, the probability of picking just the thirty triples made up of 2R and 1W is the ratio out of the total possible triples as defined by the following relation:

$$P(RRW) = \frac{\text{No. of possible (RRW) triples}}{\text{Total no. of possible triples}} = \frac{5C2 \cdot 3C1}{8C3} = \frac{30}{56} = \frac{15}{28}.$$

5.6.7 Generalized Double Combination Approach

The process of double combination may be generalized to consider any number of red and white balls in the urn of which k number of balls are red and h number of balls are white, for a total number of $(k + h)$ balls. Out of this urn, n number of balls is drawn at random without replacement.

What is the probability that exactly r of the n balls drawn will turn out to be red or alternatively $(n - r)$ will turn out to be white?

As usual, the sample space of the urn needs to be defined in terms to the n sample drawn. More precisely, the total number of subsets of size n that can be generated out of the urn contents (population) of $(k + h)$ balls need to be determined. Thus, $(k + h)Cn =$ the number of ways of choosing one n subset (sample) from the urn's contents.

On the other hand, r balls may be selected from the red balls in kCr number of ways. Similarly, h balls may be selected from the white balls in $hC(n - r)$ number of ways. Because each combination of red may be coupled to each combination of white, the ratio of the product to the total number of n subsets that can be generated represents the probability the n sample contains exactly r red balls or alternatively $(n - r)$ white balls.

The transformation of the above into a generic format requires the assignment of general definitions to the terms used specifically for the urn's content:

$(k + h)$ = urn's contents of k red balls and h white balls = population in sample space, k of whom are identified by a given characteristic and h of whom are similarly identified by a different characteristic.

n = number of balls drawn from the urn without replacement on a give trial = number of items in a random sample drawn from the population without replacement on a given trial.

r = number of red balls in drawn sample = number of item in random sample identified by their k characteristic.

$(n - r)$ = number of white balls in drawn sample = number of item in random sample identified by their h characteristic.

$(k + h)Cn$ = number of combination (subsets) of size n that can be formed out of the urn's content = number of ways of choosing a subset of size n.= number of combinations of size n that can be formed from the population = number of ways of choosing a subset of size n.

$$P(\text{of } r \text{ type in } n \text{ sample}) = \frac{\overset{\text{Population}}{\underset{\text{of } k \text{ type}}{k}} C \overset{\text{Sample's}}{\underset{k \text{ type}}{r}} \times \overset{\text{Population}}{\underset{\text{of } h \text{ type}}{h}} C \overset{\text{Sample's}}{\underset{h \text{ type}}{(n-r)}}}{\underset{\substack{\text{Population} \\ \text{of } k \text{ and } h \text{ types}}}{(k+h)} C \underset{\substack{\text{Random sample} \\ \text{of } k \text{ and } h \text{ types}}}{n}}.$$

A shipment of vials is packed in a box of twenty-four vials of which two are defective. All vials are indistinguishable and are equally likely to be selected. A sample of three vials is selected at random. What is the probability that one of the three vials is defective?

$$P(\text{one defective vial in a sample of 3}) = \frac{2C1 \times 22C(3-1)}{(2+22)C3} = \frac{2 \times 231}{2024} = \frac{21}{92} = 0.23.$$

5.6.8 Triple Combination Approach: Red, White, and Yellow Balls

An urn contains six white balls, four yellow balls, and two red balls. Four balls are drawn randomly and without replacement from the urn. What is the probability that two of the balls are white, one is yellow, and one is red?

The experiment of withdrawing four balls forces us to configure the sample space in terms of the simple events composed of four balls each. Thus, the set of all possible outcomes that make up the sample space contains $12C4 = 495$ sample points corresponding to the 495 different possible ways to choose four balls from the twelve balls in the urn.

Of the four balls randomly chosen, there are $6C2 = 15$ ways to choose two of the urn's six white balls, $4C1 = 4$ ways to choose one of the urn's four yellow balls, and $2C1 = 2$ ways to choose one of the urn's two red balls. Thus, there are $15 \times 4 \times 2 = 120$ ways to choose exactly two white balls, one yellow ball, and one red ball. The sample space, however, contains 495 sample points of which only 120 satisfy the initial restriction on the composition of the four balls chosen. The probability of such a random selection is thus the ratio noted as follows:

$$P\left(\frac{2W \times 1Y \times R}{4 \text{ balls}}\right) = \frac{6C2 \times 4C1 \times 2C1}{12C4} = \frac{15 \times 4 \times 2}{495} = \frac{8}{33} = .242 \cong \frac{1}{4}.$$

A probability of 0.24 suggests that in one of four trials, the composition of the draw fits the specified restriction.

5.7 The Sample Space Out of the Urn

The process of random selection from a group of patients, both male and female, illustrates a practical analog of the urn problem.

Given twelve male patients and nine female patients, the probability of a particular random selection must consider the number, the order, and the mix of the selection.

Sample space = {12M, 9F} $P(M) = 12/21$ $P(F) = 9/21$				
	(M, M)	(M, F)	(F, F)	
$21C6=54{,}264$ subset of six points	$12C3=220$ subsets of three M points	53,960 subsets of three MF points	$9C3=84$ subsets of three F points	$P(M_{subset}) = 220/53{,}960$ $P(F_{subset}) = 84/53{,}960$

Table 5.6. The classic Urn transposed

The following random selections may be considered:

1. P(3M from 12 and 3F from 9) = probability of selecting six patients from twenty-one of whom three are selected from the twelve males and three from the nine females.
2. P(MMM or FFF) = probability of randomly selecting three males or three females.

For the first random selection, the probability of selecting six patients from the total of twenty-one suggests that three males are to be selected from the twelve available males in $12C3$ ways. Similarly, three females may be selected from the nine female patients in $9C3$ ways. Because each selection from the male patients may be coupled to a selection from the female patients, the six patients may be chosen in $12C3 \times 9C3$ ways.

The problem, however, stipulates a random choice of six patients, which may include any number of combinations of all male or female or a combination thereof. As a matter of fact, random choice of six patients from a pool of twenty-one can be done in $21C6$ or 54,264 ways irrespective of their sex. The question then is how many subsets of six patients out of this grand total meet our query of being equally divided between the sexes. The answer is the ratio of the coupled selection from the random selection or

$$P(3M \text{ and } 3F) = \frac{\text{No.}(3M_{subset}) \times \text{No.}(3F_{subset})}{\text{No.(six pts subsets)}} = \frac{12C3 \times 9C3}{21C6} = \frac{220 \times 84}{54264} = \frac{18480}{54264} = \frac{110}{323}.$$

The probability of (MMM or FFF) is essentially the probability of no particular sequence. What is being asked can be restated as follows:

1. What is the probability of selecting the first male out of twelve males? i.e., $P(M)$
2. What is the probability of selecting a second male given that the first selection is a male? i.e., $P(M_2|M_1)$
3. What is the probability of selecting a third male, given that the second selection is a male? i.e., $P(M_3|M_2)$

The probability of the first choice = 12/21.
The probability of the second choice = 11/20.
The probability of the third choice = 10/19.

The same line of reasoning may be applied to the female selection. Thus, the probability of the first female selection is conditional on the fact that the sample space of twenty-one has been reduced by the choice of three males, leaving only eighteen to choose from. So that $P(F) = 9/18$ and the probability of a second female and third female patient, $P(F_2|F_1) = 8/17$ and $P(F_3|F_2) = 7/16$.

The probability of the particular sequence being materialized is thus the product of the individual probabilities.

$$\left(\frac{12}{21}\times\frac{11}{20}\times\frac{10}{19}\right)\left(\frac{9}{18}\times\frac{8}{17}\times\frac{7}{16}\right)=\frac{22}{133}\times\frac{7}{68}=\frac{11}{646}$$

The probability of one sequence must now be combined (added) with the probability of all possible sequences involving the permutation of six patients of two kinds, male and female. In other words, the probability of one sequence needs to be multiplied by the total number of permutations of six persons, three of whom are of one gender and the other three of the opposite gender ($6P3, 3 = 20$), or what amount to the same thing the combination of six patients taken three at a time: $6P3,3 = 6C3 = 20$.

$$\frac{11}{646} \times 20 = \frac{110}{323} = 0.3406$$

To address the second random selection of three males and there females, $P(\text{MMM or FFF})$, the same line of reasoning prevails in choosing the three males. The choice of the three females, however, is to be independently treated as an alternative choice. The probability of the choice is thus

$$\left(\frac{12}{21} \times \frac{11}{20} \times \frac{10}{19} \right) + \left(\frac{9}{21} \times \frac{8}{20} \times \frac{7}{19} \right) = \frac{22}{133} + \frac{6}{95} = \frac{8}{35},$$

or, what amounts to the same thing, the sum of the ratios of their respective number of combinations to the total possible number of combinations generated by a three-member subset,

$$\frac{\text{No.}(3M_{\text{subset}}) + \text{No.}(3F_{\text{subset}})}{\text{No.(three-point subsets)}} = \frac{12C3 + 9C3}{21C3} = \frac{220 + 84}{1330} = \frac{304}{1330} = \frac{8}{35}.$$

Note that the choice of three males or three females is mutually exclusive, allowing the probability of the choice to be added so as to obtain the final probability.

5.8 Mad Cow Disease

As a topical counterpart, consider the shipment of twenty-four head of cattle from an English farm to Europe. Of the twenty-four heads, six are infected but asymptomatic, six are carriers, and twelve are completely free of the disease. If six cattle are chosen at random, what is the probability that one will be diseased, one will be a carrier, and four will be free of the disease?

The sample space is now configured to include a total of $24C6 = 134,596$ events of six heads, each from the total of twenty-four heads, corresponding to 134,596 equally likely sample points. Of the six heads randomly chosen, there are $6C1 = 6$ ways to choose one diseased cow from the herd's six diseased cows, $6C1 = 6$ ways to choose one carrier from the herd's six carriers, and $12C4 = 495$ ways to choose four healthy cattle from the herd's twelve healthy cows. Thus, there 6 × 6 × 495 = 17,820 sample points in the compound event consisting of one diseased, one carrier, and four healthy heads. Thus,

$$P\left(\frac{1 \text{ diseased} \times 1 \text{ carrier} \times 4 \text{ healthy}}{6 \text{ heads}}\right) = \frac{6C1 \times 6C1 \times 12C4}{24C6} = \frac{6 \times 6 \times 495}{134596} = 0.132.$$

The probability of 0.132 needs to be considered unacceptable from the public health point of view.

5.9 The Probability of Being on Time

Let A be the event that the chief resident begins his rounds on time, and let B be the event that the resident likewise joins the rounds on time. The on-time probability for the chief resident was $P(A) = 0.9$, whereas the on-time probability for the resident was $P(B) = 0.7$. Given that A and B are independent (the punctuality of one doctor need not be affected by the punctuality of the other), the following is a synopsis of the possible on-time relation between the two physicians. The aim of this exercise is to consolidate in the reader's mind the innate relationship between words, symbols, and Venn diagrams in the synthesis of probability statements and or queries.

Refer to panel 5 of Figure 5.8b.

$$P(\text{both doctors begin rounds on time}) = P(E \text{ and } F) = \overset{\text{both}}{P(E \cap F)} = \overset{(0.9)}{P(E)} \times \overset{(0.7)}{P(F)} = 0.63.$$

Panel 12 of Figure 5.8b:

$$P(\text{neither doctor begins on time}) = P(\text{not } A \text{ and not } B) = \overset{\text{neither}}{P(\overline{A} \cap \overline{B})} = \overset{(0.1)}{P(\overline{A})} \times \overset{(0.3)}{P(\overline{B})} = 0.03.$$

The probability that exactly one of the two physicians begins on time may be derived in one of three ways:

Panels 5 and 12 of Figure 5.8b:

$$P(\text{exactly one}) = 1 - [P(\text{both}) + P(\text{neither})] = 1 - (0.63 + 0.03) = 0.34.$$

Panels 6 and 7 of Figure 5.8b:

$$P(\text{exactly one}) = A \bullet \bar{B} + B \bullet \bar{A} = (0.9 \times .3) + (0.7 \times 1) = 0.34.$$

Figure 5.7:

$$P(\text{exactly one}) = P(\text{either}) - P(\text{both})] = 0.97 - 0.63 = 0.34.$$

The probability of at least one of the two physicians is on time may similarly be derived by three alternate relations:

Panels 8 and 5 of Figure 5.8b:

$$P(\text{at least one}) = P\left(A \overset{\text{either}}{\cup} B \right) = P(A) + P(B) - P\left(A \overset{\text{both}}{\cap} B \right) = 0.9 + 0.7 - 0.63 = 0.97.$$

Figure 5.7:

$$P(\text{at least one}) = P(\text{exactly one}) + P(\text{both}) = 0.34 + 0.63 = 0.97.$$

Panels 8 and 12 of Figure 5.8b:

$$P(\text{at least one}) = 1 - P(\text{neither}) = 1 - 0.03 = 0.97.$$

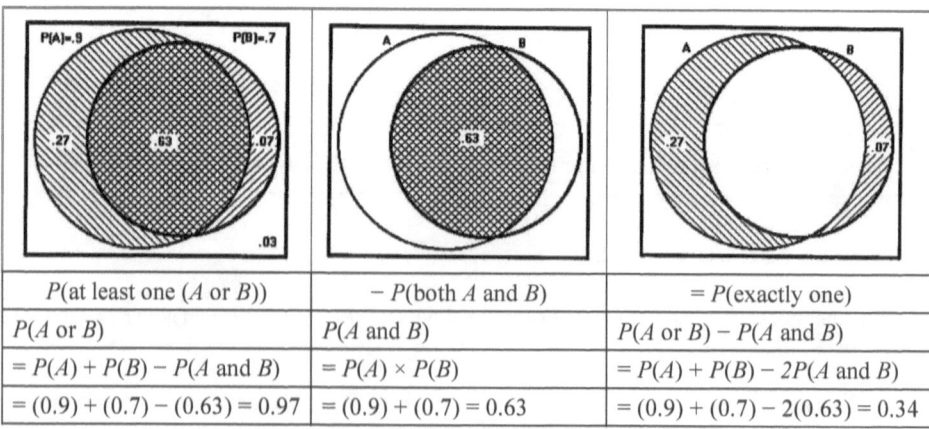

$P(\text{at least one } (A \text{ or } B))$	$- P(\text{both } A \text{ and } B)$	$= P(\text{exactly one})$
$P(A \text{ or } B)$	$P(A \text{ and } B)$	$P(A \text{ or } B) - P(A \text{ and } B)$
$= P(A) + P(B) - P(A \text{ and } B)$	$= P(A) \times P(B)$	$= P(A) + P(B) - 2P(A \text{ and } B)$
$= (0.9) + (0.7) - (0.63) = 0.97$	$= (0.9) + (0.7) = 0.63$	$= (0.9) + (0.7) - 2(0.63) = 0.34$

Figure 5.7. Probability relations in Venn diagrams, words, and symbols. Note that the crosshatched area is derived from the confluence of the diagonals of both A and B.

5.10 The Sample Space Whose Elements are not Equally Likely

What is the probability of rolling two sixes in three rolls of a die? Because each of the three rolls results in six or nonsix, we are dealing with a binary set {six, nonsix} equivalent to the basic binary set of {0, 1} or {H, T}. In the case of a die, because the six could be equally substituted by any one of the six numbers, a more appropriate designation of this binary set would be success or failure,

$$\{s, f\}$$

Because the die was rolled three times, this is equivalent to the permutation with a repetition of size three from the binary set of {six, nonsix}, resulting in $2^3 = 8$ possible permutations of the sixes and the nonsixes.

The glaring difference between the two sample spaces is the probability associated with each of the elements. In the case of the die, the probability associated with the outcome of nonsix or failure is 5/6 in contrast to the probability associated with success of 1/6.

(0, 0, 0)	(0, 0, 1)	(0, 1, 0)	(1, 0, 0)	(0, 1, 1)	(1, 0, 1)	(1, 1, 0)	(1, 1, 1)
1/8	1/8	1/8	1/8	1/8	1/8	1/8	1/8
(f, f, f)	(f, f, s)	(f, s, f)	(s, f, f)	(f, s, s)	(s, f, s)	(s, s, f)	(s, s, s)
5/6×5/6×5/6	5/6×5/6×1/6	5/6×1/6×5/6	1/6×5/6×5/6	5/6×1/6×1/6	1/6×5/6×1/6	1/6×1/6×5/6	1/6×1/6×1/6
125/216	25/216	25/216	25/216	5/216	5/216	5/216	1/216

Table 5.7. The Probability of triple roll

Because the outcomes are mutually exclusive, the probability of each triple roll is the product of the respective outcomes of the triple roll, which as noted in Table 5.7 varies from 1/216 to 125/216. Thus, the probability of two successes in three rolls can be computed as follows:

$$P[(f, s, s) \text{ or } (s, f, s) \text{ or } (s, s, f)] = P(f, s, s) + P(s, f, s) + P(s, s, f).$$

The products resulting from the permutation of two successes with one failure are, however, equally likely, so that the probability of rolling two sixes in three rolls equals $3 \times 5/216 = 15/216$.

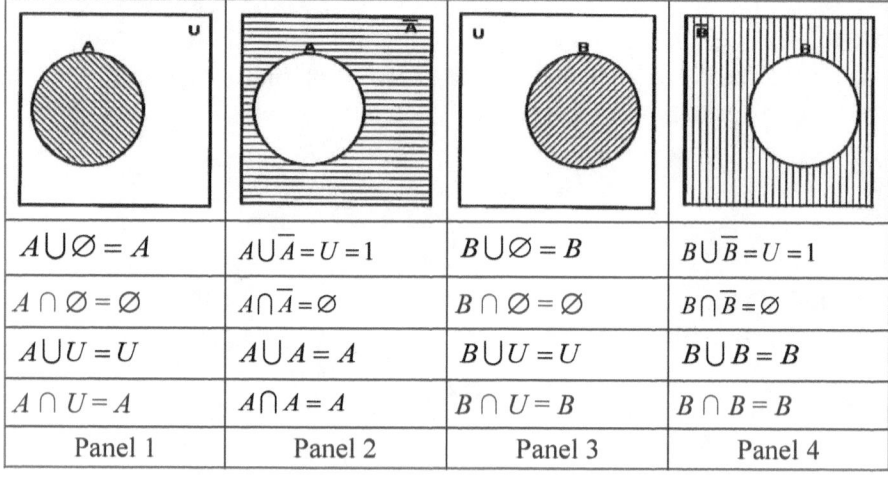

$A \cup \varnothing = A$	$A \cup \overline{A} = U = 1$	$B \cup \varnothing = B$	$B \cup \overline{B} = U = 1$
$A \cap \varnothing = \varnothing$	$A \cap \overline{A} = \varnothing$	$B \cap \varnothing = \varnothing$	$B \cap \overline{B} = \varnothing$
$A \cup U = U$	$A \cup A = A$	$B \cup U = U$	$B \cup B = B$
$A \cap U = A$	$A \cap A = A$	$B \cap U = B$	$B \cap B = B$
Panel 1	Panel 2	Panel 3	Panel 4

Figure 5.8a. Basic set operations in Venn diagrams,
symbols, and words.

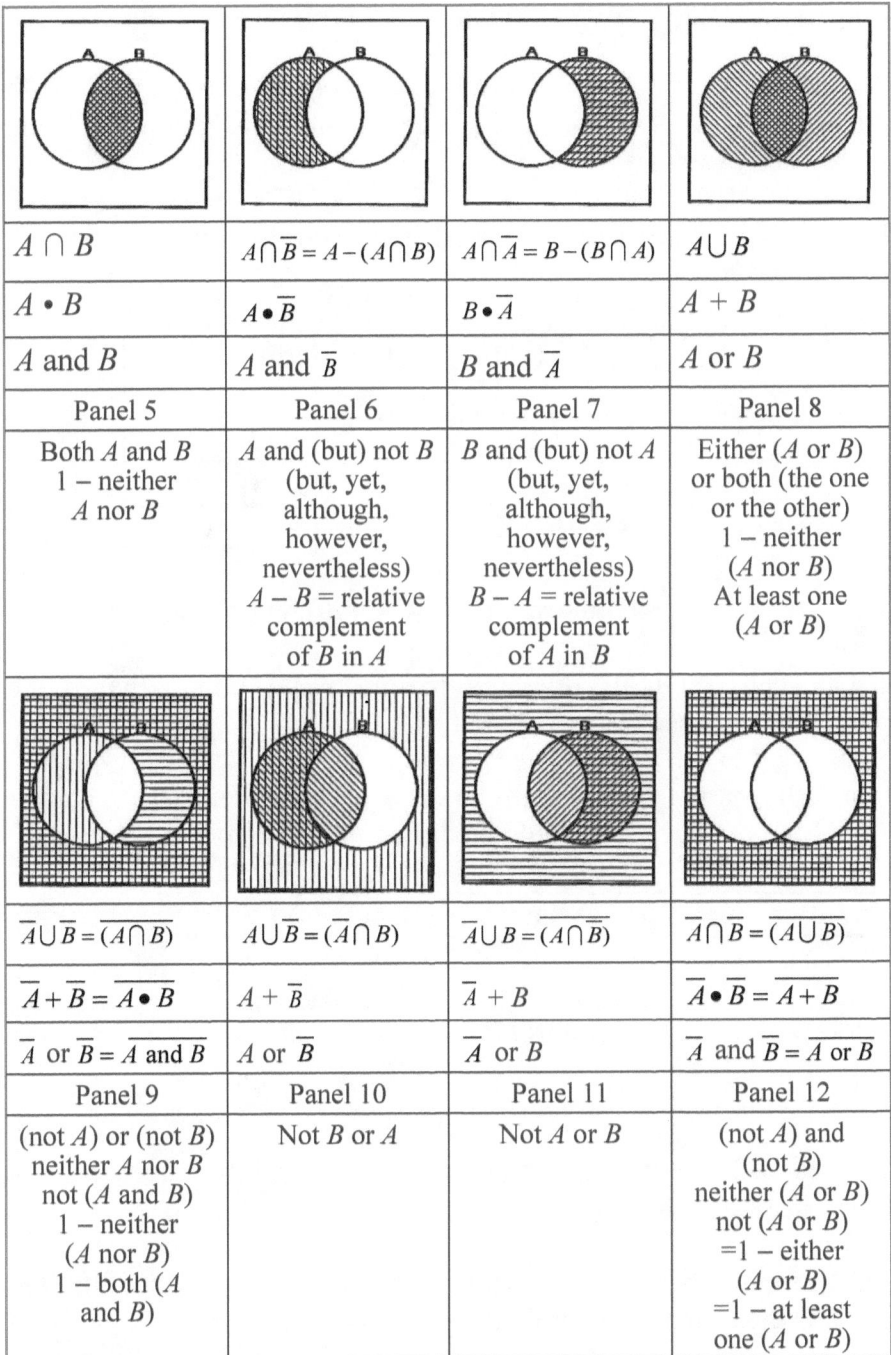

$A \cap B$	$A \cap \overline{B} = A - (A \cap B)$	$A \cap \overline{A} = B - (B \cap A)$	$A \cup B$
$A \cdot B$	$A \cdot \overline{B}$	$B \cdot \overline{A}$	$A + B$
A and B	A and $\overline{B}$	B and $\overline{A}$	A or B
Panel 5	Panel 6	Panel 7	Panel 8
Both A and B 1 − neither A nor B	A and (but) not B (but, yet, although, however, nevertheless) $A - B$ = relative complement of B in A	B and (but) not A (but, yet, although, however, nevertheless) $B - A$ = relative complement of A in B	Either (A or B) or both (the one or the other) 1 − neither (A nor B) At least one (A or B)
$\overline{A} \cup \overline{B} = \overline{(A \cap B)}$	$A \cup \overline{B} = \overline{(\overline{A} \cap B)}$	$\overline{A} \cup B = \overline{(A \cap \overline{B})}$	$\overline{A} \cap \overline{B} = \overline{(A \cup B)}$
$\overline{A} + \overline{B} = \overline{A \cdot B}$	$A + \overline{B}$	$\overline{A} + B$	$\overline{A} \cdot \overline{B} = \overline{A + B}$
$\overline{A}$ or $\overline{B} = \overline{A \text{ and } B}$	A or $\overline{B}$	$\overline{A}$ or B	$\overline{A}$ and $\overline{B} = \overline{A \text{ or } B}$
Panel 9	Panel 10	Panel 11	Panel 12
(not A) or (not B) neither A nor B not (A and B) 1 − neither (A nor B) 1 − both (A and B)	Not B or A	Not A or B	(not A) and (not B) neither (A or B) not (A or B) =1 − either (A or B) =1 − at least one (A or B)

Figure 5.8b. Basic set operations in Venn diagrams, symbols, and words.

5.11 The Double Urn Problem in Jest and Reality

The urn problem relevance to the main thesis of this monograph is illustrated by the analogous and parallel solutions of the following juxtaposed examples.

Red and white balls: two identical urns with different contents are placed side by side.

	Red balls	White balls	Row Total
Urn A	54	18	$A = 72$
Urn B	6	162	$B = 168$
Column total	$R = 60$	$W = 180$	240

Table 5.8. Duplicate Urns with different contents

□ One ball is blindly drawn from one of the urns. What is the probability it is red?

Urn A and urn B are mutually exclusive; therefore, $P(A) = P(B) = 1/2$. However, a red ball could be drawn from either A or B, so that

$$P(\text{red}) = P(\text{urn A and red}) \text{ or } P(\text{urn B and red})$$

$$P(\text{red}) = P(A) \bullet P(\text{red} \mid A) + P(B) \bullet P(\text{red} \mid B).$$
$$\underset{\frac{1}{2} \times}{} \quad \underset{\frac{54}{72} +}{} \quad \underset{\frac{1}{2} \times}{} \quad \underset{\frac{6}{168} = \frac{11}{28}}{}$$

□ A red ball was blindly drawn from one of the two urns. What is the probability that it was drawn from urn A?

The question may be rephrased to read: What is the probability that urn A is the source, given that the ball is red?

$$P(A|Red) = \frac{P(A \text{ and } Red)}{P(Red)}.$$

$P(red)$, as derived from the previous equation, may now be substituted in the denominator of the formula for the conditional event.

$$P(A|Red) = \frac{P(A \text{ and } Red)}{P(A \text{ and } Red) \text{ or } P(B \text{ and } Red)}.$$

$$P(A|Red) = \frac{P(A) \bullet P(Red|A)}{P(A) \bullet P(Red|A) + P(B) \bullet P(Red|B)}.$$

$$P(A|Red) = \frac{\dfrac{1}{2} \times \dfrac{54}{72}}{\dfrac{1}{2} \times \dfrac{54}{72} + \dfrac{1}{2} \times \dfrac{6}{168}} = \frac{\dfrac{27}{72}}{\dfrac{11}{28}} = \frac{21}{22}.$$

5.12 Lyme Disease: Proved and Unproved

A newly developed test for the detection of latent Lyme disease was administered to all the 240 patients registered at the rheumatology clinic. Prior to the test, the presence of the disease was independently confirmed in sixty patients. The final results were tabulated in a 2 × 2 contingency table (Table 5.9).

	Lyme Points (Red Balls)	Non-Lyme Points (White Balls)	Row Total
	D^+	D^-	
Urn A Positive test: T^+ (glass balls)	54	18	$T^+ = 72$

Urn B Negative test: T⁻ (plastic balls)	6	162	T⁻ = 168
Column total	D⁺ = 60	D⁻ = 180	240

Table 5.9. Duplicate Urns transposed

At the conclusion of the trial, it becomes possible to fill in the four cells of the 2 × 2 contingency table and consequently to address the four pertinent probability questions.

1. What is the (conditional) probability that the test in question turns out to be positive, T^+, given that the patient being tested has been independently confirmed to be infected with the disease, D^+?

$$P(T^+ \mid D^+) = \frac{P(T^+ \cap D^+)}{P(D^+)} = \frac{54}{60} = 0.90 = \text{probability of testing positive on a proven case} = Sn.$$

2. What is the (conditional) probability that the test in question turns out to be negative, T^-, given that the patient being tested has been confirmed to be free from the disease, D^-?

$$P(T^- \mid D^-) = \frac{P(T^- \cap D^-)}{P(D^-)} = \frac{162}{180} = 0.90 = \text{probability of testing negative on proven free case} = Sp.$$

3. What is the (conditional) probability that patient being tested is indeed infected with the disease, D^+, given that the test in question turned out to be positive, T^+? Of the seventy-two patients who reacted positively to the test, only fifty-four are proven to have Lyme disease.

$$(D^+ \mid T^+) = \frac{P(T^+ \cap D^+)}{P(T^+)} = \frac{54}{72} = 0.75 = \text{posterior probability} = \text{predictive value of a positive test probability}$$
of confirming the presence of the disease given a positive test.

4. What is the (conditional) probability that the patient being tested is indeed totally free of the disease, D^-, given that the test in question turned out to be negative, T^-? Of the 168 patients who reacted negatively to the test, only 6 are proven to have Lyme disease.

$$P(D^- \mid T^-) = \frac{P(T^- \cap D^-)}{P(T^-)} = \frac{162}{168} = 0.96 = \text{posterior probability} = \text{predictive value of a negative test}$$

probability of confirming freedom from the disease given a negative test.

□ Finally, one might ask, what is the probability of a positive test in a randomly selected patient?

$$P(\text{Lyme}) = P(\text{red}) = \frac{60}{240} = \frac{1}{4}.$$

$$P(\text{No Lyme}) = P(\text{white}) = \frac{180}{240} = \frac{3}{4}.$$

$$P(T^+) = P(\text{Lyme and } T^+) \text{ or } P(\text{no Lyme and } T^+).$$
$$\frac{60}{240} \times \frac{90}{100} \qquad + \qquad \frac{180}{240} \times \frac{10}{100} = \frac{3}{10}$$

5.13 Prostatic Cancer: Confirmed and Excluded

In the following example, the role of conditional probability in the evaluation of a diagnostic test will be examined.

A diagnostic test for the detection of prostatic cancer has reached the stage of preliminary clinical trial. A total of one hundred patients suspected on initial examination of malignant transformation were tested. Exhaustive investigations, including biopsy, were performed later to rule in or rule out the suspected malignancy. The resultant data are summarized in Table 5.10 and configured in Figure 5.9.

	Ca Confirmed Disease Present	Ca Excluded Disease Absent	Row Total
	D^+	D^-	
Positive test, T^+	24	14	$T^+ = 38$
Negative test, T^-	6	56	$T^- = 62$
Column total	$D^+ = 30$	$D^- = 70$	100

Table 5.10. Summary of data derived from the clinical trial

The correspondence between the four outlined compartments or cells in the table, referred to as two-by-two table or array, and the four disjoint subset in the associated Venn diagram bear a closer examination.

1. The sum of the left vertical column of cells = D circle = 30 = number of patients confirmed with the disease.
2. The sum of the right vertical column of cells = D^- = the complement of $D^+ = (\overline{D^+}) = 70$ = number of patients proven to be free from the disease.
3. The sum of the top horizontal cells = T^+ circle = 38 = number patients tested positive.
4. The sum of the bottom horizontal cells = T^- = the complement of $T^+ = (\overline{T^+}) = 62$ = number patients tested negative.

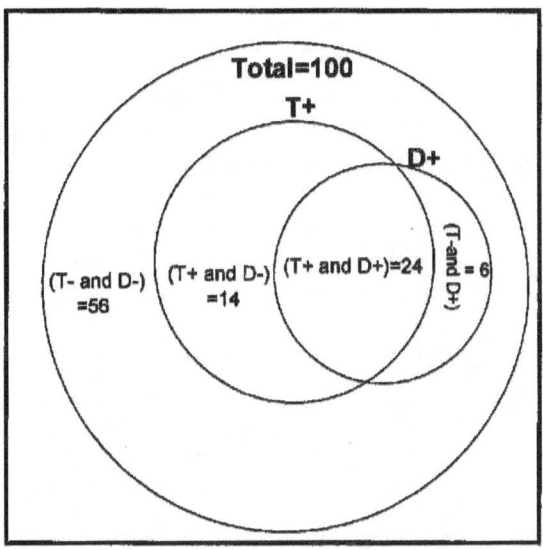

Figure 5.9. Correspondence between the four subsets
of the Venn diagram and the 2 × 2 Table 5.10.

The numbers in the individual cells correspond to the four mutually
exclusive and exhaustive subsets of the Venn diagram. Graphically,
this is reflected in the modified Table and Venn diagram where each
cell is now a distinct subset the population total comprising the
universal set of the one hundred patients (Table 5.10 and Figure 5.10).

Alternatively, each cellular compartment in the table along with its
corresponding subset in the Venn diagram is a single representative
of the four subsets that obtain from the intersection of the T^+ circle
with the D^+ circle.

The one-to-one correspondence between the four cellular
compartments of the table and the disjointed subset of the
Venn diagram renders the application of sets to either mode of
presentation equally valid. Thus, the need to designate each cellular
compartment by a letter is obviated. One only needs to remember
that the intersection area, $(T^+ \cap D^+)$, represent the subset that tested
positive and has been proven to be by other means to be correctly
diagnosed as harboring the disease now being tested.

At the other end, the balance of the universal set, $(T^+ \cap D^+)$, represent the subset that tested negative and has been equally proven to be free from the disease being tested. The two wings of the Venn diagram and their corresponding cells represent the two subsets comprising the erroneous categorization of truly diseased patients as negative and of truly free patients as positive.

	Ca Confirmed Disease Present D^+	Ca Excluded Disease Absent D^-	Row Total
T^+	$(T^+ \cap D^+) = 24$	$(T^+ \cap D^-) = 14$	$T^+ = 38$
T^-	$(T^- \cap D^+) = 6$	$(T^- \cap D^-) = 56$	$T^- = 62$
Column total	$D^+ = 30$	$D^- = 70$	100

Table 5.11. Trial results expressed in set notation and assigned to the 2 × 2 tabular array

At the conclusion of the trial, it becomes possible to fill in the four cells of the 2 × 2 contingency table and consequently to address the four pertinent probability questions:

1. What is the (conditional) probability that the test in question turns out to be positive, T^+, given that the patient being tested has been independently confirmed to be stricken with the disease, D^+?

$$P(T^+)+|D^+) = \frac{P(T^+ \cap D^+)}{P(D^+)} = \frac{24}{30} = 0.8 = \text{probability of testing positive on a proven case} = \text{Sn.}$$

2. What is the (conditional) probability that the test in question turns out to be positive, T^+, given that the patient being tested has been independently confirmed to be free the disease, D^-?

$$P(T^+|D^-) = \frac{P(T^+ \cap D^-)}{P(D^-)} = \frac{14}{70} = 0.2 = \text{probability of testing positive on a free case} = 1 - \text{Sn.}$$

3. What is the (conditional) probability that the test in question turns out to be negative, T⁻, given that the patient being tested has been confirmed to be free from the disease, D⁻?

$$P(T^- \mid D^-) = \frac{P(T^- \cap D^-)}{P(D^-)} = \frac{56}{70} = 0.8 = \text{probability of testing negative on a proven free case} = Sp.$$

4. What is the (conditional) probability that the test in question turns out to be negative, T⁻, given that the patient being tested has been confirmed to be free from the disease, D⁻?

$$P(T^- \mid D^+) = \frac{P(T^- \cap D^+)}{P(D^+)} = \frac{6}{30} = 0.2 = \text{probability of testing negative on a proven free case} = 1 - Sp.$$

A. What is the (conditional) probability that patient being tested is indeed stricken with the disease, D⁺, given that the test in question turned out to be positive, T⁺? Of the thirty-eight patients who reacted positively to the test, only twenty-four are proven to have the disease.

$$P(D^+ \mid T^+) = \frac{P(T^+ \cap D^+)}{P(T^+)} = \frac{24}{38} = 0.631 = \text{posterior probability} =$$
predictive value of a positive test = probability of confirming the presence of the disease given a positive test.

B. What is the (conditional) probability that patient being tested is indeed totally free of the disease, D⁻, given that the test in question turned out to be negative, T⁻? Of the sixty-two patients who reacted negatively to the test, fifty-six are proven not to have the disease.

$$P(D^- \mid T^-) = \frac{P(T^- \cap D^-)}{P(T^-)} = \frac{56}{62} = 0.903 = \text{posterior probability} =$$
predictive value of a negative test = probability of confirming freedom from the disease given a negative test.

$$P(D^+ \mid T^-) = \frac{P(T^- \cap D^+)}{P(T^+)} = \frac{14}{38} = 0.368 = 1 - PVT+ \quad = \text{ probability of}$$
actual disease given
a negative test.

$$P(D^- \mid T^+) = \frac{P(T^+ \cap D^-)}{P(T^-)} = \frac{6}{62} = 0.096 = 1 - PVT- \quad = \text{ probability of}$$
freedom from disease
given a positive test.

☐ Finally, one might ask, "What is the probability of a positive test in a randomly selected patient?"

$$P(Cs) = \frac{30}{100}$$

$$P(NoCa) = \frac{70}{100}$$

$$P(T^+) = P(Ca \text{ and } T^+) \text{ or } P(NoCa \text{ and } T^+)$$
$$\frac{30}{100} \times \frac{80}{100} \quad + \quad \frac{70}{100} \times \frac{20}{100} = 0.38$$

5.14 Probability in the World of Chance

In the following pages, three games of chance probably familiar to many readers will be detailed and described in terms of the probabilities associated with a given draw or roll. The avowed purpose of the exercise is to consolidate the reader's perception of the role probability plays in a common setting, thus allowing for the extrapolation of the underlying principle to a more productive arena as the case may be. In each case, the probability associated with favorable and unfavorable events is presented with sufficient detail in order to focus on the underlying principle involved. The use of odds as an alternative to probability is demonstrated in one case, to allow the reader who is more in tune with the odds mode of probabilistic thinking to be able to translate an odds statement into a probability statement and vice versa.

5.14.1 The New York Lotto

In the game of lotto as played in New York, one selects six numbers out of fifty-four positive integers listed in one panel. On drawing day, six winning numbers and an additional supplementary number are drawn. The chances of winning are listed on the back of the play card.

The derivation of the chances illustrates an interesting application of the urn problem. Consider the third prize level in the winning events, which consists of four numbers out of six having been correctly marked. The urn analogy in this case consists of six white balls and forty-eight red balls. The question then is the probability of drawing six balls at random, of which four are white and two are red.

Third prize: four winning numbers out six

$$\frac{6C4 \times 48C2}{54C6} = \frac{15 \times 1128}{54C6} = \frac{16920}{25,827,165} = 1:1,526.4 \approx 1:1,526.$$

Thus, each of the fifteen possible combinations of drawing four of six white balls needs to be coupled to 1 of the 1,128 possible combinations of drawing two of the forty-eight red balls in the urn, resulting in 16,920 possible favorable combinations. However, the total number of all possible combination of drawing six balls at random from the urn of fifty-four balls irrespective of color is given by the denominator of the equation. Recall that for the general case of a sample space of n possible outcomes, the probability of each simple event = $1 / n(\text{SS})$.

The probability of the "event of four winning numbers" is then the ratio of the number of combinations favorable for the event to the total number of possible combinations, $n(\text{E})/n(\text{SS})$.

First prize: six winning numbers out of six

$$\frac{6C6}{54C6} = \frac{1}{54C6} = \frac{1}{25,827,165} = 1:25,827,165.$$

In this case, of these twenty-five million possible combinations, only one such combination includes exclusively all the while balls.

Second prize: five winning numbers of six

$$\frac{6C5 \times 48C1}{54C6} = \frac{6 \times 48}{54C6} = \frac{288}{25,827,165} = 1:89,677.6 \approx 1:89,678 \,.$$

Fourth prize: three winning numbers plus supplementary

$$\frac{6C3 \times 47C2}{54C6} = \frac{20 \times 1081}{54C6} = \frac{21620}{25,827,165} = 1:1,194.59 \approx 1:1,195 \,.$$

Note the reduction in the number of red balls to forty-seven corresponding to the supplementary number.

The overall odds in favor of winning some prize on choosing two panels ($1 bet) is given by the following summation of the four winning probabilities:

$$\frac{1 + 288 + 16920 + 21620}{25,827,165} = \frac{38829}{25,827,165} \times 2 = 1:332.57 \approx 1:333$$

5.14.2 The Poker Game

In a standard poker games, five cards are dealt from a deck of fifty-two cards. The ace is ranked as either 1 or 14. The probability of both the favorable an unfavorable events is detailed in Table 11-2.

Rank	E = Type of Hand	Combinations of Selected Events	$n(E)$ No. of Favorable Events	$P(E) =$ $n(E) / n(U)$ probability
1	Royal flush: ten, jack, queen, king, and ace of the same suit	4	4	$P(E) =$ 0.000002
2	Straight flush: five consecutive denomination of the same suit, excluding a royal flush	$n = 14$ ranks per suit $r =$ partition number of 5 $n - r + 1 = 14 - 5 + 1 = 10 =$ Number of possible straight flushes per suit $10 \times 4 = 40 =$ number of straight flushes per deck including four royal flushes	$40 - 4 = 36$	$P(E) =$ 0.000014
3	Four of a kind: four cards of the same denomination (face value = rank)	• Face value of the four: $13C1 = 13$ • Four cards of the same face value out of 4: $4C4 = 1$ • One face value of the remaining 12 cards: $12C1 = 12$ • Face value of the card: $4C1 = 4$	$13 \times 1 \times 12$ $\times 4 = 624$	$P(E) =$ 0.00024
4	Full house: three cards of one denomination, two of another	• Face value of the three out of four: $4C3 = 4$ • Face value of the pair out of four: $4C2 = 6$ • Choosing two denominations from thirteen: $13C2 = 78$ • Permutation of two choices = 2!	$4 \times 6 \times 78$ $\times 2 = 3,744$	$P(E) =$ 0.0014
5	Flush: five cards of same suit excluding a straight and royal	$13C5 = 1,287$ $4 \times 1,287 = 5,148$ $5,148 - 36 - 4 = 5,108$	5,108	$P(E) =$ 0.0020
6	Straight: five cards of consecutive denomination not all of the same suit	$10 \times 4^5 = 10,240$ $10,240 - 36 - 4 = 10,200$	10,200	$P(E) =$ 0.0039

Table 5.12. The probability of a hand in the game of poker

Rank	E = Type of Hand	Combinations of Selected Events	$n(E)$ No. of Favorable Events	$P(E) = n(E)/$ and (U) Probability
7	Three of a kind: three cards of one denomination and one each of two other denominations	• Face value of the three: $13C1 = 13$ • Three cards of the same face value out of four: $4C3 = 4$ • Two face values of the remaining twelve cards not used in the face value of the three: $12C2 = 66$ • One card with one of the two face values: $4C1 = 4$ • One card with the other face value: $4C1 = 4$ • One card with the other face value: $4C1 = 4$	$13 \times 4 \times 66$ $\times 4 \times 4$ $= 54{,}912$	$P(E) =$ 0.0211
8	Two pairs: two cards of one denomination, two cards of another, and one card of a third denomination	• Face value of the pair: $13C1 = 13$ • Two cards of the same face value out of four: $4C2 = 6$ • Face value of the remaining twelve: $12C1 = 12$ • Two cards of the same value out of three: $3C2 = 3$ • Remaining one card not used in the two pairs: $11C1 = 11$ • Remaining card with one face value: $4C1 = 4$	$13 \times 6 \times 12$ $\times 3\ 11 \times 4$ $= 123{,}552$	$P(E) =$ 0.0475
9	One pair: two cards of one denomination, one card each from three other denominations	• Face value of the pair: $13C1 = 13$ • Two cards of the same face value out of four: $4C2 = 6$ • Three face values of the remaining twelve cards not use in the pair face value: $12C3 = 220$ • One card with one of the three face values: $4C1 = 4$ • Second card with the other face value: $4C1 = 4$ • Third card with yet another face value: $4C1 = 4$	$13 \times 6 \times$ $220 \times 4 \times$ 4×4 $= 1{,}098{,}240$	$P(E) =$ 0.4226
10	Nothing of interest		$2{,}598{,}960$ $- 1{,}296{,}420$ $= 1{,}302{,}540$	$P(E) =$ 0.5012
11	Total number of possible poker hands	$52C5 = 2{,}598{,}960$	$2{,}598{,}960$	$P(E) =$ 1.0000

The Game of Craps					
Point Number; Come Out	Combinations that Make Up the Number	Ways of Rolling the Number	P(Point)	P(Making a Point)	P(Point and Making It)
2	1-1	1	1/36		
3	2-1; 1-2	2	2/36		
4	3-1; 2-2; 1-3	3	3/36	3/9	$\frac{3}{36} \times \frac{3}{9} = \frac{1}{36}$
5	4-1; 3-2; 2-3; 1-4	4	4/36	4/10	$\frac{4}{36} \times \frac{4}{10} = \frac{2}{45}$
6	5-1; 4-2; 3-3; 2-4; 1-5	5	5/36	5/11	$\frac{5}{36} \times \frac{5}{11} = \frac{25}{396}$
7	6-1; 5-2; 4-3; 3-4; 2-5; 1-6	6	6/36		
8	6-2; 5-3; 4-4; 3-5; 2-6	5	5/36	5/11	$\frac{5}{36} \times \frac{5}{11} = \frac{25}{396}$
9	6-3; 5-4; 4-5; 3-6	4	4/36	4/10	$\frac{4}{36} \times \frac{4}{10} = \frac{2}{45}$
10	6-4; 5-5; 4-6	3	3/36	3/9	$\frac{3}{36} \times \frac{3}{9} = \frac{1}{36}$
11	6-5; 5-6	2	2/36		
12	6-6	1	1/36		

Table 5.13. The probability of a point and the probability of making it

The rules of the game of craps are the following: a player using two dice

☑ Wins if a 7 or 11 comes out on the first roll.
☒ Loses if 2, 3, or 12 comes out on the first roll.
☑ Wins if 4, 5, 6, 8, 9, or 10 comes out on the first roll, and the same sum comes out again before 7 does in succeeding throws of the dice.
☒ Loses if 4, 5, 6, 8, 9, or 10 comes out on the first roll, and 7 comes out before the sum first obtained comes out again in succeeding throws of the dice.

What is the probability of winning in the game of craps?

Rules of the game (in casino language):

On the first roll, called the "come out," the dice may "pass" or "don't pass," depending on the outcome.

☑ If the come out is 7 or 11, the dice "pass."
☒ If the come out is 2, 3, or 12, the dice "don't pass."

If the come out is 4, 5, 6, 8, 9, or 10, the shooter continues to roll the dice until either the "point" (i.e., the come-out number) or a 7 comes up.

☑ If the point comes up before a 7, the dice "pass."
☒ If the 7 comes up first, the dice "don't pass."

The object of the game from the bettor's point of view is simply to predict whether the dice will pass or not. The sample space of all possible points (sums of the face value), the combination that can produce a given point and the number of such combinations, as well as their corresponding probability are detailed in Table 11.2. The rules stipulated so far lead to the following win, loose, or wait for the disposition of the point.

The come out is 7 or 11:
$P(7) + P(11) = 6/36 + 2/36 = 8/36 =$ probability of winning on first roll.

The come out is 2, 3, or 12:
$P(2) + P(3) + P(12) = 1/36 + 2/36 + 1/36 = 4/36 =$ probability of loosing on first roll.

The come out is 4, 5, 6, 8, 9, or 10:
$P(4) + P(5) + P(6) + P(8) + P(9) + (10) = 3/36 + 4/36 + 5/36 + 5/36 + 4/36 + 3/36 = 24/36 =$ probability to be decided by continuous rolling until the cycle is broken in a pass or don't pass.

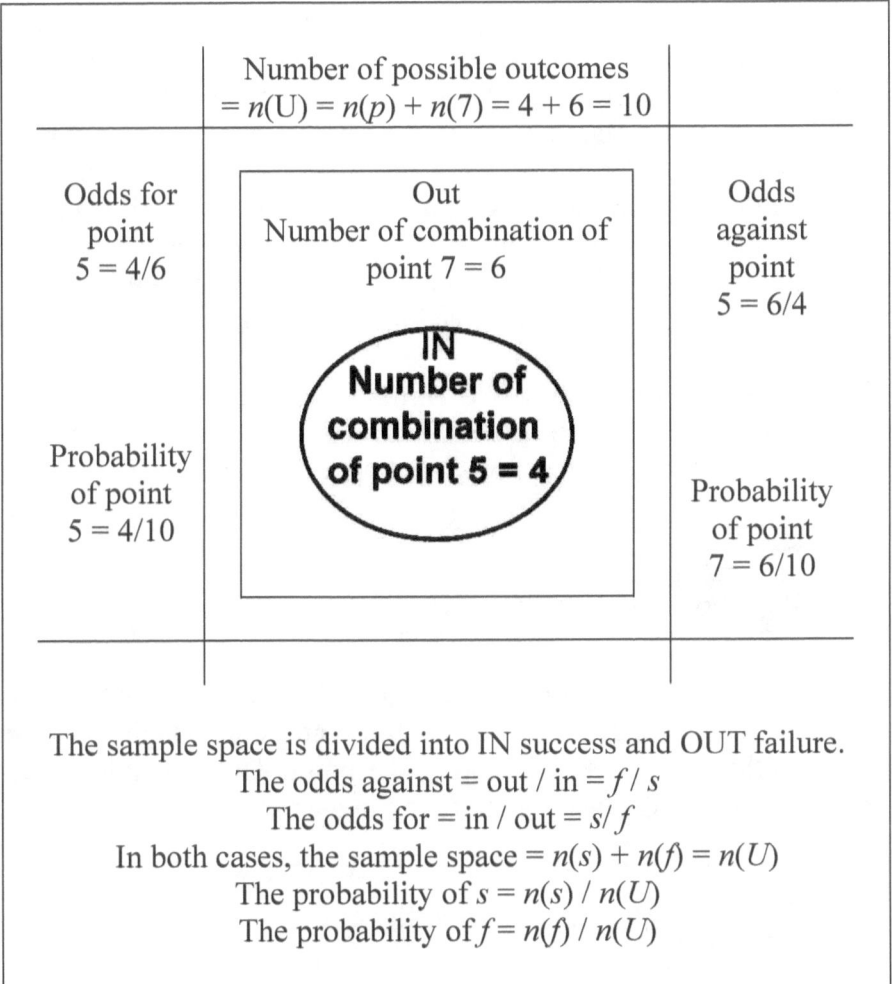

Number of possible outcomes
$= n(U) = n(p) + n(7) = 4 + 6 = 10$

Odds for point 5 = 4/6

Out
Number of combination of point 7 = 6

Odds against point 5 = 6/4

IN
Number of combination of point 5 = 4

Probability of point 5 = 4/10

Probability of point 7 = 6/10

The sample space is divided into IN success and OUT failure.
The odds against = out / in = f/s
The odds for = in / out = s/f
In both cases, the sample space = $n(s) + n(f) = n(U)$
The probability of $s = n(s) / n(U)$
The probability of $f = n(f) / n(U)$

Table 5.14. The odds for and against a point and the corresponding probability

Because the point is "made" only if it is rolled before a seven appears, the probability of "making" a point is the ratio of the probability of the point to the sum of the probabilities of 7 and the point under consideration. The sample space in this case includes both the number of unfavorable outcomes, 6 for the 7, and the number of favorable outcomes for any of the six numbers that make the other come out points. If the come out point is 4, then the sample space includes both the number of ways or combinations a 4 is rolled, namely, 3, and the number of ways or combinations a seven may be rolled, namely, 6. The probability of the point 4 is then the ratio of 3/3 + 6 or 3/9. For the point 5, the probability is similarly calculated to equal the ratio of number of ways the point itself appear to the total number of ways both 5 and 7 appear, which equals 4/4 + 6 = 4/10. Because the make number and the come-out number should match for the point to pass and because both numbers are independent, the probability of the come out and the probability of the make is equal to the probability of the come out multiplied by the probability of the make, as noted in Table 5.14.

The probability of passing by coming out on any one of the six points and then making the point is equal to the sum of the probabilities of passing (winning) through any point.

$$\frac{1}{36} + \frac{2}{45} + \frac{25}{396} + \frac{25}{396} + \frac{2}{45}\frac{1}{36} = \frac{134}{495}$$

The probability of winning in the game of craps must include the probability of rolling a 7 or 11 on the come out, which must be added to the probability of making the point. The probability that the dice will pass is given by the following sum.

$$\frac{8}{36} + \frac{134}{495} = \frac{244}{495} = 0.4929 = \text{probability of pass.}$$

The probability that the dice will fail to pass is then

$$1 - \frac{244}{495} = \frac{251}{495} = 0.5071.$$

The odds against a pass is then 251:244, just a hair less than even.

The New York Times: Opinionator
April 25, 2010
Chances Are
by Steven Strogatz

The right answer is 9 percent. *How can it be so low?*

Gigerenzer's point is that the analysis becomes almost transparent if we translate the original information from percentages and probabilities into natural frequencies:

Eight of every 1,000 women have breast cancer. Of these 8 women with breast cancer, 7 will have a positive mammogram. Of the remaining 992 women who don't have breast cancer, some 70 will still have a positive mammogram.

Because a total of 7 + 70 =77 women have positive mammogram, and only seven of them truly have breast cancer, the probability of having breast cancer given a positive mammogram is 7 of 77, which is 1 in 11, or about 9 percent.

End of the excerpted article.

Based on the data given above, results are tabulated in a 2 × 2 contingency table as follows:

	Ca Confirmed Disease Present D^+	Ca Excluded Disease Absent D^-	Row Total
Positive mammogram, T^+	7	70	$T^+ = 77$
Negative mammogram, T^-	1	922	$T^- = 923$
Column total	$D^+ = 8$	$D^- = 992$	1,000

Table 5.15. Contingency table based on data

Based on the data in Table 5.15, probability questions may be phrased as follows:

What is the probability of a positive or negative test (T^+ or T^-) (mammogram) given the presence or absence of disease (D^+ or D^-) (breast cancer)?

1. $P(T^+ | D^+) = \dfrac{7}{8} = 0.875$ = sensitivity $-$ Sn

2. $P(T^- | D^-) = \dfrac{922}{992} = 0.929$ = specificity $-$ Sp

3. $P(T^+ | D^-) = \dfrac{70}{992} = 070 = 1 - Sp$

4. $P(T^- | D^+) = \dfrac{1}{8} = 0.125 = 1 - Sn$

The second set of probability questions are phrased as follows:

What is the probably of actual disease D^+ or its absence D^- (breast cancer) given a positive or negative test result (T^+ or T^-)?

1. $P(D^+ | T^+) = \dfrac{7}{77} = 0.090 = 9\%$ = posterior probability = predictive value of a positive test.

2. $P(D^- | T^-) = \dfrac{922}{992} = 0.999 = 99\%$ = posterior probability = predictive value of a negative test.

3. $P(D^- | T^+) = \dfrac{70}{77} = 0.909 = 91\% = 1 - PVT[+]$.

4. $P(D^+ | T^-) = \dfrac{1}{923} = 0.001 = 1 - PVT[-]$.

Note that the predictive value of a positive test was the sole question posed by Dr. Gerd Gigerenzer.

Chapter 6

Dependence versus Independence

This chapter considers the dual relationship of events: first, as to their timing with respect to their sequential or simultaneous occurrence; and second, as to their interdependence with respect to their effect on the likelihood of each other.

With respect to timing, events can be categorized as either mutually exclusive and disjoint or mutually nonexclusive and conjoint. Within each of the two categories, the interrelationship between the events may be further classified as dependent or independent (Table 6.1).

6.1 Mutually Exclusive Case

In the mutually exclusive case, events A and B are disjoint in that they could not occur concurrently because the given occurrence of B precludes the occurrence of A. Furthermore, the sets do not overlap, that is, they did not intersect; they share no element in common, which translates the probability of the intersection to be 0, denoting that the two events are disjoint nonintersecting (Table 6.1, 1a).

As noted in Table 6.1 (1b), two mutually exclusive events cannot be independent because mutual exclusiveness requires the product to be zero, as dictated by the dependence of one on the other. Because independence rules out any necessary relation between the two events that reduces the probability of the excluded event to zero and because independence may assign any positive probability to any one of the two events, it is obvious that independence and mutual exclusiveness are contradiction in terms. Because by definition, the occurrence of one event precludes the other event from occurring.

$$P(A \cap B) = P(A) \times (B) \neq P(\emptyset) \neq 0.$$

Similarly, as noted in Table 6.1 (1a), two events are said to be disjoint if the outcome of the experiment is exclusively derived from either one of the two nonoverlapping sets that define the outcomes of the two events. Thus, an outcome derived from one of the sets automatically rules out its occurrence from the other set, confirming the dependence of either event on the other. As in the case of the complements, if either of the two events occurs, the other cannot, implying that the positive probability associated with the occurring event automatically reduces the probability of the nonoccurring event to zero. In this sense, the two events are mutually exclusive if the product of their respective probabilities is zero.

$$P(A \cap B) = P(A) \times P(B) = P(\emptyset) = 0.$$

Therefore, either $P(A) = 0$ or $P(B) = 0$, which in fact contradicts the assumption of nonzero probability and thus confirms that A and B are disjoint, nonoverlapping, and share no elements in common.

Given the separate probability of two mutually exclusive events A and B, the probability of their union, however, projects an element of simplicity unique to disjoint sets.

In the case of disjoint sets, and in the absence of an intersecting subset, the probability of their union is simply reduced to the sum of their individual probabilities (Table 6.1, 3a).

Conversely, an event is said not to occur if the actual outcome lies outside the subset that defines the event, although still within the same sample space. Consequently, if the event does not occur, its complement does occur, which by necessity includes all the elements within the same sample space, but outside the particular subset of the event in question. Obviously, the event and its complement are disjoint or mutually exclusive because they cannot possibly occur concurrently.

Thus, the union of the event and its mutually exclusive complement accounts for the total or universal sample space, and the sum of their probabilities adds up to 1 (Table 6.1, 3a).

$$P(A \cup \overline{A}) = P(A) + P(\overline{A}) = 1 = P(\text{sample space}).$$

6.2 Mutually Nonexclusive Case

In the mutually nonexclusive case, two events A and B are said to be conjoint or synchronous, if one or the other of the two events occurs such that the outcome of either A or B lies within their union ($A \cup B$). On the other hand, when both A and B occur, one of the elementary events they have in common must occur so that the actual outcome common to both lies within, their intersection ($A \cap B$).

As noted in Table 6.1 (4a), the general formula for the union of two intersecting sets must make allowance for the double inclusion of the intersecting subset by subtracting it from the proposed union.

$$P(A \cup B) = P(A) + P(B) - P(A \cap B).$$

If only $P(A)$ and $P(B)$ are known, there is no simple general formula for finding the probability of $A \cap B$. However, if A and B are independent, that is, the occurrence of one has no effect on the likelihood of the other so that the value of $P(A)$ is the same whether or not we know that the actual outcome of the experiment lies in B, then A and B are independent events. Stated otherwise, in the case of concurrent events, independence by definition implies the negation or denial of the tie up between the events A and B as expressed by the conditional probability notation, so that

$P(A|B) = P(A)$ And $P(B|A) = P(B)$ (Table 6.1, 5b).

And in such a case, the probability of the intersection becomes the product of the respective probabilities of A and B (Table 6.1, 6b).

$P(A \cap B) = P(A \mid B) \times P(A) \Rightarrow\Rightarrow P(A \cap B) = P(A) \times P(B).$
$P(B \cap A) = P(B \mid A) \times P(A) \Rightarrow\Rightarrow P(A \cap B) = P(A) \times P(B).$

This unique simplification is possible if the independence of the two events is proven to be the case.

The concept of independence is best illustrated by reference to a modified Venn diagram of A and B (Figure 6.1), where the precondition for independence, $P(A|B) = P(A)$, could be quantitatively and graphically evaluated

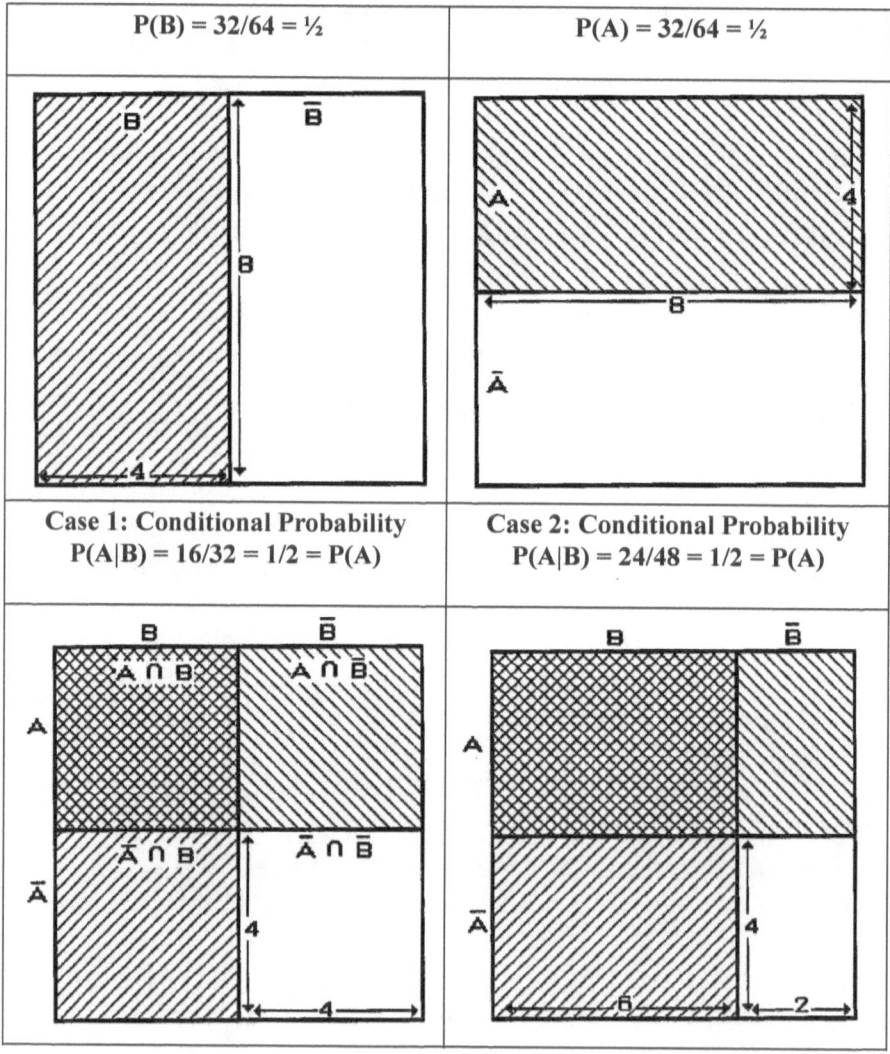

Figure 6.1. Conditional probability of independent events

Given the basic definition of conditional probability,

$$P(A \mid B) = \frac{P(A \cap B)}{P(B)}.$$

In the first case, the graphic answer as to how much of A is in B is obviously the area of intersection as a fraction of the B area, both calculated as noted previously in terms of the universal set. In a similar fashion, the probability of B refers to the area occupied by B as a fraction of the total area. The ratio of the intersection to that of the B area now becomes the area shared by A and B as fraction of B area alone.

$$P(A \mid B) = \frac{\dfrac{16}{64}}{\dfrac{32}{64}} = \frac{16}{32} = \frac{1}{2} = P(A).$$

Note that because both terms share the same denominator, that is, both are ratios of the universal set, the common denominator cancels out in the process so that the result gives the proportion of the intersection as a fraction of the B area.

In the second case (Figure 6.1), B now occupies 48/64 or 3/4 of the total area. The intersection is now 24/64 or 3/8 of the total area (instead of the original 1/4 of case 1). The ratio, however, remains essentially unchanged so that 24/48 = 1/2. In other words, one-half the area of B is shared by A so that the area shared by A and B is still the same fraction of the absolute B area.

$$P(A \mid B) = \frac{\dfrac{24}{64}}{\dfrac{48}{64}} = \frac{24}{48} = \frac{1}{2} = P(A).$$

From cases 1 and 2, it is graphically and numerically evident that the probability of A remained unchanged irrespective of the area of B because in both cases

$$P(A|B) = P(A) = 1/2.$$

A more direct approach to prove independence is based on the definition noted earlier that A and B are independent, if and only if

$$P(A \cap B) = P(A) \times P(A) \times P(B).$$

Rapid verification of the condition for independence is readily achieved by the construction of a 2×2 matrix (Table 6.2).

		Event B		Row Sums
		B	B'	
Event A	A	$P(A \cap B)$	$P(A \cap B')$	$P(A \cap B) + P(A \cap B') = P(A)$
	A'	$P(A' \cap B)$	$P(A' \cap B')$	$P(A' \cap B) + P(A' \cap B') = P(A')$
Column sums		$P(A \cap B) +$ $P(A' \cap B)$	$P(A \cap B') +$ $P(A' \cap B')$	Total = 1
		$=P(B)$	$=P(B')$	

Table 6.2. Verification of the condition for independence
using a 2×2 array

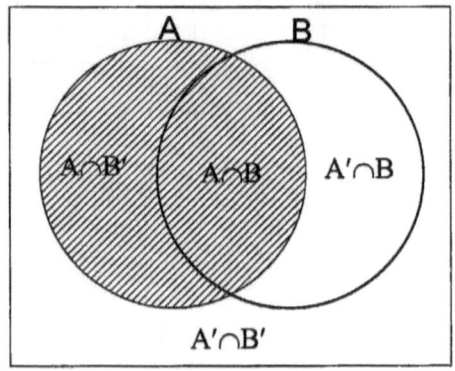

Figure 6.2

$$P(A \mid B) = \frac{P(A \cap B)}{P(B)} = \frac{P(\text{Cell})}{P(\text{Column})}.$$

$P(A \cap B) = P(A|B) \bullet P(B) \Rightarrow P(A \cap B) =$
$P(A) \bullet P(B) = P(\text{row}) \times P(\text{column})$

$$P(B \mid A) = \frac{P(A \cap B)}{P(A)} = \frac{P(\text{cell})}{P(\text{row})}.$$

$P(A \cap B) = P(B|A) \bullet P(A) \Rightarrow P(A \cap B) =$
$P(B) \bullet P(A) = P(\text{column}) \times P(\text{row})$

It becomes readily apparent that if $P(A \cap B)$ is indeed equal to $P(A)$ $\bullet$ $P(B)$, then the numerical value in any one cell of the four cells must actually be the product of the corresponding row and column.

If, as noted in Table 6.3, this is actually the case, then A and B are independent.

		Event B		
		B	B'	
Event	A	$1/2 \times 1/2 = 1/4$	$1/2 \times 1/2 = 1/4$	$1/4 + 1/4 = P(A) = 1/2$
	A'	$1/2 \times 1/2 = 1/4$	$1/2 \times 1/2 = 1/4$	$1/4 + 1/4 = P(A') = 1/2$
		$1/4 + 1/4 =$ $P(B) = 1/2$	$1/4 + 1/4 =$ $P(B') = 1/2$	Total = 1

Table 6.3. Confirmation of independence using the data in a 2 × 2 array

The product function in case of independence is the product of the two fractions of the probability of A and B. Note that ½ of ½ = ¼: ½ × ½ = ¼. The fraction of a fraction is the product of the two fractions, so that one-half of one-half equals one-quarter (an apple cut in half, then half of the half is a quarter of apple).

The third case is shown in Figure 6.3.

Conditional Probability $P(A\|B) = 24/32 = 6/8$ $P(A) = 24/64 + 16/64 = 40/64 = 5/8$	Conditional Probability Case 1: Alternative notation and symbols for defining the joint probabilities
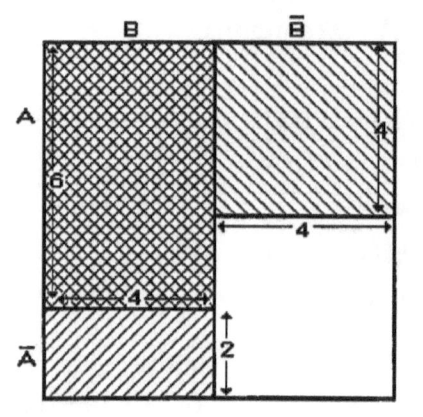 Figure 6.3. Conditional probability of dependent events	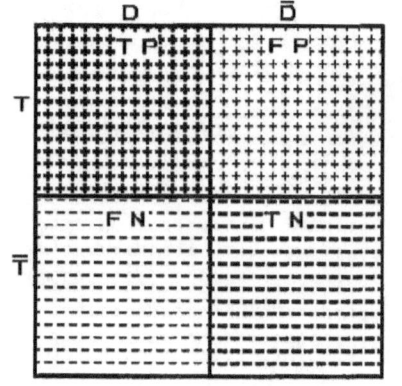 Figure 6.1a. Conditional probability of independent events in alternative notation

$$P(A|B) = \frac{\dfrac{24}{64}}{\dfrac{32}{64}} = \frac{24}{32} = \frac{6}{8}$$

$$P(A) = \frac{24}{64} + \frac{16}{64} = \frac{40}{64} = \frac{5}{8}$$

In this case, $P(A|B) \neq P(A)$. Note that the Venn diagram is divided by more than two intersecting lines such that the area of intersection and the A area are not identical. When the data are entered in the 2 × 2 matrix, application of the product rule proves that the values in the individual cells do not equal the product of the corresponding row and column (Table 6.4).

		Event *B*		Row sums
		B	*B'*	
Event *A*	*A*	$1/2 \times 3/4 = 3/8$	$1/2 \times 1/2 = 2/8$	$3/8 + 2/8 = P(A) = 5/8$
	A'	$1/2 \times 1/4 = 1/8$	$1/2 \times 1/2 = 2/8$	$1/8 + 2/8 = P(A') = 3/8$
Column sums		$3/8 + 1/8 = P(B)$ $= 1/2$	$2/8 + 2/8 = P(B')$ $= 1/2$	

Table 6.4. Verification of dependence using
the data from case 3 of Figure 6.1

In the clinical example cited previously, the data are transcribed
in the probability format. Note specifically that in every case, the
product $P(A) \bullet P(B)$ does not equal the cell probability in every
instance. The relationship between the given test and the disease in
question is certainly not independent of each other (Table 6.5).

	Ca Confirmed Disease Present	Ca Excluded Disease Absent	*P* (row)
	D^+	D^-	
T^+	$P(T^+ \cap D^+) = 0.24$ $(P(T^+) \bullet P(D^+) = 0.38 \times 0.3 = 0.114$	$P(T^+ \cap D^-) = 0.14$ $P(T^+) \bullet P(D^-) = 0.38 \times 0.7 = 0.266$	$P(T^+)$ $=$ 0.38
T^-	$P(T^- \cap D^+) = 0.06$ $(P(T^-) \bullet P(D^+) = 0.62 \times 0.3 = 0.186$	$P(T^- \cap D^-) = 0.56$ $(P(T^-) \bullet P(D^-) = 0.62 \times 0.7 = 0.434$	$P(T^-)$ $=$ 0.62
P (column)	$P(D^+) = 0.3$	$P(D^-) = 0.7$	1

Table 6.5. Verification of dependence using the clinical data

Mutually exclusive $A \cap B = \varnothing$ Disjoint (or) asynchronous	Dependent Events	Independent Events
	Events A and B cannot occur simultaneously. If A occurs, then B does not occur, and vice versa. Therefore, disjoint events are automatically dependent because the occurrence of one event provides information about the occurrence of the other. Thus, the occurrence of one event affects the probability of the occurrence of the other event.	Independence means that knowledge of one event does not provide knowledge of the other event. In fact, if A and B are two independent events, then they cannot be mutually exclusive. Thus, the occurrence of one event does not affect the probability of the occurrence of the other event. The probability of A is not affected by (not conditional upon) the occurrence of the second event B.
	1a. Intersection (conjunction)	**1b. Intersection (conjunction)**
	$\boxed{P(A \cap B) = P(A) \times P(B) = P(\varnothing) = 0}$ Then A and B are disjoint (non-overlapping)	If A and B are independent, $\boxed{P(A \cap B) = P(A) \times P(B) \neq P(\varnothing) \neq 0,}$ then $(A \cap B) \neq \varnothing$ Therefore, A and B are not mutually exclusive
	2a. Conditional	**2b. Conditional**
	$P(A|B) \neq P(A)$ or $P(B\}A) \neq P(B)$ $P(A|B) = 0$ Occurrence of B, precludes A from occurring	Probability A is conditional upon the occurrence of B The two events cannot be independent
	3a. Union (disjunction)	**3b. Union (disjunction)**
	$P(\varnothing)=0$ $P(A \cup B) = P(A) + P(B) - P(A \cap B)$ $\boxed{P(A \cup B) = P(A) + P(B)}$ $P(A \cup \overline{A}) = P(A) + P(\overline{A}) = 1$	Independent events are never mutually exclusive
Mutually nonexclusive $A \cap B \neq \varnothing$ Conjoint (and) synchronous	**4a. Union (disjunction)**	**4b. Union (disjunction)**
	$\boxed{P(A \cup B) = P(A) + P(B) - P(A \cap B)}$ $\Rightarrow\Rightarrow\Rightarrow$	$P(A \cup B) = P(A) + P(B) - P(A) \times P(B)$ $P(\overline{A \cap B}) = P(\overline{A}) \times P(\overline{B})$
	5a. Conditional	**5b. Conditional**
	$\boxed{P(A \mid B) = \dfrac{P(A \cap B)}{P(B)}}$ $\Rightarrow\Rightarrow\Rightarrow$ $\boxed{P(B \mid A) = \dfrac{P(A \cap B)}{P(A)}}$ $\Rightarrow\Rightarrow\Rightarrow$	$\boxed{P(A \mid B) = \dfrac{P(A) \times P(B)}{P(B)} = P(A)}$ $\boxed{P(B \mid A) = \dfrac{P(B) \times P(A)}{P(A)} = P(B)}$
	6a. Intersection (conjunction)	**6b. Intersection (conjunction)**
	$P(A \cap B) = P(B) \times P(A \mid B)$ $\Rightarrow\Rightarrow\Rightarrow$ $P(A \cap B) = P(B) \times P(B \mid A)$ $\Rightarrow\Rightarrow\Rightarrow$	$P(A \cap B) = P(B) \times P(A)$ $P(B \cap A) = P(A) \times P(B)$

Table 6.1. Relationship between the timing of events and their subsequent independence

The mutually exclusive or disjoint events are as follows:

1. They cannot happen at the same time.
2. Sets do not overlap: no intersection.
3. They have no point in common.
4. The intersection of two mutually exclusive sets = empty set 1a, which contradicts the assumption of nonzero probability and thus confirms that A and B are disjoint and nonoverlapping (Table 6.1, 1b).
5. Nonoverlapping sets are not independent because they share no point in common (Table 6.1, 3b).
6. All complementary events are mutually exclusive, so the A and A' partitions the SS into two mutually exclusive and exhaustive subsets (Table 6.1, 3a).

Events A and B are independent if and only if

1. There is simultaneous membership in two sets.
2. Of A and B are subsets of an SS, then A and B is their intersection.
3. A and B contain those sample points that belong to both.
4. If A and B are independent then.
5. The product function in case of independence is the product of the two fractions of the probability of A and B.

Note that ½ of ½ = ¼: ½ × ½ = ¼ The fraction of a fraction is the product of the two fractions.

So that one-half of one-half equals one-quarter (an apple cut in half, then half of the half is a quarter of apple).

If the two events are independent, then their simultaneous membership in the shared SS = intersection is a fraction of a fraction of the SS, which translates into a fraction × fraction.

6. Because it implies that both $P(A)$ and $P(B)$ have nonzero probabilities, therefore they must have a point in common.

Within each of the two categories, the interrelationship between the events may be classified as dependent and independent (Table 6.1).

In the Mex case the sets do not overlap, that is, they did not intersect. They share no element in common; thus, $\cap B = \emptyset$, which translates the probability of the intersection to 0, denoting that the two events are disjoint nonintersecting.

To round off the other possibility, note the case of the second Mex. In the case of where the events are conjoint, the classification into dependent and independent assumes a particular relevance.

Chapter 7

Clinical versus Diagnostic Conditional Probability

In the preceding chapter, the concept of conditional probability was approached via the simple framework of a 2 × 2 matrix. In this chapter, and all the discussion to follow, the same concept will be amplified to serve as the infrastructure on which all further discussion will be based. The component cells of the matrix will be standardized and predefined in terms of probability while its relationship to the corresponding set will be graphically depicted by a Venn diagram.

Table 7.1 is the prototype table under discussion. Events A and B are now replaced by any one test and any given disease. In this setting, the sample space for D (disease) is partitioned between those that carry the disease, D^+ (disease present), and those proven free from the disease, D^- (disease absent), such that the total number of individuals in the sample space under consideration, so-called sample universe $n(U)$, is the sum of the two mutually exclusive and exhaustive events, $n(D^+)$ and $n(D^-)$. This is graphically depicted in Figure 7.1, where a sample universe of 1,000 individuals is considered, of which D^+ comprise 300 individuals. Note that the relative areas of D^+ and its complement D^- are drawn to be quantitatively representative such that the D^+ circle area is actually 0.3 of the U circle area.

In probabilistic terms, the numerical data are readily converted into probability fractions of the sample universe, which in graphic terms is the equivalent of the area percentage occupied by the D^+ circle, so that $P(D^+) = n(D^+)/n(U) = 300/1,000 = 30$ percent $= 0.3$.

The division of the sample universe for disease into D^+ and D^- happens to define a major epidemiological concept normally stated as follows:

$$\text{Prevalence} = \frac{\text{Number of persons with a disease}}{\text{Total number of individuals (population)}} @ t_0 (\text{Point in time})$$

The group in this case is our sample universe. This definition is to be differentiated from the concept of Incidence normally defined as follows:

$$\text{Incidence} = \frac{\text{Number of persons developing a disease}}{\text{Total number of individuals at risk of developing the disease}} \text{ per unit of time.}$$

Prevalence thus reflects an instantaneous evaluation of an existing situation at a given point in time. In clinical terms, one might say that the prevalence of coronary artery disease (CAD) at a cardiac clinic in men older than 50 years is estimated to be 30 percent of the total number of patients registered at the clinic, whereas the incidence of myocardial infarction (MI) in the same group is roughly less than 1 percent per year.

The concept of prevalence and prior probability may appear on casual examination to be unrelated. On closer reflection, the appraisal of prevalence in a given sample, either statistically or subjectively perceived, is in fact a probabilistic statement of the existing situation at a point in time.

Similarly, the T event (test) partitions the same sample universe into a T^+ (positive or abnormal test) and its complement T^- (negative or normal test) (Figure 7.2), such that out of the 1,000 individuals tested, 380 were found to be positive, whereas the balance of 620 individuals tested negative. Note that the relative areas of T^+ and its complement T^- are drawn to be quantitatively representative with the T^+ circle area occupying 0.38 of the U circle area.

The concurrence of the two events and the subsequent partition of the sample universe into four mutually exclusive and exhaustive subsets is detailed Table 7.1 and graphically illustrated in Figure 7.3, where each of the disjoint areas and their corresponding cubicles in the 2 × 2 table reflect their actual quantitative distribution through corresponding area allocation or alternatively their joint probabilities.

For each cell, the joint probability is the product of a predetermined conditional probability and the probability assigned to the prevalence of disease for the case under consideration:

$$\underset{\text{Total probability}}{P(T^+ \cap D^+)} = \underset{\text{Conditional probability}}{P(T^+ \mid D^+)} \times \underset{\text{Prior probability}}{P(D^+)}$$

$$\underset{\substack{\text{Experimentally determined} \\ \text{Sensitivity}}}{P(T^+ \mid D^+)} = \frac{P(T^+ \cap D^-)}{\underset{\text{Prevalence}}{P(D^+)}}$$

Recall what is being referred to here as the joint probability is the equivalent of the intersection area shared between two overlapping events as detailed in the chapter on conditional probability (chapter 5). The numerical value associated with the magnitude of the intersection (the joint probability) can only be obtained if the other two variables of the equation are available.

The conditional probability associated with each of the four cells is the actual clinically determined probability of a positive or negative test, given the presence or absence of a disease. In the first quadrant, $P(T^+|D^+)$ represents the conditional probability of a positive test, given the fact that the patient is known to have the disease. It is in fact a question concerning the reliability and sensitivity of the test in detecting the presence of disease.

On the opposite side, bottom right quadrant, the clinical probability $P(T^-|D^-)$ represents the conditional probability of a negative test, given the fact that the patient is known to be free of the disease. It is in fact a query as to how reliable and specific is the test in confirming the absence of disease.

The other conditional probabilities are what might be described as the error probabilities. In the top right quadrant, $P(T^+|D^-)$ is the probability of obtaining a positive test result in the absence of disease. In the bottom left quadrant, the question is the flip side of the former, where $(PT^-|D^+)$ addresses the probability of a negative test result in the presence of confirmed diagnosis.

The two conditional probabilities and their counterpart the error probabilities are simply the controlled evaluation derived from clinical trials as to how reliable is a given test as marker of a given disease. These probabilities are in effect the clinical parameters of the test in question.

Such being the case, the two clinical conditional probabilities, $P(T^+|D^+)$ and $P(T^-|D^-)$, are usually referred to by the more descriptive and informative terms of sensitivity and specificity.

Remember that the sensitivity (and the specificity) of the test is empirically derived based on data experimentally determined. From the trial results, the joint probability (i.e., How many D^+ tested positive? $= P(D^+ \cap T^+)$) is then divided by the $P(D^+)$ of the trial (i.e., the total number of independently proven patients that tested both positive and negative, D^+), to arrive at the desired conditional probability $p(T^+|D^+)$/ sensitivity, unique to the particular test being evaluated.

$$\underset{\substack{\text{Under investigation}\\ P(T^+|D^+)\\ \text{Sensitivity}}}{} = \frac{\overset{\text{Experimentally determined}}{P(T^+ \cap D^+)}}{\underset{\text{Experimentally determined}}{P(D^+)}}.$$

Experimentally, the two basic conditional probabilities of sensitivity and specificity are the ratios of the corresponding joint probability to the marginal probability, which under the experimental conditions is the total number of D^+ and D^- patients that tested both positive and negative, which in this case is the sum of the joint probabilities of the respective column (Table 7.1, bottom two rows).

Thus, to determine the sensitivity of a particular test, both the joint probability and the probability of the disease in the trial population are experimentally determined a priori in order to evaluate the desired sensitivity of the test.

The $P(D^+)$, the prior probability, includes subsets of patients that tested both positive and negative but were independently proven to harbor the disease. Accordingly, D^+ value is the sum of the two areas within the D^+ circle, that is, TP + FN.

Graphically, $P(T^+|D^+)$ or sensitivity represents the ratio of the intersection area ($T^+ \cap D^+$), that is, the TP subset to the total area occupied by the D^+ circle. $P(T^- \mid D^-)$ or specificity is the ratio of the outer ring area encircling both T and D circles ($T^- \cap D^-$), that is, the TN subset to the total D^- area, namely, the area outside the D^+ circle, which is the complement of D^+ (Figures 7.1 and 7.3).

This circuitous definition of joint probability and conditional probability is unavoidable, considering that sensitivity and specificity for any particular test are clinically derived under a controlled condition, which determines their corresponding magnitude. In routine clinical situations, the given magnitudes of sensitivity and specificity together with the prevalence are used to calculate the joint probabilities in the individual case.

Given the three variables of sensitivity, specificity, and prevalence, the relevant question that the clinician needs to answer is, however, a unique conditional probability, which is in turn a function of the three other variables, namely, the all important posterior or diagnostic probability.

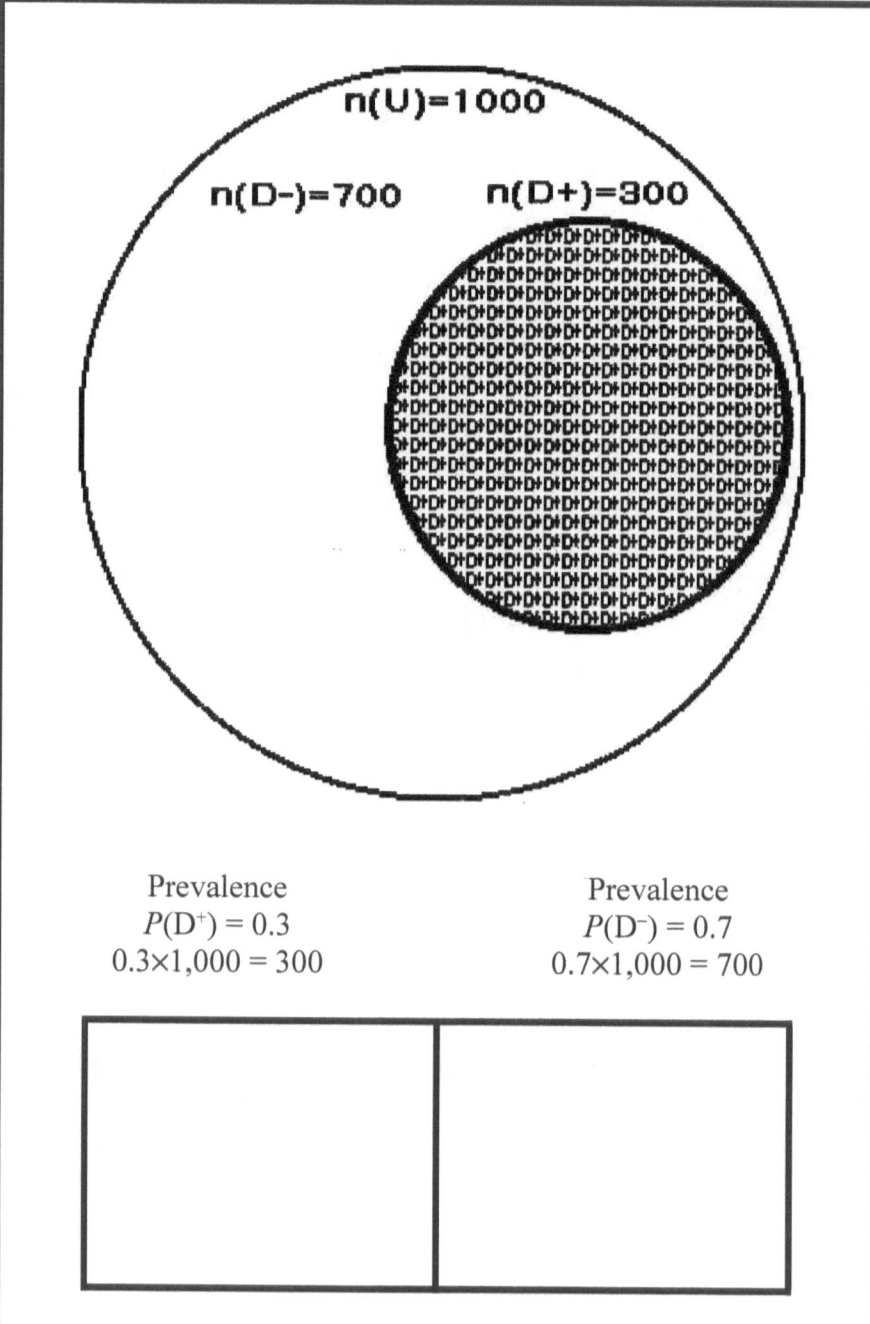

Figure 7.1. Venn diagram of the partition of the sample universe into two mutually exclusive and exhaustive subsets

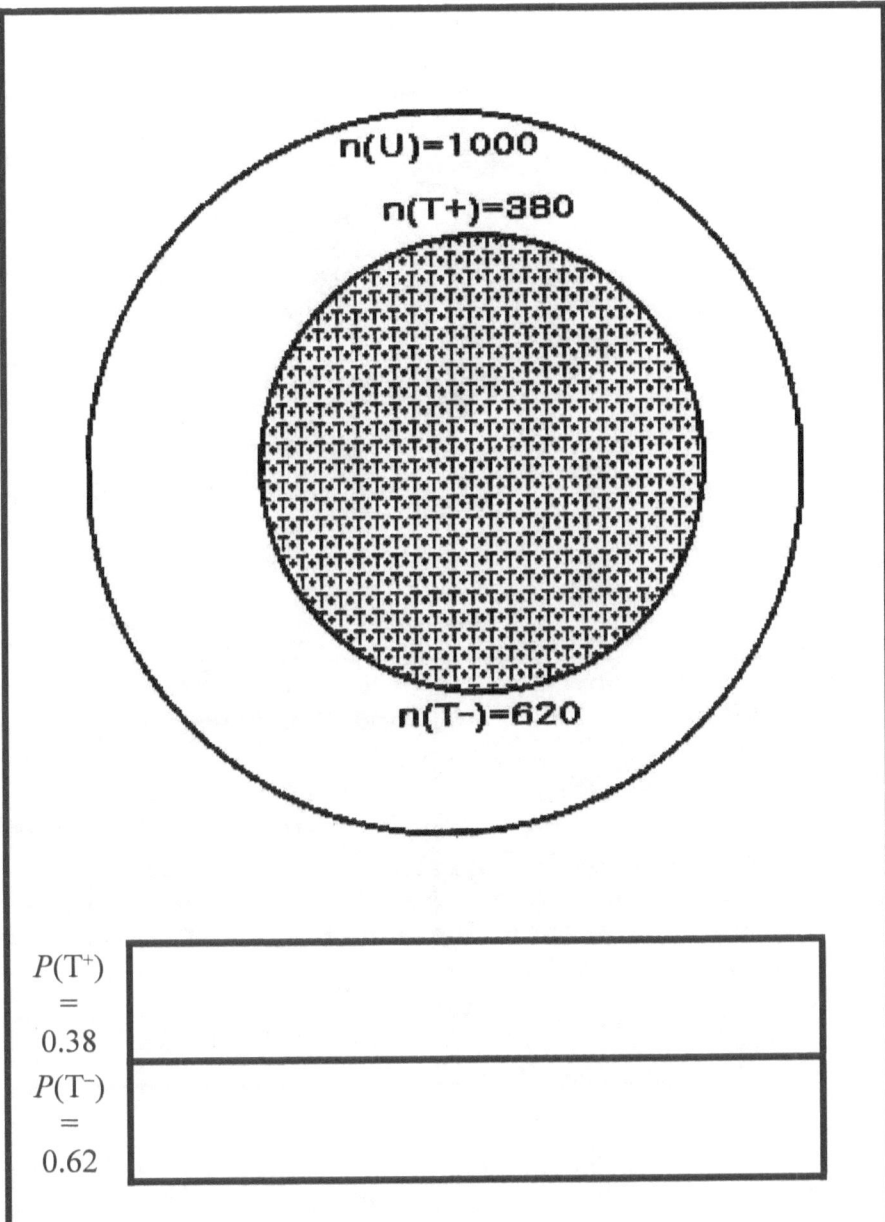

Figure 7.2. Venn diagram of the partition of the sample universe into a mutually exclusive and exhaustive subsets

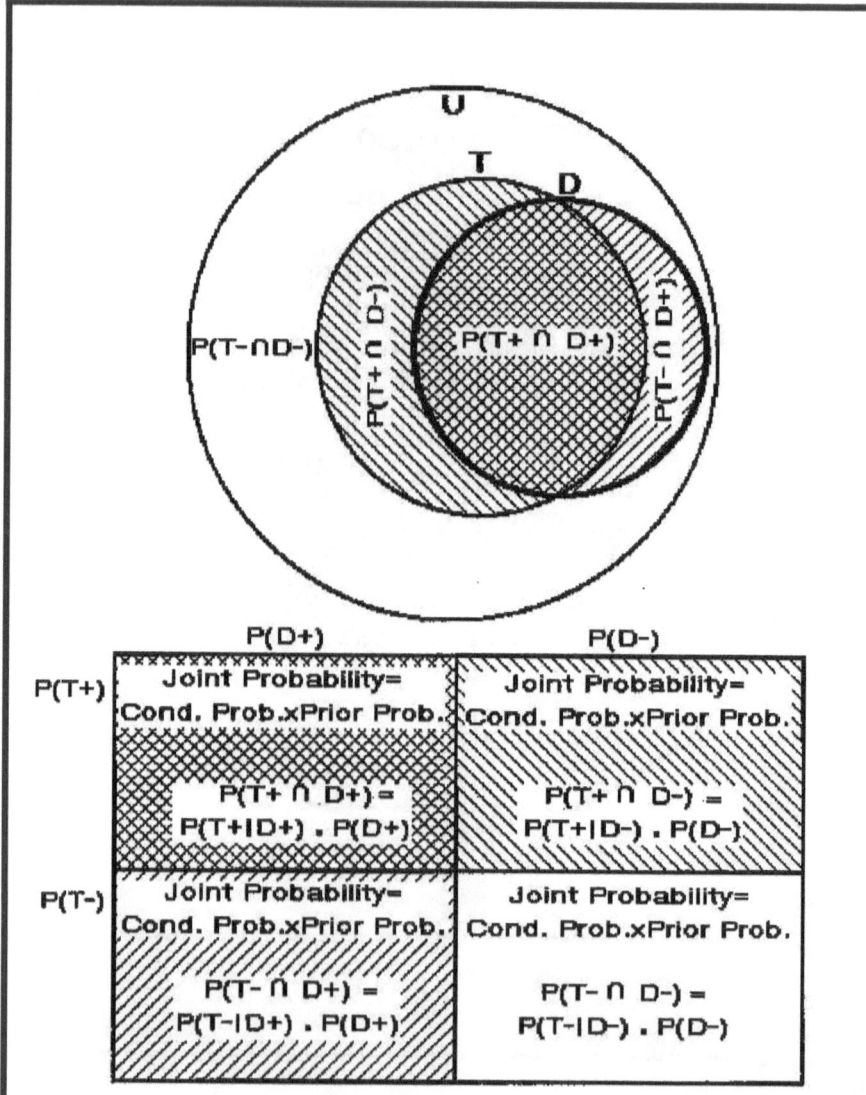

Figure 7.3. Venn diagram of the correspondence between the probabilities of the Venn subsets and the cells of the 2 × 2 table

$P(D^+ | T^+)$, the probability of disease given a positive test, is exactly the inverse of the $P(T^+ | D^+)$, the probability of a positive test given the presence of disease, that is, the sensitivity of the test.

In this context, the clinician faced with a positive or negative test result may opt to accept the result as final or elect to proceed into a more definitive workup in order to confirm or rule out the disease in question irrespective of the rest result.

To address the critical diagnostic decision, the conditional probability, $P(D^+|+ | T^+)$, that is, the degree of certainty in confirming the diagnosis of having the disease on the strength of a reported positive test, or $P(D^- | T^-)$, the certainty of ruling out the disease once a negative test result is reported, needs to be answered in specific quantitative terms.

The other two conditional probabilities, as in the case of the clinical conditional probabilities, involve the diagnostic error incurred in each decision that will permit the diagnosis to be entertained despite a negative test $(PD^+|P(D^+ | T^-)$ or to be ruled out despite a positive test $P(D^-|T^+)$.

The diagnostic probabilities are best designated as the posterior or revised probabilities. This term is in effect the classical terminology used in mathematical parlance. It is in a sense more appropriate than diagnostic probability because it is assigned on the basis of a given prior probability, $P(D^+)$.

Here again we are dealing with a ratio, but once the cells in the 2 × 2 matrix are filled out through our knowledge of the prevalence $P(D^+)$ and the sensitivity/specificity of the test, the numerator and the denominator are easily determined from the clinical data (Table 7.1).

$$
\underset{\text{Posterior drobability}}{\underset{\text{To be determined}}{P(T^+ | D^+)}} = \frac{\overset{\text{Clinically derived}}{P(T^+ \cap D^+)}}{\underset{\text{Clinically determined}}{P(D^+)}}
$$

The table may look somewhat unnecessarily complicated; however, if one concentrates on a single cell (e.g., Upper left) and compare the Venn areas with the cell, the cross relationship becomes obvious.

Each posterior conditional probability is defined as the ratio of the corresponding joint probability to the marginal probability of the respective row which in effect is the sum of the joint probabilities for that row, which in turn is the probability assigned to the total number of positive test results, T^+.

Graphically, $P(D^+|T^+)$ or the posterior probability of disease given a positive test result represents the ratio of the intersection area $(T^+ \cap D^+)$ to the total area occupied by T^+. Similarly, $P(D^-|T^-)$ or the posterior probability of freedom from the disease, given the a negative test result, is the ratio of the outer ring area encircling both T and D $(T^- \cap D^-)$ to the ring area of T^-, which is the complement of T^+ (Figures 7.3. and 7.4).

To recapitulate, the posterior probability $P(D^+|T^+) = \dfrac{P(T^+ \cap D^+)}{P(T^+)}$ is simply a shorthand expression for determining how much of D^+ is in the reduced sample space of T^+. The answer is the intersection area $(T^+ \cap D^+)$ as a fraction of the T^+ area, which numerically is equal to the ratio of the number in the top left cell to the marginal number T^+, which is the sum of the two numbers in the adjoining cells.

This simplified version is not comprehensive enough to accommodate the conditional probabilities associated with each of the four cells.

Note, however, that the multiplication format of the conditional probability has been entered in each of the cells. For the top left cell, the expression is

$$P(T^+ \cap D^+) = P(T^+|D^+) \times P(D^+).$$

For the top right cell, the expression is

$$P(T^+ \cap D^-) = P(T^+|D^-) \times P(D^+).$$

Substituting for the intersection, $P(T^+ \cap D^+)$, in the posterior probability equation yields the simplest formulation of the diagnostic conditional probability expressed in terms of three variables:

1. The clinical probability of positive test given the certainty of disease (sensitivity)
2. The prior probability of disease or its prevalence in the universe under consideration (prior probability or prevalence)
3. The probability of a positive test, $P(T^+)$

$$P(D^+|T^+) = \frac{P(T^+ \cap D^+)}{P(T^+)} = \frac{P(T^+|D^+) \bullet P(D^+)}{P(T^+)} = P(T^+|D^+) \times \frac{P(D^+)}{P(T^+)}.$$

Substituting for $P(T^+)$ in the above-noted abbreviated formula for posterior probability yields the following expanded version for positive T. Note that the probability of T^+ is in effect the sum of its probability across the top two cells of the 2×2 array.

$$P(D^+|T^+) = \frac{P(T^+ \cap D^+)}{P(T^+)} = \frac{P(T^+|D^+) \bullet P(D^+)}{P(T^+|D^+) \bullet P(D^+) + P(T^+|D^-) \bullet P(D^-)}.$$

Similarly, the expanded version for negative T is

$$P(D^-|T^-) = \frac{P(T^- \cap D^-)}{P(T^-)} = \frac{P(T^-|D^-) \bullet P(D^-)}{P(T^-|D^+) \bullet P(D^+) + P(T^-|D^-) \bullet P(D^-)}.$$

The expanded format is essentially a restatement of what has already been said in terms of the conditional probabilities involved. This simple manipulation, however, yields the classical Bayes' formulation of inverse or posterior probability. Note that in each of the above formulae, the prior probabilities, $P(D^+)$ and $P(D^-)$, are factors in the numerator.

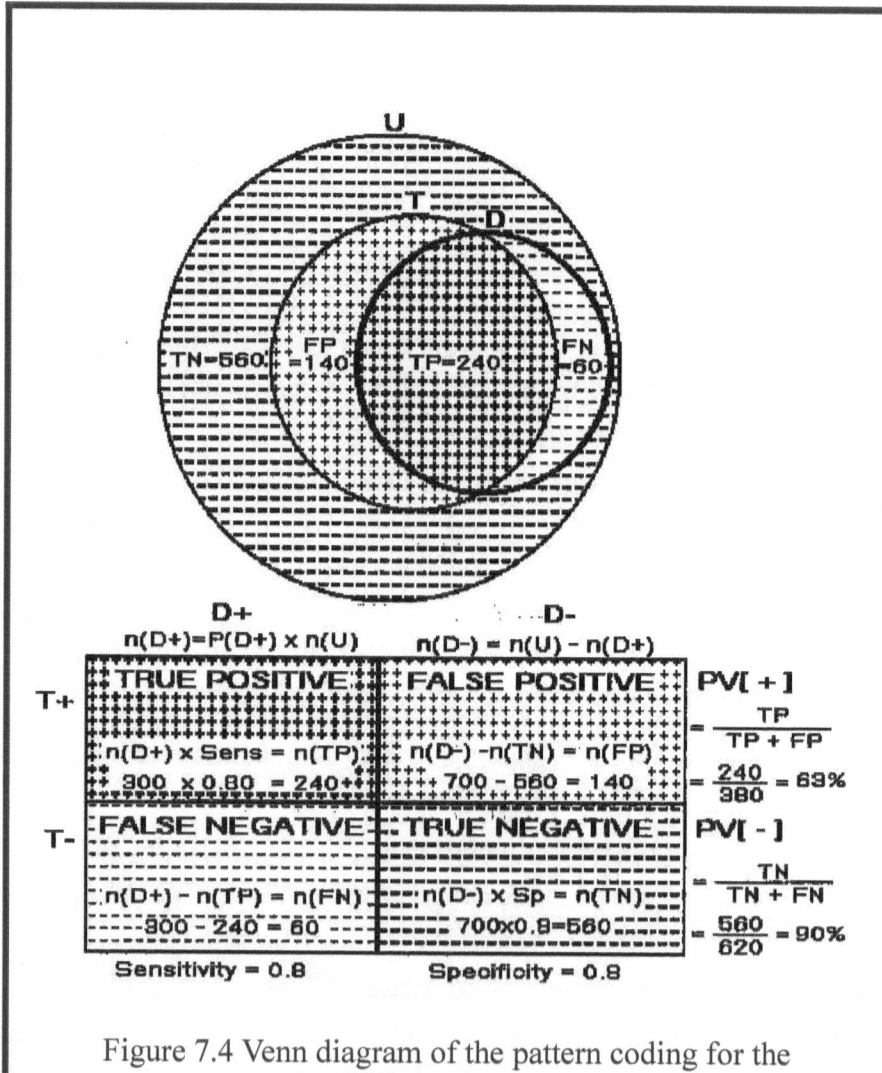

Figure 7.4 Venn diagram of the pattern coding for the identification of clinical subsets

The above presentation is an attempt to illustrate the theoretical underpinning of the conditional probabilities both graphically and mathematically. However, the terminology and the set notation used make such a presentation ineffective as a practical tool for routine application.

Recall that the partitions of the sample space were previously designated as subsets of the sample space using set notation to identify the individual subset. The same notation is retained in the labeling of the four main cells in previous tables.

In terms of the joint probabilities, the four areas may be appropriately renamed to reflect the actual numerical value of the subset rather than its joint probability expressed as a fraction.

$P(T^+ \cap D^+) \Rightarrow$ True positive (TP)
$P(T^+ \cap D^-) \Rightarrow$ False positive (FP)
$P(T^- \cap D^+) \Rightarrow$ False negative (FN)
$P(T^- \cap D^-) \Rightarrow$ True negative (TN)

The correspondence between the set notation and the clinical notation is depicted in the disjointed Venn diagram (Figure 7.5).

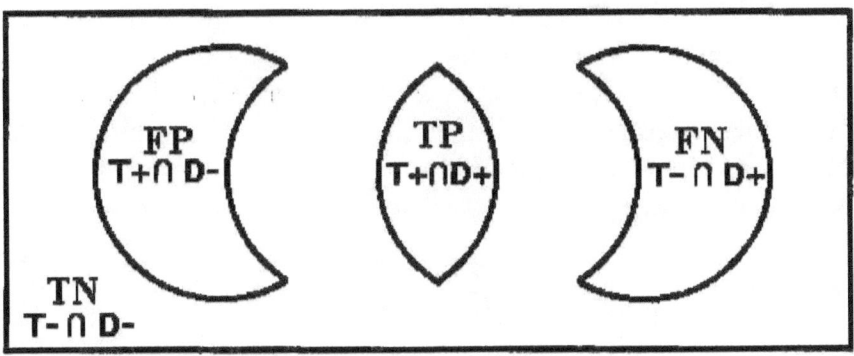

Figure 7.5. Venn diagram of the correspondence between set notation and clinical notation

Note that the terms true and false reflect the actual correspondence between the result of the test and the extant state of disease or absence of disease.

The graphic Venn diagram is then "pattern coded" for visual identification (Figure 7.6):

Bold + for TP; normal + for FP
Bold − for TN; normal − for FN

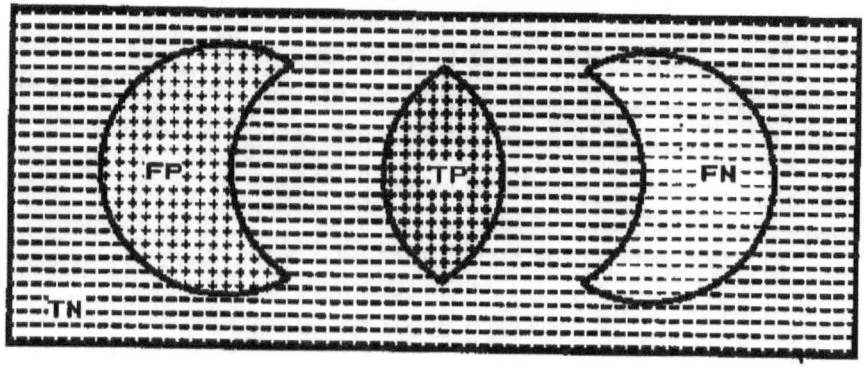

Figure 7.6. Venn diagram of the pattern coding for the identification of clinical subsets.

The four cells are now correspondingly designated. Given the new designation, we are now in a position to convert the clinical probabilities (sensitivity and specificity) as well as the posterior probabilities into a simpler formulation incorporating the new designation. Thus,

$$\text{Sensitivity} = P(T^+ \mid D^+) = \frac{P(T^+ \cap D^+)}{P(D^+)}.$$

$$\overset{\text{Sensitivity}}{P(T^+ \mid D^+)} \times P(D^+) = P(T^+ \cap D^+).$$

Substituting the new term of TP for the probability of intersection $P(T^+ \cap D^+)$ and denoting $P(D^+)$ by its numerical counterpart in the above relation, the cell can now be assigned a numerical value given the sensitivity of the test in question and the prevalence of the disease under discussion:

$$\text{Sensitivity} \times n(D^+) = n(\text{TP}).$$

The specificity designation in probabilistic notation was given in the initial presentation as follows:

$$\text{Specificity} = P(T^- \mid D^-) = \frac{P(T^- \cap D^-)}{P(D^-)}.$$

$$\overset{\text{Specificity}}{P(T^- \mid D^-)} \times P(D^-) = P(T^- \cap D^-).$$

Substituting TN for the probability of intersection $P(T^- \cap D^-)$ and $n(D^-)$ for the complement of the prevalence,

$$\text{Specificity} \times n(D^-) = n(\text{TN}).$$

For the posterior probability, yet another term, *predictive value*, is introduced intended to emphasize the diagnostic accuracy of the test result:

$$\text{Posterior probability} = P(D^+ \mid T^+) = \frac{P(T^+ \cap D^+)}{P(T^+)}.$$

Substituting TP for the numerator and TP +FP for the denominator, we obtained the revised formula for the predictive value of a positive test (Table 7.2):

$$\text{Posterior probability} = P(D^+ \mid T^+) = \frac{\text{TP}}{\text{TP} + \text{FP}} = \text{PV}[+] = \text{Predictive value of positive test.}$$

The predictive value of a negative test is similarly derived as follows:

$$\text{Posterior probability} = P(D^- \mid T^-) = \frac{P(T^- \cap D^-)}{P(T^-)}.$$

Substituting TN for the numerator and TN + FN for the denominator, the revised formula for the predictive value of a negative test result is obtained (Table 7.2):

$$\text{Posterior probability} = P(D^- \mid T^-) = \frac{TN}{TN + FN} = PV[-] = \text{Predictive value of negative test.}$$

The table is now configured in terms of three basic parameters, two of which (sensitivity and specificity) need to be derived a priori through carefully executed trials and or experiments. The third parameter (prevalence) is the one parameter that can be subjectively entertained or experimentally derived, depending on the situation under consideration.

	Any given disease			
	Prevalence Prior probability $P(\mathrm{D+}) = \dfrac{n(\mathrm{D+})}{n(\mathrm{U})}$	Prevalence Prior probability $P(\mathrm{D}^-) = \dfrac{n(\mathrm{D}^-)}{n(\mathrm{U})}$	Universe $P(\mathrm{U}) = 1$ $P(\mathrm{D}^+) + P(\mathrm{D}^-) = 1$	
T^+	Joint probability = Conditional probability × Prior probability $P(\mathrm{T}^+ \cap \mathrm{D}^+) =$ $P(\mathrm{T}^+\|\mathrm{D}^+) \times P(\mathrm{D}^+)$	Joint probability = Conditional probability × Prior probability $P(\mathrm{T}^+ \cap \mathrm{D}^-) =$ $P(\mathrm{T}^+\|\mathrm{D}^-) \times P(\mathrm{D}^+)$	T^+ row total Marginal $P(\mathrm{T}^+)$ $P(\mathrm{T}^+\|\mathrm{D}^+) +$ $P(\mathrm{T}^+ \cap \mathrm{D}^-)$	Posterior probability = $P(\mathrm{D}^+ \| \mathrm{T}^+) = \dfrac{P(\mathrm{T}^+ \cap \mathrm{D}^+)}{P(\mathrm{T}^+)}$
T^-	Joint probability = Conditional probability × Prior probability $P(\mathrm{T}^- \cap \mathrm{D}^+) =$ $P(\mathrm{T}^-\|\mathrm{D}^+) \times P(\mathrm{D}^+)$	Joint probability = Conditional probability × Prior probability $P(\mathrm{T}^- \cap \mathrm{D}^-) =$ $P(\mathrm{T}^-\mathrm{D}^-) \times P(\mathrm{D}^-)$	T^- row total Marginal $P(\mathrm{T}^-)$ $P(\mathrm{T}^-\|\mathrm{D}^+) +$ $P(\mathrm{T}^- \cap \mathrm{D}^-)$	Posterior probability = $P(\mathrm{D}- \| \mathrm{T}-) = \dfrac{P(\mathrm{T}-\cap \mathrm{D}-)}{P(\mathrm{T}-)}$
	D^+ Column total Marginal $P(\mathrm{D}^+)$ $P(\mathrm{T}^+ \cap \mathrm{D}^+) +$ $P(\mathrm{T}^- \cap \mathrm{D}^+)$	D^- Column total Marginal $P(\mathrm{D}^-)$ $P(\mathrm{T}^+ \cap \mathrm{D}^-) +$ $P(\mathrm{T}^- \cap \mathrm{D}^+)$	Total	
	Clinical probability = sensitivity = Sensitivity $P(\mathrm{T}^+ \| \mathrm{D}^+) = \dfrac{\text{Joint probability}\ P(\mathrm{T}^+ \cap \mathrm{D}^+)}{P(\mathrm{D}^+)\ \text{Marginal probability}}$	Clinical probability = specificity = Specificity $P(\mathrm{T}^- \| \mathrm{D}^-) = \dfrac{\text{Joint probability}\ P(\mathrm{T}^- \cap \mathrm{D}^-)}{P(\mathrm{D}^-)\ \text{Marginal probability}}$		

Table 7.1. Basic conditional probability table, which may be interpreted in two ways:

1. Determine sensitivity/specificity by experimentally filling the four cells
2. Fill in the numerical values of the cells, given the experimentally derived sensitivity and specificity

	Any Given Disease			
	Prevalence $P(D^+) = \dfrac{n(D^+)}{n(U)}$	1 − Prevalence $P(D^-) = \dfrac{n(D^-)}{n(U)}$	Sample universe $P(U) = 1$ $P(D^+) + P(D^-)$ $= 1$	
	$P(D^+) = \dfrac{119}{119 + 836} = 0.12$	$P(D^-) = \dfrac{836}{119 + 836} = 0.88$	$0.12 + 0.88 = 1$	
	Disease present $n(D^+) = P(D^+) \times n(U)$	Disease absent $n(D^-) = P(D^-) \times n(U)$	Sample universe $n(U) = n(D^+) +$ $n(B^-)$	
	119	836	955	
T^+	True positive $n(D^+) \times Sn = n(TP)$	False positive $n(D^-) - n(TN)$ $= n(FP)$	T^+ row total $n(T^+) = n(FN) +$ $n(TN)$	Predictive value of positive test $PV[+] = \dfrac{TP}{TP + FP}$
	109	92	$109 + 92 = 201$	$PV[+] = \dfrac{109}{201} = 54\%$
T^-	False negative $n(D^+) - n(TP) =$ $n(FN)$	True negative $n(D^-) \times Sp = n(TN)$	T^- row total $n(T^-) = n(FN) +$ $n(TN)$	Predictive value of negative test $PV[-] = \dfrac{TN}{TN + FN}$
	10	744	$10 + 744 = 754$	$PV[-] = \dfrac{744}{754} = 98.6\%$
	D^+ column total $= 110$ $n(D^+) = n(TP) +$ $n(FN)$	D^- column total $= 836$ $n(D^-) = n(FP) +$ $n(TN)$	U total $n(U) = 955$ $n(TP) + n(FP) +$ $n(FN) + n(TN)$	
	Sensitivity $Sn = \dfrac{TP}{TP + FN}$	Specificity $Sp = \dfrac{TN}{TN + FP}$		
	$= \dfrac{109}{119} = 0.916$	$= \dfrac{744}{836} = 0.899$		

Table 7.2. Practical probability table: constructed from the data of the cooperative study whose abstract is presented in chapter 7.1

7.1 Diagnostic Marker Cooperative Study for the Diagnosis of Myocardial Infarction

Janice Zimmerman, MD; Robert Fromm, MD, MPH;
Denise Meyer, MT(ASCP); Ann Boudreaux, MD;
Chuan-Chuan C. Wun, PhD; Richard Smalling, MD, PhD;
Barry Davis, MD, PhD; Gabriel Habib, MD; Robert Roberts, MD

Background: Millions of patients present annually with chest pain, but only 10% to 15% have myocardial infarction. Lack of diagnostic sensitivity and specificity of clinical and conventional markers prevents or delays treatment and leads to unnecessary costly admissions. Comparative data are lacking on the new markers, yet using all of them is inappropriate and expensive.

Methods and Results: The Diagnostic Marker Cooperative Study was a prospective, multicenter, double-blind study with consecutive enrollment of patients with chest pain presenting to the emergency department. Diagnostic sensitivity and specificity and frequency of increase in patients with unstable angina were determined for creatine kinase-MB (CK-MB) subforms, myoglobin, total CK-MB (activity and mass), and troponin T and I on the basis of frequent serial sampling for ≤24 hours. Of 955 patients with chest pain, 119 (12.5%) had infarction identified by use of CK-MB mass, and 203 (21%) had unstable angina. CK-MB subforms were most sensitive and specific (91% and 89%) within 6 hours of onset, followed by myoglobin (78% and 89%). For late diagnosis, total_CK-MB activity (derived from subforms) was the most sensitive and specific (96% and 98%) at 10 hours from onset, followed by troponin I (96% and 93%), but not until 18 hours, and troponin T (87% and 93% at 10 hours). In unstable angina, CK-MB subforms were increased in 29.5%, myoglobin in 23.7%, troponin I in 19.7%, and troponin T in 14.8%. All markers were increased in 99 patients. With each marker as the diagnostic standard, CK-MB subforms and myoglobin remained the most sensitive for early diagnosis.

Conclusions: The CK-MB subform assay alone or in combination with a troponin reliably triages patients with chest pain and should lead to improved therapy and reduced cost. (*Circulation.* 1999;99:1671-1677.)

7.2 Timed Conditional Probability: Risk Assessment

The subject of risk occupies a prominent role in the era of environmental concern, mass screening, and preventive therapy. Even in the routine practice of medicine, every medical decision is associated with some degree of risk to the patient. Thus, the determination of risk factors and its accurate stratification in the symptomatic and asymptomatic individual followed by the appropriate therapeutic and preventive measures is of major concern in the practice of medicine.

Consider the excerpts from the following literature: Preoperative Risk Assessment; Risk Stratification and Triage in the Context of the ER or in the Field; Prediction of Outcome and/or Survival; Prognosis in the Post Hospital Phase; and Risk/Benefit Ratio of Preventive Intervention. Needless to say, a quantitative appreciation of the generic term of risk is of paramount importance in the decision-making process and the art and format of communication with the average patient.

7.2.1 Definition

At the basic level, risk is a probability that a person will develop a disease or an adverse outcome over a specified period. Often, the probability is conditional on the associated presence of risk factors, as such risk may be considered a conditional probability over a specified period.

	(D^+) MI at t_1	(D^-) No MI at t_1	
Risk factor: hyperlipidemia RF^+ (T^+)	$a = 25$	$b = 975$	$a + b = 1,000$: points at risk at t_0
Risk factor: Normal lipid profile RF^- (T^-)	$c = 10$	$d = 990$	$c + d = 1,000$: points at no risk at t_0
	$a + c = 35$ MI at t_1	$b + d = 1,965$ No MI at t_1	$a + b + c + d = 2,000$

	Cumulative incidence risk	
	$\text{Incidence}_{\text{Exposed}} = \dfrac{a}{a+b} = \dfrac{25}{1000} = 0.025 \;/\; 5 \text{ years}$	
	$\text{Incidence}_{\text{Unexposed}} = \dfrac{c}{c+d} = \dfrac{10}{1000} = 0.01 \;/\; 5 \text{ years}$	
	$\underset{\text{Relative risk}}{\text{RR}} = \dfrac{I(E)}{I(\overline{E})} = \dfrac{al(a+b)}{cl(c+d)} = \dfrac{0.025}{0.01} = 2.5$	
	$\underset{\text{Attributable risk}}{\text{AR}} = \dfrac{a}{a+b} - \dfrac{c}{c+d} = I(E) - I(\overline{E})$	
	$0.025 - 0.01 = 0.015 = 1.5 \text{ percent}$	

Table 7.1. A hypothetical cohort (prospective) study of 1,000 hyperlipidemic and 1,000 normolipidemic patients, tested at time zero (t_0) and followed over a period of five years. At the conclusion of the time period (t_1), thirty hyperlipidemic patients developed myocardial infarct (MI), whereas only ten with the normal lipid profile developed MI.

7.2.2 Cohort Study

A hypothetical cohort (prospective) study of 1,000 hyperlipidemic and 1,000 normolipidemic patients, tested at time zero (t_0) and followed over a period of five years, is displayed in the contingency table. The follow-up in this study is perfect (extremely rare occurrence), uninterrupted by what epidemiologists refer to as *censored observations* (withdrawals, deaths).

For the 1,000 hyperlipidemic patients, with normal ECG at time zero, the risk of developing MI is defined by the following relation:

$$\underset{\text{Exposure}}{\text{Absolute risk}} = \frac{\text{No. of MIs developed on exposure to RF}^+ \text{ from } t_0 \Rightarrow t_1}{\text{Total no. (at risk = susceptible), exposed to RF}^+ \text{ at } t_0} = \underset{\text{Exposure}}{\text{Incidence}}.$$

Thus, the probability of developing an MI over the specified period is simply a risk of MI in hyperlipidemics =

$$P(\text{MI} \mid \text{RF}^+) = \frac{a}{a+b} = \frac{25}{1000} = 0.025/5 \text{ years} = \underset{\text{Exposure}}{\text{Incidence}}.$$

Note that of the 1,000 hyperlipidemic patients at time zero (t_0), twenty-five sustained an MI at (t_1). Applying the same line of reasoning to the normal lipidemic group, the corresponding risk of developing an MI is defined as follows:

$$\text{Absolute risk}_{\text{Unexposure}} = \frac{\text{No. of MIs developed in the unexposure to } RF^+ \text{ from } t_0 \Rightarrow t_1}{\text{Total no. (at risk = susceptible), unexposed to } RF^+ \text{ at } t_0} = \text{Incidence}_{\text{Unexposure}}.$$

Thus, the probability of developing an MI over the specified period is simply Risk of MI in normolipidemics =

$$P(MI \mid RF^-) = \frac{c}{c+d} = \frac{10}{1000} = 0.010/5 \text{ years} = \text{Incidence}_{\text{Unexposure}}.$$

Note that of the 1,000 normolipidemic patients at time zero (t_0), only 10 sustained an MI at (t_1).

7.2.3 Relative Risk (Risk Ratio)

The correlation between the risk factor and the disease outcome, that is, the relative risk, is portrayed in this hypothetical example as the risk ratio of the two probabilities. Essentially, it is a ratio of the incidence of disease in the exposed subjects divided by the incidence in the unexposed subjects.

$$\text{Relative risk}_{\text{Risk ratio (RR)}} = \frac{\text{Exposure risk}}{\text{Unexposure risk}} = \frac{\text{Incidence of } D^+ \text{ in exposed subjects}}{\text{Incidence of } D^+ \text{ in unexposed subjects}} / \text{time period.}$$

In this prospective study, the relative risk ratio of 2.5 is a concise way of stating the relative probabilities between the hyper- and normolipidemic as to the likelihood of developing an MI.

$$\text{Relative risk}_{\text{Risk ratio (RR)}} = \frac{P(D^+) + RF^+}{P(D^+) \mid RF^-} = \frac{a/(a+b)}{c/(c+d)} = \frac{0.025}{0/01} = \underset{\text{more likely to develop MI}}{2.5 \text{ times}}.$$

A ratio of 1 would have implied that hyperlipidemia is not a risk factor as such, whereas a ratio of 10 would have been a conclusive evidence of the adverse relationship. As a measure of the association between risk factor and outcome, relative risk (in contrast to absolute risk) determines the ratio of the likelihood of sustaining the outcome in question for those exposed compared with the unexposed.

7.2.4 Attributable Risk

Attributable risk is the risk difference in exposed persons that can be directly attributed to the exposure to the risk factor. Attributable risk is determined by subtracting the incidence of the disease in the exposed from that of the unexposed. It is assumed that the cause of the disease had an equal chance of causing the disease in both the exposed and nonexposed individuals.

$$\text{Attributable Risk} = P[\text{MI} \mid \text{RF}^+] - P[\text{MI} - \text{RF}^-] = \frac{a}{a+b} = \frac{c}{c+d} = I(E) - I(\overline{E}).$$

7.2.5 Case-Control Study

As noted in the previous example, the key element in a cohort study is the time span required for the follow-up of the cohort. Witness the Framingham Study, which started in 1949 and was concluded after a time span of thirty years. The gigantic effort involved in such a study, although of major epidemiologic impact, is certainly beyond the resources of the average research facility.

The case-control study, essentially a retrospective study in contrast to the prospective cohort study, offers a practical alternative. In a hypothetical construct of such a study, a hundred case of proven MI are selected and matched to a hundred normal controls.

The historical data of both groups are then researched over a past period to provide the relevant presence or absence of the risk factors, in this case the lipidemic profile.

The data thus researched are tabled in a similar contingency table that differs from the previous prospective table by its choice of the independent variable. Patients with predetermined lipid profile (hyper- and normolipidemic) in the cohort study whose outcome is to be determined by its future association with the relevant risk factor, in contradistinction to patients in the case-control study (MI and non-MI points) whose outcome has been determined by its past association with a relevant risk factor.

In the absence of the time factor in the case-control study, the relative risk ratio as defined and applied to a cohort study is not applicable in this case. However, a good approximation to the relative risk ratio may be derived from another ratio, which is independent of time, namely, the odds ratio.

	MI	No MI	Probability odds of disease
Hyperlipidemia: RF$^+$	$a = 65$	$b = 45$	$\dfrac{P(D^+)}{P(D^-)} = \dfrac{a}{b} = \dfrac{65}{45}$
Normal lipid profile: RF$^-$	$c = 35$	$d = 55$	$\dfrac{P(D^+)}{P(D^-)} = \dfrac{c}{d} = \dfrac{35}{55}$
	$a + c = 100$	$b + d = 100$	
	Exposure odds among MI and no MI		
	$\text{Odds}_{\text{Exp/MI}} = \dfrac{a}{c} = \dfrac{65}{35}$	$\text{Odds}_{\text{Exp/NoMI}} = \dfrac{b}{d} = \dfrac{45}{55}$	
	$\text{Odds ratio}_{\text{Exp}} = \dfrac{\frac{a}{c}}{\frac{b}{d}} = \dfrac{a \times d}{b \times c} = \dfrac{3575}{1575} = 2.27$		$\text{Odds ratio}_{\text{Exp}} = \dfrac{\frac{a}{b}}{\frac{c}{d}} = \dfrac{a \times d}{b \times c} = \dfrac{3575}{1575} = 2.27$

Table 7.2. A hypothetical case control (retrospective) study of one hundred proven MI cases and one hundred matched controls with normal coronary circulation. Note that lipid data are historical in the sense of having been documented to exist over the past five years.

Recall that the definition of odds lacks the time element because it is simply a numerical ratio.

$$\text{Odds for event } S = \frac{\text{No. of successes}}{\text{No. of failures}} = \frac{\text{No. of times event occurred}}{\text{No. of times event did not occure}}.$$

The perusal of the table reveals an interesting relationship regarding the odds of disease versus the odds of exposure.

Consider first the odds of exposure to the lipidemic factor given the presence of MI:

Odds of exposure to lipidemic factor in the presence of $MI = \dfrac{RF^+ \mid D^+}{RF^- \mid D^+} = \dfrac{a}{c} = \dfrac{65}{35}$.

Similarly, the odds of exposure to the lipidemic factor given the absence of MI is calculated follows:

Odds of exposure to lipidemic factor in the absence of $MI = \dfrac{RF^+ \mid D^-}{RF^- \mid D^-} = \dfrac{b}{d} = \dfrac{45}{55}$.

The odds ratio is thus defined as:

$$\text{Odds ratio} = \frac{\text{Odds of exposure to risk factor given disease}}{\text{Odds of exposure to risk factor given no disease}} = \frac{RF^+ \mid D^+}{RF^+ \mid D^-}.$$

The odds ratio in this case, as derived in the following equation, asserts that the risk of being exposed to the lipidemic factor is 2.27 times higher in the sample with MIs than for those without MIs.

$$OR = \frac{\text{Odds of disease given exposure to risk factor}}{\text{Odds of disease given no exposure to risk factor}} = \frac{a/b}{c/d} = \frac{ad}{bc} = \frac{3575}{1575} = 2.27.$$

The odds of lipidemia given the presence or absence of MI is not as clinically relevant as the odds of MI given the presence or absence of the lipidemic factor.

As noted in the last column of Table 7.2, consider now the odds of MI given the exposure to the lipidemic factor,

Odds of MI in the presence of the lipidemic factor $= \dfrac{D^+ \mid RF^+}{D^- \mid RF^+} = \dfrac{a}{b} = \dfrac{65}{45}$,

and the odds of MI given the absence of exposure to the lipidemic factor,

Odds of MI in the absence of the lipidemic factor $= \dfrac{D^+ \mid RF^-}{D^- \mid RF^-} = \dfrac{c}{d} = \dfrac{35}{55}$.

The odds ratio is defined as

$$OR = \frac{\text{Odds of MI given exposure to the lipidemic factor}}{\text{Odds of MI given lack of exposure to the lipidemic factor}} = \frac{D^+ \mid RF^+}{D^+ \mid RF^-}.$$

Similarly, the odds ratio as derived below asserts that the risk of MI is 2.27 times higher in the sample exposed to the risk factor than those unexposed.

$$OR = \frac{\text{Odds of disease given exposure to risk factor}}{\text{Odds of disease given no exposure to risk factor}} = \frac{a/b}{c/d} = \frac{ad}{bc} = \frac{3575}{1575} = 2.27.$$

This surprising finding as related to the case control study asserts that the odds ratio of having the risk factor is equivalent to the odds ratio of having the disease.

$$\text{Odds ratio (exposure)} = \frac{\dfrac{a}{c}}{\dfrac{b}{d}} = \text{Odds ratio (disease)} = \frac{\dfrac{a}{b}}{\dfrac{c}{d}} = \frac{ad}{bc}.$$

As a measure of the degree of association, the odds ratio in this case serves as fairly good estimate of the relative ratio derived from the cohort study, 2.37 versus 2.5.

7.3 Prevalence, Incidence, and Risk

These three terms, often misunderstood, are of paramount importance in the critical appreciation of medical literature. The key element that binds the three terms is the time factor that ties what is essentially a proportion or probability to a time scale. Recall that by definition, a proportion/probability is fraction, which relates the part to the whole as noted in the relations illustrated in Tables 7.1 and 7.2.

$$\text{Proportion} = \frac{a}{a+b} = \frac{\text{No. of MIs}}{\text{No. of MIs} + \text{No. of Non-MIs}} = \frac{\text{Subset of denominator}}{\text{Denominator sample space}} = \frac{\text{Part}}{\text{Total}}.$$

7.3.1 Prevalence

The term prevalence is also called point prevalence to underscore its brief encounter with time defined as follows:

$$\underset{\text{Proportion}}{\text{Prevalence}} = \frac{\text{No. of individuals with a given disease at a point in time (time zero, } t_0)}{\text{Population with and without the disease at the same point in time}}.$$

Thus, prevalence is the frequency of a condition or disease at a point in time. It is in fact a snap shot of the health state of a particular group or population at a given point in time. Thus, prevalence may be defined as the probability of a given disease/condition at t_0.

7.3.2. Prevalence: Prostate Cancer*

$$\text{Prevalence } (1,985) = \frac{\text{No. of autopsy Dx of prostate Ca in men} > 50 \text{ years}}{\text{No. of men (US)} > 50 \text{ (population)}} = \frac{8,193,000}{27,310,000} = 0.3.$$

Incidence, on the other hand, as noted from the discussion of risk, is intimately associated with the prospective cohort study in which the number events are cumulatively added over the specified period ending with a time limited proportion as defined below:

$$\underset{\text{Cumulative/time}}{\text{Incidence}} = \frac{\text{No. of new cases during a specified interval of time from } t_0 \Rightarrow t_1}{\text{Population at risk at the beginning of the time interval, } t_0}.$$

7.3.3 Incidence: Prostate Cancer

$$\text{Incidence of clinical Ca./year} = \frac{\text{No. of clinical Ca / year}}{\text{Male population} > 50 \text{ at risk}} = \frac{86,000}{27,310,000} = 0.0031 = 0.31\% / \text{year}.$$

$$\frac{1}{0.00093} = 1071 : 1 \text{ clinical Ca in 321 males} > 50.$$

$$\text{Mortality rate} = \frac{\text{No. of deaths / year}}{\text{Male population} > 50 \text{ at risk}} = \frac{25,000}{27,310,000} = 0.00093 = 0.093\% / \text{year}.$$

$\frac{1}{0.00093} = 1071$: 1 in 1,071 males > 50 per year.

Similarly, the definition of risk follows an identical format noted as follows:

$$\underset{\text{Probability/time}}{\text{Absolute risk}} = \frac{\text{No. new cases (events, outcome) over a specific time interval } (t_0 \Rightarrow t_1)}{\text{Total no. free of disease but at risk (susceptible to the outcome) at } t_0}.$$

In both instance, the final result is probability-proportion/time units where persons at risk are the basic measure evident from the structure of the cohort study. Such time is an implicit factor although not an integral part of the equation. An alternative approach of measuring the incidence rate of an event adopts person-time unit as the basic measure.

$$\text{Incidence rate} = \frac{\text{No. of events}}{\text{Person - years}}.$$

A person-year is defined as one person surviving for one year. In the hypothetical cohort study noted previously, twenty-five events (MIs) occurred during the follow-up period of five years.

$$\text{Incidence rate} = \frac{25 \text{ events (MIs)}}{5 \text{ person - years}} = 5 \text{ per person-year.}$$

The distinctive feature of this formulation of incidence is the flexibility of the denominator. The five person-years could be reconfigured as sixty person-months because the number of subjects is not included in the formulation.

7.3.4 Interrelation of Incidence and Prevalence

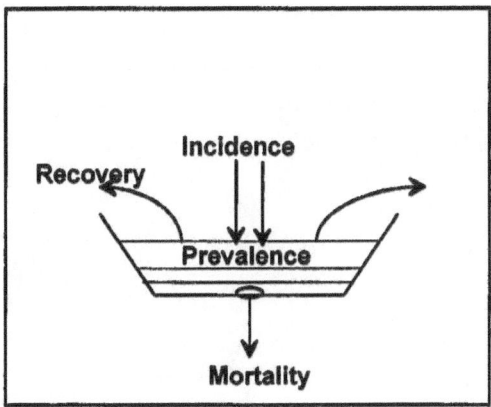

Figure 7.1. Flow Diagram of the variants affecting Prevalence

In a steady state, the relationship between prevalence and incidence can be shown to be mathematically related:

$$\frac{\text{Prevalence}}{1-\text{Prevalence}} = \frac{P(D^+)}{P(D^-)} = \text{Incidence} \times \text{Duration of disease.}$$

When prevalence is below 0.1 (10 percent), the denominator approaches 1, and the relationship can now be simplified to read

$$\text{Prevalence} \approx \text{Incidence} \times \text{Duration.}$$

AS noted in the classic figure, the level of prevalence is directly proportional to the incidence rate as well as the duration of the disease in question. A shorter duration (accelerated recovery or death) would result in a lower level of prevalence.

Over the past decade, the impact of randomized trials on the practice of medicine has been to say the least revolutionary. With this in mind, the interpretation of the trial outcomes needs to consider the format in which it is presented. As noted previously, the risk format, both absolute and relative, are derivatives of the same basic data.

The exclusive use of the relative format in presenting the benefit of a particular therapy may lead the casual observer to overestimate the associated risk or benefit.

To put the relevant data in perspective and to avoid "cognitive bias," the use of the reciprocal of the absolute risk reduction has been recommended as the perfect adjunct to both the absolute risk and the relative risk reduction.

Risk	Type	Illustration Using the Helsinki Heart Study Result[5]
Absolute risk reduction	(Risk of an event without Rx)– (Risk of an event with Rx)	Over five years 3.9 percent of untreated persons had an event (MI) – 2.5 percent of treated persons had an event = 1.4 percent is the absolute risk reduction with Rx. "In the treated group, 1.4 percent fewer persons had MI"
Relative risk	$\dfrac{\text{Risk of an event with Rx}}{\text{Risk of an event without Rx}}$	$RR = \dfrac{2.5\% \text{ of treated persons had an event}}{3.9\% \text{ of untreated persons had an event}} = 0.64$ The risk of Event with Rx is 2/3 the risk if untreated
Relative risk reduction	$1 - \dfrac{\text{Risk of an event with Rx}}{\text{Risk of an event without Rx}}$	$1 - \dfrac{2.5\% \text{ of treated persons had an event}}{3.9\% \text{ of untreated persons had an event}} = 0.34$ 34 percent is the relative risk reduction with Rx
Number needed to treat NNT	$\dfrac{1}{\text{Absolute risk reduction}}$	$\dfrac{1}{1.4\%} \; 71\%$ 71 persons had to be treated for five years to prevent one Mississippi

Table 7.3
Equivalent expressions of therapeutic benefit: risk reduction

[5] Hux, J. E. and N. C. David. 1995. In the eye of the beholder "commentary." Archives of Internal Medicine 155 (Nov. 27).
Frick, M. H., O. Elo, K. Haapa, et al. 1987. Helsinki heart study: Primary-prevention trial with gemfibrozil in middle-aged men with dyslipidemia. New England Journal of Medicine 317:1237-1245.

$$RR = \frac{2.5\% \text{ of treated persons had an event}}{3.9\% \text{ of untreated persons Had an event}} = 0.64 = 2/3 \text{ risk reduction.}$$

The risk of event in the period studied for persons given the treatment is two-thirds the risk of the event for persons who remained untreated.

$$RR = \frac{3.9\% \text{ of untreated persons had an event}}{2.5\% \text{ of treated persons had an event}} = 1.56 \text{ higher risk.}$$

Part II

Bayes' Theorem

Chapter 8

Bayes' Theorem: Descriptive and Graphic Approach

A reverse or retrograde reconstruction and analysis of the logical steps involved in the diagnostic process seem to be the ideal port of entry into the format of decision theory given the intuitive familiarity with the process honed through years of apprenticeship by the practicing physician.

This is best illustrated by what might be considered a variant of the diagnostic process, which begins when a patient contacts his physician for a particular symptom or sign suffered and/or noted by the patient. Under normal routine circumstance, the patient's presenting symptom and/or sign elicits from the examining physician a sequence of differential diagnostic probabilities that need to be ruled in or ruled out.

Assume for this hypothetical case that the patient is referred to the cardiac clinic of a university hospital because of atypical chest pain (ACP). It would be reasonable to suggest that of the many diagnostic possibilities, the probability of coronary artery disease (CAD) is high on the list.

The question that needs to be addressed and answered is an estimate of the diagnostic probability that the patient might have CAD despite the atypical presentation of the symptoms.

In probabilistic terms, the question is phrased: $P(CAD|ACP)$, that is, probability of CAD given the symptom of ACP.

The answer to this outwardly simplistic question is at the heart of the Bayesian statistical decision theory. In assessing a given probability, the physician may not have been aware that in doing so, he subconsciously or intuitively answered correctly or otherwise three implicit questions needed for the final answer. Stated in terms of the Bayes' theorem in its simplest form, the above-noted question results in the following equation:

$$P(\text{CAD} \,|\, \text{ACP}) \overset{\text{Predictive value}}{=} P(\text{ACP} \,|\, \text{CAD}) \overset{\text{Clinical sensitivity}}{\times} \frac{P(\text{CAD})}{P(\text{ACP})}. \quad (8.1a)$$

Three separate probability statements are involved and need to be answered if the final diagnostic probability is to be correctly estimated.

In symbolic generic format, the equation can be abbreviated to read as follows:

$$P(\text{disease|symptom}) \overset{\text{Predictive value}}{=} P(\text{symptom} \,|\, \text{disease}) \overset{\text{Clinical sensitivity}}{\times} \frac{P(\text{disease})}{P(\text{symptom})}.$$

The equation may be further modified to yield the original conditional diagnostic probability format:

$$P(\text{CAD} \,|\, \text{ACP}) = P(\text{ACP} \,|\, \text{CAD}) \times \frac{P(\text{CAD})}{P(\text{ACP})}.$$

Substituting D^+ for CAD and S^+ for ACP, the equation may be rewritten in the probabilistic format

$$P(D^+ \,|\, S^+) = P(S^+ \,|\, D^+) \overset{\text{Sensitivity}}{\times} \frac{\overset{\text{Prior probility}}{P(D^+)}}{P(S^+)}. \quad (8.1b)$$

Finally, the relationship may be restructured into its conditional format:

$$P(D^+ \,|\, S^+) \overset{\text{Posterior probability}}{=} \frac{\overset{\text{Joint probability}}{P\left(S^+ \,|\, D^+\right) \times P(D^+)}}{P(S^+)} = \frac{\overset{\text{Intersection}}{P(S^+ \cap D^+)}}{\underset{\text{Marginal probability}}{P(S^+)}}.$$

8.1 Numerical and Graphic Equivalents of the Diagnostic Procedure

The first factor that must be addressed is the prior estimate of the prevalence of the particular disease $P(D^+)$ in the subset of population under consideration. The prior probability of a particular disease in a given subset of population varies with the characteristics of the subset as well as the nature of the disease.

In the present context, $P(D^+)$ refers to the probability of CAD in the totality of patients frequenting the cardiac clinic of this particular institution. In epidemiological parlance, $P(D^+)$ refers to the prevalence of D, CAD in this instance, in the active patients files of the clinic. Note that the prevalence of a given disease in the population at large (epidemiologically considered to be 100,000) is certainly different from its prevalence at the cardiac clinic or any other clinic for that matter because we are dealing here with a subset of the general public. What has to be emphasized is that the unconditional probability of a given disease, that is, its prevalence, needs to be considered in the context of the subset of population under consideration rather than the population at large. In essence, the idea of prevalence aims to categorize a given patient within a particular sample universe as probable carrier of a given disease and to assign a certain probability to this fact, prior to any objective or subjective data supporting or contradicting the prior probability for the disease. To reiterate, the concept of prevalence implies that a randomly selected chart from the clinic current active files would turn out to be that of a patient with CAD.

Assume that in the opinion of the cardiologist, 30 percent of the patients registered at the clinic suffer from CAD in its various manifestation, such that a randomly selected chart will turn out to be that of a patient with CAD. In probabilistic notation, $P(D^+) = 0.3$ (30 percent).

Assuming that the total number of patients registered at the clinic is 1,000, using a modified quantitative Venn diagram, the situation at the clinic may be graphically illustrated as in Figure 8.1. Note that the 700 patients free from CAD are registered at the clinic for other reasons. Thus, $P(\text{non-CAD}) = P(D^-) = 0.7$, so that $P(1 - D^+) = 0.7$.

These two events are then mutually exclusive and complementary, for the obvious reason that they cannot happen at the same time, and the sum of their probabilities equals 1 (0.3 + 0.7 = 1.0). They are also exhaustive because they include the totality of the patient population at the cardiac clinic.

The second question that needs to be addressed and answered relates to the unconditional probability of the presenting symptom $P(S^+)$ in the clinic sample universe of total files. This is a question that cannot be answered offhand. Again, based on the clinical experience of the resident cardiologist, the symptom of ACP is rather common and may account for as much as 20 percent of the patients count such that a randomly selected chart would include an ACP symptom with a probability of two out of ten, or $P(S^+) = 0.2$.

Graphically, the situation is illustrated in Figure 8.2. Note the 800 patients that present with other symptoms. Thus, $P(S^-) = 0.8$ includes the rest of the patients population that present with symptoms other than the ACPs. Thus, $P(\text{non-ACP}) = P(S^-) = 0.8$, so that $P(1 - S^+) = 0.8$.

The third factor in the equation, $P(S^+ \mid D^+)$, is an estimate of what might be considered a textbook clinical fact; the physician is likely to remember or look up if pressed, as to the probability of ACP given CAD. State differently, the question that needs to be addressed is how often a patient with CAD presents with ACP.

The answer to $P(S^+ \mid D^+)$ is not something that can be estimated offhand. As was the case with the sensitivity of a test, it must be based on prior statistical study accepted in the current literature. The literature suggested estimate of $P(S^+ \mid D^+) = 0.2$, such that only 20 percent of patients with proven CAD present with ACP.

Solving for the diagnostic probability $P(D^+|S^+)$ by substituting for the given unknowns, the probability of CAD, given the presenting symptom of ACP at this particular clinic, is 0.3. Thus,

$$\underset{\text{Predictive value}}{P(D^+ \mid S^+)} = \underset{\text{Clinical sensitivity}}{P(S^+ \mid D^+)} \times \frac{P(D^+)}{P(S^+)} = 0.2 \times \frac{0.3}{0.2} = 0.3.$$

This is the revised or posterior probability that the patient presenting with ACP may be a carrier of CAD.

In this case, the revised probability, $P(D^+ \mid S^+)$, is not different from the prior probability, $P(D^+)$, which was assumed to be the equivalent of the prevalence of the disease at the clinic. In other words, the patient presented with ACP did not alter the initial probability based only on the prevalence of the disease among the clinic population. The implication is that in this case, only three of ten cases with similar presentation are true CAD patients, whereas seven of ten similarly presenting cases may prove to be false positive and therefore free from CAD.

From the above equation, note that because $P(D^+) = 0.3$, the actual number of patients known to have CAD may be calculated given the total number of patients at the clinic; thus,

$0.3 \times 1{,}000 = 300 =$ number of patients presumed to have CAD at the clinic.

Similarly, the actual number of patients presenting with ACP may be calculated given the total number of patients and ratio of those presenting with ACP; thus,

$0.2 \times 1{,}000 = 200 =$ number of patients presenting with ACP at the clinic.

Additionally, because the clinical probability, $P(S^+ \mid D^+)$, suggested by the clinical literature is said to equal 0.2, which is actually the percentage of patients who are both symptomatic and carrier of the disease from the total of diseases patients, one may also calculate the actual number of patients from those known to have CAD, as calculated previously, $n(D^+) = 300$ patients who also concurrently present with the complaint of ACP. Thus,

$P(S^+ \mid D^+) \times P(D^+) = 0.2 \times [0.3 \times 1{,}000] = 0.2 \times 300 = 60$ patients.

These 60 patients are at once CAD patients whose presenting symptom is ACP.

The Venn diagram can now be completed because the extent of the intersection of the D⁺ circle with the S⁺ circle accurately defines the intersection area and thus subdivides the universe circle into four mutually exclusive and exhaustive partitions designated as follows and graphically portrayed in Figure 8.3:

$P(S^+ \mid D^+)$ = sensitivity = true-positive rate (TP)

$P(S^- \mid D^+)$ = 1 − sensitivity = false-negative rate (FN)

$P(S^- \mid D^-)$ = specificity = true-negative rate (TN)

$P(S^+ \mid D^-)$ = 1 − specificity = false-positive rate (FP)

The graphical representation includes all the conditional and unconditional probabilities in a graphic quantitative form, where all derived relationship and probabilities can be visually appreciated (Figure 8.3).

This diagram supplemented by the standard binary table (Table 8.1) represents the basic skeleton on which all future discussion will be based. Accordingly, the dimensions of the diagram will be drawn to represent the estimated probability ratio or its numerical counterpart as follows:

1. U circle area: representing the total number of patient in the sample universe

$$n(U) = \overset{P(U)}{1.0} \times 1000 = 1000.$$

2. D⁺ circle area: representing the number of patients estimated to have the disease

$$n(D^+) = \overset{P(D^+)}{0.3} \times 1000 = 300.$$

3. S⁺ circle area: representing the number of patients estimated to present with a chief complaint of ACP

$$n(S+) = \overset{P(S+)}{0.2} \times 1000 = 200$$

4. Intersection area: representing the number of patients whose presenting symptom is that of ACP given that they do actually suffer from CAD

$$n(S^+ \cap D^+) = \overset{P(S^+|D^+)\ P(D^+)}{0.2\ \times\ 300} = 60.$$

5. Area inside the U circle and outside both S^+ and D^+ circles: representing the number of patients presenting with other symptom and known to be free from CAD

$$n(S^- \cap D^-) = \overset{P(S^-|D^-)\ P(D^-)}{0.8\ \times\ 700} = 560.$$

Give the above numerical and graphic data, the essential diagnostic conditional probability can now be implemented as follows:

$$P(D^+|S^+) = P(S^+|D^+) \times \frac{P(D^+)}{P(S^+)} = 0.2 \times \frac{0.3}{0.2} = 0.3. \quad (8.1c)$$

The final derived Bayes' diagnostic conditional probability, $P(D^+|S^+)$, can be graphically appreciated as the ratio of the intersection area to the reduced sample space of the S^+ circle. Note again that the diagnostic conditional probability $P(D^+|S^+)$ now reverses the sequence of the clinical conditional probability, $P(S^+|D^+)$, by restricting the probability of the disease to the defined subset S^+ instead of D^+ of the original sample universe, U.

With the three factors now defined numerically and graphically, the answer to the diagnostic conditional probability, $P(D^+|S^+)$, needs to be reevaluated in view of the arbitrary numerical values assigned to the factors.

Numerically, the answer noted in the previous equation, 0.3, refers to the percentage or ratio of patients who are true CAD patients from the total number presenting with the chief complaint of ACP. Of the three factors required for the solution of equation 8.1c, two, $P(S^+ \mid D^+)$ and $P(S^+)$, were arbitrarily assigned numerical values unsupported by controlled trials thus rendering the validity of the result of questionable merit. The third factor, $P(D^+)$, remains valid because it is based on the known frequency of the disease in this particular population.

Graphically, the answer sought is the converse of the conditional probability, $P(S^+ \mid D^+)$, which requires the evaluation the intersection area as a fraction of the reduced sample space S^+ area alone instead of its former relation to the reduced sample space of D^+ area.

Considering equation 8.1c again in light of the above-mentioned statements, it is obvious that graphical or numerical solution of the equation requires a numerator that defines the size of the intersection area, $P(S^+ \mid D^+) \times P(D^+)$, and a denominator that defines the size of S^+ circle area. As stated previously, neither $P(S^+)$ nor $P(S^+ \mid D^+)$ or their numerical or area equivalents are readily available; therefore, the solution of the equation is not possible unless $P(S^+)$ and $P(S^+ \mid D^+)$ or their equivalents could be indirectly determined.

This hypothetical scenario portrays the necessary background data needed to answer the initial diagnostic differential. Of the three factors needed for solution, the second factor is the most problematic because the $P(S^+)$ ratio is not readily available so that the number of patients with the given presenting symptom in the sample universe under consideration remains nonquantifiable.

It becomes obvious that a quantitative solution requires the use of data derived from controlled experimental evaluation that can be readily substituted for the missing factors in the simplified Bayes' equation. With this in mind, a standardized evaluation process covering a possible diagnostic test needs to be designed so as to provide the necessary numerical data needed for the diagnostic probability given the test results.

This backdoor introduction and demonstration of the structural ingredients necessary for assessing the diagnostic probability of disease given a particular symptom/sign/test provides the necessary frame for the controlled trial. Indirectly replacing the essential two factors needed for the solution is the conditional probability $P(S^- \mid D^-)$ of specificity in addition to the conditional probability $P(S^+ \mid D^+)$ of sensitivity and the unconditional probability $P(D^+)$ of prevalence.

8.2 Evaluation of the Operating Characteristics of Diagnostic Test

In general, the evaluation process for any test or procedure involves the uniform application of the test to two well-defined and complementary subsets comprising the sample universe, a disease subset, D^+, and a nondiseased subset, D^- (Figure 8.1).

Because the subject is CAD, let us consider briefly the acceptable criteria of disease from the hemodynamic point of view and its validation by what is considered to be the nearest approximation to physical reality, that is, coronary angiocardiography. Note that the relationship of diameter to area is such that a reduction in diameter by 50 percent of its normal results in a reduction of the area to 25 percent, and a decrease in diameter to 25 percent of its normal value results in the critical reduction of the area to 6 percent of its normal area.

Two subsets of population are then chosen, one with 75 percent luminal narrowing of one or more arteries demonstrated on angiography and the other with perfectly normal arteries angiographically validated. (A detailed treatment of the subject will be considered in chapter 16.)

Both sets are then given a stress test. A cutoff point is assigned, whereby 1 mm of ST segment depression in the left precordial leads is considered to be a positive response to graded exercise test (GXT).

A study along the same lines has been conducted by several investigators. For the sake of consistency in this presentation, a hypothetical trial is conducted on 500 proven CAD patients and 500 normals. The results are entered in the 2 × 2 binary table and then used for the calculation of sensitivity and specificity of the applied test (Table 8.2). Once derived, these two characteristics of any given test together with the prevalence factor constitute the triad required to solve the expanded Bayes' equation and to answer the all important clinical question of the probability of disease in a particular patient given the positive or negative result of a given test:

Probability of disease | given a positive test = $P(D^+ \mid T^+)$
Probability of disease | given a negative test = $P(D^+ \mid T^-)$

8.3 Posttest Diagnostic Procedure

The impact of probability theory on the diagnostic process comes into focus by the selective use of testing procedure designed to enhance or further attenuate the estimated initial clinical diagnostic probability (a dead end value of 0.3 was obtained in this case). A test is then undertaken to confirm or exclude a given disease entity, which the patient's presenting signs/symptoms suggest to be the most likely diagnosis. To this end, the patient is then advised that a cardiac graded exercise stress test is indicated.

The question that needs to be readdressed is, given the result of a GXT, what is the probability of CAD in a particular patient? In other words, how confident one can be in confirming or excluding the first diagnosis on the differential list? The focus of interest in this case is therefore the conditional posttest probability of CAD.

	Coronary Artery Disease			
	Prevalence	1 – Prevalence	Universe	
	$P(D^+) = 0.3$	$P(D^-) = 0.7$	$P(U){=}0.3 + 0.7{=}1$	
	Disease present	Disease absent	Sample universe	
	$n(D^+) = P(D^+)$ $\times n(U)$	$n(D^-) = P(D^-)$ $\times n(U)$	$n(D^+) + n(D^-) =$ $N(U)$	
	$0.3 \times 1{,}000 =$ 300	$0.7 \times$ $1{,}000{=}700$		

Symptoms/ signs	ACP	True positive	False positive	S^+ row total	Predictive value of positive test
	S^+	$P(S^+\|D^+) \times$ $P(D^+) =$	$P(S^+\|D^-) \times$ $P(D^-) =$	$P(S^+) = 0.2$	$P(D^+\|S^+) =$
					$\dfrac{P(S+\|D+) \times P(D+)}{P(S^+)}$
				$0.2 \times 1{,}000 =$	
		$0.2 \times 300 = 60$	$700 \times 0.2 = 140$	200	
					$0.2 \times 300 / 200$ $= 60 / 200 = 0.3$
	Other symptoms S^-	False negative $P(S^-\|D^+) \times$ $P(D^+)=$	True negative $P(S\text{-}\|D^-) \times$ $P(D^-)=$	S^- row total $P(S\text{-}) = 0.8$	Predictive value of negative test $P(D^-\|S\text{-}) =$
				$240 + 560 =$	$\dfrac{P(S\text{-.}\|D-) \times P(D-)}{P(S\text{-})}$
		$300 \times 0.8 = 240$	$0.8 \times 700 = 560$	800	$0.8 \times 700/800 =$ $560/800$ $= 0.7$
		D^+ column total $= 300$	D^- column total $= 700$	U total $= 1{,}000$	
		$=$			
		$P(S^+\|D^+) =$ sensitivity $= 0.2$	$P(S^-\|D^-) =$ specificity $= 0.8$		

Table 8.1. Binary probability table representing the basic prototype for all subsequent 2 × 2 tables. The bold bordered cells partition the sample space under consideration into four mutually exhaustive and exclusive subsets corresponding to the four subsets of the equivalent Venn diagram. The double-ruled bordered cells represent the marginal values associated with the main four cells. The two cells in the outermost right border are reserved for the predictive values, whereas the two cells at the bottom are reserved for the sensitivity and specificity of the test under consideration. The two cells on the left subdivide the symptom/sign into binary values dictated by the cutoff point assigned by the examiner. The top three cells represent the subdivision of the sample universe into two subsets representing those in whom the disease is assumed to be present and those assumed to be free of the disease in question. The order of deployment of each cell shall remains constant throughout this monograph.

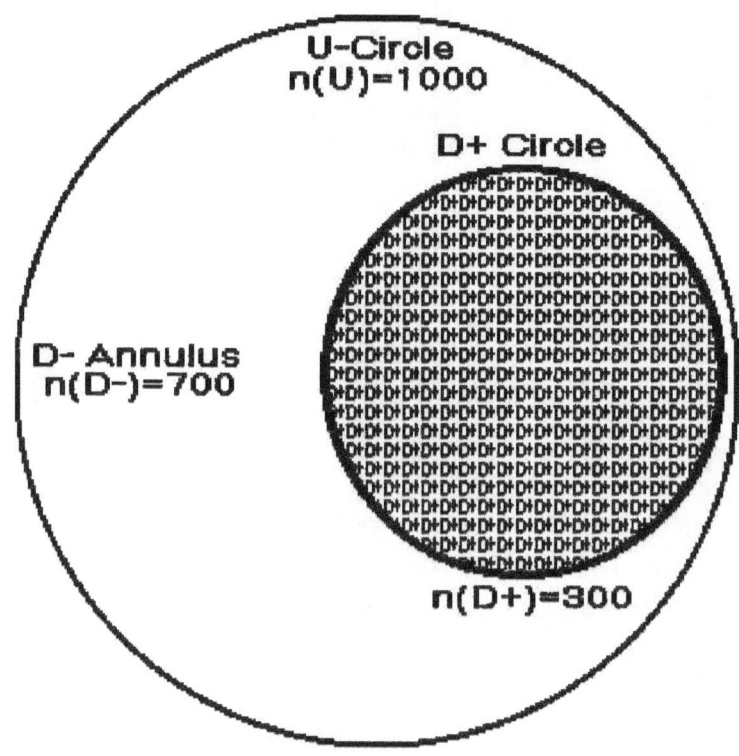

Figure 8.1. Venn diagram of the partition of the sample universe into two mutually exclusive and exhaustive subsets comprising patients assumed to carry the disease and patients assumed to be free from the disease. Note that the relative area of the D⁺ circle corresponds to the actual prevalence of the disease in the sample universe. Graphically, the D⁺ area is made equal to 300 units in comparison to the U circle of 1,000 units.

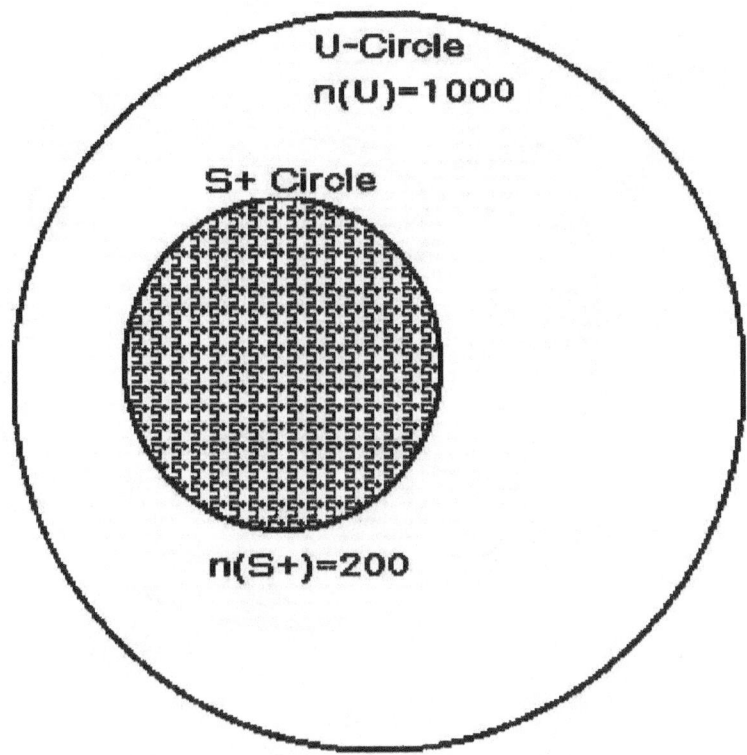

Figure 8.2 Venn diagram of the partition of the sample universe of 1,000 patients into two mutually exhaustive and exclusive subsets. The S⁺ circle area is numerically proportional to the number of patients reporting to the clinic with ACP. The S⁺ area together with its complement, the S⁻ area (i.e., patients presenting with other than ACP), constitute the sample universe at this clinic.

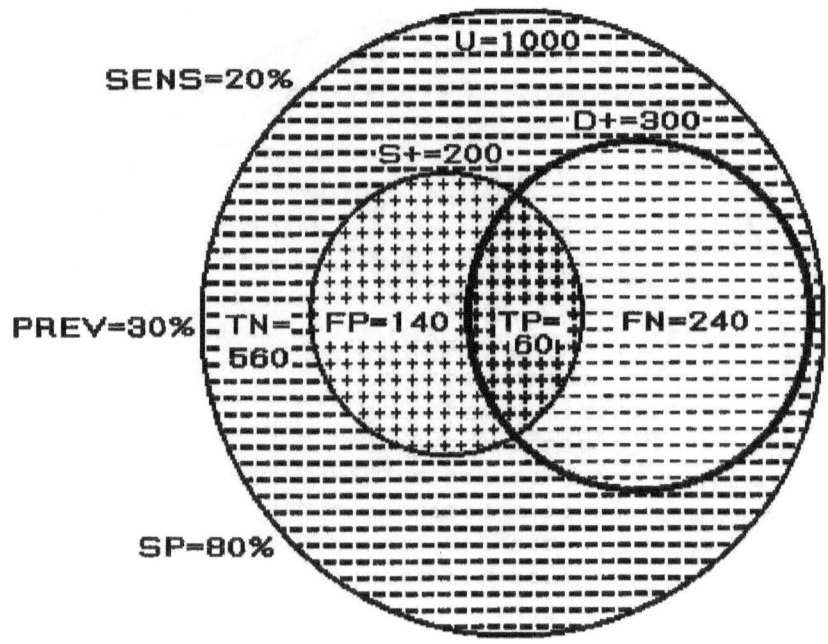

Figure 8.3. Venn diagram representation of the partition of the sample space into four mutually exclusive and exhaustive subsets corresponding to the binary 2 × 2 table. The diagram is drawn to scale such that the area of each subset relative to the universal area is correctly proportioned. In addition, the ratio of the two conditional probabilities may be visually estimated.

For the sensitivity, $P(S^+|D^+)$, the estimated ratio could be intuitively appreciated by comparing the intersection area to the D^+ circle area. Similarly, the predictive value, $P(D^+|S^+)$, could be appreciated by noting the ratio of the intersection area to the S^+ area.

Chapter 9

Bayes' Theorem: Formal Approach

Bayes' theorem is essentially a statement of conditional probabilities. This is best illustrated by reexamining the result of the diagnostic trial reproduced below (Table 9.1).

	Ca Confirmed Disease present	Ca Excluded Disease absent	Row Total
	D^+	D^-	
Positive test, T^+	24	14	$T^+ = 38$
Negative test, T^-	6	56	$T^- = 62$
Column total	$D^+ = 30$	$D^- = 70$	100

Table 9.1. A concise and simplified spreadsheet
of a hypothetical trial results

As it stands, the table is simply a mini spreadsheet of the trial results in which thirty proven cases and seventy excluded cases were subjected to a given test.

What is not readily discernible from the simple framework is that the table provides the necessary background from which two crucial questions of interest may be addressed and answered:

1. How good is the test in minimizing the erroneous or false test results both on the positive and negative side?
2. How accurate is the test result in differentiating the correctly identified and proven case from the falsely categorized?

The answer to these queries is of course the subject matter of this monograph.

To address these questions, we begin by recasting the numerical table in the equivalent probabilistic mode (Table 9.2). Obviously, given the sample space of the universe of one hundred cases, each cubicle represents the joint probability of its corresponding T and D elements, such that the sum of the probabilities of the four cubicles equals 1. The joint probability in each of the cells is of course the fraction of the area occupied by the particular subset from the total area of the universe set, which is also the disjointed area that issued from the fragmentation of the universe set as a result of the intersection of the T^+ and D^+ subsets (Figures 5.6 and 7.4).

Similarly, the marginal probabilities are now expressed as the sum of the joint probabilities of their respective column and row.

	Ca Confirmed Disease Present	Ca Excluded Disease Absent	P(row)
	D^+	D^-	
Positive test, T^+	$P(T^+ \cap D^+) = 0.24$	$P(T^+ \cap D^-) = 0.14$	$P(T^+) = 0.38$
Negative test, T^-	$P(T^- \cap D^+) = 0.06$	$P(T^- \cap D^-) = 0.56$	$P(T^-) = 0.62$
P(column)	$P(D^+) = 0.3$	$P(D^-) = 0.7$	1

Table 9.2. Joint and marginal probabilities of the trial results

The joint probabilities may now be individually expressed in terms of their corresponding conditional and marginal prior probability (Table 9.3 and Figure 9.1). With this transformation, it now becomes possible to address the first question, namely, how good is the test? Which, in terms of the probability notation, is succinctly expressed to read $P(T^+ \mid D^+)$ for the first equation, which rephrases the question by asking to address the probability of a positive test given the certainty of disease?

	Ca Confirmed Disease Present	Ca Excluded Disease Absent	P(row)
	D^+	D^-	
Positive test, T^+	Joint probability = conditional probability × prior probability Joint probability $P(T^+ \cap D^+) = 0.24$ Sensitivity $P(T^+ \mid D^+) \times P(D^+)$	Joint probability = conditional probability × prior probability Joint probability $P(T^+ \cap D^-) = 0.14$ $=$ 1–Sp $P(T^+ \mid D^-) \times P(D^-)$	Marginal $P(T^+) =$ $0.24 + 0.14$ $= 0.38$
Negative test, T^-	Joint Probability = Cond. Prob. × Prior Prob. Joint probability $P(T^- \cap D^+) = 0.06$ $=$ 1-Sn $P(T^- \mid D^+) \times P(D^+)$	Joint Probability = Cond. Prob. × Prior Prob. Joint Probability $P(T - \cap D-) = 0.56$ $=$ Specificity $P(T^- \mid D^-) \times P(D^-)$	Marginal $P(T^-) =$ $0.06 + 0.56$ $= 0.62$
P(column)	Marginal $P(D^+) =$ 0.3	Marginal $P(D^-)$ $= 0.7$	1

Table 9.3. Joint probabilities expressed in terms of their conditional and marginal probabilities

The four distinct joint probability equations may now be rearranged and expressed in terms of their respective conditional probability as follows:

$$P(T^+ | D^+) = \frac{P(T^+ \cap D^+)}{P(D^+)} = P(\text{positive test} | \text{given the presence of Ca}) \quad (9.1a)$$

$$P(T^+ | D^-) = \frac{P(T^+ \cap D^-)}{P(D^-)} = P(\text{positive test} | \text{given the absence of Ca}) \quad (9.1b)$$

$$P(T^- | D^+) = \frac{P(T^- \cap D^+)}{P(D^+)} = P(\text{negative test} | \text{given the presence of Ca}) \quad (9.1c)$$

$$P(T^- | D^-) = \frac{P(T^- \cap D^-)}{P(D^-)} = P(\text{negative test} | \text{given the absence of Ca}) \quad (9.1d)$$

The four conditional probabilities are actually two because equations 9.1a and 9.1c are complements of each other, whereas equations 9.1b and 9.1d are similarly related.

From the data in the basic table, the corresponding numerical values that may be assigned to the conditional probability are as follows:

$$P(T^+ | D^+) \frac{24/100}{30/100} = \frac{24}{30} = 0.8 = \text{sensitivity} = \text{true-positive rate}$$

$$P(T^+ | D^-) \frac{14/100}{70/100} = \frac{14}{70} = 0.2 = (1 - \text{specificity}) = \text{false-positive rate}$$

$$P(T^- | D^+) \frac{6/100}{30/100} = \frac{6}{30} = 0.2 = (1 - \text{sensitivity}) = \text{false-negative rate}$$

$$P(T^- | D^-) \frac{56/100}{70/100} = \frac{56}{70} = 0.8 = (\text{specificity}) = \text{true-negative rate}$$

Equations 9.1a and 9.1d thus define the characteristics of the test in question by noting its discriminating capacity in separating the true from the false for both the positive and the negative results. In this case, the test has been able to correctly identify 80 percent of the cases when positive or negative.

To address the second question as to how accurate are the test results, a change in perspective in viewing the basic data is required.

Suppose a person is selected at random from this population comprising the universal set of one hundred cases. What is the probability that this individual has the disease? Because 30 percent of the population have the disease and it is equally likely that any individual would be selected, we assign a probability of 0.3 to the event "disease present and confirmed" (Figure 9.2).

This probability $P(D^+) = P$(disease present) = 0.3 is referred to as *prior probability* in the sense that it is assigned prior the observation of any empirical information. Of course, $P(D^-) = 0.7$ is the corresponding prior probability that the individual "is free from the disease."

Assume that through repeated trials, it was determined that the new but imperfect diagnostic test T actually resulted in the sets of conditional probabilities noted previously that the test indicates the disease is present, that is, the test is positive, given that the person has the disease, 80 percent of the time,

$$P(T^+ \mid D^+) = 0.8 \text{ (sensitivity = TP rate)},$$

and the corresponding conditional probability that the test indicates the disease is absent, that is, the test is negative, given that the person does not have the disease, 80 percent of the time,

$$P(T^- \mid D^-) = 0.8 \text{ (specificity = TN rate)}.$$

If now, from the vantage point of this perspective where the test's sensitivity and specificity (conditional probabilities) have been defined together with the prevalence (prior probability) of the disease in question in the sample universe under consideration, a person is selected at random and given the test, the question that needs to be addressed is how accurate is the result in confirming or denying the actual presence or absence of the disease in this particular person?

In probability notation, the question is rephrased to read $P(D^+ \mid T^+)$, the conditional probability of confirmed disease given the test result as positive.

Verbally expressed as the probability, P(disease is present | positive test indicates the disease is present) = $P(D^+ \mid T^+)$ is referred to as a *posterior probability* or a *revised probability* because it is assigned after the observation of empirical or additional information.

As in the case of the conditional probabilities concerning sensitivity and specificity, two pairs of equations (two equations and their complements) may be derived from the basic definition of conditional probability and the application of probability rules.

$$\underset{\text{Posterior probability}}{P(D^+ \mid T^+)} = \frac{\overset{\text{Joint probability}}{P(T^+ \cap D^+)}}{P(T^+)} \qquad (9.2\text{a})$$

$$\underset{\text{Posterior probability}}{P(D^- \mid T^+)} = \frac{\overset{\text{Joint probability}}{P(T^- \cap D^+)}}{P(T^+)} \qquad (9.2\text{b})$$

$$\underset{\text{Posterior probability}}{P(D^- \mid T^-)} = \frac{\overset{\text{Joint probability}}{P(T^- \cap D^-)}}{P(T^-)} \qquad (9.2\text{c})$$

$$\underset{\text{Posterior probability}}{P(D^+ \mid T^-)} = \frac{\overset{\text{Joint probability}}{P(T^+ \cap D^-)}}{P(T^-)} \qquad (9.2\text{d})$$

The joint probability of $P(T^+$ and $D^+)$ in the numerator of equation 9.2a is computed by the multiplication rule, as follows:

$$P(T^+ \cap D^+) = P(D^+)P(T^+|D^+) \quad (9.\text{A})$$

Substituting in equation 9.2a, we obtain Bayes' theorem in its simplest form as follows:

$$P(D^+ | T^+) = \frac{P(T^+ | D^+) \bullet P(D^+)}{P(T^+)}.$$

$$\underset{\text{Posterior probability}}{P(D^+ | T^+)} = \underset{\text{Sensitivity}}{P(T^+ | D^+)} \times \frac{P(D^+)}{P(T^+)}. \qquad (9.3a)$$

Note that the posterior conditional probability is now a function of three variables, two of which were included in the initial conditions stipulated: $P(T^+ | D^+)$ being the sensitivity of the test in question and $P(D^+)$ assumed to be the accepted prevalence of the disease.

To compute the denominator, we observe that

$$P(T^+) = P(T^+ \cap D^+) \cup P(T^+ \cap D^-).$$

Hence,

$$P(T^+) = P(T^+ \cap D^+) + P(T^+ \cap D^-) \qquad (9.B)$$

because the two joint events (T^+ and D^+) and (T^+ and D^-) are mutually exclusive.

When the joint probabilities $P(T^+$ and $D^+)$ and $P(T^+$ and $D^-)$ are expressed in terms of their multiplication product, equation 9.B becomes

$$P(T^+) = P(T^+D^+) \times P(D^+) + P(T^+|D^-) \times P(D^-) \,(9.C)$$

Now substituting into the numerator of equation 9.3a the expression for the joint probability given in equation 9.A, and substituting into the denominator the marginal probability $P(T^+)$ given in equation 9.C, the expanded version of Bayes' theorem is obtained as follows:

$$P(D^+ | T^+) = \frac{P(T^+ | D^+) \bullet P(D^+)}{P(T^+ | D^+) \bullet P(D^+) + P(T^+ | D^-) \bullet P(D^-)}. \qquad (9.4a)$$

The substitution process used in the derivation of equation 9.4a could be repeated for equations 9.4b-9.4d, resulting in two pairs of equations, as follows:

$$P(D^- \mid T^+) = \frac{P(T^+ \mid D^-) \bullet P(D^-)}{P(T^+ \mid D^+) \bullet P(D^+) + P(T^+ \mid D^-) \bullet P(D^-)}.$$

(9.4b)
(complement of equation 9.4a)

$$P(D^+ \mid T^+) = \frac{P(T^- \mid D^-) \bullet P(D^-)}{P(T^- \mid D^+) \bullet P(D^+) + P(T^- \mid D^-) \bullet P(D^-)}.$$

(9.4c)

$$P(D^+ \mid T^+) = \frac{P(T^- \mid D^+) \bullet P(D^-)}{P(T^- \mid D^+) \bullet P(D^+) + P(T^- \mid D^-) \bullet P(D^-)}.$$

(9.4d)
(complement of equation 9.4c)

The derivation of Bayes' formulae (equations 9.4a and 9.4d) is reproduced in the classic binary format to delineate the relationship of the individual cellular components of the table to the variable factors that constitute the expanded version noted previously (Table 9.4 and Figure 9.2).

In terms of the disease example, substituting the known values into Bayes' theorem formula in equation 9.3a, we find that

$$P(D^+ \mid T^+) = \frac{(0.8)(0.3)}{(0.8)(0.3) + (0.2)(0.7)}.$$

$$P(D^+ \mid T^+) = \frac{0.24}{0.38} = 0.6316.$$

Hence, the posterior probability that the individual has the disease given that the test indicated the presence of the disease is 0.63 or 63 percent (Table 9.5 and Figure 9.3).

In summary, if a person was selected at random from this given population, the prior probability that the individual would have the disease is 0.3 or 30 percent. On the other hand, after we have the empirical information that the test indicated the disease is present, we revise the probability that the individual has the disease upward to 0.63 or 63 percent.

Although the posterior probability (0.63) is two times as large as the prior probability (0.3), 0.63 is still a fairly high probability, although not compelling, that the individual has the disease given that the test indicated the disease was present. This result, from the fact that there are large numbers of persons in this population who do not have the disease but for whom the test would (falsely), indicates that the disease is present.

In this chapter, two conditional probabilities were derived and illustrated. The critical difference between the two needs to be further emphasized.

The clinical conditional probability associated with sensitivity is the ratio of the intersection area to the D^+ area, which is another way of relating T^+ to the reduced sample space D^+

$$P(D^+ \mid T^+) = \frac{P(T^+ \cap D^+)}{P(D^+)} = \frac{\text{Intersection area}}{\text{Disease circle area}} = \frac{24}{30} = 0.8.$$

In the table format, this relationship may be equally translated to the ratio of the contents of the first main cell (bold bordered) to the marginal column at the bottom.

The diagnostic conditional probability associated with the posterior probability, on the other hand, relates the same intersection area to the T^+ circle by asking how much of D^+ is in the T^+ domain. In this case, the reduced sample space is T^+.

$$P(D^+ \mid T^+) = \frac{P(T^+ \cap D^+)}{P(T^+)} = \frac{\text{Intersection area}}{\text{Test circle area}} = \frac{24}{38} = 0.63.$$

Similarly, in the table format, this relationship may be equally translated to the ratio of the contents of the first main cell (bold bordered) to the marginal column at the left side of the bold bordered cells.

As we have seen, Bayes' theorem weighs prior information with empirical evidence. The manner in which it does this may be seen by laying out the calculations in table form (Table 9.4 and Figure 9.2).

The first row of the table addresses the key question of prevalence or prior probability. In practice, the answer to this question need not be restricted to data from epidemiological surveys, although they must be taken into consideration. In modern Bayesian decision theory, subjective prior probability assignments are made in many applications. Bayes' theorem is then a means of revising these probability assignments. For any one patient, the assigned probability is basically a reflection of the physician's tentative diagnosis in the case, prior to any definitive testing procedure. This means that subjective judgments and current quantitative knowledge are captured in the form of prior probabilities. The ratio $P(D^+)$ may thus be translated into the probability that the patient is tentatively believed to have the disease, whereas $P(D^-)$ signifies the probability that the patient is believed to be free of the disease

The second row is simply a numerical translation of the given probabilities for the number assigned to the sample set.

The third row, within the bold borders, gives the joint probabilities of the joint events as function of the conditional probability and the prior probability; namely, the conditional probabilities of the additional information given the basic events, in this case, $P(T^+ \mid D^+) = P$(test indicates disease is present given that the patient has the disease) = (sensitivity), and $P(T^+ \mid D^-) = P$(test indicates disease is present given that the patient does not have the disease) = $(1 -$ specificity), in conjunction with prior probabilities of $P(D^+)$ and $P(D^-)$.

Note that as indicated in equation 9.C, the sum of these joint probabilities is the marginal probability $P(T^+)$. When the joint probability in the first cell is divided by the sum of the joint probabilities of the corresponding row, $P(T^+)$, the results are the posterior or revised probability shown in the last cell of the last column.

The same procedure applied to each of the four cells results in the four posterior probabilities noted previously (equations 9.4a-9.4d).

The fifth row, first cell, is the equivalent marginal probability $P(D^+)$ for the first column, which is the sum of the joint probabilities of the corresponding column. When the joint probability in the first cell is divided by the sum of the joint probabilities of the corresponding column, $P(D^+)$, the result is the sensitivity shown in the first cell of the last row.

The same procedure is applicable to each of the four cells resulting in the four conditional probabilities of sensitivity and specificity and their corresponding complements.

Reviewing Bayes' formula again, we note that in this instance the following:

The basic format:

$$P(D^+ \mid T^+) = \frac{P(D^+) \times P(T^+ \mid D^+)}{P(T^+)}. \quad (9.3a)$$

The expanded format:

$$P(D^+ \mid T^+) = \frac{P(D^+)P(T^+ \mid D^+)}{P(D^+)P(T^+ \mid D^+) + P(D^-)P(T^+ \mid D^-)}. \quad (9.4a)$$

The expanded format translated into the equivalent conditional probabilities of sensitivity and specificity and nonconditional probability of prevalence or prior probability, as follows:

$$P(D^+ \mid T^+ = \frac{(\text{Prevalence})(\text{Sensitivity})}{(\text{Prevalence})(\text{Sensitivity}) + (1 - \text{prevalence})(1 - \text{specificity})}.$$

Where the variables may be defined as follows:

1. $P(D^+)$: the prevalence, same as originally estimated
2. $P(D^-)$: the complement of prevalence
2. $P(T^+)$: the T^+ circle area, which is a function of both sensitivity and specificity as well as the prevalence
3. $P(T^+ \mid D^+)$: sensitivity, calculated from the experimentally derived binary table entries
4. $P(T^+ \mid D^-)$: complement of specificity $(1 - \text{specificity})$ calculated from the experimentally derived binary table entries

The various formats of the two main posterior probability formulae and their corresponding complements are tabled and individually graphed in order to avert the possible confusion that may arise from the use of the complement of any formula (see Appendix for additional detail).

9.1 Bayes' Theorem: Odds and Likelihood Alternative

As noted in Figure 12.1, the probability of D^+ in a given population that constitute the sample universe is the ratio of the number of persons with the disease to the total number of individuals in the sample population both with and without the disease.

$$P(D^+) = \frac{n(D^+)}{n(U)} = \frac{n(D^+)}{n(D^+) + n(D^-)} = \frac{s\,(\text{successes})}{s\,(\text{successes}) + f\,(\text{failures})}.$$

Similarly, the probability of D^- in a given population is the ratio of the number of persons without the disease to the total number of individuals in the sample population both with and without the disease.

$$P(D^-) = \frac{n(D^-)}{n(U)} = \frac{n(D^-)}{n(D^+)+n(D^-)} = \frac{f\,(\text{failures})}{s\,(\text{successes})+f\,(\text{failures})}.$$

By contrast, the odds in favor of D^+ is the ratio of the number of persons with the disease to the number of persons without the disease.

$$\text{Odds in favor of } D^+ = \frac{P(D^+)}{P(D^-)} = \frac{P(D^+)}{1-P(D^+)} = \frac{n(D^+)}{n(D^-)} = \frac{s}{f}.$$

Similarly, the odds against D^+ is the ratio of the number of persons without the disease to the number of persons with the disease.

$$\text{Odds against } D^+ = \frac{P(D^-)}{P(D^+)} = \frac{1-P(D^+)}{P(D^+)} = \frac{n(D^-)}{n(D^+)} = \frac{f}{s}.$$

The conversion from one format to the other, as noted in the following equations, is in accordance with the standard conversion formulae detailed earlier.

Convert probability $\Rightarrow$ Odds in favor

$$\frac{P}{1-p} = \frac{P(D+)}{1-P(D+)} = \frac{P(D+)}{P(D-)} = \text{Odds (F)}.$$

Convert Probability $\Rightarrow$ Odds against

$$\frac{1-P}{p} = \frac{P(D+)}{1-P(D+)} = \frac{P(D-)}{P(D+)} = \text{Odds (A)}.$$

Convert odds in favor $\Rightarrow$ Probability

$$\frac{\text{Odds(F)}}{\text{Odds(F)}+1} = P(\text{D}+).$$

Convert odds against $\Rightarrow$ Probability

$$\frac{1}{\text{Odds}(A)+1} = P(\text{D}+).$$

Posterior Probability: The Odds Alternative

One need not be reminded that the goal of the exercise whether using classical probability or its variant of odds and likelihood is essentially identical. In both cases, one is interested in the final diagnostic probability or odds of disease given the results of the test. Thus, instead of the desired predictive value of a positive test (posterior or revised probability given a positive test), the concept of posterior odds for disease given a positive test result is substituted. In terms of the conditional probability notation, the difference between the two variants is formulated as follows:

Posterior probability for D^+, given a positive test $= P(\text{D}^+|T^+)$

Posterior odds in favor of D^+ given a positive test $= \dfrac{P(\text{D}+\,|\,\text{T}+)}{P(\text{D}-\,|\,\text{T}+)}$

The odds variants are therefore a statement of the ratio of probability of disease to the absence of disease given a positive test result. Graphically, this can be demonstrated using the following transformation.

Graphically then, the posterior odds for disease given a positive test result reflects the division of the T^+ circle into its complementary subsets of TP and FP as expressed by the ratio for/against the disease in the presence of T^+.

Similarly, the posterior odds for the presence of disease against its absence in the presence of negative test result is graphically denoted by the subdivision of the T-ring into the subsets of FN and TN. The ratio of these two complementary subsets is then the graphic equivalent of the odds ratio.

Missing from this formulation is the intermediate step that bridges the gap between the prior odds and the posterior odds. This is now furnished by the innovative introduction of the likelihood ratio.

$$\frac{P(T^+ \mid D^+)}{P(T^+ \mid D^-)} = \frac{\text{Probability of } T^+ \text{ in a person with } D^+}{\text{Probability of } T^+ \text{ in a person with } D^-} = \text{Likelihood ratio for a positive } T^+ : LR^+.$$

Thus, as can be readily noted, the likelihood ratio for a positive test (T⁺) translates as the ratio of true-positive rate (Sens) to that of false-positive rate (1 − Sp), such that

$$\frac{P(T^+ \mid D^+)}{P(T^+ \mid D^-)} = \frac{\text{Sensitivity}}{1-\text{Specificity}} = \frac{TP}{TP+FN} \times \frac{TN+FP}{FP} = \frac{TP}{D^+} \times \frac{D^-}{FP} = \left[\frac{D^-}{D^+} \times \frac{TP}{FP} \right] = LR + \text{ for } T^+.$$

And the likelihood ratio for a negative test (T⁻) is similarly defined by the following relationship:

$$\frac{P(T^- \mid D^+)}{P(T^- \mid D^-)} = \frac{\text{Probability of } T^- \text{ in a person with } D^+}{\text{Probability of } T^- \text{ in a person with } D^-} = \text{Likelihood ratio for negative } T^- : LR^-.$$

Similarly, the likelihood ratio for a negative (T⁻) translated as the ratio of false-negative rate (1 − Sens) to that of the true-negative rate (Sp), such that

$$\frac{P(T^- \mid D^+)}{P(T^- \mid D^-)} = \frac{1-\text{Sensitivity}}{\text{Specificity}} = \frac{FN}{TP+FN} \times \frac{TN+FP}{TN} = \frac{FN}{D^+} \times \frac{D^-}{TN} = \left[\frac{D^-}{D^+} \times \frac{FN}{TN} \right] = LR^- \text{ for } T^-.$$

When the likelihood ratio for positive T⁺ is multiplied by the prior odds for D⁺, the posterior odds of D⁺ given T⁺ is obtained as follows:

$$\underset{\text{Prior odds}}{\left[\frac{D^+}{D^-}\right]} \times \underset{\text{Likelihood ratio}}{\left[\frac{D^-}{D^+} \times \frac{TP}{FP}\right]} = \frac{TP}{FP} = \text{Posterior odds for } D^+ \text{ given } T^+.$$

The posterior odds for D^+ and T^- and a prior odds for D^+ are obtained in a similar fashion.

$$\underset{\text{Prior odds}}{\left[\frac{D^+}{D^-}\right]} \times \underset{\text{Likelihood ratio}}{\left[\frac{D^+}{D^-} \times \frac{FN}{TN}\right]} = \frac{FN}{TN} = \text{Posterior odds for } D^+ \text{ given } T^-.$$

Finally, the intrinsic relationship between the two variant of posterior probability is made distinctly clear from the following equality:

$$\text{Posterior odds for } D^+ \text{ given } T^+ = \frac{P(D^+ \mid T^+)}{P(D^- \mid T^+)} = \frac{PV[+]}{1 - PV[+]} = \frac{TPIT^+}{FPIT^+} = \frac{TP}{FP}.$$

And

$$\text{Posterior odds for } D^+ \text{ given } T^- = \frac{P(D^+ \mid T^-)}{P(D^- \mid T^-)} = \frac{1 - PV[-]}{PV[-]} = \frac{FNIT^-}{TNIT^-} = \frac{FN}{TN}.$$

	Pretest probability = Prevalence	Pretest probability = 1 − Prevalence	Prior odds = Prevalence + 1 − Prevalence	
	$P(D^+) = \dfrac{n(D^+)}{n(D^+)+n(D^-)}$	$P(D^-) = \dfrac{n(D^-)}{n(D^+)+n(D^-)}$	Prior odds $= \dfrac{P(D^+)}{P(D^-)}$	
	Disease present $= P(D^+) \times n(U) = n(D^+)$	Disease absent $P(D^-) \times n(U) = n(D^-)$	Sample universe $n(D^+) + n(D^-) = n(U)$	
T^+	Conditional Probability — Sensitivity $P(T^+ \mid D^+) = \dfrac{P(T^+ \cap D^+)}{P(D^+)}$	Conditional Probability — 1−Specificity $P(T^+ \mid D^-) = \dfrac{P(T^+ \cap D^-)}{P(D^-)}$	Likelihood ratio for T^+ $LR^+ = \dfrac{P(T^+\mid D^+)}{P(T^+\mid D^-)} = \dfrac{Sn}{1-Sp}$	Posterior odds for D^+ — Prior odds for D^+ × LR for T^+ $\dfrac{P(D^+\mid T^+)}{P(D^-\mid T^+)} = \dfrac{P(D^+)}{P(D^-)} \times \dfrac{P(T^+\mid D^+)}{P(T^+\mid D^-)}$
T^-	Conditional Probability — 1−Sensitivity $P(T^- \mid D^+) = \dfrac{P(T^- \cap D^+)}{P(D^+)}$	Conditional Probability — Specificity $P(T^- \mid D^-) = \dfrac{P(T^- \cap D^-)}{P(D^-)}$	Likelihood ratio for T^- $LR^- = \dfrac{P(T^-\mid D^+)}{P(T^-\mid D^-)} = \dfrac{1-Sn}{Sp}$	Posterior odds for D^+ — Prior odds for D^+ × LR for T^- $\dfrac{P(D^+\mid T^-)}{P(D^-\mid T^-)} = \dfrac{P(D^+)}{P(D^-)} \times \dfrac{P(T^-\mid D^+)}{P(T^-\mid D^-)}$
	Sensitivity $P(T^+ \mid D^+) = \dfrac{TP}{TP+FN}$ $\quad$ 1 − Sensitivity $P(T^- \mid D^+) = \dfrac{FN}{TP+FN}$	Specificity $P(T^- \mid D^-) = \dfrac{TN}{TN+FP}$ $\quad$ 1 − specificity $P(T^+ \mid D^-) = \dfrac{FP}{TN+FP}$		

Table 9.4. Basic odds table

Any Given Disease

	Pretest probability	Pretest probability	Prior odds	Posterior odds
	$P(D^+) = \dfrac{n(D^+)}{n(D^+)+n(D^-)}$	$P(D^-) = \dfrac{n(D^-)}{n(D^+)+n(D^-)}$	Prior odds $= \dfrac{P(D^+)}{P(D^-)}$	
	$P(D^+) =$	$P(D^-) =$	Prior odds $=$	
	Disease present $= P(D^+) \times n(U) = n(D^+)$	Disease absent $P(D^-) \times n(U) = n(D^-)$	Sample universe $n(D^+) + n(D^-) = n(U)$	
	$n(D^+) =$	$n(D^-) =$	$n(U) =$	
T^+	True positive $n(D^+) \times Sn = n(TP)$	False positive $n(D^-) - n(TN) = n(FP)$	Likelihood ratio for T^+ $\boxed{LR^+ = \dfrac{Sn}{1-Sp}}$	Posterior odds for D^+ Prior odds for $D^+ \times LR^+ =$ Post odds for T^+ $\boxed{\dfrac{P(D^+)}{P(D^-)} \times LR^+ = \text{Post odds}}$
	$n(TP) =$	$n(FP) =$	$LR^+ =$	Post odds $=$
	False negative $n(D^+) - n(TP) = n(FN)$	True negative $n(D^-) \times Sp = n(TN)$		
	$n(FN) =$	$n(TN) =$		
T^-	Sensitivity $\boxed{P(T^+ \mid D^+) = \dfrac{TP}{TP+FN}}$	Specificity $\boxed{P(T^- \mid D^-) = \dfrac{TN}{TN+FP}}$	Likelihood ratio for T^- $\boxed{LR^- = \dfrac{1-Sn}{Sp}}$	Posterior odds for D^+ Prior odds for $D^+ \times LR^- =$ Post odds for T^- $\boxed{\dfrac{P(D^+)}{P(D^-)} \times LR^- = \text{Post odds}}$
	$Sn =$	$Sp =$	$LR^- =$	Post odds $=$
	1 − Sensitivity $\boxed{P(T^- \mid D^+) = \dfrac{FN}{TP+FN}}$	1 − Specificity $\boxed{P(T^+ \mid D^-) = \dfrac{FP}{TN+FP}}$		
	$1 - Sn =$	$1 - Sp =$		

Table 9.5. Practical Odds Table

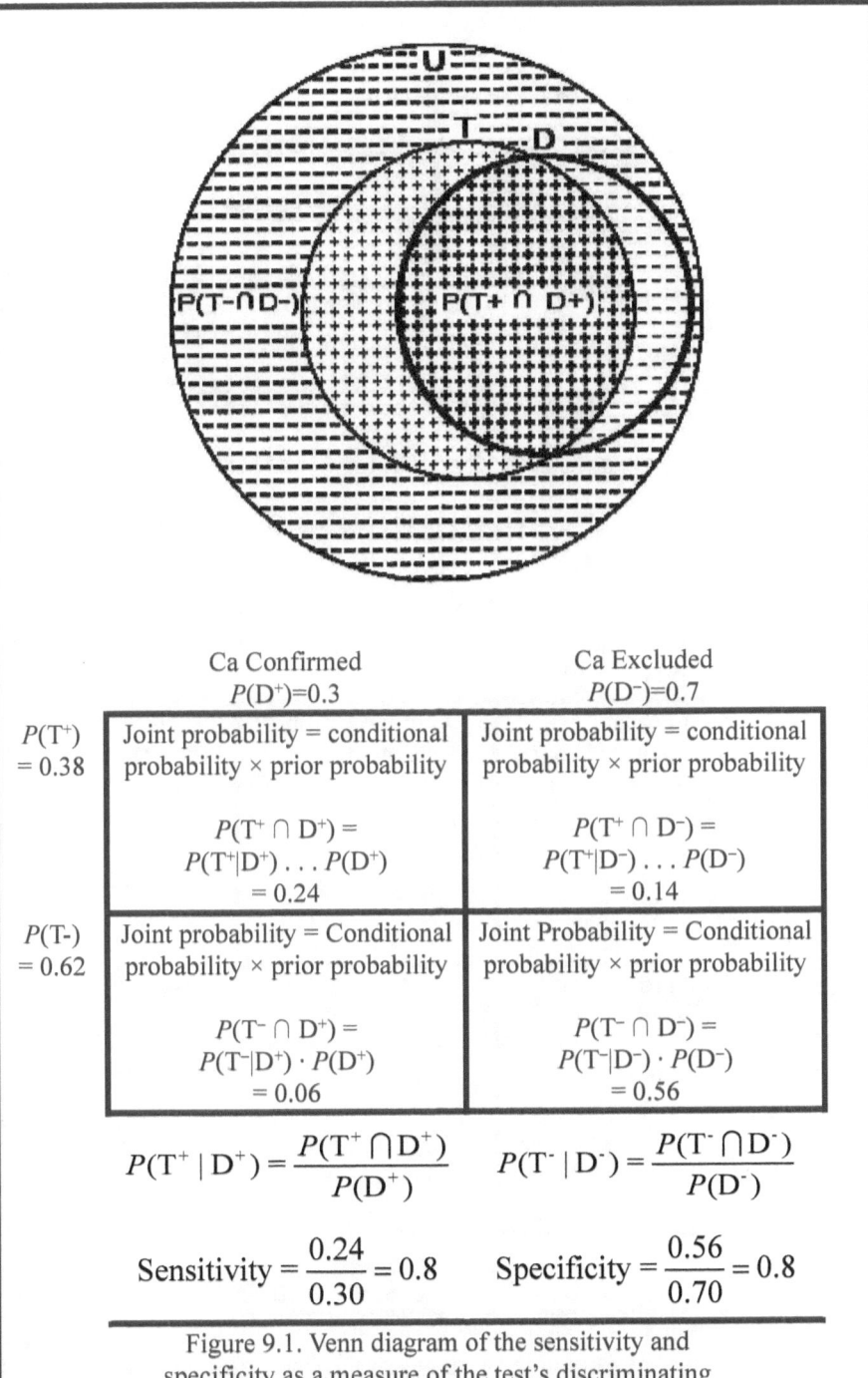

	Ca Confirmed $P(D^+)=0.3$	Ca Excluded $P(D^-)=0.7$
$P(T^+)$ = 0.38	Joint probability = conditional probability × prior probability $P(T^+ \cap D^+) =$ $P(T^+\|D^+) \dots P(D^+)$ = 0.24	Joint probability = conditional probability × prior probability $P(T^+ \cap D^-) =$ $P(T^+\|D^-) \dots P(D^-)$ = 0.14
$P(T\text{-})$ = 0.62	Joint probability = Conditional probability × prior probability $P(T^- \cap D^+) =$ $P(T^-\|D^+) \cdot P(D^+)$ = 0.06	Joint Probability = Conditional probability × prior probability $P(T^- \cap D^-) =$ $P(T^-\|D^-) \cdot P(D^-)$ = 0.56

$$P(T^+ \mid D^+) = \frac{P(T^+ \cap D^+)}{P(D^+)} \qquad P(T^- \mid D^-) = \frac{P(T^- \cap D^-)}{P(D^-)}$$

$$\text{Sensitivity} = \frac{0.24}{0.30} = 0.8 \qquad \text{Specificity} = \frac{0.56}{0.70} = 0.8$$

Figure 9.1. Venn diagram of the sensitivity and specificity as a measure of the test's discriminating capacity in separating the true from the false.

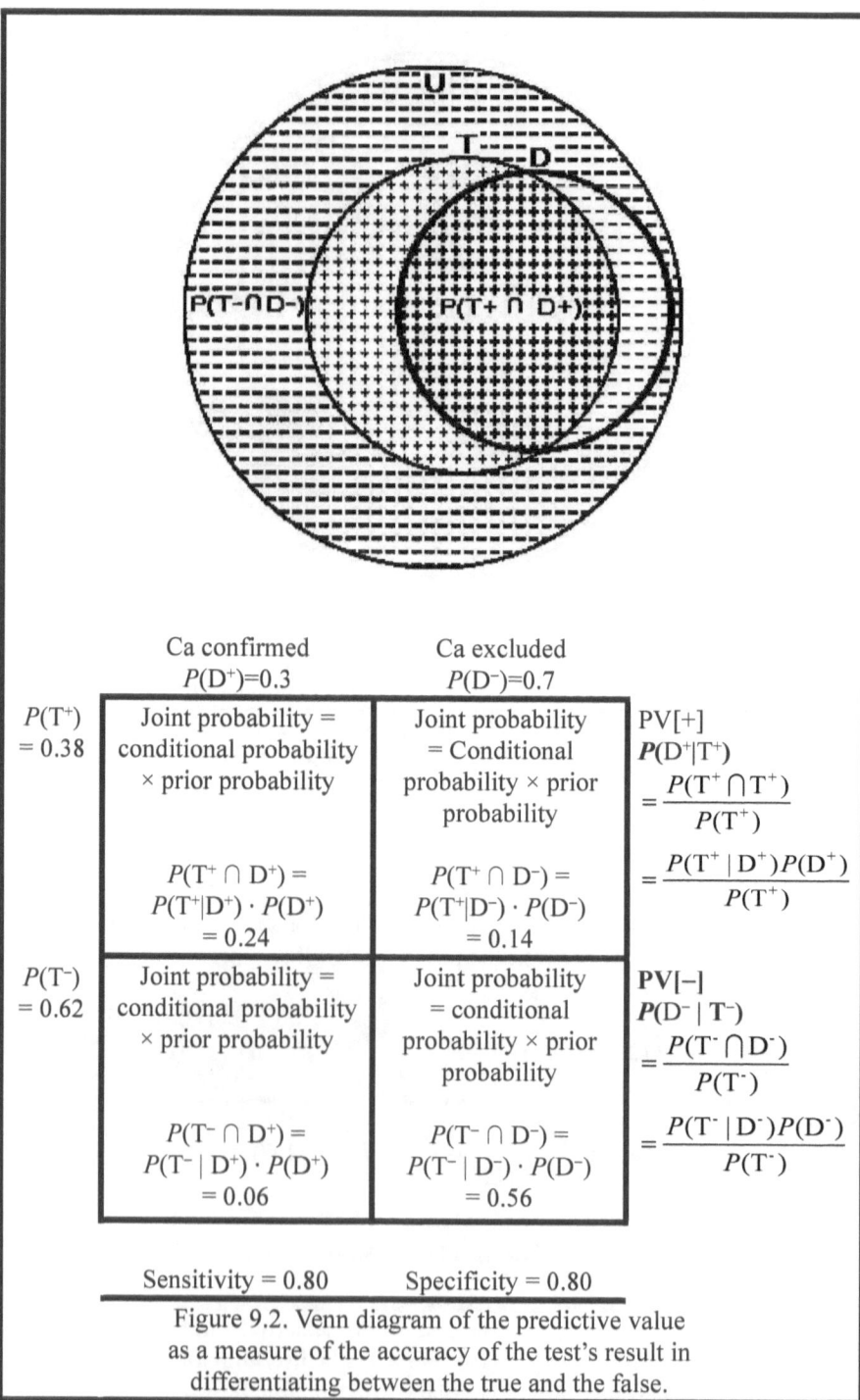

	Ca confirmed $P(D^+)=0.3$	Ca excluded $P(D^-)=0.7$	
$P(T^+)$ $= 0.38$	Joint probability = conditional probability × prior probability $P(T^+ \cap D^+) =$ $P(T^+|D^+) \cdot P(D^+)$ $= 0.24$	Joint probability = Conditional probability × prior probability $P(T^+ \cap D^-) =$ $P(T^+|D^-) \cdot P(D^-)$ $= 0.14$	PV[+] $P(D^+|T^+)$ $= \dfrac{P(T^+ \cap T^+)}{P(T^+)}$ $= \dfrac{P(T^+ \mid D^+)P(D^+)}{P(T^+)}$
$P(T^-)$ $= 0.62$	Joint probability = conditional probability × prior probability $P(T^- \cap D^+) =$ $P(T^- \mid D^+) \cdot P(D^+)$ $= 0.06$	Joint probability = conditional probability × prior probability $P(T^- \cap D^-) =$ $P(T^- \mid D^-) \cdot P(D^-)$ $= 0.56$	PV[−] $P(D^- \mid T^-)$ $= \dfrac{P(T^- \cap D^-)}{P(T^-)}$ $= \dfrac{P(T^- \mid D^-)P(D^-)}{P(T^-)}$

Sensitivity = 0.80   Specificity = 0.80

Figure 9.2. Venn diagram of the predictive value
as a measure of the accuracy of the test's result in
differentiating between the true and the false.

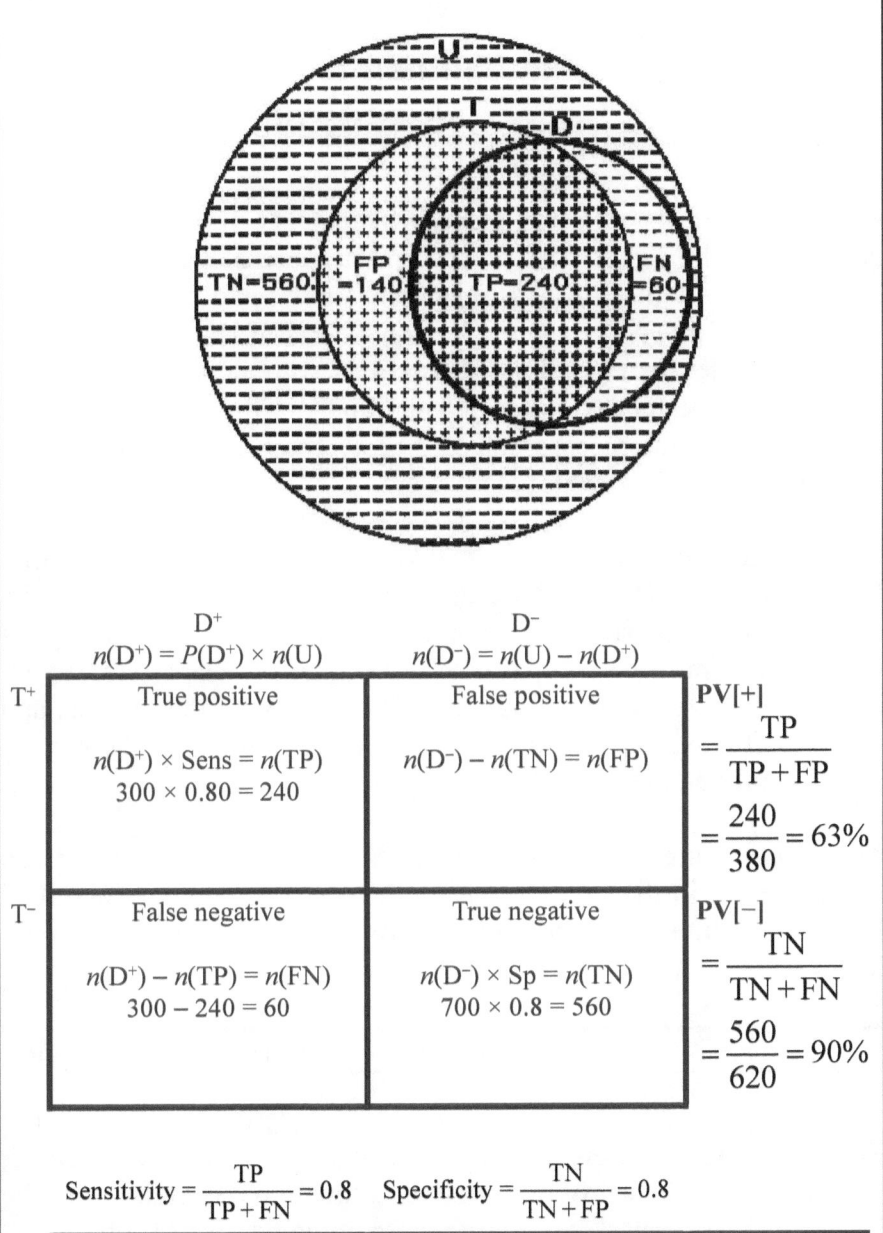

Figure 9.3. Venn diagram of the partition of the sample universe into true- and false-positive and true- and false-negative subsets corresponding to the joint probabilities. The conditional probabilities denoted by the predictive value, sensitivity, and specificity may also be expressed in the alternative notation.

Chapter 10

Prevalence, Sensitivity, Specificity, and Predictive Value

10.1 Graphic Overview

Graphical representation of the basic elements of Bayes' theorem begins with the assignment of specific number of individuals with and without the disease to the sample universe to be individually tested for the given disease by the application of test T. The sample universe circle, the U circle, is then drawn with an area numerically representing the total number of individuals in the sample universe known to have the disease and to be free from the disease that are being tested for the specific disease entity.

The disease circle, D^+ circle, is then drawn with an area representing the actual number of individuals who were known to have the disease prior to the administration of the test. The D^+ circle partitions the U circle into two compartments: an inner disease circle, the D^+ circle to include the actual number of patients with the disease, and an outer D^- ring that includes the balance of patients in the sample universe proven to be free from the disease in question (Figure 8.1).

The D^+ circle area, therefore, represents the prevalence of the given disease entity in the sample universe under consideration, assumed to number 1,000 in this presentation, multiplied by the total number in the sample universe so that (Table 9.4)

$$D^+ \text{ circle area} = n(D^+) = \text{prevalence} \times n(U) = P(D^+) \times n(U).$$

The outer ring or the annulus, the D^- ring surrounding the D^+ circle, includes the balance of individuals known to be free from the disease. The D^- ring is of course the complement of D^+ circle and includes all those proven to be free of the disease, such that

$$n(D^+) + n(D^-) = n(U) = \text{total number in the sample universe}$$

$$n(D^-) = (1 - \text{prevalence}) \times n(U) = P(D^-) \times n(U)$$

302

The sample universe circle with both its subsets of D^+ and D^- is then tested for the disease in question, again subdividing the sample universe into two different and complementary compartments, an inner T^+ circle compartment to include all those who tested positive and an outer T^- ring to include all those who tested negative (Figure 8.2).

The area of the T^+ circle may be considered as a composite of fusion of the two disjointed subsets: $(T^+ \cap D^+) + (T^+ \cap D^-)$ as noted in the disjointed Venn diagram (Figure 10.2.). The T^+ circle area may thus be calculated given the probability of each subset, that is, the probabilities associated with the top two cells of the binary table. The sum of these probabilities is of course the marginal probability $P(T^+) = P(T^+ \cap D^+) + (T^+ \cap D^-)$ (Table 9.4). The T^+ circle area may now be calculated as in the case of the D^+ circle area in the following manner:

$$T^+ \text{ circle area} = \text{marginal } P(T^+) \times n(U).$$

The area of the T^+ circle and the extent of its intersection with the D^+ circle are determined by interplay of the three independent variables of sensitivity, specificity, and prevalence, as noted in the following equation, in which the two joint probabilities are depicted in terms of the sensitivity and specificity as well as the prevalence:

$$T^+ \text{ circle area} = n(T^+) = [(\text{prevalence})(\text{sensitivity}) + (1 - \text{prevalence})(1 - \text{specificity})] \times n(U).$$

As noted in Figure 8.3, the intersection of the T^+ circle with the D^+ circle, however, subdivides each of the intersecting circles into two compartments, with one compartment shared in between the intersecting circles, resulting in the subdivision of the U circle into four compartments, with three of these remaining within the D^+ and T^+ circles and the fourth occupying the space left over outside the intersecting circles and the U circle. Given a sample universe with a given disease prevalence, the deciding factor in the size allocation of the compartments within the U circle depends on the size and extent of intersection of the T^+ circle with the D^+ circle, which as noted earlier is a function of the several parameters that comprise the operating characteristics of the test under consideration.

10.2 Sensitivity

Ideally, sensitivity is best defined as the conditional probability of a positive test result given the presence of a true disease condition,

$$\underset{\text{Sensitivity}}{P(T^+ \mid D^+)} = \frac{\overset{\text{Joint probability}}{P(T^+ \cap D^+)}}{\underset{\text{Prevalence}}{P(D^+)}}.$$

Sensitivity may be equally defined using the numerical equivalent of the ratio of the joint probability and the marginal probability of D^+ (prevalence). Alternatively, the areas depicted in the Venn diagram as tabled and entered in the corresponding binary table are equally valid equivalent (Figures 7.4 and 7.5 and Tables 7.1 and 7.2).

$$\text{Sensitivity} = \overset{\text{Sensitivity}}{P(T^+ \mid D^+)} = \frac{TP}{TP + FN} = \text{TP rate} = \text{TP\%}.$$

In descriptive and graphic terms, sensitivity may be depicted as follows:

♦ The percentage of patients with the disease that are correctly labeled and identified by the test as positive (TP) from the total number of diseased patients labeled both as truly positive and mislabeled as false negative (TP + FN)
♦ The percentage of T^+ results in patients with the disease
♦ The proportion of patients with disease in whom the test is positive
♦ T^+ circle intersection with D circle (TP) as a percentage of the full D circle area (TP + FN)

10.3 Levels of Sensitivity: Diagnostic Implication

In actual practice, the probability assigned to a particular test is the result of the clinical assessment of the ratio of a true-positive result to the total of both the correctly labeled and interpreted true positive and the falsely interpreted and labeled as negative (i.e., positive, but misinterpreted and labeled negative) test result under controlled field conditions.

$$\uparrow Sn = \frac{TP}{TP + FN \downarrow} = <1 = <100\%.$$

As noted in the preceding relation, sensitivity of a given test is inversely proportional to its FN component. Thus, the sensitivity of a given test rests essentially on its discriminating power to avoid miscalling or labeling a proven disease entity test result as negative (i.e., false negative).

$$\uparrow\uparrow Sn = \frac{TP}{TP + \underset{\to 0}{FN}} = \frac{TP}{TP} = \to 1 = \to 100\%.$$

A highly sensitive test implies a small number of FN so that in the limit as the number of FN approaches 0, sensitivity as defined by the ratio TP / (TP + FN) approaches 1 or 100 percent, implying maximum sensitivity. A theoretical sensitivity of 100 percent (FN = 0) stipulates the absence of false-negative results so that the presence of disease is never falsely mislabeled as negative, but it (100 percent sensitivity) implicitly guarantees the authenticity of true-negative result. Stated differently, a negative test outcome, in the context of maximal sensitivity, is 100 percent true negative,

$$FN \to 0, TN \to 100 \text{ percent.}$$

Simultaneously, it allows the test to detect all proven disease entities under consideration (Figures 10.1 and 10.4).

Thus, a positive test with maximal sensitivity is capable of correctly labeling and identifying all patients with the disease because 100 percent or all true-positive patients encompassed by the D^+ circle are now a proper subset of the T^+ circle. Note, however, that the T^+ circle includes in addition a false-positive subset surrounding the D^+ circle. Thus, a maximally sensitive test is unable to exclude a certain percentage of patients that were mislabeled as positive although they are actually free from the disease (FP).

The previously mentioned obvious relations lead to the following conclusions:

1. Positive test, T^+, detects all proven disease entities, D^+ (100 percent), although it also mislabels a certain percentage of disease free as false positive.
2. Negative test T^-, detects all truly negative cases (i.e., it never miscalls a real case disease, D^+, as negative (FN = 0).

The surprising corollary of the previously mentioned conclusions is not the obvious conclusion that a highly sensitive test as the name implies is ideally suited for the detection of proven cases such that a T^+ confirms the presence of D^+, which carries the mnemonic PID (positivity in disease), but the not-so-obvious fact that a negative test rules out the presence of the disease being tested, that is, a true-positive case; thus,

$\therefore$ $T^- \Rightarrow$ 100 percent TN $\Rightarrow$ rules out D^+ (the disease in question).

	Prevalence $P(D^+)$	1 − Prevalence $P(D^-)$	
T^+	$1 \times n(D^+) = n(D^+)$ $= TP$	FP = 0	Predictive value $PV[+] = P(D^+\mid T^+) = \dfrac{TP}{TP + \underset{=0}{FP}} = \dfrac{TP}{TP} = 1$
			Predictive error $1 - PV[+] = P(D^-\mid T^+) = \dfrac{\overset{=0}{FP}}{TP + FP} = 0$
$T-$	FN = 0	$1 \times n(D^-) = n(D^-)$ $= TN$	Predictive value $PV[-] = P(D^-\mid T^-) = \dfrac{TN}{TN + \underset{=0}{FN}} = 1$
			Predictive error $1 - PV[-] = P(D^+\mid T\_) = \dfrac{\overset{=0}{FN}}{TN + FN} = 0$

Sensitivity $$P(T^+ \mid D^+) = \frac{P(T^+ \cap D^+)}{P(D^+)}$$	**Specificity** $$P(T^- \mid D^-) = \frac{P(T^- \cap D^-)}{P(D^-)}$$
$$Sn = \frac{TP}{\underset{=0}{TP + FN}} = 1$$	$$Sp = \frac{TN}{\underset{=0}{TN + FP}} = 1$$
1-Sensitivity $$P(T^- \mid D^+) = \frac{P(T^- \cap D^+)}{P(D^+)}$$	**1-Specificity** $$P(T^+ \mid D^-) = \frac{P(T^+ \cap D^-)}{P(D^-)}$$
$$1 - Sn = \frac{\overset{=0}{FN}}{TP + FN} = 0$$	$$1 - Sp = \frac{\overset{=0}{FP}}{TN + FP} = 0$$

Table 10.1. Theoretical results of maximal sensitivity and specificity

The previous equation is the basis of the mnemonic Sn/N/out (sensitivity/negative/R/out the presence of the disease under investigation). The implication of this unexpected conclusion translates that a highly sensitive test is not the ideal test for mass testing in order to detect and confirm the presence of disease on a population cohort, but rather as diagnostic tool in the differential Dx where the R/out result helps to narrow the field of inquiry.

Moreover, the higher the sensitivity, the less the false negative and the greater the predictive value of negative test (not the positive) and thus the more likely a negative test will correspond to the absence of the disease in question, thus excluding it from the differential (Figures 10.1 and 10.4).

Finally, note given the theoretical assumption of 100 percent sensitivity, the predictive value of a negative test, T⁻, is equivalently 100 percent, "PV[−] = 1," because the false negative is now assumed to be absent (FN = 0), which further confirms the screening potential of a highly sensitive test (Table 10.1).

A positive test is thus not fully predictive of disease because of the admixture of false-positive results. Thus, the disease cannot be ruled in with certainty.

Positive T⁺: ◆ Implies very high probability that the patient is correctly identified and classified as diseased, although with less than 100 percent certainty because of the admixture of the FP in the positive results.

A negative test with maximal sensitivity identifies all patients known to be free from the disease because no false negative is possible given 100 percent sensitivity. A negative test is thus fully predictive of the absence of disease. A test that turns out to be negative is a true negative, which now encompasses the total area outside the T⁺ circle, that is, the complement of T⁺.

Negative T⁻:   ◆ Absolutely rules out the disease in question with 100 percent certainty (FN = 0)
       ◆ Excludes a given diagnostic possibility

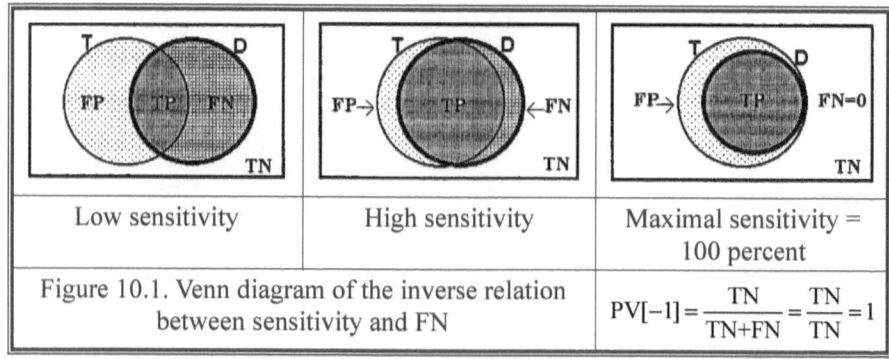

Low sensitivity	High sensitivity	Maximal sensitivity = 100 percent
Figure 10.1. Venn diagram of the inverse relation between sensitivity and FN		$PV[-1] = \dfrac{TN}{TN+FN} = \dfrac{TN}{TN} = 1$

10.4 Indication for High-Sensitivity Tests

Maximum sensitivity is required under the following conditions:

◆ To rule out the disease in question with 100 percent certainty (no FN)
◆ To screen for the absence of disease at large given that a false-negative result is rare
◆ To exclude the disease from the differential

The corollary of maximal sensitivity, given an FN value of 0 percent, is a maximal predictive value for negative test, $P(D^-|T^-)$ = 100 percent, which attests to the exclusion reliability of the test result such that the probability of no disease given the negative result is 100 percent or, alternatively, the probability of disease given a negative test, $P(D^+|T^-)$, is 0 percent (Table 10.1).

The implication of the previously mentioned conditions suggests that maximal sensitivity is essential where false-negative results are not to be tolerated and the suspected diagnosis needs to be ruled out with certainty. A false-negative (FN) result may be catastrophic in the presence of an acute MI or dissecting aneurysm of the aorta. In essence, maximal sensitivity is required to rule out critical but manageable diseases or disorders. On the other hand, a false-negative diagnosis may be tolerated when dealing with a serious but incurable disease because a negative result, while delaying the final diagnosis, is unlikely to change the course of the disease.

10.5 The Complement of Sensitivity

The complement of sensitivity, the insensitivity, is the variant used with the emphasis placed on the error involved in the sensitivity measure rather than the actual measure. It can be defined using the numerical equivalents of areas depicted in the Venn diagram as tabled and entered in the corresponding binary table,

$$\text{Insensitivity} = P(T^- | D^+) = \frac{FN}{TP + FN} = FN\,\text{rate} = 1 - \text{Sensitivity}.$$

In descriptive terms, insensitivity may be described as follows:

- ♦ The percentage of patients with the disease mislabeled and falsely identified as negative
- ♦ The percentage of patients with the disease included in the negative sift out and falsely ruled out to be free of the disease
- ♦ D^+ circle area outside the T^+-D^+ intersection as a percentage of the total D^+ circle area
  In the limit, complementary sensitivity = 0, as FN approaches 0.

10.5.1 Predictive Value

Predictive value is defined using the numerical equivalent of the areas depicted in the Venn diagram or, alternatively, as tabulated in the corresponding binary table (Figures 10.6A, 10.6B, 10.7A, 10.7B),

$$\text{Predictive value of negative test: } PV[-] = P(D^- \mid T^-) = \frac{TN}{TN + FN}.$$

In descriptive and graphic terms, the predictive value of negative test, PV[−], may be depicted as follows:

- The area outside both T circle and D circle as a percentage of the T^- ring area (area outside the T^+ circle, i.e., the complement of the T^+ circle)
- The percentage of correctly labeled T^- (TN) results in patients negatively labeled
- The percentage of correctly labeled and identified patients without the disease (TN) from total number of negatively labeled patients
- The probability that the patient is actually free from the disease given the negative test results
- The lack of confidence in the diagnosis for which the test was performed and found to be negative
- The degree of denial that the patient is actually free from the disease given the negative result
- All the above verbal definition of a negative predictive value, which is elegantly summarized by the simple notation $P(D^-|T^-)$ (i.e., probability of D^- given T^-)

Similarly, the predictive error of negative test is similarly defined using the numerical equivalent of the areas depicted in the Venn diagram or, alternatively, as tabulated in the corresponding binary table (Figures 10.6A, 10.6B, 10.7A, 10.7B),

$$\text{Predictive error of negative test: } 1 - PV[-] = P(D^+ \mid T^-) = \frac{TN}{TN + FN}$$

In descriptive terms, predictive error may be described as follows:

♦ The D^+ circle area outside intersection with T^+ circle as a percentage of the T^- ring
♦ The percentage of falsely labeled results in the negatively labeled patients
♦ The percentage of falsely labeled patients with the disease from total number of negatively labeled patients.

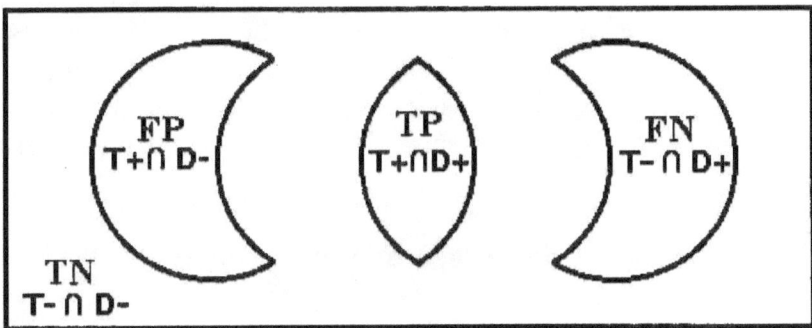

Figure 10.2. Disjointed Venn diagram depicting
the relation between D and T

10.6 Specificity

Ideally, specificity is best defined as the conditional probability of a negative test result given the absence of a true disease condition,

$$\underset{\text{Specificity}}{P(T^- \mid D^-)} = \dfrac{\overset{\text{Joint probability}}{P[T- \mid D-]}}{\underset{\text{1-Prevalence}}{P(D-)}}.$$

Specificity may be equally defined using the numerical equivalent of the ratio of the joint probability and the marginal probability of D^- (prevalence). Alternatively, the areas depicted in the Venn diagram as tabled and entered in the corresponding binary table are equally valid equivalent (Figures 7.4 and 7.5 and Tables 7.1 and 7.2),

$$\text{Specificity} = P(\overset{\text{Specificity}}{T^- \mid D^-}) = \frac{TN}{TN + FP} = TN \text{ rate} = TN\%.$$

In descriptive and graphic terms, specificity may be depicted as follows:

- ♦ The number of patients without the disease correctly cleared by the test as negative (TN) from the total number of patients known to be free from the disease (TN + FP)
- ♦ The area outside both T circle and the D circle as the percentage of the ring area surrounding the D circle (area outside the D circle, i.e., the complement of the D circle)
- ♦ The percentage of T⁻ results in patients without the disease
- ♦ The proportion of patients without the disease in whom the test is negative

10.7 Levels of Specificity: Diagnostic Implication

In actual practice, the probability assigned to a particular test is the result of the clinical assessment of the ratio of true-negative result to the total of both correctly labeled and interpreted true negative and falsely interpreted and labeled positive (i.e., negative misinterpreted and labeled positive) test results under controlled field conditions.

$$\uparrow Sp = \frac{TN}{TN + FP \downarrow} = < 1 = < 100\%.$$

As noted in the preceding relation, specificity of a given test is inversely proportional to its FP component. Thus, the specificity of a given test rests essentially on its discriminating power to avoid miscalling or labeling the proven absence of disease entity test result as positive test result (i.e., false positive).

$$\uparrow\uparrow Sp = \frac{TN}{TN + \underset{\to 0}{FP}} = \to 1 = \to 100\%.$$

A highly specific test implies a small number of FP so that in the limit, as the number of FP approaches 0, specificity approaches 1 or 100 percent, implying maximum specificity. A theoretical specificity of 100 percent (FP = 0) stipulates the absence of false-positive results so that the absence of disease is never falsely mislabeled as positive, although it guarantees the authenticity of true-positive result. Stated differently, a positive outcome, in the context of maximal specificity, is 100 percent true positive,

$$FP \rightarrow 0, TP \rightarrow 100 \text{ percent.}$$

Simultaneously, it allows the test to detect all unproven disease entities under consideration (Figures 10.3 and 10.4).

Thus, a negative test with maximal specificity is capable of correctly labeling and identifying all patients without the disease because 100 percent of all true-negative patients are encompassed by the ring surrounding the D circle (true negative being the complement of the D circle). Note, however, that the D⁻ ring is unable to exclude a percentage of patients with the disease falsely identified and mislabeled as negative (FN).

The previously shown obvious relations lead to the following conclusions:

1. Negative test, T⁻, detects all proven cases free from the disease entity, D⁻ (100 percent), although it also mislabels a certain percentage of disease carriers as false negative.
2. Positive test, T⁺, detects all truly positive cases (i.e., it never miscalls a negative case, D⁻, as positive (FP = 0).

The surprising corollary of the previously mentioned conclusions is not the obvious conclusion that a highly specific test as the name implies is ideally suited for the detection of the absence of the disease such that a T⁻ confirms the negation of disease, D⁻, which carries the mnemonic NIH (negativity in health), but the not-so-obvious fact that a positive test rules in the presence of the disease being tested, that is, true-positive case; thus,

∴ $T^+ \Rightarrow 100$ percent TP $\Rightarrow$ Rules in D^+ (the disease in question),

which is the basis of the mnemonic Sp/P/In (specificity/positive/*R*/in the presence, D^+, of the disease under investigation). The implication of this unexpected conclusion translates that a highly specific test is the ideal diagnostic tool to detect and confirm the presence of disease, but not as the diagnostic tool designed to rule out a disease in question in a differential Dx.

Finally, note that given the theoretical assumption of 100 percent specificity, the predictive value of a positive test, T^+, is equivalently 100 percent (PV[+] = 1) because the false positive is now assumed to be absent (FP = 0), which further confirms the diagnostic potential of a highly specific test (Table 10.1).

Thus, the higher the specificity, the less the false positive and the greater the predictive value of a positive result and the more likely that a positive result corresponds to the presence of disease, thus confirming the actual disease.

A negative test is thus not fully predictive of the absence of disease because of the admixture of false-negative results. Therefore, the disease cannot be ruled out with certainty.

Negative T^-: ♦ Implies very high probability that the patient is correctly identified and classified as nondiseased, although with less than 100 percent certainty because of the admixture of the FN in the negative results. A negative test does not rule out the disease in question with absolute certainty.

A positive test with maximal specificity identifies all patients with the disease. Because no FP is possible given 100 percent specificity, a test that turns out to be positive is a true positive, which now encompassed the total positive results inside the T^+ circle. A positive test is thus fully predictive of the presence of disease.

Positive T^+:♦ Confirms and establishes the diagnosis of the disease in question with 100 percent certainty (FP = 0)
♦ Rules in the disease in question

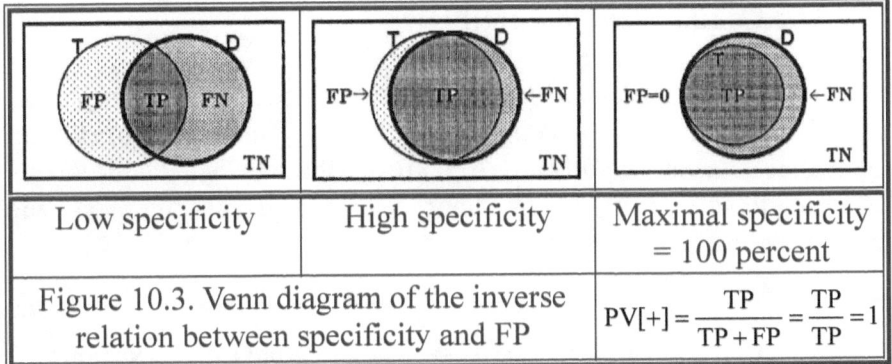

Low specificity	High specificity	Maximal specificity = 100 percent
Figure 10.3. Venn diagram of the inverse relation between specificity and FP		$PV[+] = \dfrac{TP}{TP + FP} = \dfrac{TP}{TP} = 1$

10.8 Indication for High-Specificity Tests

Maximum specificity is required under the following conditions:

- ♦ To rule in the disease in question with 100 percent certainty (no FP)
- ♦ To confirm the disease from the differential
- ♦ To screen for the absence of disease at large, given that a false-positive result is rare

The corollary of maximal specificity is the predictive value of positive test, $P(D^+|T^+) = 100$ percent, which attests to the reliability of the test result such that the probability of disease given the positive result is 100 percent or, alternatively, the probability of disease given a negative test, $P(D^+|T^-)$, is 0 percent.

The implication of the previously mentioned conditions suggests that maximal specificity is essential where false-positive results are not to be tolerated and the suspected diagnosis needs to be ruled in with certainty. A false-positive diagnosis of MI is extremely traumatic for obvious psychological and economic effects. On the other hand, a false-positive diagnosis that may require unnecessary and life-threatening surgery is to be avoided. In essence, maximal specificity is required to establish the diagnosis with confidence when the disease is critical but may or may not be curable (e.g., cancer, Amyotrophic Lateral Sclerosis (ALS)).

10.9 The Complement of Specificity

The complement of specificity is the variant used with the emphasis, placed on the error involved in the specificity measure rather than the actual measure. It can be defined using the numerical equivalents of areas depicted in the Venn diagram as tabled and entered in the corresponding binary table,

$$\text{Nonspecificity} = P(T^+ \mid D^-) = \frac{FP}{TN + FP} = FP \text{ rate} = 1 - \text{specificity}.$$

In descriptive terms, nonspecificity may be described as follows:

- ◆ The percentage of patients without the disease mislabeled and falsely identified as positive
- ◆ The percentage of patients without the disease falsely labeled positive
- ◆ The T^+ circle area outside the T^+-D^+ intersection as a percentage of the total T^+ circle
  In the limit, the complement of specificity $= 0$, as FP approaches 0.

10.9.1 Predictive Value

Predictive value is defined using the numerical equivalent of the areas depicted in the Venn diagram or, alternatively, as tabulated in the corresponding binary table (Figures 10.6A, 10.6B, 10.7A, 10.7B),

$$\text{Predictive value of positive test: } PV[+] = P(D^+ \mid T^+) = \frac{TP}{TP+FP}.$$

In descriptive language, the predictive value (PV) of a positive test, PV[+], is depicted as follows:

- ◆ The T circle intersection area with the D circle as a percentage of the T circle area
- ◆ The percentage of correctly labeled and identified patients with the disease from total number of positively labeled patients

♦ The probability that the patient actually has the disease given that the test is positive

♦ The percentage of confidence in the diagnosis for which the test was found to be positive

♦ The degree of confirmation and ruling in of the disease given that the test is positive

The predictive error can be similarly defined using the numerical equivalent of the areas depicted in the Venn diagram or, alternatively, as tabulated in the corresponding binary table (Figures 10.6A, 10.6B, 10.7A, 10.7B),

$$\text{Predictive error of positive test: } 1 - PV[+] = P(D^- \mid T^+) = \frac{FP}{TP + FP}$$

In descriptive and graphic terms, predictive error may be described as follows:

♦ The T^+ circle area excluding the intersection area with the D^+ circle as a percentage of the total T^+ circle area

♦ The percentage of mislabeled T^+ results in the positively labeled patients

♦ The percentage of patients without the disease that are mislabeled and falsely identified by the test as positive from the total number of positively labeled patients

10.10 Sensitivity versus Specificity

Nonspecific (in contradistinction to highly specific) sign, symptom, or test implies a higher proportion of FP. A positive sign, symptom, or test cannot rule in the Dx because often it is associated with the absence of disease, which may be categorized appropriately as in the technical literature as false alarm (false positive). The ubiquitous nonspecific ST-T changes are simply statements that imply questionable association with myocardial ischemia.

A highly specific test is ideal as a diagnostic tool. A positive test confirms the Dx of the target disease.

Insensitive (in contradistinction to highly sensitive) test implies a higher proportion of FN. A negative test cannot exclude the target disease with certainty, thus giving false assurance (false negative) that those presumed free of disease are not so free.

A highly sensitive test is ideal to screen or sift the "healthy" patient (non-D$^+$: free of D$^+$) from the sample being screened for D$^+$, and a negative test eliminates the Dx from the differential.

Sensitivity: Positivity in Disease (PID)	Specificity: Negativity in Health (NIH)
To exclude Dx	To confirm Dx
To rule out Dx	To rule in Dx
To disprove Dx	To prove Dx
To eliminate Dx	To clinch Dx
You need a negative test result (T$^-$) from a test with high sensitivity so that FN will be minimal	You need a positive test result (T$^+$) from a test with high specificity so that FP will be minimal
$\uparrow Sn = \dfrac{TP}{TP + FN \downarrow} = <1 = <100\%$	$\uparrow Sp = \dfrac{TN}{TN + FP \downarrow} = <1 = <100\%$
SnNout: Sn(T$^-$) $\Rightarrow$ rule out	SpPIn: Sp(T$^+$) $\Rightarrow$ rule in
$\uparrow\uparrow Sn = \dfrac{TP}{TP + \underset{=0}{FN}} = \dfrac{TP}{E} = 1 = 100\%$	$\uparrow\uparrow Sp = \dfrac{TN}{TN + \underset{=0}{FP}} = 1 = 100\%$
Sn = 100 percent $\therefore$ T$^-$ $\Rightarrow$ excludes Dx $\Rightarrow$ rule out	Sp = 100 percent $\therefore$ T$^+$ $\Rightarrow$ confirms Dx $\Rightarrow$ rule in
Given a highly sensitive test: T$^-$ excludes the target disease	Given a highly specific test: T$^+$ is diagnostic of the target disease
$\downarrow Sn = \dfrac{TP}{TP + FN \uparrow} =$ Insensitive test ($\uparrow$ FN)	$\downarrow Sp = \dfrac{TN}{TN + FP \uparrow} =$ Nonspecific test ($\uparrow$ FP)
Given an insensitive test: T$^-$ often misinterprets the positive as negative (false assurance)	Given a nonspecific test: T$^+$ is often misinterprets the negative as positive (false alarm)

Table 10.2. Indications and pitfalls of sensitivity and specificity

Nonspecific (in contradistinction to highly specific) sign, symptom, or test implies a higher proportion of FP. A positive sign, symptom, or test cannot rule in the Dx because often it is associated with the absence of disease, which may be categorized appropriately as in the technical literature as false alarm (false positive). The ubiquitous nonspecific ST-T changes are simply statements that imply questionable association with myocardial ischemia.

Insensitive (in contradistinction to highly sensitive) test implies a higher proportion of FN. A negative test cannot exclude the target disease with certainty, thus giving false assurance (false negative) that those presumed free of disease are not so free.

A highly specific test is ideal as a diagnostic tool. A positive test confirms the Dx of the target disease.

A highly sensitive test is ideal to screen or sift the "healthy" patient (non-D^+: free of D^+) from the sample being screened for D^+, and a negative test eliminates the Dx from the differential.

Screen: (verb) to separate or sift out or by means of a sieve or screen; (noun) a coarse sieve used for sifting out fine particles as of sand, gravel, or coal.

Sift: (verb) to put through a sieve in order to separate the fine from the coarse.

It would have been the ideal point to end the chapter on the assumption that all clinical biochemical and physiologic test results can be categorized on a binary scale of normal/abnormal, positive/negative, and so on, and that both sensitivity and specificity are independent of each other in the context of a given test. The fact is that most clinical laboratory data are normally cited in conjunction with a normal range provided by the laboratory. Furthermore, far from being independent, both are inversely related and together with prevalence determine the final predictive value of a given test. The balance of this chapter aims to clarify these two critical facets of relevant clinical tests.

The Reference Interval: Arbiter of the Test Result

Consider The Fasting Blood Sugar level in Normal men, 30 years or more in age, Graph 10-1(22-1).

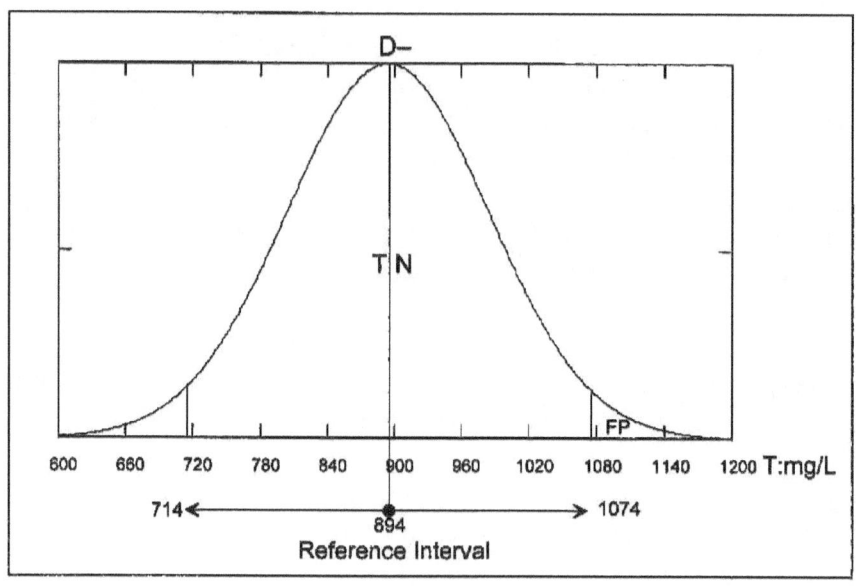

Figure 10.4. Graph of fasting blood sugar levels obtained form 106 normal men older than thirty years using the hexokinase method. A mean value of 894 mg/L was obtained. The 95 percent range is given at 714-1,074 (Geigy Scientific Tables).

The normal distribution was obtained by plotting the frequency of a given value of blood sugar level on the continuous scale of mg/L. The reference range posted at 714-1,074 embracing 95 percent (95.4) of the 106 men tested was set as the norm for the nondiabetic population. This arbitrary definition of the reference range left five normal nondiabetic subjects outside the range either on hyperglycemic or hypoglycemic sides. Leaving for the moment the lower tail end of the curve, a normal nondiabetic subject whose fasting blood sugar level turns out to be 1,140 for example would be classified as a potential diabetic, a false-positive result given the imposed reference range.

The normal distribution of fasting blood sugar in a sample of equal number of diabetic patients whose mean was calculated at 1,200 mg/L superimposed on the same scale of the nondiabetic sample is shown in Figure 10.5 (Figure 22.4).

The cutoff level of 1,074, the level determined for the normal sample, resulted in a crossover marked by a significant false negative, in contrast to the relatively smaller false-positive area for the nondiabetic subject.

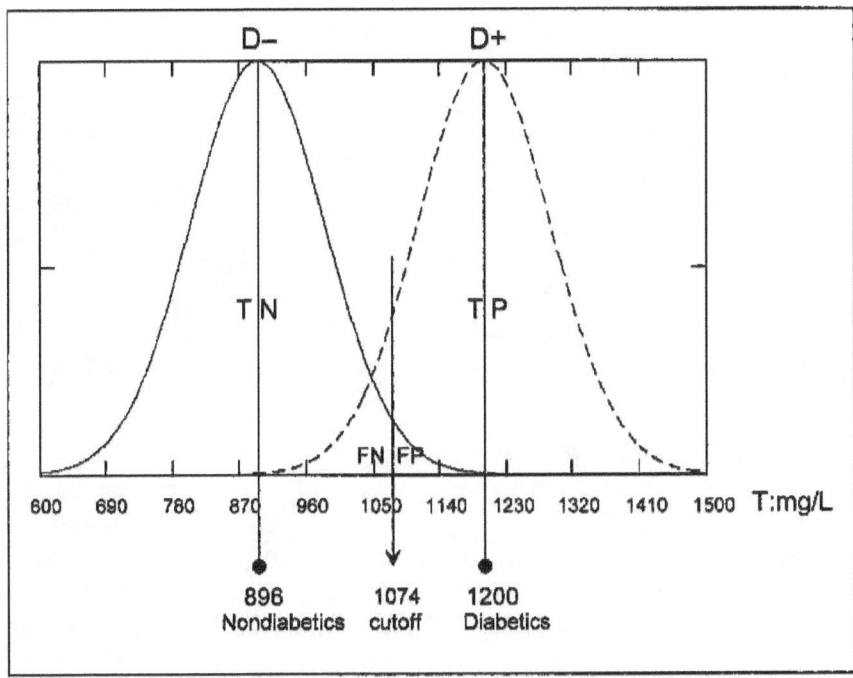

Figure 10.5. Graph of the normal distribution of fasting blood sugar in an equivalent sample of diabetic patients whose mean was calculated at 1,200 mg/L, superimposed on the same scale of the nondiabetic sample

The normal distribution of fasting blood sugar in a sample of equal number of diabetic patients whose mean was calculated at 1,500 mg/L, superimposed on the same scale of the nondiabetic sample, is shown in Figure 10.6 (Figure 22.5).

In this case, the crossover is practically eliminated, resulting in a clear demarcation at the 1,200 level between the diabetics and the nondiabetics. Recall, however, that both the solid curve and the dashed curve extend underneath each other territory, so that rate possibility of a false positive and false negative can never be eliminated.

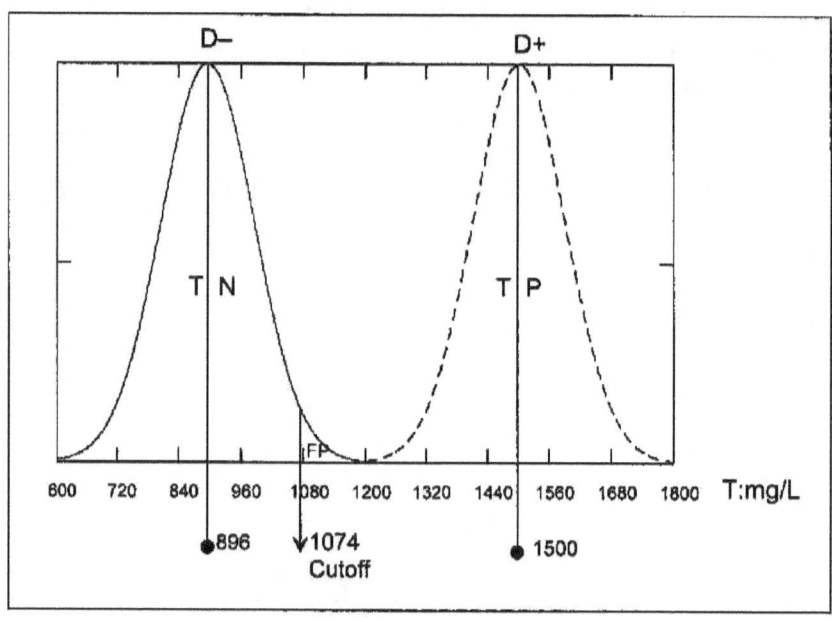

Figure 10.6. Graph of the normal distribution of fasting blood sugar in an equivalent sample of diabetic patients whose mean value was calculated at 1,500 mg/L, superimposed on the same scale of the nondiabetic sample

The key factor in the determination of the reference interval is the arbitrary selection of the cutoff points and thus the placement of the cutoff vertical axis ideally marking off the true negative (nondiabetics) from the true positive (diabetics), allowing nonetheless for the unavoidable minimal percentage of false positive in case of the nondiabetics and false negatives in the case of the diabetics. From Figure 22.4, it is graphically obvious that the placement of the vertical decision axis at the cutoff point determines the extent of the FP and FN on either side. A shift of the cutoff axis to the left or right results in a different proportion of the false results, thus altering the sensitivity and specificity of the test.

The critical role of the cutoff axis in defining the limiting characteristics of a given is best visualized by translating the annotated Venn diagram into the equivalent distribution.

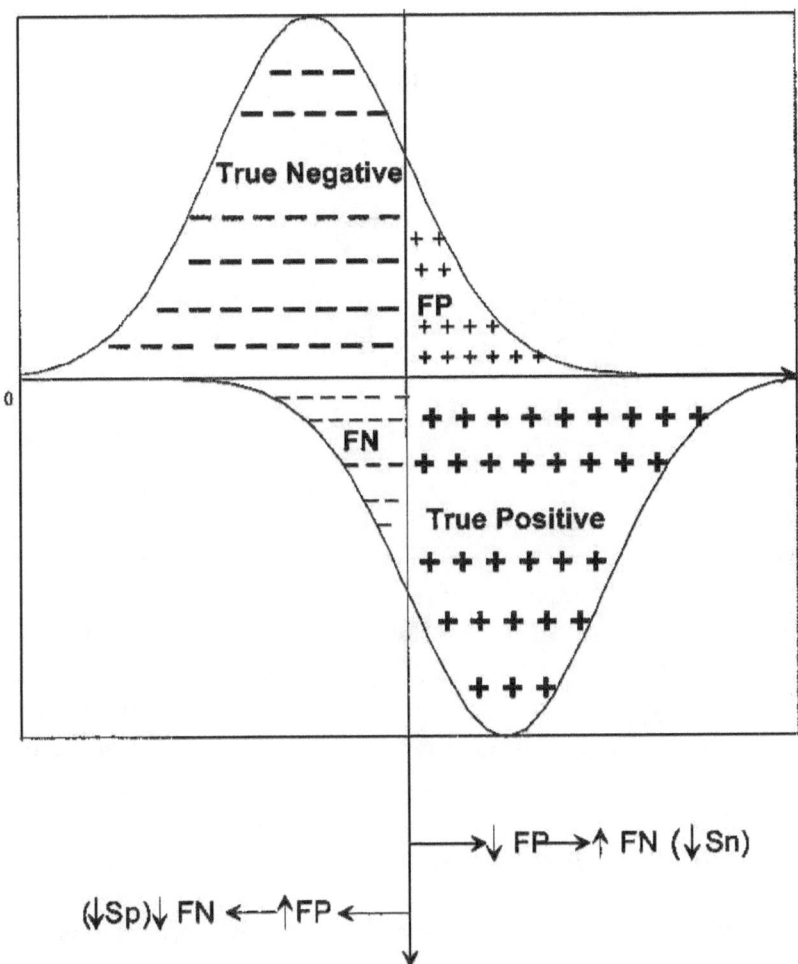

Figure 10.7. Graph of a universal view of the partition of overlapping distribution by the placement of the vertical cutoff axis

$$\uparrow \text{Specificity} = \uparrow \left(\frac{\text{TN}}{\underbrace{\text{TN} + \text{FP} \downarrow}_{\text{Cutoff} \rightarrow}} \right) \Rightarrow \uparrow \text{FN} \rightarrow \downarrow \left(\frac{\text{TP}}{\text{TP} + \text{FN} \uparrow} \right) \rightarrow \downarrow \text{Sensitivity}$$

$$\uparrow \text{Sensitivity} = \uparrow \left(\frac{\text{TP}}{\underbrace{\text{TP} + \text{FN} \downarrow}_{\leftarrow \text{Cutoff}}} \right) \Rightarrow \uparrow \text{FP} \downarrow \left(\frac{\text{TP}}{\text{TP} + \text{FN} \uparrow} \right) \rightarrow \downarrow \text{Specificity}$$

The area under the right-hand D^+ curve is divided into two parts by the vertical line, namely, a TP area and an FN area to the left of the vertical line. These two areas add up to 100 percent (TP + FN = 1). Likewise, the left-hand distribution curve (D^-) is divided into two areas, namely, a TN area and an FP area to the right of the vertical line. The two areas add up to 100 percent (TN + FP = 1).

The key factor to note is the obvious inverse relationship of the FN area to the FP area associated with the displacement of the cutoff vertical axis to the left or right. Clearly, the arbitrary positioning of the cutoff axis is the determining factor of the operating characteristics of any given test because the TP rate and the FP rate are sufficient to determine the test's sensitivity and specificity (TP + FN = 1; TN + FP =1). In the blood sugar level test cited previously, every shift of the decision axis results in a different pair of FP and TP rates. When FP value of each pair is plotted against the TP value of the same pair, a curve called *receiver operating characteristic* (ROC) is generated, which represents the inverse relationship associated with the shifting placement of the vertical axis (Graph 10-4). Note that the each axis of the graph ranges from 0 to 1, corresponding for the vertical axis to 0 to 100 percent TP rate and similarly for the horizontal axis representing 0 to 100 percent FP rate.

Each point on the ROC curve corresponds to the placement on the x axis of the vertical line, which divides the two overlapping population curves into a subgroup relationship of TP, FN, TN, and FP.

For a given test, variation on the position of the vertical line (decision axis) results in the displacement of the critical point on the same ROC curve. The adoption of a different test results in a different ROC curve with its own decision axis and ROC curve.

The conservative critical point produces very few FP but at the cost of a low TP rate. The risky critical point identifies most TP, but at the cost of relatively high FP rate. The intermediate critical point results midway between the two extremes.

The discriminative ability is a function of its position with respect to the diagonal. In the ROC, the decision matrix has only two degrees of freedom, not four; that is, only two members can be entered freely in the matrix and the other two numbers will follow.

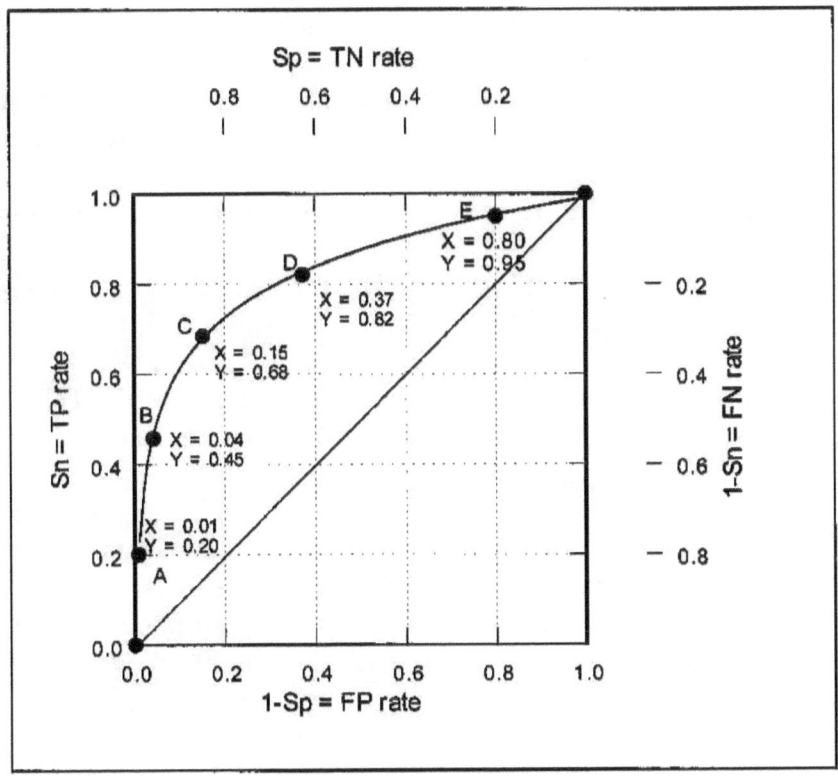

Hypothetical ROC curve
Figure 10.8. Graph of the hypothetical ROC curve
that depicts the placement of the cutoff point (i.e., the vertical
decision axis) over five decision criteria (A → E)

$$\text{Lilelihood ratio} = \frac{\text{Sensitivity}}{1-\text{Specificity}} = \frac{\text{TP rate}}{\text{FP rate}} = \frac{Y}{X}:$$

$$\text{LR at } A = \frac{0.20}{0.01} = 20; \quad \text{LR at } B = \frac{0.45}{0.04} = 11.5; \quad \text{LR at } C = \frac{0.68}{0.15} = 4.53; \quad \text{LR at } D = \frac{0.82}{0.37} = 2.21; \quad \text{LR } E = \frac{0.95}{0.80} = 1.19$$

The perusal of Figure 10.8 reveals the following points:

1. The diagonal line is the locus of a point whose $x = y$ (i.e., TP rate = FP rate) and therefore represents the likelihood ratio of 1.
2. The upper right point terminating the diagonal line represents 100 percent sensitivity and 0 percent specificity.
3. The lower left point terminating the diagonal line represents FP rate of 0 (100 percent specificity) and 0 percent sensitivity.
4. The left upper corner represents the ultimate ideal test: a TP rate of 1 (100 percent sensitivity) and an FP rate of 0 (100 percent specificity).
5. The points on the ROC curves A to D all share a likelihood ratio greater than 1.
6. The greater the TP rate (sensitivity), the smaller the FN rate. At the limit, a TP rate of 1 (100 percent sensitivity) coincides with 0 percent FN rate.
7. The smaller the FP rate (1 − specificity), the greater the TN rate. At the limit A, FP rate of 0 coincides with a TN rate of 1 (100 percent specificity).
8. As point A moves up the curve on its locus to E, there is a gradual decrease in the FN rate and simultaneous increase in the FP rate. At point A, the FN rate is maximal (FN rate = 0.8) and FP rate is minimal (FP rate = 0.01). At point C, the FN rate is intermediate (FN rate = 0.32) and the FP rate is likewise intermediate (FP rate = 0.15). At point E, the FN rate is minimal (FN rate = 0.05) and the FP rate is maximal (FP rate = 0.95).

In terms of the overlapping distribution of Figure 22.4, points A to E on the ROC curve correspond to a stepwise displacement of the vertical cutoff axis from the extreme right at A to the extreme left at E, slicing the overlapping curves into a thin slice of FP and a much larger slice of FN at A and gradually reallocating the slices to maximum of FP and a minimum of FN at E.

This chapter began by defining the cutoff point for a test with a continuous scale of values on a statistical basis embracing the norm of 95.4 percent of the 106 men tested, leaving five subjects known to be normal outside the arbitrarily defined range of values.

The previously mentioned consideration, however, has made it clear that every cutoff point is associated with a reciprocal proportion of FP and FN results. What is not readily apparent is that these are testing and diagnostic errors and, in the context of the health care environment, costly errors both in terms of health and economics. Consider for a moment an MI patient discharged from the ER on the basis of a false-negative CK-MB and equivocal ECG. Which brings us to the final question of this elaborate presentation as to the optimal choice of a cutoff point in the context of a diagnostic workup that would minimize the cost of false results inherent in all testing and diagnostic procedures?

The answer to this dilemma requires a detour into the realm of decision and information theory, which is beyond the scope of this primary presentation. A brief outline will be presented to round up the all important issue of diagnosis.

The health costs, mortality and morbidity, sustained through an FP or FN errors, are measured by person-years, where one person survives one year. Irrespective of this technical measure, the health costs of a diagnostic error are all too visible to ignore.

$$k \left(\underset{\text{Cost ratio}}{\frac{FP_{Cost}}{FN_{Cost}}} \right) \times \left(\underset{\text{Pretest odds}}{\frac{P(D^-)}{P(D^+)}} \right) = \underset{\text{optimal cutoff point}}{\text{Slope of}}$$

As noted earlier, because FP error is inversely related to FN error through the placement of the cutoff axis, this ratio becomes key component of the formula for the optimal cutoff point.

Minimal FN $\Rightarrow$ High Sensitivity	Minimal FP $\Rightarrow$ High Specificity
Critical but manageable	Life-threatening intervention
Acute MI	Unnecessary surgery
Dissecting aneurysm	Treatable malignant infectious disease
Potentially fatal but treatable	Treatable malignant neoplastic disease
Blood donors	
Acceptable high FP $\Rightarrow$ low specificity	Acceptable high FN $\Rightarrow$ low sensitivity
MI: traumatic impact	Incurable serious disease
$\left(\dfrac{FP_{Cost} \downarrow}{FN_{Cost} \uparrow} \right)$ Low cost ratio $\downarrow \times$ $\left(\dfrac{P(D^-)}{P(D^+)} \right)$ High prevalence $\downarrow =$ Slope of optimal cutoff point	$\left(\dfrac{FPCost \uparrow}{FNCost \downarrow} \right)$ High relative cost $\uparrow \times$ $\left(\dfrac{P(D^-)}{P(D^+)} \right)$ Low prevalence $\uparrow =$ Slope of optimal cutoff point

Table 10.3.

Thus, in the case of an emergent MI, an FN error is far more costly that the opposite error of FP. The ratio in this case tends to be small. The second element in the formula is the pretest odds of the disease. The product of the two elements is the slope of the tangent to the desired cutoff point on the curve. Note the reversal of order in this formula. In elementary geometry, a point is designated on a curve, and its tangent is then calculated. In this case, the tangent is given, and its point of origin or contact is to be found. The slope as defined by the previously mentioned formula for an emergent MI turns out to be small, which puts the tangent to the ROC curve at an optimal cutoff point near point E, where a highly sensitive test is required to rule out FN errors, a fact made abundantly obvious early in the discussion of sensitivity and specificity. The difference being the exact quantitative placement of the cutoff point in conformity with restriction placed on the test parameters.

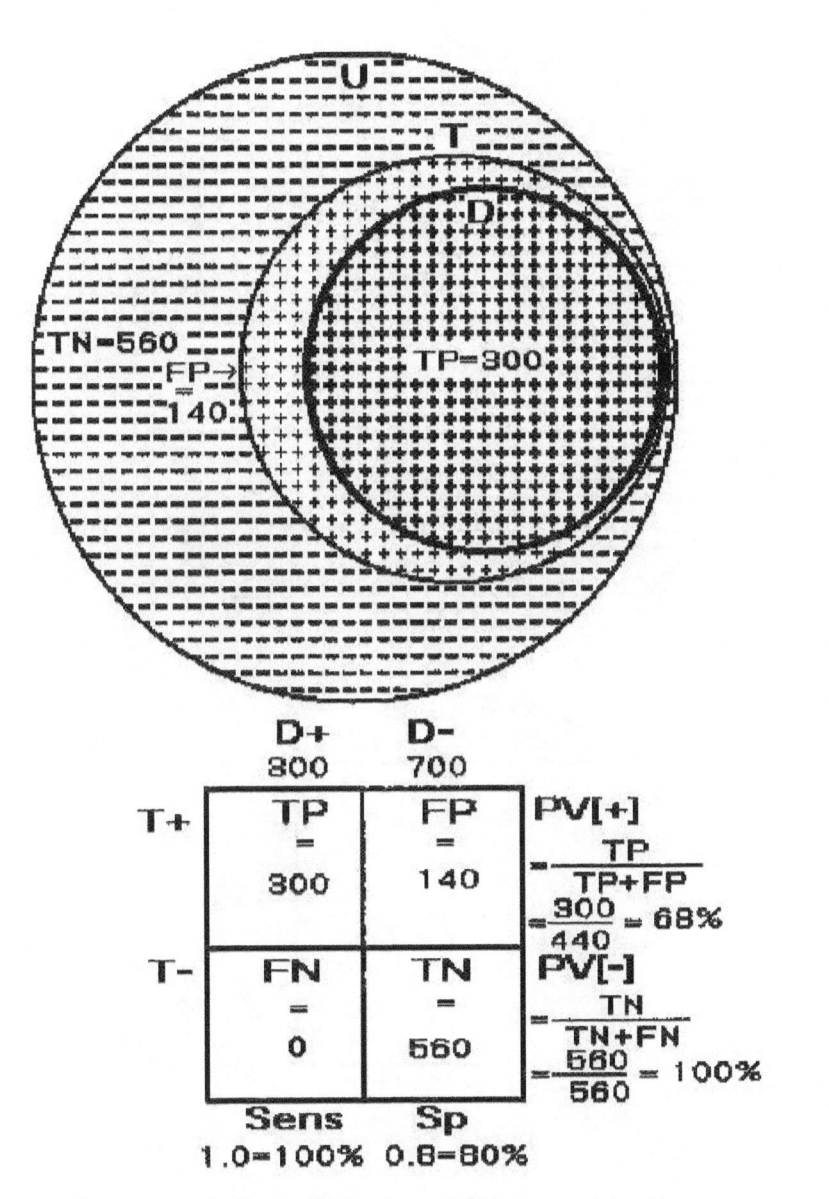

Figure 10.9. Venn diagram of the partition of the sample universe at maximal sensitivity. A negative test result rules out the disease in question with absolute certainty.

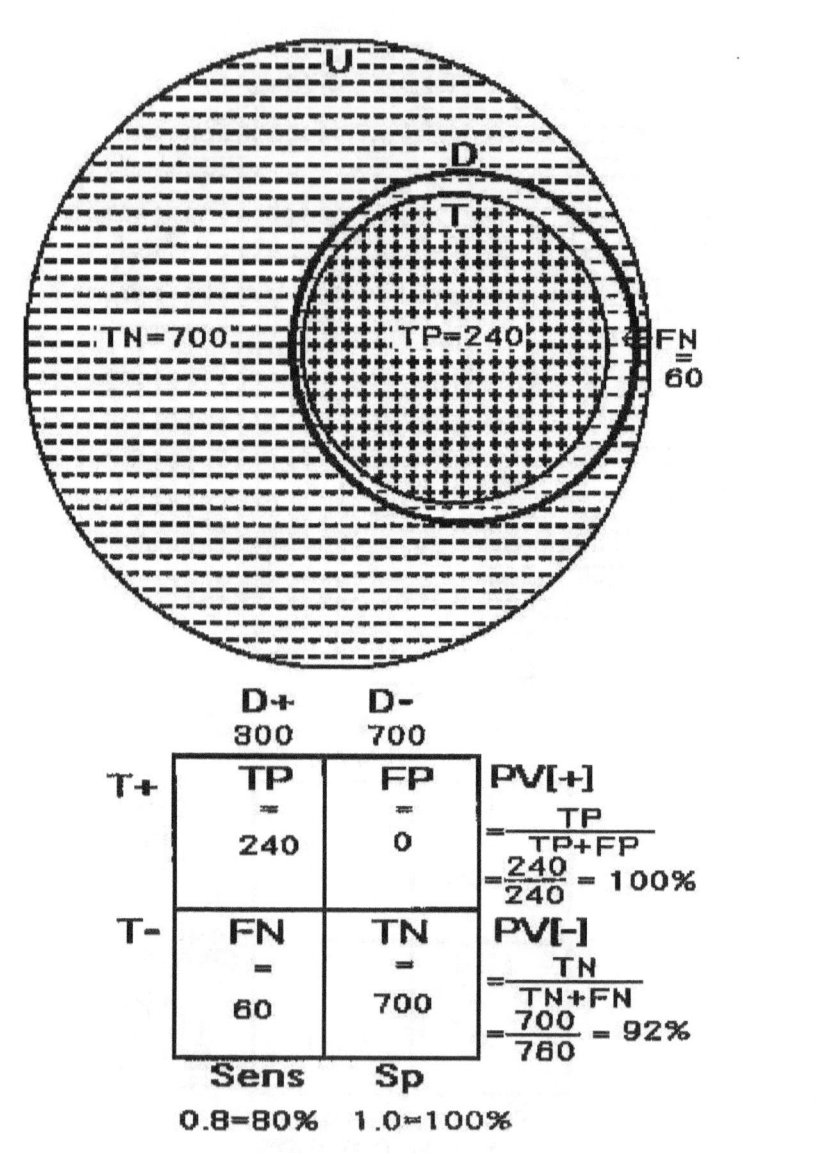

Figure 10.10. Venn diagram of the partition of the sample universe at maximal specificity. A positive test result confirms the disease in question with absolute certainty.

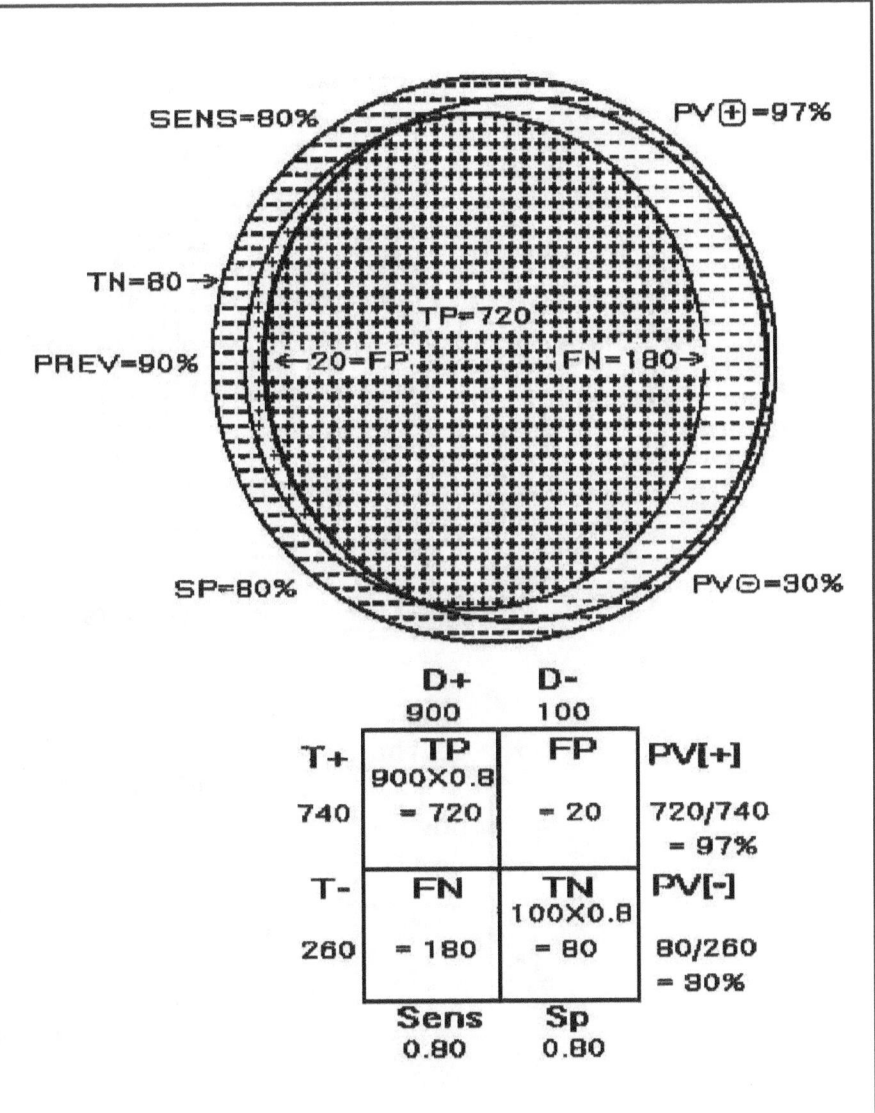

Figure 10.11. (A and B) Venn diagram of the dominant effect of a change in prevalence (90-10 percent) on the predictive values for a given sensitivity and specificity (80 percent)

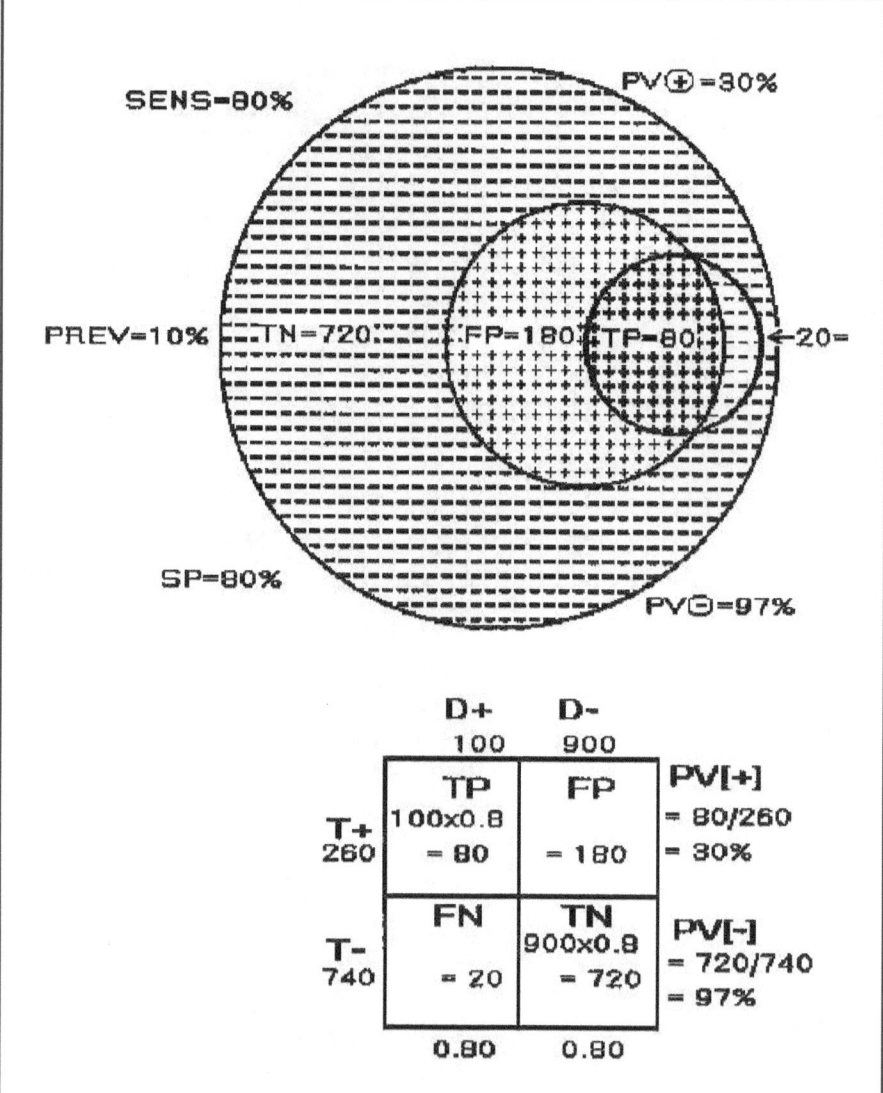

Figure 10.11. (A and B) Venn diagram of the dominant effect of a change in prevalence (10-90 percent) on the predictive values for a given sensitivity and specificity (80 percent)

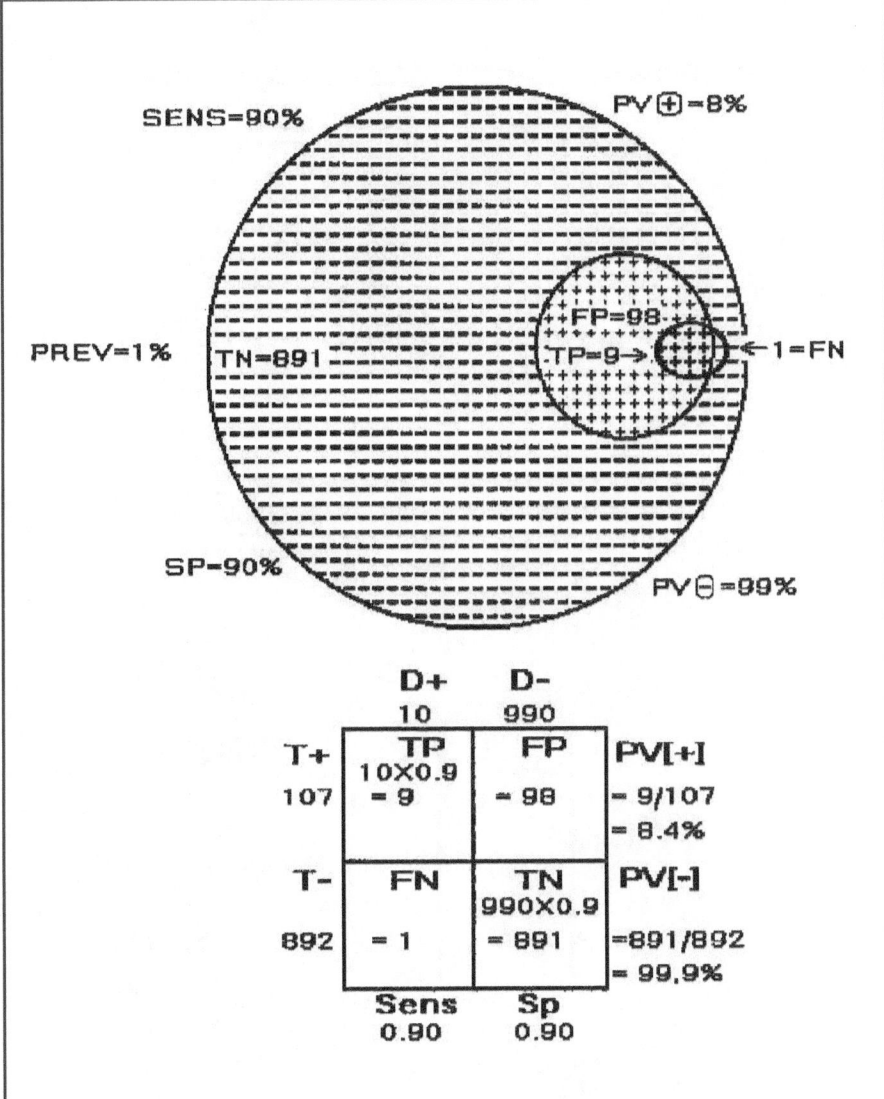

Figure 10.12 (A and B) At a prevalence of 1 percent, an increase in sensitivity and specificity to 99 percent is required in order to boost the positive predictive value to the 50 percent threshold

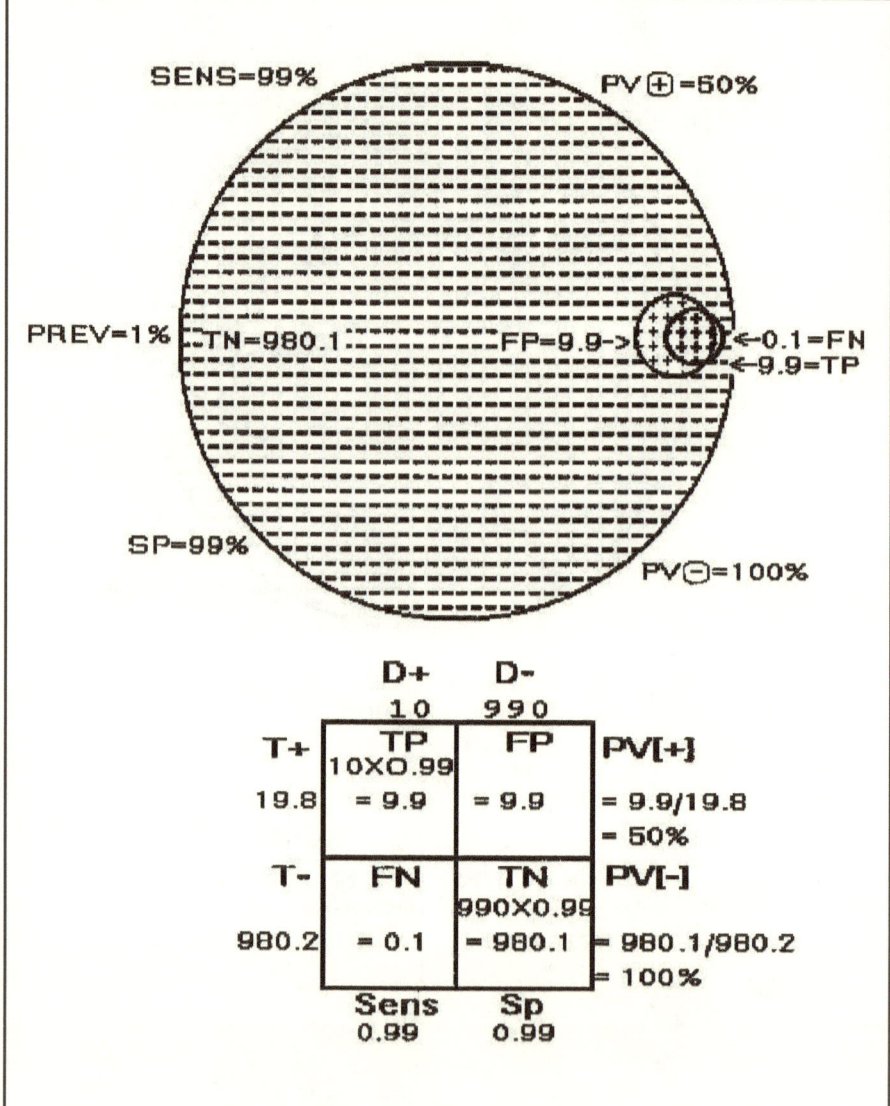

Figure 10.12. (A and B) At a prevalence of 1 percent, an increase in sensitivity and specificity to 99 percent is required in order to boost the positive predictive value to the 8 percent threshold

Chapter 11

The Discrete Random Variable Distribution: An Overview

The concept of distribution is central to both probability and statistics. As in all distributions, physical or hypothetical, the concept involves the apportionment of a specific number of quantifiable elements or data to each of the given items, individuals, categories, or classes, making up the recipient population under consideration.

The division of a set of quantifiable elements or data (sum of measurements or statistics) and their subsequent allocation to the individuals, categories, or classes constitute the frequency of observations or measurements of a particular variable allocated (distributed) to each member unit.

To fully appreciate this concept, one needs to have a precise notion of the elements involved in the making of a given distribution. The key element to be considered in this context is that of the variable. A random variable (RV) in statistics is any attribute or characteristic that may take different values, which distinguishes one subject (animate, physical, or conceptual) from another.

The data are generally based on individual observation or measurement taken on the smallest sampling unit. The set of numbers so derived are related in one-to-one correspondence to the subjects or items comprising the sample space whose members share a common characteristic that is being measured or observed, which determines the nature of the variable being used in the actual measurement or observation.

In general, a variable may be quantitative or qualitative in nature. A nominal variable, as the name suggests, is a qualitative variable where categories are labeled or named but not assigned a number. The simplest nominal scale is the dichotomous nominal scale, where the variable in this case assumes two well-defined, exclusive, and exhaustive attributes for example, present/absent and cured/ not cured. The ordinal variable is similarly a qualitative variable possessing an inherent rank, qualifying it a semiquantitative measure. for example, grades I-IV/VI murmur, 1+ → 4+ acetone.

The quantitative variable data are numerical and may be either discrete, for example, heart rate in beats per minute, or continuous as in the determination of a chemical or physiological value, for example $PO_2 = 65$ mm Hg.

In the discrete case, the possible values are clearly demarcated, so that a process of enumeration (tally) is required for the final count. In the continuous case, on the other hand, the process of quantitative measurement whereby numbers are assigned to specify the different characteristic of a variable is implied, as in the measurement of length, mass, or time. However, although a variable is continuous, the process of measurement always reduces it to a discrete one. Numerical data thus result from the process of measurements that assign numbers to observations.

In statistics, the set of the observed characteristics or scores is referred to as the population. Population is thus defined as the complete set of observations, measurements, or scores from which conclusions are drawn. In this sense, the definition becomes an abstraction that also includes groups of persons or objects, although not exclusively.

The variation among members of the sample regarding a particular characteristic makes the variable of interest, the score for the subject being measured. The variable of interest in medicine may range over all the physiological and clinical parameters. In other fields, the variables of interest are unlimited in scope. The following is a selective sample of variables that may serve as practical or theoretical examples:

- Number of heads on tossing six coins
- Sum of numbers on rolling a pair of dice
- Test score (outcome) of proficiency test
- Height of the male freshmen class of college A
- Weight of newborn babies
- Cholesterol level in juvenile diabetics

- Vital capacity in smokers of different age
- RR interval (time interval between two adjacent R waves) in 100,000 beats in the ECG of a patient with atrial fibrillation.
- Resting heart rate in ninety marathon runners

In the context of distribution, the concept of frequency of a single event, measurement, or range of values or measurement is defined as the number of observation measurements associated with a particular value or class of values. Frequency distribution ensues when both the frequency, that is, the number of instances that fall in each event or class of the data, and the events or classes of data it refers to are portrayed graphically or in a tabular format.

Frequency distribution thus addresses the question of how to summarize and display large masses of ungrouped data in a way that makes it possible to draw relevant inferences by showing the frequency with which each score or variable occur.

Initially, the mass of data obtained from a random sample is unorganized and unordered. Consider, for example, the resting heart rate of ninety marathon runners. As presented in Table 11.1, no obvious conclusion may be inferred from the scattered numerical data other than the overall low rate in the group.

60	61	52	66	62	60	63	58	65	57	56	59	66	54	55	66	63	57
59	64	55	58	57	60	56	61	57	62	61	65	63	63	53	60	59	62
56	57	58	66	54	58	64	58	65	60	64	59	67	60	61	58	55	57
53	60	62	57	58	59	62	61	59	61	65	61	61	58	55	67	56	65
60	63	55	56	65	62	55	60	69	63	67	64	54	67	68	60	64	62

Table 11.1. Resting heart rate of ninety marathon runners obtained from the ECG in the upright sitting position

Confronted with such an array of mixed data, the most common approach at summarizing the different numbers, with the objective of providing a representative score that mirrors the aggregate of the scores, is to derive the arithmetic mean by summing up the individual measurements (the resting heart rates in this instance) and by dividing the sum by the number of the rates (subjects) measured.

$$\overline{X} = \frac{1}{n}\sum_{i=1}^{n} X_i = \frac{\text{Sum of all scores}}{\text{Number of scores}} = \frac{5426}{90} = 60.289 = \text{Arithmetic mean} = \text{Average resting HR.}[6]$$

The need to supplement the derived mean by additional details is essentially an attempt to portray the manner of the distribution of the ninety distinct numbers.

Figure 11.1 shows a preliminary simple graphic illustration of the distribution of the different resting heart rates among the sample of ninety runners. As noted in Figure 11.1, a distribution pattern is now evident in the obvious clustering of ten identical rates at the resting frequency of 60 bpm, whereas only one unique rate was observed at the extremes of the resting heart rates of 52, 68, and 69 bpm exhibited by the runners.

---

[6] To write the sum of the n numbers X_1, X_2, X_3, . . . X_n in a compact format, the summation notation Σ (Sigma) surrounded by the necessary notations is used to represent the sum

$$X_{1+}X_{2+}X_{3+}...X_n = \sum_{i=1}^{n} X_i,$$

which simply reads that the values of Xi should be summed from the lower limit of i = 1, the subscript of Σ, to the upper limit of the superscript of Σ, n, meaning that Xi is to be summed from i = 1 to i = n.

Note that if X was identically the same for all runners, that is, (X = a constant), then $\sum_{n=1}^{n} X = nx$. In this case, both the summation and the product are identical.

The symbol $\overline{x}$ (read X-bar) is used to represent the mean, so that the mean of the n is

$$\overline{X} = \frac{X_1 + X_2 + X_3 + ...X_n}{n} = \frac{\sum_{i=1}^{n} X_i}{n} = \frac{\text{Sum of all scores of } X}{\text{Number of scores, } n} = \frac{5426}{90} = \text{Arithmetic mean} = \text{Average resting HR} = 60.289.$$

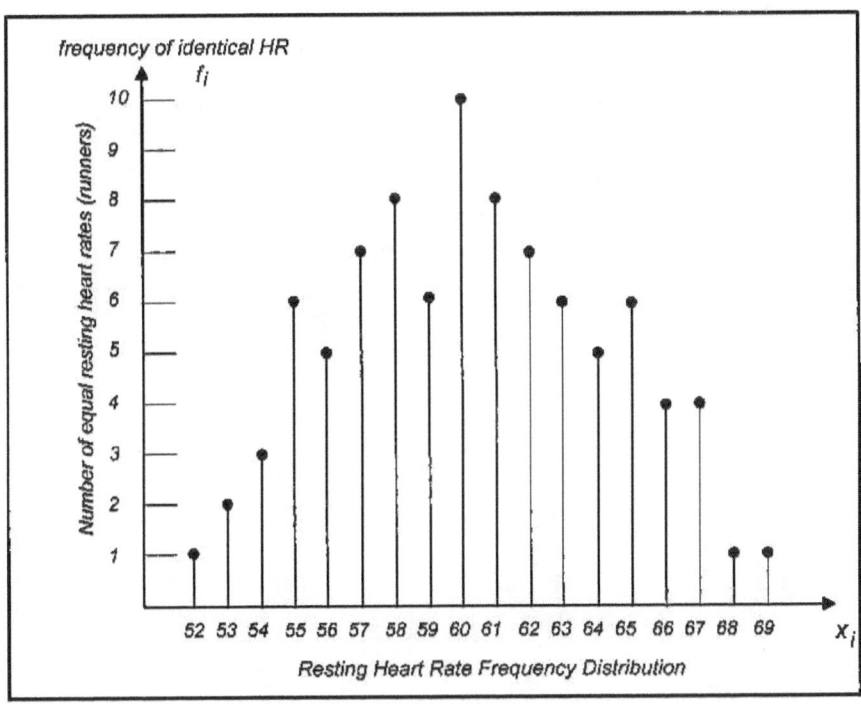

Figure 11.1. Line chart of the resting heart rates ranging from 52 to 69 bpm were plotted on the x axis. The frequency of occurrence associated with each heart rate was plotted on the y axis.

Note that the chart displays the frequency of the observed rates associated with each of the individual recorded rates. Indirectly, the frequency may be associated with the number of the runners exhibiting the same rate.

A simple frequency histogram may be made to replace Figure 11.1 in a one-to-one exchange. As in the construction of Figure 11.1, the vertical axis is assigned to the frequency, and the horizontal axis displays the outcome of individual measured variable or heart rate of the eighteen different classes comprising the spectrum of variation obtained.

In a similar way, the height of each vertical bar in the histogram represents the number of observations in each different class comprising the eighteen different resting heart rates obtained from the ninety runners.

The histogram displays an additional feature not readily apparent in Figure 11.1. In this presentation, given a base of one unit in width, the area of each rectangle is numerically identical to the frequency associated with it. This is another way of saying that the total area enclosed by the eighteen rectangles is actually the sum of the product of the resting heart rates and their corresponding frequency. The implication of this fact will become apparent later in the discussion.

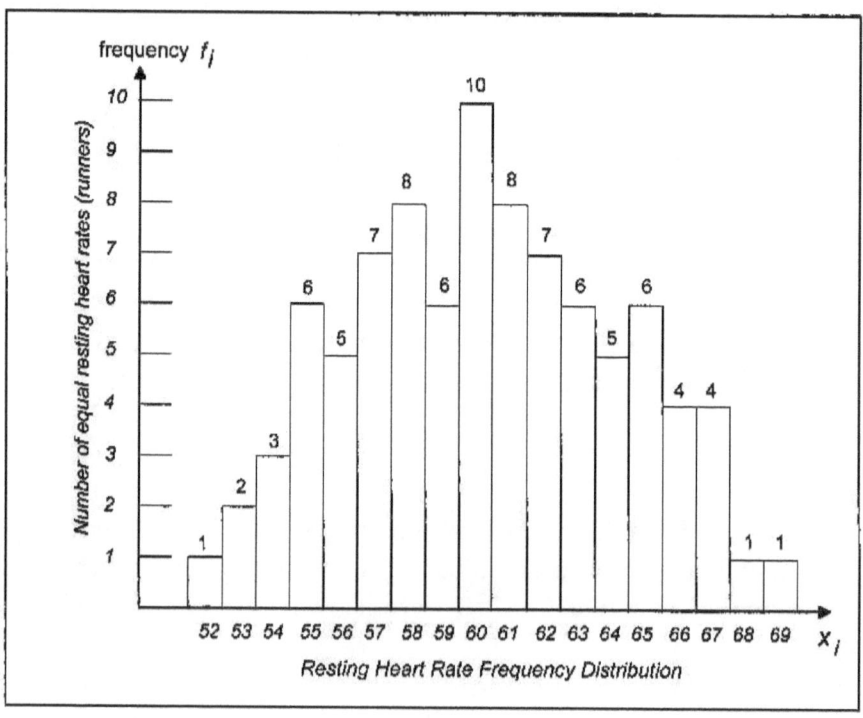

Figure 11.2. The height of each rectangle corresponds to the frequency associated with the individual heart rate. In this case, because the base of each rectangle is a unit width, its area corresponds similarly to the same frequency

The more meaningful approach at organizing the data is to tabulate the frequency of occurrence of the individual numbers in any order, preferably in a descending or ascending order.

A table showing the scores and their frequency of occurrence is called a *frequency distribution*.

HR X_i	Frequency f_i	$\sum_{i=1}^{n} x_i f_i = 2747$	Relative frequency $\left(\dfrac{f_i}{n}\right)$	HR X_i	Frequency f_{i_s}	$\sum_{i=n}^{n} x_i f_i = 2679$	Relative frequency $\left(\dfrac{f_i}{n}\right)$
52	1	52 × 1 = 52	1/90 = 0.011	61	8	61 × 8 = 488	8/90 = 0.088
53	2	53 × 2 = 106	2/90 = 0.022	62	7	62 × 7 = 434	7/90 = 0.077
54	3	54 × 3 = 162	3/90 = 0.033	63	6	63 × 6 = 378	6/90 = 0.066
55	6	55 × 6 = 330	6/90 = 0.066	64	5	64 × 5 = 320	5/90 = 0.055
56	5	56 × 5 = 280	5/90 = 0.055	65	6	65 × 6 = 390	6/90 = 0.066
57	7	57 × 7 = 399	7/90 = 0.077	66	4	66 × 4 = 264	4/90 = 0.044
58	8	58 × 8 = 464	8/90 = 0.088	67	4	67 × 4 = 268	4/90 = 0.044
59	6	59 × 6 = 354	6/90 = 0.066	68	1	68 × 1 = 68	1/90 = 0.011
60	10	60 × 10 = 600	10/90 = 0.111	69	1	69 × 1 = 69	1/90 = 0.011
	Σfi = n				n = 90		

Table 11.1. Frequency and relative frequency distribution of the resting heart rates in ninety marathon runners

As previously noted, the multiplication of each heart rate by its corresponding frequency determines the area of the unit rectangle. The total area, which is the sum of all the unit rectangles, $\sum_{i=1}^{n} x_i f_i$, when divided by the total number of the frequencies, $\sum_{i=1}^{n} f_i$ (total number of runners), gives the same arithmetic mean obtained earlier.

$$\overline{X} = \frac{\overset{n}{\underset{i=1}{\sum}} x_i \overset{\text{HR frequency}}{f_i}}{\underset{\text{Ttotal number of frequencies}}{\overset{n}{\underset{i=1}{\sum}} f_i}} = \frac{5426}{90} = 60.289 \text{ mean resting heart rate of the 90 runners.}$$

Two factors of importance emerge from the manipulation of the raw data, as follows:

1. The arithmetic mean derived from the raw data can be seen to be identical to the mean derived from the frequency distribution as noted in the following equation. Note that by adding a total of twenty numbers instead of the initial ninety, an identical result was obtained; hence,

$$\overline{X} = \frac{\overset{n}{\underset{i=1}{\sum}} x_i}{n} = \frac{\overset{n}{\underset{i=1}{\sum}} \overset{\text{Area of rectangle}}{x_i f_i}}{\underset{\text{Height of rectangle}}{\overset{n}{\underset{i=1}{\sum}} f_i}}$$

2. This identity between the two relations may not be apparent at first sight. However, as noted in Figure 11.2, it is easy to appreciate that the area enclosed by the rectangles when divided by the number of rectangles is actually the sum of the variable rates divided by the total number of their frequencies, which in this case corresponds to the number of subjects n, so that

$$\overline{X} = \frac{\sum_{i=1}^{n} x_i}{n} = \frac{\sum_{i=1}^{n} x_i \times 1(f_i) \quad \text{Unit base}}{\sum_{i=1}^{n} f_i = \quad n \quad \text{number of units}}$$

Frequency, as defined so far, is the number of repeated measurements associated with a subject, individual, or a class interval of the same rate.

The different heart rates may be conveniently grouped into a superclass of three contiguous rates, thus reducing the number of classes from eighteen to six. By reducing individual scores to a smaller number, it becomes easier to display and to grasp the overall pattern of distribution and spread. However, once the scores have been placed in class intervals, they lose their specific identity because the midpoint of the interval is assumed to represent the scores within.

HR X_i	Frequency f_i	$\sum_{i=1}^{n} x_i f_i = 2742$	Relative frequency $\left(\dfrac{f_i}{n}\right)$	HR X_i	Frequency f_i	$\sum_{1=n} x_i f_i = 2685$	Relative frequency $\left(\dfrac{f_i}{n}\right)$
53	6	53 × 6 = 318	6/90 = 0.0667	62	21	62 × 21 = 1,302	21/90 = 0.2333
56	18	56 × 18 = 1,008	18/90 = 0.2	65	15	65 × 15 = 975	15/90 = 0.1667
59	24	59 × 24 = 1,416	24/90 = 0.2667	68	6	68 × 6 = 408	6/90 = 0.0667

Table 11.2. Frequency and relative frequency distribution
of the resting heart rates in ninety marathon runners
grouped into six classes of three contiguous rates

When data are grouped together in class intervals as in Figure 11.2, then all values in the class are assumed to be equal to the class mark. The frequency of the class is written as f_i; with this notation, the mean can be computed for grouped data as follows:

$$\overline{X} = \frac{\overset{n}{\underset{i=1}{\sum}} \overset{\text{Area of class rectangle}}{x_i f_i}}{\underset{i=1}{\overset{n}{\sum}} \underset{\text{Height of class rectangle}}{f_i}} = \frac{x_1 f_1 + x_2 f_2 + \cdots + x_n f_n}{f_1 + f_2 + \cdots f_n} = \text{frequency} \times \text{class marks}$$

In this case, however, note that the total area of the six rectangles is slightly different from the area obtained when each rectangle represented a unique heart rate. This discrepancy, small in this case, may be significant when dealing with larger and more spread out array. Such being the case, the mean differs from that obtained earlier. The equality sign between the two derivation is now replaced with the almost equal sign as noted in the following relation:

$$\overline{X} = \frac{\overset{n}{\underset{i=1}{\sum}} x_i}{n} \cong \frac{\overset{n}{\underset{i=1}{\sum}} \overset{\text{Area of class rectangle}}{x_i f_i}}{\underset{i=1}{\overset{n}{\sum}} \underset{\text{Height of class rectangle}}{f_i}} = \frac{5427}{90} = 60.300 \ \text{mean resting heart rate of the runners.}$$

The histogram is now converted to the grouped data distribution interval with a width of three units.

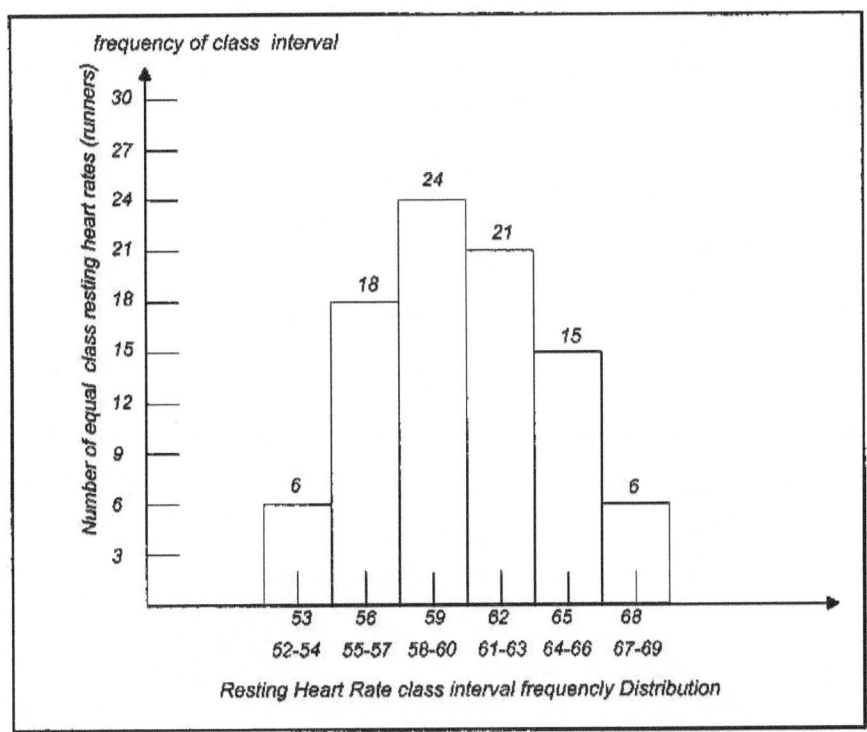

Figure 11.3. The height of each rectangle corresponds to the frequency. In this case, the base of each rectangle is a class unit instead of individual unit width, and its area now corresponds to the product of the frequency and the class mid rate.

The question of proportion rather than how many is answered by computing the relative frequency, which is the proportion or percentage of the different classes from the total number of cases.

By dividing each frequency of the class intervals by the total number of cases in the distribution, the proportion of cases in the interval is obtained, expressed as decimal fraction. The use of relative frequency is essential when comparing two or more frequency distribution.

In a relative frequency histogram, the height of each vertical bar in the histogram represents the proportion of observations is each class. Note that the sum of the relative frequencies equals 1 or 100 percent. In this case, the product of the class heart rate and the relative frequency, $\dfrac{f_i}{n}$, when summed over all the classes yields the same mean heart rate as obtained earlier.

$\sum x_i \times$ Relative frequency $= \overline{X} =$ Mean resting heart rate.

$53 \times 0.0667 + 56 \times 0.2 + 59 \times 0.2667 + 62 \times 0.2333 + 65 \times 0.1667 + 68 \times 0.0667 = 60.3061.$

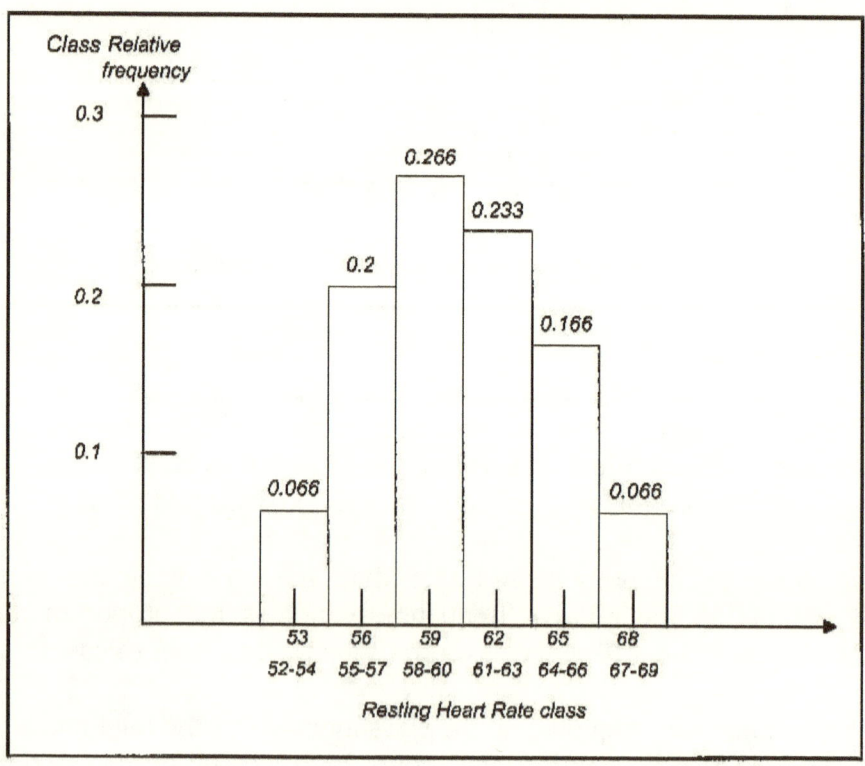

Figure 11.4. The height of each rectangle corresponds to the relative frequency. In this case, the base of each rectangle is a class unit instead of individual unit width, and its area now corresponds to the product of the relative frequency and the class mid rate.

The three relations may now be combined in order to bring forth a point that is equally relevant when dealing with probabilities and which in final analysis is the purpose of this presentation, as follows:

$$\overline{X} = \frac{\displaystyle\sum_{i=1}^{n} x_i}{\underset{\text{number of scores}}{n}} \cong \frac{\displaystyle\sum_{i=1}^{n} \overset{\text{HR}}{x_i} \times \overset{\text{frequency}}{f_i}}{\displaystyle\sum_{i=1}^{n} f_i} = \sum_{i=1}^{n} x_i \overset{\text{Relative frequency}}{\left(\frac{f_i}{n}\right)} = \text{Arithmetic mean of all observations.}$$

The practical equivalence of the three relations is of theoretical importance, as will be seen later.

Chapter 12

The Odds Paradigm as the Popular Mode

The odds approach, essentially a variant of probability, may be easier to comprehend, being the favored mode of predicting the outcome in sporting and gaming events. The concept is intuitive in its evaluation of success versus failure, as applied in the gambling jargon. The relationship between what is essentially two approaches to probability is not always firmly connected. One usually tends to think in terms of odds or probability, depending on habit, training, or experience.

In simple terms, the odds may be defined as the ratio of two mutually exclusive and exhaustive subsets of a given sample universe (e.g., ratio of number of persons with disease to those without in a given defined population universe). Thus, by splitting all possible outcomes of the sample universe into two distinct and complementary categories that are mutually exclusive and exhaustive, comprising as the situation warrants success versus failure, have versus have not, disease versus no disease, and so on, the concept of odds pits one subset against its complement in the form of a simple ratio or fraction. By contrast, probability is the ratio of a given subset to the total sample universe of which it is only one subset.

$P(S) = \dfrac{n(s)}{n(s)+n(f)} = \dfrac{n(s)}{n(U)}$	Number of possible outcomes $= n(U) =$ $n(s) + n(f)$	$P(\bar{S}) = \dfrac{n(f)}{n(s)+n(f)} = \dfrac{n(f)}{n(U)}$
Conversion to odds: Odds for event S $\dfrac{P(S)}{P(\bar{S})} = \dfrac{P(S)}{1-P(S)}$ Conversion to probability: Probability of S $= \dfrac{\text{Odds for S}}{1+\text{Odds for S}}$		Conversion to odds: Odds against event S $\dfrac{P(\bar{S})}{P(S)} = \dfrac{1-P(S)}{P(S)}$ Conversion to probability: Probability of $\bar{S}$ $= \dfrac{\text{Odds against S}}{1+\text{Odds against S}}$
Odds for event $S = \dfrac{n(s)}{n(f)}$	Sample Space $= U = S + \bar{S}$	Odds against event $S = \dfrac{n(f)}{n(s)}$

Table 12.1. Reciprocal conversion of odds and probability

Using success or failure as the defining outcome of a given event (craps, thoroughbred racing, or clinical trials), the odds for (in favor of) an event and against an event (usually given as a ratio rather than a fraction, which is normally used in probabilistic estimates) are stated as follows:

$$\text{Odds for Event S} = \frac{n(s)}{n(f)} = \frac{\text{number of successes}}{\text{number of failures}} = \frac{\text{Event S}}{\text{Complement } \overline{S}}$$

Event S is to be differentiated from the simple event s for success, which contains exactly one element in the subset S. Similarly, the complement of event S, $\overline{S}$, is to be differentiated from its constituent elements designated as f for failure. The sum of all the simple elements, both s and f, constitutes the sample space under consideration,

$$\text{Odds against Event S} = \frac{n(f)}{n(s)} = \frac{\text{number of failures}}{\text{number of successes}} = \frac{\text{Complement } \overline{S}}{\text{Event S}}.$$

Note that event S and its complement, $\overline{S}$, are mutually exclusive and exhaustive such that the total number of possible outcomes is the sum of all the simple events within the sample space, U.

In probabilistic terms, the number of successes or failures is related as a fraction to the total number of possible outcomes of both s and f,

$$P(S) = \frac{n(s)}{n(s)+n(f)} = \frac{n(s)}{n(U)} = \frac{\text{number of successes}}{\text{number of possible outcomes (both } s \text{ and } f)}$$

$$p(\overline{S}) = \frac{n(f)}{n(s)+n(f)} = \frac{n(f)}{n(U)} = \frac{\text{number of failures}}{\text{number of possible outcomes (both } s \text{ and } f)}$$

The conversion from one format to another is entered in the side panels for an overview of the inherent relationship. As a memory aid, the transition from odds to probability and vice versa may be envisaged as noted in the Venn diagram in terms of the elements and subsets comprising the sample space. Thus, odds is the ratio of the elements within the subset (circle), which are favorable for a particular event to those outside the circle, which are against the event in question. By contrast, the probability is the ratio of a given subset for or against to the total sample space. The conversion from one approach to another is simply a matter of adjusting by subtracting or adding the components of the sample space to fit the mode adopted.

The relationship between probability and odds is perhaps best appreciated using the classical throw of a fair die such that the probability of an ace (a successful event in the old literature) is the event in question. The relationship between the probability of an ace and the odds in favor of an ace is illustrated by the following example of forward and reverse conversion:

1s	2f	3f	4f	5f	6f

Converting to odds: read left to right.

$$P(S) = P(\text{Ace}) = \frac{1}{6} = \frac{s}{s+f} \rightarrow \left[\frac{P(S)}{1-P(S)}\right] \rightarrow \frac{1/6}{1-1/6} = \frac{1/6}{5/6} = \frac{1}{5} = \text{Odds in favor of } S$$

Converting to probability: read right to left.

$$P(S) = P(\text{Ace}) = \frac{1}{6} = \frac{1/5}{6/5} = \frac{1/5}{1+1/5} \leftarrow \left[\frac{\text{Odds}}{1+\text{Odds}}\right] \leftarrow \frac{s}{f} = \frac{1}{5} = \text{Odds in favor of } S \,(\text{Ace}).$$

Similarly, the relationship between the probability of no ace and the odds against an ace is illustrated by the following example of forward and reverse conversion:

$$P(\bar{S}) = P(\text{no Ace}) = \frac{5}{6} = \frac{s}{s+f} \rightarrow \left[\frac{1-P(S)}{P(S)}\right] \rightarrow \frac{5/6}{1-5/6} = \frac{5}{1} = \text{Odds against an Ace.}$$

$$P(\bar{S}) = P(\text{no Ace}) = \frac{5}{6} = \frac{5/1}{1+5/1} \leftarrow \left[\frac{\text{Odds against}}{1+\text{Odds against}}\right] \leftarrow \frac{f}{s} = \frac{5}{1} = \text{Odds against an Ace}$$

In converting from probability to odds, the numerator is subtracted from the denominator so as to reduce the denominator to the exact complement of the numerator. The reverse process of converting odds to probability involves restoring the denominator to include both subsets of the sample universe. In this case, the numerator is added to the denominator in order to restore the odds ratio to its original probability ratio.

In general, the denominator of the ratio is adjusted by adding or subtracting the necessary factor, f or s, to accommodate the desired conversion.

For the ace in question, the arithmetic involved is the addition or subtraction of 1 for the event under consideration and 5 for its complement,

$$P(S) = \frac{s}{s+f} = \frac{1}{6} = \frac{\left[\dfrac{s}{(s+f)-s}\right] \rightarrow}{\left[\dfrac{1}{5+1} = \dfrac{s}{s+f}\right] \leftarrow} = \frac{1}{6-1} = \frac{1}{5} = \frac{s}{f} = \text{Odds for S}$$

$$P(\overline{S}) = \frac{f}{s+f} = \frac{5}{6} = \frac{\left[\dfrac{s}{(s+f)-f}\right] \rightarrow}{\left[\dfrac{5}{5+1} = \dfrac{f}{s+f}\right] \leftarrow} = \frac{5}{6-5} = \frac{5}{1} = \frac{f}{s} = \text{Odds against S}$$

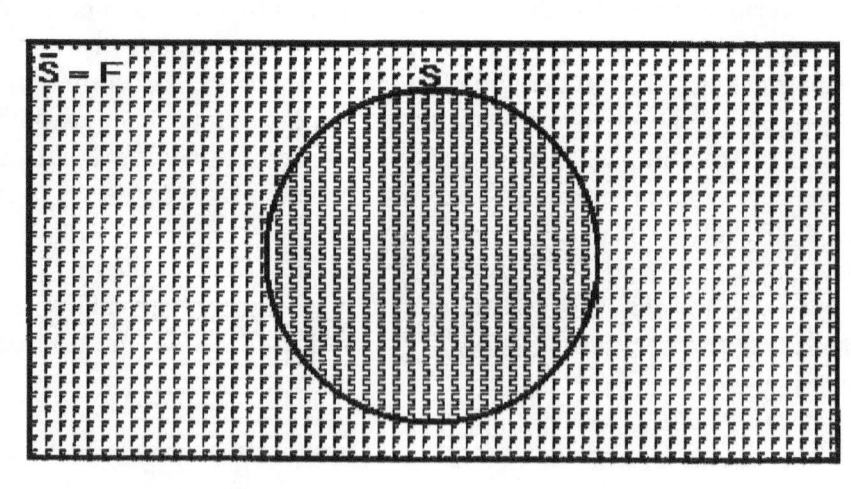

Odds in favor of S	Odds against S
$\dfrac{P(S)}{P(\overline{S})} = \dfrac{P(S)}{1-P(\overline{S})}$	$\dfrac{P(\overline{S})}{P(S)} = \dfrac{1-P(\overline{S})}{P(S)}$
Probability of S	Probability of $\overline{S}$
$\dfrac{\text{Odds in favor of S}}{1+\text{Odds in favor of S}}$	$\dfrac{\text{Odds against S}}{1+\text{Odds against S}}$

Figure 12.1. Venn diagram of the odds alternative to probability: reciprocal conversion formulae.

Part III
Clinical Application

Chapter 13

HIV Infection

The HIV epidemic continues to grow worldwide. As of September 1992, it is estimated that the number of AIDS cases in the United States exceeds one-fourth million, with more than a million infected with HIV-1. The increased number of cases and their broad dispersion require the active involvement of primary care physician. Physicians, however, usually tend to refer HIV-infected patients to specialty centers once seropositivity is identified. Clearly, all primary physicians must be able to assess risk of HIV-1 and, when indicated, initiate appropriate testing.

The clinical situation may involve asymptomatic patients with or without clear risk factors, or symptomatic patients with clinically active HIV-1 infection. Seroprevalence rates for HIV range from less than 0.1 percent (0.001) for the low-risk group to more than 20 percent for high-risk population.

Currently, the debate persists whether mass HIV screening should be initiated and whether health care providers should be tested. To answer these questions, a clear understanding of Bayes' theorem and its diagnostic implication is mandatory.

The current standard is to use an enzyme-linked immunosorbent assay (ELISA) to screen initially for HIV antibodies. The sensitivity and specificity of ELISA are reported to be 0.98 and 0.99, respectively. Given this unsurpassed sensitivity and specificity, the feasibility of universal screen seems to be logically obvious. In fact, what seems to be intuitively obvious will appear to be otherwise on closer scrutiny (Table 13.1). In this case, as in all testing procedure, the possibility of a false-positive result carries with it the need for further diagnostic procedures with its associated medical, economic, and social hazards, which in this case precludes, in particular, the need for mass screening.

If the ELISA is positive, the Western blot method is then used to confirm the diagnosis. The Western blot is positive when one of several patterns of colored bands is present; otherwise, in the absence of such pattern, the test is considered negative (neglect for the moment the indeterminate result). When done in sequence, ELISA and Western blot have a combined sensitivity of 99.9 percent and a combined specificity of 99.5 percent (Table 13.2).

13.1 HIV Screen in Blood Banks: Excerpts from a Debate in the Literature

The critical application of sensitivity and specificity in screening for what in 1985 was referred to as human T-cell lymphotropic virus type III (HTLV-III) was highlighted in the "Status Report on the Acquired Immunodeficiency Syndrome"[7] from the Council on Scientific Affairs of the American Medical Association. Referring to the recent introduction of ELISA testing by the three manufacturers listed in Table 13.3 for the screening of blood and plasma, the report states,

Table 13.3. Sensitivities, specificities, and expected false-positive rates for three HTLV-III antibody test kits

Manufacturer	Sensitivity	Specificity	Expected False Positive (Antibody Prevalence)	
			0.1 percent	1.0 percent
Abbott Laboratories	93.4 percent	99.8 percent	68	17
Electro-Nucleonics Inc.	99.6 percent	99.2 percent	89	44
Litton Bionetics	98.9 percent	99.6 percent	80	29

"At the present time approximately 20 million units of blood and plasma are processed annually in the nation in blood banking and plasma collection facilities. Assuming a 0.1% prevalence of HTLV-III antibody in the general population, and with the sensitivity

---

[7] Council on Scientific Affairs, "Status Report on the Acquired Immunodeficiency Syndrome," *Journal of the American Medical Association* 254 (1985): 1342-1345.

and specificity of the Abbott Laboratories HTLV-III ELISA kit, for example, it can be estimated that, on a national level, this would translate into approximately 20,000 positive test results, of which 13,600 (20,000 × 0.68) may be false-positive results."

In the February 14, 1986, issue, under the title "AIDS and Testing for AIDS," Dr. Michael Kanter,[8] in a letter to the editor responding to the Status Report, writes,

"The Council on Scientific Affairs calculated that testing blood components for human T-cell lymphotropic virus type III (HTLV-III) using Abbott Laboratories' enzyme linked immunosorbent assay kit would result in 20,000 positive results annually. This calculation assumed there are 20 million blood donors annually and a prevalence rate of HTLV-III antibody in the general population of 0.1%. Unfortunately, the number of donors (D) multiplied by the prevalence of the antibody (P) equals the number of persons with HTLV-III antibody, *not the number of positive test results* (Italics mine), as these authors concluded."

After a brief note on the derivation of true-positive and false-positive numbers, Dr. Kanter concludes that

"The number of positive test results will be 58,640, 179,760, and 99,700 using the kits by Abbott Laboratories, Electro-Nucleonics, Inc, and Litton Bionetics, respectively. The ratio of false-positives to true positives for a prevalence of 0.1% is 2.1, 8.0, and 4.0 and the *predictive value of a positive test result is 32%, 89%, and 80%* [Italics mine] using the kits by Abbott Laboratories, Electro-Nucleonics, Inc. and Litton Bionetics, respectively."

---

8   Letters; "Aids and Testing for Aids," *Journal of the American Medical Association* 255 (1986): 743.

In the June 6, 1986, issue, in a letter to the editor under the title "Testing for AIDS: More Problems with Predictive Values," Dr. Robert S. Wallis[9] writes, commenting on the letter by Dr. Kanter,

"While I agree with the thrust of the letter, it appears to contain two mathematical errors. The correct predictive values for the three assays (Abbott Laboratories, Electro-Nucleonics, Inc., and Litton Bionetics) should be 32%, 11%, and 20%, respectively (not 32%, 89%, and 80% as stated)" (Tables 4, 5, and 6).

Immediately, underneath the letter, a framed correction was inserted by the journal; quoted in part, it reads

---

CORRECTION

Incorrect Percentages—An error occurred in the Letter to the Editor entitled "AIDS and Testing for AIDS . . ." by Michael Kanter, MD, . . .

and the predictive value of a positive test result is 32%, 11%, and 20% (not '32%, 89%, and 80%') . . .

As noted in the attached tables, both Dr. Michael Kanter and Dr. Robert S. Wallis were correct in their calculation. Furthermore, the thrust of Dr. Kanter regarding the distinction between prevalence and true positives suggests that these basic concepts may not be always appreciated even at the highest level of erudition.

---

9   Letters; "Testing for Aids," *Journal of the American Medical Association* 255 (1986): 2900.

		HIV			
		Prevalence $P(D^+) =$	1-Prevalence $P(D^-) =$	Sample universe $P(U) = 1$	
		Disease present $n(D^+) = P(D^+) \times n(U)$ =2	Disease absent $n(D^-) = P(D^+) \times n(U)$ =998	Sample universe $n(U) = n(D^+) + n(D^-)$ =1,000	.
ELISA test	Positive test, T^+ Abnormal test	True positive $= n(D^+) \times$ Sens $=2 \times 0.98 = 1.96$	False positive $= n(D^-) = n(TN)$ =9.98	T^+ row total $= 11.94$	Predictive value of positive test, posterior probability $PV[+] = \dfrac{TP}{TP + FP}$ 1.96 / 11.94 = 16.4 percent
	Negative test, T^- Normal test	False negative $= n(D^+) - n(TP)$ =0.04	True negative $= n(D^-) \times SP$ $= 998 \times 0.99 = 988.02$	T^- row total $= 988.6$	Predictive value of negative test, posterior probability $PV[-] = \dfrac{TN}{TN + FN}$ 988.02 / 988.06 = 99.9 percent
		D^+ column total $= 2$ Sensitivity $= 0.98$ $= \dfrac{TP}{TP + FN}$	D^- column total $= 998$ Specificity $= 0.99$ $= \dfrac{TN}{TN + FP}$	U total	

Table 13.1. The sensitivity of the ELISA screening test for the HIV has been described to be as high as 0.98 (98 percent) and the specificity as high as 0.99 (99 percent). In a population in which 2 in 1,000 persons have been infected with the virus, a positive test result has a predictive value of 16.4 percent.

This is another way of saying "That only 16.4% of those reported positive, are truly positive and infected." The patient in question may or may not be truly positive. In fact, the chance of his being truly positive is one in six, whereas the chance of his being false positive, that is, free of infection but branded as positive, is five out of six or 83.6 percent.

These consideration apply with equal measure to all clinical and laboratory tests, of which the above is only one example.

		HIV			
		Prevalence	1-Prevalence	Sample universe	
		$P(D^+) = 0.164$	$P(D^-) = 0.836$	$P(U) = 1$	
		Positive Western blot	Negative Western blot	Sample universe	
		$n(D^+) = P(D^+) \times n(U)$	$n(D^-) = P(D^-) \times n(U)$	$n(U) = n(D^+) + n(D^-)$	
		=164	=836	=1,000	
ELISA test	Positive test, T$^+$ \ Abnormal test	True positive, ++ \ $=n(D^+) \times$ Sens \ $=164 \times 0.999 =$ 163.8	False positive, +− \ $=n(D^-) = n(TN)$ \ =3.2	T$^+$ row total \ \ 167	Predictive value of positive test, posterior probability \ $PV[+] = \dfrac{TP}{TP + FP}$ \ 1.96 / 11.94 = 16.4 percent
	Negative test, T$^-$ \ NORMAL TEST	False negative, −+ \ $=n(D^+) - n(TP)$ \ =0.2	True negative, − − \ $=n(D^-) \times SP$ \ $= 836 \times 0.995 =$ 831.8	T$^-$ row total \ \ =832	Predictive value of negative test, posterior probability \ $PV[-] = \dfrac{TN}{TN + FN}$
		D$^+$ column total = 164	D$^-$ column total = 836	U total = 1,000	
		Sensitivity = 0.999 \ $= \dfrac{TP}{TP + FN}$	Specificity = 0.995 \ $= \dfrac{TN}{TN + FP}$		

Table 13.2. The predictive value of 16.4 percent for the positive result derived in Table 13.1 may now be considered the prior probability or prevalence in this case because the positive result of the ELISA has increased the initial or prior probability of 0.02 percent to a posterior probability of 16.4 percent.

When this value is entered as the updated prevalence in the contingency 2×2 table, and the result of the Western blot is then juxtaposed to the results of ELISA, four possible sequence of results may be obtained: $+\,+$, $+\,-$, $-\,+$, and $-\,-$. In case both tests turn out to be positive, the predictive value soars to 98 percent, leaving little doubt as to the validity or accuracy of the result. On the other hand, a negative Western blot following a positive ELISA reduces the predictive value to a mere 2 percent ($1 - 0.98 = 0.02$).

		HIV			
		Prevalence $P(D^+) = 0.001$	1-Prevalence $P(D^-) = 0.999$	Sample universe $P(U) = 1$	
		Disease present $n(D^+) = P(D^+) \times n(U)$ =20,000	Disease absent $n(D^-) = P(D^-) \times n(U)$ =19,980,000	Sample universe $n(U) = n(D^+) \times n(D^-)$ =20,000,000	
ELISA test	Positive test, T⁺ Abnormal test	True positive $=n(D^+) \times$ Sens = 18,680	False positive $=n(D^-) = n(TN)$ =39,960	T⁺ row total = 58,640	Predictive value of positive test, posterior probability $PV[+] = \dfrac{TP}{TP + FP}$
	Negative test, T⁻ Normal test	False negative $=n(D^+) - n(TP)$ =1,320	True negative $= n(D^-) \times SP$ = 19,940,040	T⁻ row total =	Predictive value of negative test, posterior probability $PV[-] = \dfrac{TN}{TN + FN}$
		D⁺ column total	D⁻ column total	U total	
		Sensitivity = 93.4 percent $= \dfrac{TP}{TP + FN}$	Specificity = 99.8 percent $= \dfrac{TN}{TN + FP}$		

Table 13.4. Assuming a 0.1 percent (0.001) prevalence of HTLV-III among twenty million blood donors implies that the number of donors who are actually HTLV-III carriers is 20,000 (20 million × 0.001 = 20,000).

The number of true-positive test results given a sensitivity of 93.4 percent is 18,680 (20,000 × 0.934= 18,680), while the number of false-positive results given a **specificity** of 99.8 percent is 39,960 (19,980,000 × 0.002 = 39,960). The total number of positive test results (both true and false), using the Abbott kit, is then equal to 58,640 (18,680 + 39,960).

The predictive value of a positive test is then calculated as follows:

$$\frac{18,680}{18,680+39,960} = 0.318 = 32\%$$

		HIV			
		Prevalence $P(D^+) = 0.001$	1-Prevalence $P(D^-) = 0.999$	Sample universe $P(U) = 1$	
		Disease present $n(D^+) = P(D^+)$ $\times n(U)$ $=20,000$	Disease absent $n(D^-) = P(D^+)$ $\times n(U)$ $=19,980,000$	Sample universe $n(U) = n(D^+) +$ $n(D^-)$ $=20,000,000$	
ELISA test	Positive test, T^+ Abnormal test	True positive $=n(D^+) \times$ Sens $= 19,920$	False positive $=n(D^-)$ $- n(TN)$ $=159,840$	T^+ row total $= 179,760$	Predictive value of positive test, posterior probability $PV[+] = \dfrac{TP}{TP + FP}$
	Negative test, T^- Normal test	False negative $=n(D^+) - n(TP)$ $=80$	True negative $=n(D^-) \times$ SP $= 19,820,160$	T^- row total $=$	Predictive value of negative test, posterior probability $PV[-] = \dfrac{TN}{TN + FN}$
		D^+ column total	D^- column total	U total	
		Sensitivity = 99.6 percent $= \dfrac{TP}{TP + FN}$	Specificity = 99.2 percent $= \dfrac{TN}{TN + FP}$		

Table 13.5. Assuming a 0.1 percent (0.001) prevalence of HTLV-III among twenty million blood donors.

The number of true-positive test results given a sensitivity of 99.6 percent is 19,920, whereas the number of false-positive results given a specificity of 99.2 percent is 159,840. The total number of positive test results (both true and false), using the Electro-Nucleonics kit, is then equal to 179,760. The predictive value for a positive test is calculated at 11 percent.

		HIV			
		Prevalence	1-Prevalence	Sample universe	
		$P(D^+) = 0.001$	$P(D^-) = 0.999$	$P(U) = 1$	
		Disease present	Disease absent	Sample universe	
		$n(D^+) = P(D^+) \times n(U)$	$n(D^-) = P(D^+) \times n(U)$	$n(U) = n(D^+) + n(D^-)$	
		=20,000	=19,980,000	=20,000,000	
ELISA test	Positive test, T$^+$ Abnormal test	True positive $=n(D^+) \times$ Sens $= 19,780$	False positive $=n(D^-) - n(TN)$ =79,920	T$^+$ row total = 99,700	Predictive value of positive test, posterior probability $PV[+] = \dfrac{TP}{TP + FP}$
	NEGATIVE TEST, T$^-$ Normal test	False negative $=n(D^+) - n(TP)$ =220	True negative $=n(D^-) \times$ SP = 19,900,080	T$^-$ row total =	Predictive value of negative test, posterior probability $PV[-] = \dfrac{TN}{TN + FN}$
		D$^+$ column total	D$^-$ column total	U total	
		Sensitivity = 98.9 percent $= \dfrac{TP}{TP + FN}$	Specificity = 99.6 percent $= \dfrac{TN}{TN + FP}$		

Table 13.6. Assuming a 0.1 percent (0.001) prevalence of HTLV-III among twenty million blood donors.

The number of true-positive test results given a sensitivity of 98.9 percent is 19,780, whereas the number of false-positive results given a specificity of 99.6 percent is 79,920.

The total number of positive test results (both true and false), using the Litton Bionetics kit, is then equal to 99,700. The predictive value for a positive test is calculated at 20 percent.

Chapter 14

Tumor Markers

Tumor markers are assuming an increasingly prominent role in the screening, diagnosis, staging, and monitoring of cancer treatment. Established markers currently in use include carcinoembryonic antigen for colon cancer, human chorionic gonadotropin for trophoblastic cancer in women and testicular cancer in men, and α-fetoprotein for hepatocellular carcinoma and germ-cell tumors.

The prostate-specific antigen (PSA) as a serum marker for adenocarcinoma of the prostate represents at once a significant advance in the screening, diagnosis, and staging of the disease while simultaneously presenting a dramatic picture of confrontation between the advocates and the opponents of universal screening for the disease. To better appreciate the screening controversy, a brief note on the pathophysiology of prostate cancer is necessary.

Prostate cancer begins as a small focus within the peripheral portion of the gland (stage A). In most cases, this small cancer remains focal. It is estimated that the prevalence of this clinically insignificant prostate cancer for men fifty years or older ranges from 35 percent to 45 percent. An active focal cancer that grows into a prostate nodule enters stage B. Both stages A and B are usually asymptomatic and may or may not be detected on digital rectal examination (DRE). The cancer enters symptomatic stage C when the nodule perforates the prostate capsule. In stage D, the cancer spreads beyond the confines of the gland to involve the pelvic lymph nodes and/or bone.

A rational approach to this debate must consider the natural history of the disease as well as the parameters of the screening test under consideration. In order to put the natural history of the disease in perspective, one needs to begin, paradoxically, with the outcome rather than the inception of the disease.

Numerous studies have consistently documented that approximately 30 percent of men between fifty and seventy-five years have subclinical so-called latent prostate cancer. This is an averaging process that obliterates the age-dependent frequency one needs to be aware of in assessing the real frequency in a given patient, considering that the prevalence rate in men aged seventy-five years (bracket of seventy to seventy-nine years) is approximately 42 percent, far in excess of the average for men older than fifty years.

Because prevalence defines the number of men who actually harbor histologically recognizable disease rather than the number who will actually develop it, the magnitude of this percentage is best appreciated when translated into the staggering number of approximately nine million men, representing approximately one-third of the more than fifty male population in the United States (28,038,000 men >50/3 = 9,346,000). This bleak picture is partially alleviated by the fact that the number of men who will develop the clinical disease in one year (1993) is relatively small accounting for 135,000 patients for the year, or 1.4 percent (135,000/9,346,000 = 1.4 percent) of the estimated subclinical total to be found in men older than fifty years.

The incidence of prostate cancer, which reflects the probability that an individual older than fifty years will develop the clinical disease, is estimated at 0.48 percent per year.

Estimated number of more than fifty men in the United States: 28,038,000

Prevalence of latent prostate cancer in the more than fifty men in the United States = 30 percent

Estimated number of more than fifty men in the United States with latent cancer = 28,038,000 / 3 = 9,346,000

Prostate cancer incidence = 135,000 patients/year (1993)

Incidence in men older than fifty years: 135,000/28,038,000 per year = 0.48 percent

Prostate cancer mortality = 35,000 patients/year (1993)

Mortality rate in men older than fifty years: 35,000 / 28,038,000 per year = 0.12 percent

Prevalence-to-death ratio: 9,346,000 / 35,000 = 267:1

Similarly, the expected number of deaths from metastatic prostate cancer for 1993 is estimated at 35,000 for the year, which translates into a probability of death from the disease in men older than fifty years of 0.12 percent per year.

The high prevalence-to-death ratio of 267:1 is unique to this most common malignancy in men, which further emphasizes the extreme divergence between prevalence on the one hand and incidence or mortality on the other hand.

The divergence between incidence and prevalence would have been a mitigating factor except for the fact that once the malignancy escapes its capsular confines, its potential for cure is almost eliminated, and because this picture represents most cases at presentation, the need to detect the malignancy while still in its intracapsular confines is paramount. Alternatively, the identification of the pathological factors responsible for the crossover of the malignant focus from its intracapsular to its extracapsular phase may serve equally well to isolate those who are most likely to benefit from surgical intervention while sparing those presumed to remain in the subclinical phase from unnecessary intervention. The prevalence of these potentially invasive foci is estimated at 6 to 9 percent of the total.

The PSA is normally secreted by the epithelial cells into the prostate duct system as a normal constituent of human semen with a minimal reflux into the circulation. The disruption of the prostate architecture by inflammation or infiltration leads to an increase reflux into the circulation, with resulting greater concentration of PSA in the serum. In addition, because PSA is exclusively the product of both normal hyperplastic and neoplastic prostatic tissues, its concentration in the serum is in direct proportion to the tissue mass or volume, both normal or neoplastic. With this in mind, elevation beyond the normal range may be equally the result of benign prostate hypertrophy (BPH) or malignant increase in tissue mass.

Metpath (*Metpath Reference Manual*, 1994) quotes the reference range for men older than 40 years using an enhanced monitoring assay as 0.5-4.0 MCG/L.[10]

Prostate cancerous tissue, however, produces considerably higher levels of PSA per unit volume than BPH. In fact, it has been calculated that serum PSA is elevated on average 3.6 ng/mL (Yang assay) for every gram of prostate cancer (compared with 0.3 ng/mL for every gram of BPH).

---

[10] Values between 4 and 11.8 are more likely to be secondary to BPH than to cancer, whereas values between 11.8 and 22 are just as likely to be cancer as BPH. Values higher than 22 are highly suggestive of cancer. There is no single value of PSA that is diagnostic of cancer. Cancer may be found in association with low or high levels of PSA.

These differential data in PSA levels per unit volume form the background of the concept of PSA density, defined as the ratio of serum PSA concentration to prostate volume as measured by transrectal ultrasonography. Statistically significant differences between mean PSA density values for BPH and cancer (e.g., 0.044 and 0.581, respectively) have been reported as fairly accurate in distinguishing between BPH and cancer.

In patients with PSA density higher than 0.15 and a serum PSA between 4.1 and 10, the risk for prostate cancer is estimated at a minimum of 15 percent, which makes it possible to identify the high-risk subset that should be further evaluated (i.e., with direct biopsy).

Moreover, in the advanced stage of prostate cancer, PSA correlates closely with the prostatic cancer volume, thus making PSA a valuable staging tool in untreated patients. Alternatively, PSA may serve as a marker for the complete elimination of cancerous tissue, so that following a successful radical prostatectomy, serum PSA levels tend to fall to zero. Failure to recede to the zero level implies residual metastatic foci.

A second corollary of the differential secretion rate per unit volume between cancerous and hyperplastic tissue is the concept of the rate of change of PSA over a specified period. The concept is of course an extension of the fact that doubling the cancerous volume would result in a steeper rate of increase in the level of PSA as compared with the same hyperplastic volume. Thus, the difference in the rate of increase has been shown to be of diagnostic import in distinguishing benign hyperplastic tissue from intracapsular cancerous tissue.

In order to evaluate statistically the role of PSA as a screening tool, a MEDLINE search for screening studies was conducted by Dorr et al.[11] No conclusive set of parameters emerged from the search.

---

[11] V. J. Dorr, et al., "An Evaluation of Prostate-Specific Antigen as a Screening Test for Prostate Cancer," *Archives of Internal Medicine* 153 (1993): 2529-2537.

However, when these studies were averaged, a sensitivity of 71 percent (81-43 percent range) and a specificity of 75 percent (93-59 percent range) were obtained for PSA value greater than 4.0 ng/dL.

Dr. Dorr concludes, "To date, there is no evidence that screening with PSA will result in a better outcome. PSA, in these studies, failed to prove itself as a clinically effective screening test."

Using the reported prevalence of 30 percent and the averaged values of sensitivity and specificity calculated by Dorr et al., Table 14.1. is constructed to delineate the unacceptable range of false positive and false negative associated with the three parameters.

		Prostate Carcinoma			
		Prevalence P(D⁺)=300	1 − Prevalence 1-P(D⁺)=700	Sample universe	
PSA	Positive test, T⁺ >4 µg/L Abnormal test	True positive = 213	False positive = 175	T⁺ row total = 388	PV[+] = 54.9 percent 1 − PV[+] = 45.1 percent = 45.2 percent
	Negative test, T− <4 µg/L Normal	False negative =87	True negative =525	T⁻ row total =612	1 − PV[−] = 14.3 percent PV[−] = 85.7 percent
		D⁺ column total = 300	D⁻ column total = 700	U total = 1,000	
		Sensitivity = 71 percent	Specificity = 75 percent		

Table 14.1. Predictive values for PSA of >4.0 ng/dL in men older than 50 years. Based on the averaging of data from available studies[2]

If the prevalence of prostatic cancer in the male population of the United States older than fifty years is assumed to be 30 percent, then with a sensitivity of 71 percent and a specificity of 75 percent, the probability is more than 50 percent that a randomly selected man older than 50 years, with a positive, test does in fact harbor an occult form of prostate cancer. In the face of 30 percent prevalence, a specificity of 75 percent is totally inadequate to separate the true positive from the false positive, thus rendering such a screening enterprise inadequate to the task.

From Table 14.1, a positive predictive value of 54.8 is obtained associated with a predictive value for a false-positive result, that is, a predictive value of the complement of 45.1 percent. In view of the unique pathophysiology associated with cancer of the prostate, the unqualified use of PSA as a screening test is untenable because it is the product of normal hyperplastic as well as cancerous prostate tissue. As a result, benign conditions such as BPH and prostatitis can be associated with abnormal levels of serum PSA. However, given the direct correlation between prostate tissue volume and PSA level, it seems logical to ascertain that the rate of change of PSA level over time from a baseline value rather than the baseline value per se is of diagnostic import. This indeed was the subject of a paper by Carter et al.[12] on what is aptly termed the longitudinal evaluation of PSA levels with and without prostate disease. In this study, Carter et al. was able to document that consecutive yearly tests can significantly increase the ability to differentiate between patients with BPH and those with prostatic cancer even before the diseases are clinically evident. PSA elevation tends to be gradual up to the time of diagnosis in men with BPH, whereas PSA levels increase exponentially 5 to 10 years prior to a diagnosis of prostate cancer.

To quote from the comment at the end of the article, "The increasing prevalence of prostate disease that occurs with age is the most important factor affecting PSA level in men. In men thought to have no evidence

---

[12] H. B. Carter et al., "Longitudinal Evaluation of Prostate-Specific Antigen Levels in Men with and without Prostate Disease," *Journal of the American Medical Association* 267 (1992): 2215-2220.

of prostate disease (control group), the rate of change in PSA was lower than in subjects with prostate disease and was not significantly different from 0.0 µg/L per year." Dr. Carter concludes, "Therefore, PSA elevations are not specific for prostate cancer, and a normal PSA level does not exclude the presence of cancer. This is reflected in the 78.7% sensitivity and 59.2% specificity using PSA of 4.0 µg/L or greater as a detection criterion in a recent prostate screening study."[4]

Table 14.2 was constructed from the data of serum PSA concentrations in 235 men in the comparison group studied by Catalona et al.[13]

		Prostate carcinoma			
		Prevalence $P(D^+) = 61$	$1 - \text{Prevalence}$ $1 - P(D^+) = 174$	Sample universe	
PSA	Positive test, T^+ >4 µg/L Abnormal test	True positive $= 48$	False positive $= 71$	T^+ row total $=119$	PV[+] = 48/119 = 40 percent
	Negative test, $T-$ <4 µg/L Normal test	False negative $= 13$	True negative $= 103$	T^- row total $= 116$	PV[−] = 103/116 = 89 percent
		D^+ column total	D^- column total	U total = 235	
		Sensitivity = 48/61 = 78.7 percent	Specificity = 103/174 = 59.2 percent		

Table 14.2. Sensitivity and specificity of PSA as a detection criterion for prostate cancer screening using a cutoff point of >4 µg/L. Reconstructed Table based on sample data of 235 men studied by Catalona et al.[4]

13   W. J. Catalona et al., "Measurement of Prostate-Specific Antigen in Serum as a Screening Test for Prostate Cancer," *New England Journal of Medicine* 324 (1991): 1156-1154.

Dr. Carter concludes his comment, "Using the same criterion for prostate cancer detection we found a 78% sensitivity and a 60% specificity in this case control study. When we used a prostate cancer detection criterion based on the average rate of change in PSA between three consecutive visits (PSAR2 $\geq$0.75 µg/L per year, we found no difference in the sensitivity of prostate cancer detection compared with the use of PSA of 4.0 µg/L or greater. However, the use of this rate of change criterion in prostate cancer detection significantly increased the ability to differentiate between subjects with BPH and prostate cancer (specificity, 90%)."

Screening Criteria	Sensitivity at Diagnosis	Specificity at Diagnosis	
		BPH Cases	Controls
Single measurement (µg/L) PSA $\geq$ 4.0	0.78	0.6	0.94
Average rate of change (µg/L per year)[#] PSAR2 $\geq$ 0.75 in total sample	0.72	0.9	0.94
PSAR2 $\geq$ 0.75 when PSA< 4µg/L	0.11	1	1
[#]Rate of change in PSA levels over three consecutive visits.			

Table 14.3. Sensitivity and specificity with various screening criteria. Excerpted from Table 4 of Carter et al.[4]

The criteria for evaluating tumor markers are no different from the basic criteria applicable to all diagnostic tests. The basic parameters of sensitivity, specificity, and prevalence dictate as always the predictive values of a given result relative to the presence or absence of the marker target.

In this setting, the high sensitivity is crucial if the number of false negatives (FN) is to be kept within acceptable limits. Similarly, high specificity is essential if the number of false positives (FP) is to be restricted to an acceptable minimum. The third parameter of prevalence is of course the clinically and often subjectively derived variable of the trio that is population dependent (advanced age, benign prostatic hypertrophy, a prior history of sexually transmitted disease, and black race) that will impact the predictive value of the test.

For diagnostic purpose in symptomatic patients, specificity is favored over sensitivity. A high specificity guarantees low false-positive rate (neglecting for the moment other factors that contribute to the false-positive rate such as cross-reactivity to other tumor types), thus avoiding as much as possible the costly invasive procedures in cancer free patients. For screening purposes, however, a high level of sensitivity is required in order to reduce the number of false negatives, thus minimizing the chance of missing a true cancer patient.

In an editorial in the same issue by Joseph E. Oesterling[14] of the Mayo Clinic, we quote selectively to focus on the issue of screening:

"Although the routine use of PSA is associated with an increased prostate cancer detection rate, it is not sufficiently specific to be used alone as a screening test for prostate cancer."

Referring to the article by Carter et al. in the same issue that was quoted previously, Dr. Oesterling comments,

"To this end, Carter and associates in their paper in this issue have examined the concept of "rate of change in serum PSA." In this unique study, they demonstrated that the rate of change was more useful than the actual serum PSA level for detecting prostate cancer. When using a cutoff of 0.75 µg/L or higher per year for the rate of change, the specificity was 90% as compared with 60% for the cutoff of 4.0 µg/L or higher for the serum PSA concentration. The sensitivity for the rate of change, however, was not significantly better than that for the serum PSA concentration. Nevertheless, the increase specificity will undoubtedly have valuable implications

---

[14] J. E. Osterling, "Prostate-Specific Antigen: Improving the Ability to Diagnose Early Prostate Cancer," *Journal of the American Medical Association* 267 (1992): 2236-2238.

as more and more patients return annually for a serum PSA determination and DRE. Thus, the serum PSA level going from 1.8 µg/L to 2.9 µg/L in 1 year's time would be significant and may lead to the detection of potentially curable prostate cancer, even though both values are well within the reference range."

In response to the article by Carter et al. and the editorial by Oesterling, seven letters to the editor were printed in the December issue of the journal. Again, in order to focus on the necessity of acquiring an intuitive appreciation of the subject matter of this monograph that extends beyond the mechanistic and numerical definition of terms and variables associated with probability, a selective quote may be in order.

Dr. Thomas E. Lindow of Amesbury, Massachusetts, writes,

"As a nonresearcher clinician, I get confused enough already by statistical terms such as specificity, sensitivity, false-positive, and true-negative. I don't need to be made more confused by those who write the editorials, such as Oesterling in his *JAMA* editorial on PSA testing. The study by Carter et al. in the same issue demonstrated an improved specificity, but unimproved or worsened sensitivity of the PSA test for detecting prostate cancer by using its rate of change per year rather than its absolute value.

Oesterling, in referring to that study, states, "The sensitivity of the rate of change (of PSA) was not significantly better than that for serum PSA concentration." He then contradicts himself with the statement, "Thus, the serum PSA level going from 1.8 µg/L to 2.9 µg/L in 1 year's time would be significant and may lead to detection of potentially curable prostate cancer, though the values are well within the reference range." In the first statement, he acknowledges that such a change is the PSA level is no better (in fact, worse; 11 percent sensitivity for changes below the level of 4 mg/L) at detecting prostate cancer than the absolute PSA value would be. He seems to be muddling the concept of specificity with that of sensitivity because the sentence he writes directly between the above two is, "Nevertheless, the increased specificity will undoubtedly have valuable implications as more and more patients return annually for a serum PSA determination and DRE."

These are astute remarks by a "nonresearcher clinician" that addresses the crucial difference in the often misused and misinterpreted terms sensitivity and specificity.

To date, the prevailing clinical judgment advocates the annual determination of PSA to be followed by the determination of the PSA density for PSA $\geq$ 4 µg/L. A transrectal ultrasonography-guided sextant biopsy is indicated if the PSA density exceeds 0.15. Once the biopsy results are confirmed, surgical intervention (radical prostatectomy or external beam irradiation) is advised. One must ponder the implication of this scenario when applied to nine million men presumed to harbor the latent form of prostate cancer. The paradox becomes even more problematic when one considers the alternative for the individual patient, notwithstanding the statistical facts of incidence.

The multicenter trial under way will hopefully resolve the conflict by the turn of the century.

Chapter 15

Myocardial Infarction in the Emergency Department

Of the multitude of emergent conditions, the diagnosis of acute or evolving myocardial infarction (MI) remains a challenging encounter in clinical medicine. The challenge in question is not involved in the classical presentation of acute MI. What is being referred to is the case that precludes all the classical manifestation of acute MI, both electrocardiographic and clinical, together with all associated findings that may account for the presence of ACP in a hemodynamically stable patient considered to be potentially at risk.

In the setting of the emergency department (ED), the "R/O MI" dictum carries with it logistic, economical, and medicolegal implications. Irrespective of the final disposition of such a case (intensive care, intermediate care, or continued observation in the ED), the need for additional diagnostic testing, immediate or longitudinal, is obviously required. Of the many available options that may be considered (echocardiographic wall motion analysis, Tc 99mm pyrophosphate scan), given an inconclusive initial ECG finding, vital signs monitoring in conjunction with serial electrocardiography and serial CK-MB measurements seem to present a rational alternative in the current ED setting.

This was the subject of a study on the comparative role of serial electrocardiogram and serial CK-MB determination in confirming or ruling out the presence of acute MI conducted in the Department of Emergency Medicine at Oregon Health Science University.[15]

The study included 261 hemodynamically stable patients presenting with ACP described as chest discomfort associated with inconclusive initial ECG findings. Concurrent or parallel serial ECGs and CK-MB determinations were performed in accordance with a fixed protocol

---

[15] J. R. Hedges et al., "Serial ECGs Are Less Accurate than Serial CK-MB Results for Emergency Department Diagnosis of Myocardial Infarction," *Annals of Emergency Medicine* 21 (1992): 1445-1450.

(hourly CK-MB assay following initial sample at presentation and a repeat ECG concurrent with the fourth blood sample, three hours after the initial ECG tracing). Using set criteria for the assessment of evolving ECG changes (ECG-Δ), a total of thirty-eight patients (26+12) were identified as exhibiting significant serial ECG-Δ changes of whom eleven patients (3+8) were documented MI patients. In a similar vein, using a cutoff level ≥8 ng/mL of blood anytime during the three-hour period of observation as the criterion of significant change, thirty patients (11+7+8+4) were identified of whom nineteen were true MI. The derived sensitivities, specificities, and predictive values of both ECG-Δ and CK-MB are listed together in Table 15.1.

The sensitivity and the specificity of CK-MB are shown to be superior to that of ECG-Δ, given a nondiagnostic initial ECG. CK-MB is of course far more sensitive after eight to twelve hours from the onset of chest pain than during the first few hours.

In the previously mentioned analysis, each test was separately evaluated with reference to the diagnosis in question. The concurrent performance of two different tests with different sensitivities and specificities allows the parallel evaluation of sensitivity when either one of the two tests or both is positive. Similarly, the parallel evaluation of specificity is made possible when neither one nor the other is positive, that is, when both are concurrently negative (Table 15.2).

	MI	Rule Out MI	Row Total
Evolving ECG-Δ, negative CK-MB	3	23	26
Nonspecific ECG-Δ, positive CK-MB	11	7	18
Evolving ECG-Δ, positive CK-MB	8	4	12
	TP = 3 + 11 + 8 = 22	FP = 23 + 7 + 4 = 34	56
Nonspecific ECG-Δ, negative CK-MB	FN = 6	TN = 199	205
	No. of MIs = 28	No. of ruled out MIs = 233	No. of patients = 261
	Combined sensitivity 22 / 28 = 78.5 percent	Combined specificity 199 / 233 = 85 percent	

Table 15.2. Sensitivity and specificity of either an evolving ECG (ECG-Δ) or a CK-MB value above a cutoff level of ≥8 ng/mL or both as a parallel or concurrent criterion during a three-hour observation period in stable patients presenting with ACP

Compared with the sensitivity of either ECG-Δ or CK-MB, the parallel and concurrent evaluations of both, as noted in Table 15.2, yield a distinctly superior sensitivity of 79 percent.

Compared with their respective specificities of 95 and 96 percent, the parallel specificity of 85 percent is distinctly inferior.

Parallel combination unlike serial combination tends to favor sensitivity at the expense of specificity. In this format, the use of the concurrent results made possible the identification of twenty-two true-positive MI patients out of a total of twenty-eight proven cases. In comparison, serial ECG changes, ECG-Δ, correctly identified eleven of twenty-eight proven cases, whereas CK-MB alone was capable of correctly identifying nineteen of twenty-eight proven cases.

	Myocardial Infarction			
	Prevalence $P(D^+)$	1-Prevalence $P(D^-)$	Sample universe $P(U) = 1$	
	Disease present	Disease absent	Sample universe	
	$n(D^+) = P(D^+)$ $\times\, n(U)$ $= 28$	$n(D^-) = P(D^-)$ $\times\, n(U)$ $= 233$	$n(U) = P(D^+) +$ $n(D^-)$ $= 261$	
Positive ECG-Δ	True positive = $n(D^+) \times$ Sens $= 11$	False positive = $n(D^-) - n(TN)$ $= 27$	T^+ row total $= 38$	Predictive value of positive test $$PV[+] = \frac{TP}{TP+FP} = \frac{11}{11+27} = 29\%$$
CK-MB ≥8 ng/ mL	True positive $= 19$	False positive $= 11$	T^+ row total $= 30$	Predictive value of positive test $$PV[+] = \frac{TP}{TP + FP} = \frac{19}{19+11} = 63\%$$
Negative ECG-Δ	False negative $= n(D^+) - n(TP)$ $= 17$	True negative = $n(D^-) \times$ SP $= 206$	T^- row total $= 223$	Predictive value of negative test $$PV[-] = \frac{TN}{TN+FN} = \frac{206}{206+17} = 92\%$$
CK-MB <8 ng/ mL	False negative $= 9$	True negative $= 222$	T^- row total $= 231$	Predictive value of negative test $$PV[-] = \frac{TN}{TN + FN} = \frac{222}{222+9} = 96\%$$
	ECG-Δ sensitivity $11 / 28 = 0.39$ CK-MB sensitivity $19 / 28 = 0.68$	ECG-Δ sensitivity $206 / 233 = 0.88$ CK-MB specificity $222 / 233 = 0.95$		

Table 15.1. Sensitivity and specificity of evolving ECG changes (ECG-Δ), as the sole criterion of evolving MI during a three-hour period of observation compared with the sensitivity and specificity of CK-MB using a cutoff level ≥8 ng/mL of blood, during the same three-hour period as an alternative criterion

Chapter 16

Stress Test

Of all the hemodynamic and electrocardiographic variables associated with exercise stress test, the ST segment depression has been documented to be the best quantitative predictor of the severity of coronary artery disease (CAD).

Normally, for routine diagnostic consideration, the cutoff level of ST segment depression is usually set at 1 mm, effectively splitting the continuous spectrum of ST segment depression into a binary format, thus dividing the tested population set into a nominal dichotomous categories of positive (both true positive and false positive) and negative (both true negative and false negative) subsets.

It is important to be cognizant at all time of the diagnostic impact of a change in the cutoff level of the variable being measured. The adoption of a different cutoff effectively changes the numerical values in each subset for the same set by altering the sensitivity and specificity of the test; in a sense, it is the equivalent of adopting a different protocol for each instituted change in the level. The numerical values obtained in each subset of the binary table thus become a function of the sensitivity and specificity associated with the adoption of a lenient or stringent criterion as the current cutoff level assigned to the protocol.

Consider the effect on the false-positive and false-negative results in going from a stringent cutoff level, set at 2.5 mm, designated as T2, to a more lenient cutoff level, set at 0.5 mm, designated as T1 (Figure 16.1). In this theoretical example, starting with the stringent cutoff level, the specificity attains a value of 0.81. The perusal of the binary table reveals marked decrease in the false positives, ↓FP, such that a positive test is much more likely to be true positive than when the ST level is set at 0.5 mm. The price for the increased specificity is the concomitant decrease in the sensitivity to 0.55 as noted from the commensurate and unavoidable increase in the number of the false negatives, ↑FN.

This is a logical corollary of the accepted clinical dictum, that a good diagnostic test carries with it a very high degree of specificity, whereas the inflated false-negative subset now includes what may be considered as unacceptable numbers of missed diagnosis labeled as negative, which in reality would be classified as true positive by reference to the gold standard.

It is obvious that while tightening the criteria for positivity by setting the cutoff level at 2.5 mm is ideally suited for establishing the diagnosis when positive, it may prove to be counterproductive if the intended purpose to screen for CAD.

At the other end of the spectrum, the designated lenient level of T1 reverses the sensitivity-specificity ratio. The resultant increase in sensitivity to 0.81 cuts down the level of false negative, $\downarrow$FN, so that very few truly positive cases would remain undiagnosed.

The price, of course, is the commensurate and unacceptable increase in the number of false positives, $\uparrow$FP, with its unavoidable consequence of unnecessary and costly workup needed to undo what might have been in the first place a misplaced decision. The highly sensitive test, however, does qualify as a screening net through which very few persons falsely labeled as negative will escape being ensnared. On the other hand, a negative test in this setting carries with it a very high probability of being free of the disease.

The alternate graphic technique to the Venn diagram is the use of the classic "normal" frequency distribution curve to demonstrate the effect of the cutoff level. In general, the continuous variables associated with chemical or pathophysiological test results assumes a normal (bell-shaped) frequency distribution for both normal and diseased subjects. When the frequency distribution of the variable in question is plotted simultaneously for both normal and disease subjects, the result takes the form of normal overlapping distribution curves as seen in Figure 16.2A-16.2C. The x axis in this case covers the range assumed by the variable under normal and pathological conditions.

The distinct separation between the mean of the variable in the diseased and healthy population is clearly demarcated, whereas the degree of overlap delineates the fact that the demarcation between the normal and the pathological is never a clear-cut separation but rather a gradual spread from a common shared boundary. The positioning of the vertical cutoff line thus splits the area under the two bell-shaped curves into four separate areas.

The T1 line corresponds to the cutoff level associated with maximum sensitivity. Because the range of the normal response curve covered by the dotted area of the curve extends deep under the disease curve, a patient exhibiting ≥ 0.5 mm ST segment depression will be considered positive, irrespective of the fact that the point on the x axis that identifies the magnitude of $\downarrow$ST may actually belong to either of the two overlapping curves, implying that the result may prove to be true or false positive.

At the other end of the spectrum, the T2 line corresponding to the cutoff level associated with maximum specificity assumes that a patient exhibiting $\downarrow$ST <2.5 mm must be considered as a negative responder, again ignoring the fact that the point in question may belong to either of the two overlapping curves (Figure 16.2B).

For any given cutoff line, the values on the positive side falling simultaneously under either one of the overlapping curves may be either true or false positive. Similarly, values on the negative side of the line may be either true or false negative.

Although the respective areas under the distribution curves corresponding to the binary table may also be quantitatively demarcated, the resultant change when the two cutoff values are simultaneously plotted may not be readily appreciated. In Figure 16.1, by contrast, the four subsets are clearly demarcated for any one cutoff level. The resultant change in the numerical value of each subset as reflected by the expansion and contraction of the allocated area is visually appreciated.

The correspondence between the subsets of the Venn diagram and the areas bounded by the normal frequency distribution curves is emphasized through the use of identical fill in pattern for the corresponding subsets. The common pattern shared by the two graphic displays serves to emphasize the unity of the Bayesian and statistical approach to probability, a subject that will be touched upon later.

The above graphic example underline the need to relate quantitatively the changing cutoff level in a continuous variable to the resulting change in the true-positive and false-positive rates (i.e., sensitivity and specificity) over the whole range of the observed continuum because the same relationship applies to any test result that ranges over a set of quantitative values that could be depicted on an interval or ratio scale.

The resulting curve (Figure 16.3) defines each point on the ST segment depression continuum in terms of its corresponding true-positive and false-positive rates, euphemistically referred to as the ROC curve. For any given point (i.e., for any level of ST segment cutoff), the y coordinate defines the true-positive rate (sensitivity), whereas the x coordinate defines the false-positive rate (1 − specificity). Alternatively, the point in question could be equally defined in terms of false-negative rate (1 − sensitivity) for its y coordinate and true-negative rate (specificity) for its x coordinate. As noted in the graph, each alternate pair of x and y parameters is the complement of the corresponding pair. Thus, the inverse relationship between sensitivity and specificity is readily apparent from the plotted cutoff values by moving upward and rightward and downward and leftward along the curve and noting the change in the respective coordinates.

In this case, setting the cutoff level at the most lenient level of ↓ST ≥ 0.5 mm resulted in boosting the sensitivity into the 90s level at the expense of cutting the specificity to 24 percent. At the other end of ↓ST ≥ 2.5 mm, the specificity is boosted to the high 90s while curtailing the sensitivity into the 20s.

It is important to note that any change in the technique, method of computation, or selection of the variables defining the changes associated with the intervention will have a direct impact on the shape and limits of the ROC curve (Figure 16.3), as might be obtained when the ST segment depression is evaluated without any specific adjustment.

Equally apparent in any given ROC curve is the way the cutoff point subdivides the tested population into a subset of positive results, denoting the presumed presence of disease, and a subset of negative results, denoting the presumed absence of disease.

The importance of the ROC curve in defining the cost-benefit ratio of a given cutoff point must be fully appreciated in the context of decision-making process in order to maximize or optimize a desired end point. The choice of the cutoff level then becomes an instrument of decision applicable to the situation on hand, namely, screening versus diagnosis.

Thus, in the selection of the cutoff point, both economic and health costs inherent in the associated error need to be carefully considered. When the well-being of the patient is paramount, the psychological and often the crippling effect of being branded falsely as a carrier of the disease need to be balanced by failure to detect treatable or life-threatening condition. When financial considerations are important, the cost associated with disproving a false positive needs to be balanced by the future cost of progressive morbidity.

Viewed in this light, a body of literature now exists concerned with the precise quantitative choice of the cutoff level specially tailored to meet the need of the given situation. The cutoff level now becomes a variable designed to meet specific conditions. Furthermore, based on the designated cutoff level, a dichotomous process of decision making may be constructed to elicit the cost-benefit ratio of the alternative courses of action available.

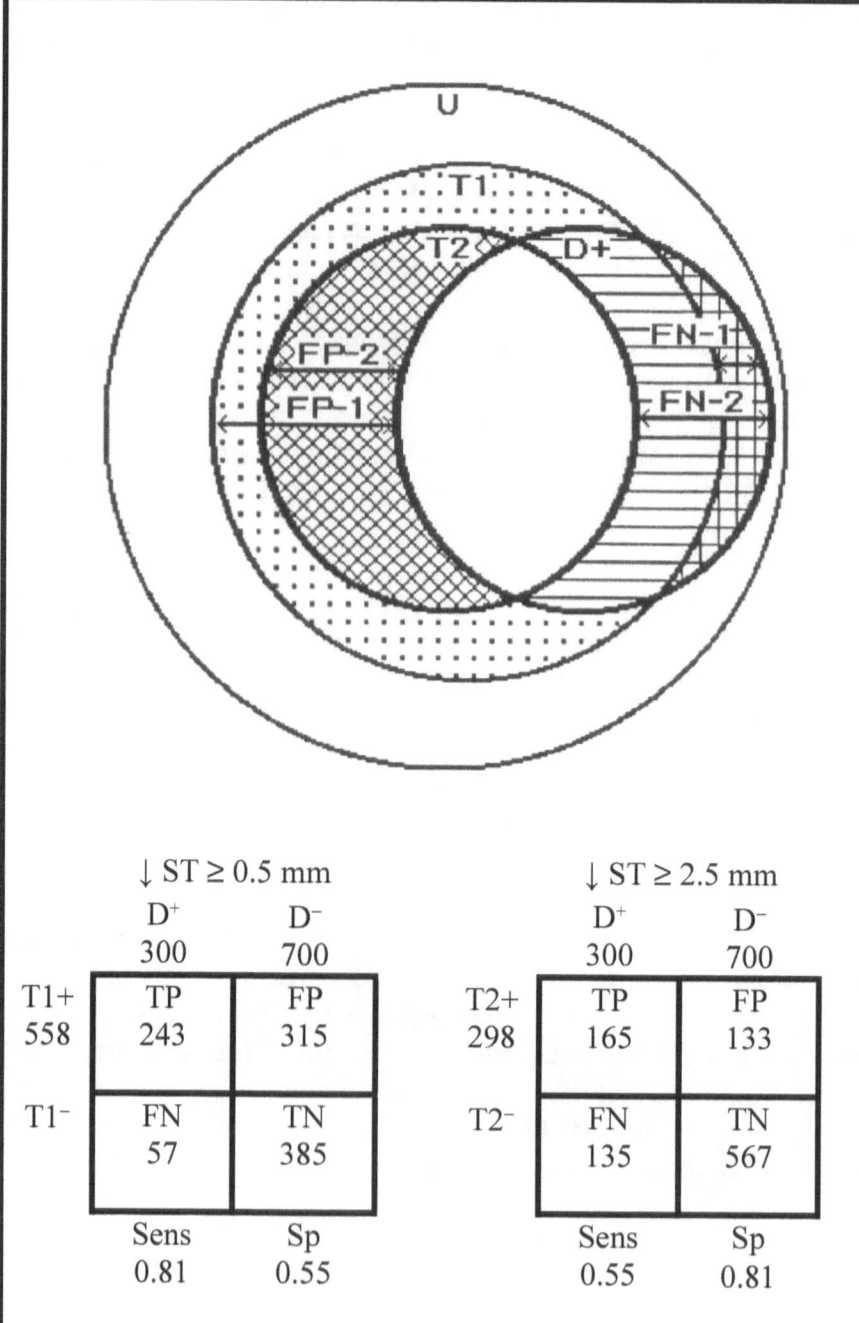

<table>
<tr><td colspan="5">↓ ST ≥ 0.5 mm</td></tr>
</table>

	D⁺ 300	D⁻ 700
T1+ 558	TP 243	FP 315
T1⁻	FN 57	TN 385
	Sens 0.81	Sp 0.55

	D⁺ 300	D⁻ 700
T2+ 298	TP 165	FP 133
T2⁻	FN 135	TN 567
	Sens 0.55	Sp 0.81

↓ ST ≥ 0.5 mm

	D^+ 300	D^- 700
T1+ 558	TP 243	FP 315
T1⁻	FN 57	TN 385
	Sens 0.81	Sp 0.55

↓ ST ≥ 2.5 mm

	D^+ 300	D^- 700
T2+ 298	TP 165	FP 133
T2⁻	FN 135	TN 567
	Sens 0.55	Sp 0.81

Figure 16.1. Venn diagram of the primary change in the cutoff level reflected in the binary tables and the Venn subsets

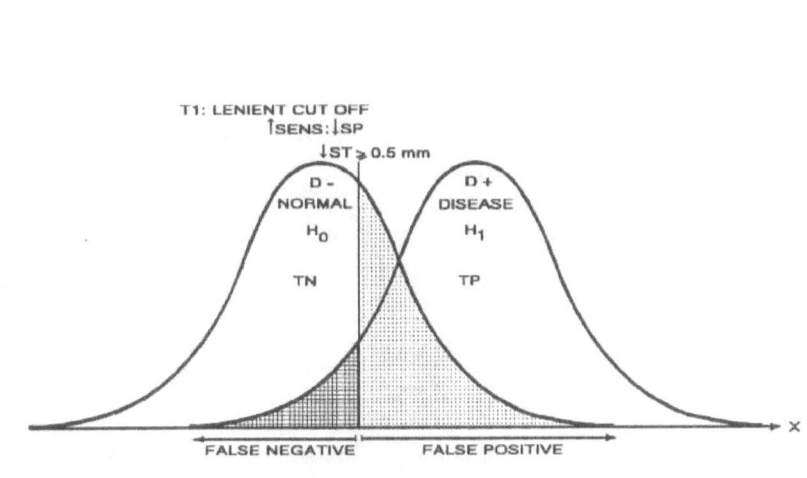

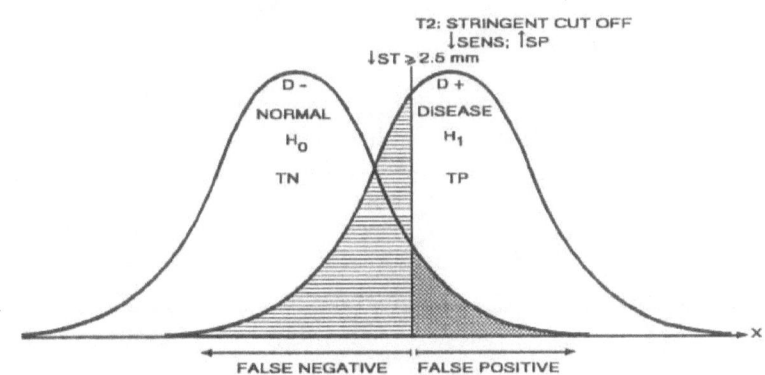

Figure 16.2. (A and B) Graph of the partition of the
distribution into four subsets by the cutoff line

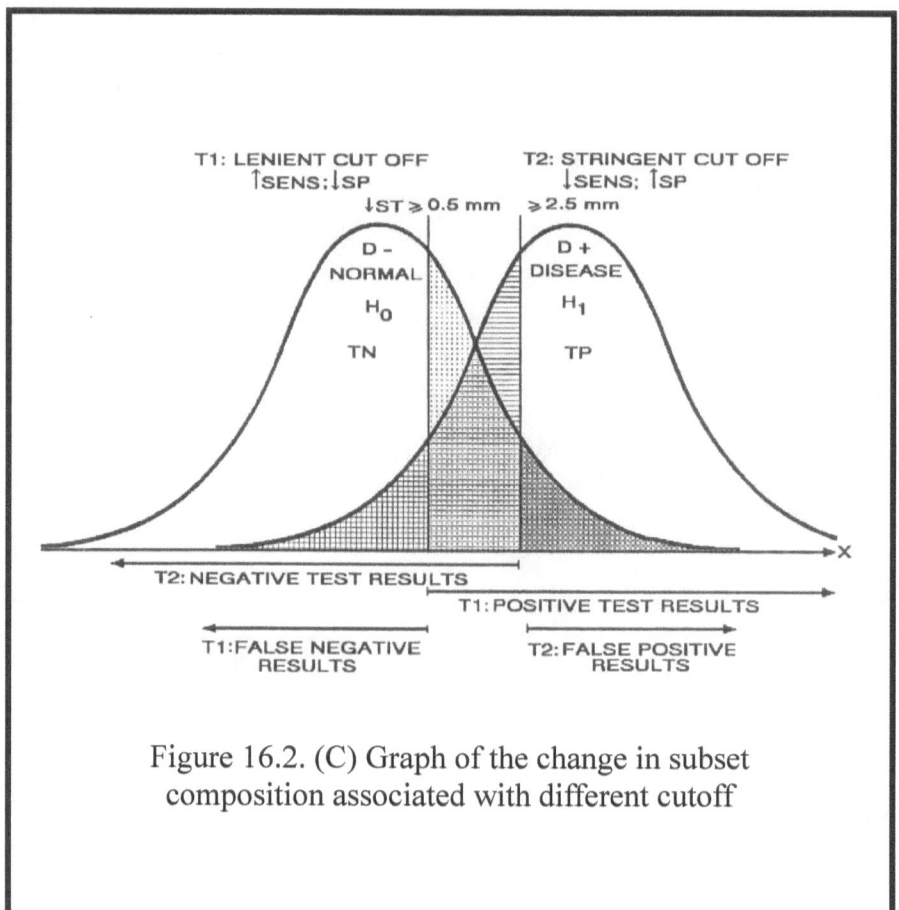

Figure 16.2. (C) Graph of the change in subset
composition associated with different cutoff

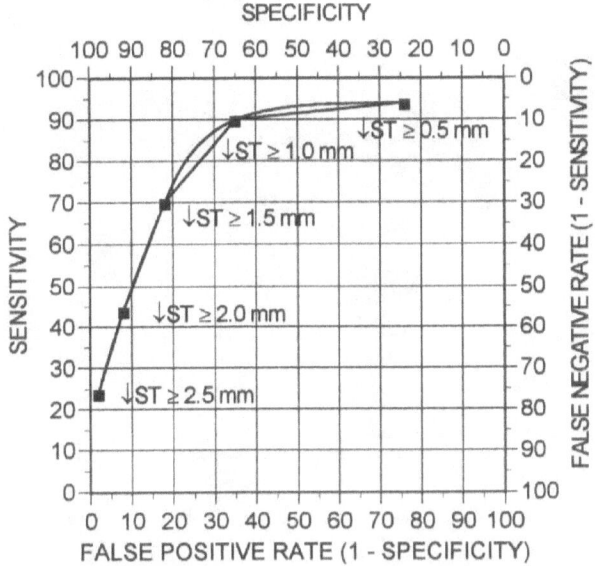

Figure 16.3. Graph of the ROC curve defining the slope-adjusted ST segment depression in the Exercise Stress Test as a function of sensitivity and specificity.

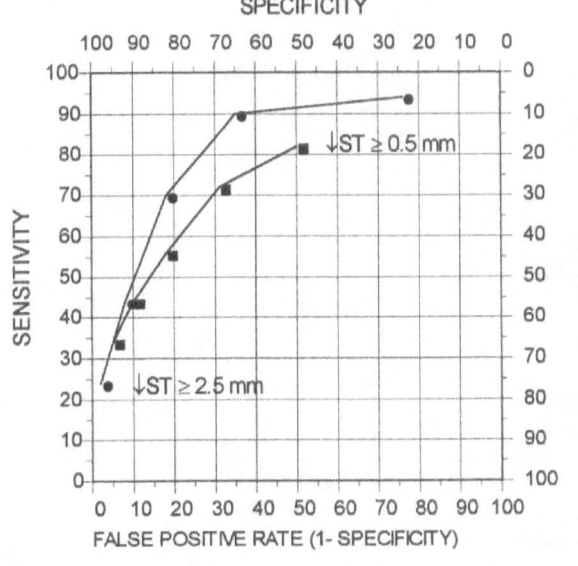

Figure 16.4. Graph of the significant change in the initial ROC curve to a less discriminating function incidental to a change in the choice of the variables.

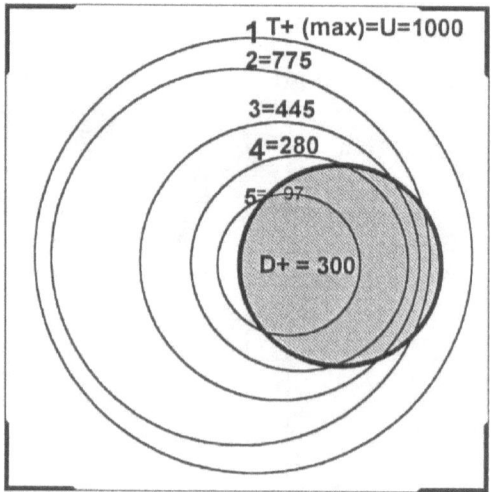

Venn presentation of the cutoff points in a hypothetical ROC curve derived from a population universe of 1,000 patients in whom D$^+$=300. A hypothetical cutoff point of 100 percent sensitivity and 0 percent specificity, (1 − specificity) = 100 percent, is included as a limiting point. At this point, circle T$^+$ encloses TP and FP with no FN or TN.

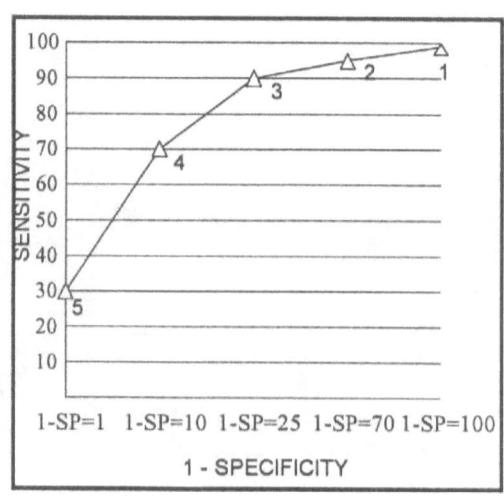

Figure 16.5. Venn diagram of the relationship of the T$^+$ circle to the D$^+$ circle for each cutoff point

Stress test		CAD			
		Prevalence $P(D^+) =$	1 – Prevalence $1 - P(D^+) =$	Sample universe	
Stress test	Positive test T^+	True positive 1 = 300 2 = 285 3 = 270 4 = 210 5 = 90	False positive = 700 = 490 = 175 = 70 = 7	$T^+ = U = 1{,}000$ = 775 = 445 = 280 = 97	Points 1-5 correspond to the cutoff points plotted in the ROC curve and graphed in the Venn diagram
	Negative test T^-	False negative = 0 = 15 = 30 = 90 = 210	True negative = 0 = 210 = 525 = 630 = 693	T^+ row	
		D^+ column total = 300	D^- column total = 700	U total = 1,000	
		Sensitivity 1 = 1 2 = 0.95 3 = 0.9 4 = 0.7 5 = 0.3	Sensitivity = 1 = 0.7 = 0.25 = 0.1 = 0.01		

Table 16.1. Change in sensitivity and the complement of specificity (1 – specificity), associated with the choice of five cutoff points in a hypothetical ROC curve reflected in the numerical values of the four resultant subsets

16.1 Coronary Artery Disease

CAD offers a unique opportunity for an in-depth critique of the of Bayesian analysis as applied to the electrocardiographic response to exercise in patients and healthy subjects. The relevance of the critique stems from the fact that the introduction of probability theory into the medical literature was derived in no small measure from its exhaustive and extensive application to the exercise stress test in an effort to provide a solid probability anchor for decision making based on the test's result. The exercise stress test, often referred to a graded exercise test (GXT), the Exercise Treadmill

Test, remains to date as one of the main primary noninvasive tools in the evaluation of CAD.

As in all Bayesian analysis, the construction of a binary table of positive and negative, normal or abnormal, and 0 or 1, required a binary definition of the disease under consideration, such that a yes or a no answer clearly demarcates the boundary between health and disease. To this end, CAD needs to be defined in strict pathophysiological and hemodynamic parameters that may be translated into the required dichotomy.

Generically, however, CAD may be considered a continuum with purely fixed static obstructive atherosclerotic lesions at one end and purely spastic dynamic vascular abnormality at the other end. Because in most cases reduction in blood flow through a given artery is derived from the additive effect of static and vasospastic components in varying proportion, the definition of CAD on purely mechanical obstructive lesions is not pathophysiologically valid.

In this bimodal obstructive pattern of occlusive coronary disease, a third critical variable is added to the atherogenesis process in the form of intramural thrombus formation superimposed on a plaque fissure or ulcer, leading to a further progressive narrowing (unstable angina) or complete occlusion (MI).

Notwithstanding the above dynamic factors in CAD, an arbitrary definition limited to a static pathological rather than pathophysiologic correlates is required for the implementation of a binary probability table as the final common pathway.

Thus, it is logical for our purpose to define CAD in terms of the severity of resulting stenosis, calculated as a percent reduction in the luminal cross-sectional area and to postulate a critical area reduction as the demarcation boundary between the presence and the absence of CAD.

The relationship of sequential reduction in arterial diameter to cross-sectional area from a baseline of unity is governed by the following relation: $\left(\dfrac{D}{2}\right)^2 \times p$ and calculated in Table 16.3.

As noted in the relationship of diameter, D, to absolute area, 50 percent reduction in D results in 75 percent reduction in area, assuming of course a concentric circular obstructive process. This static pathologic definition precludes acute or labile manifestation of CAD, including variant angina, microvascular anginal, or symptom X.

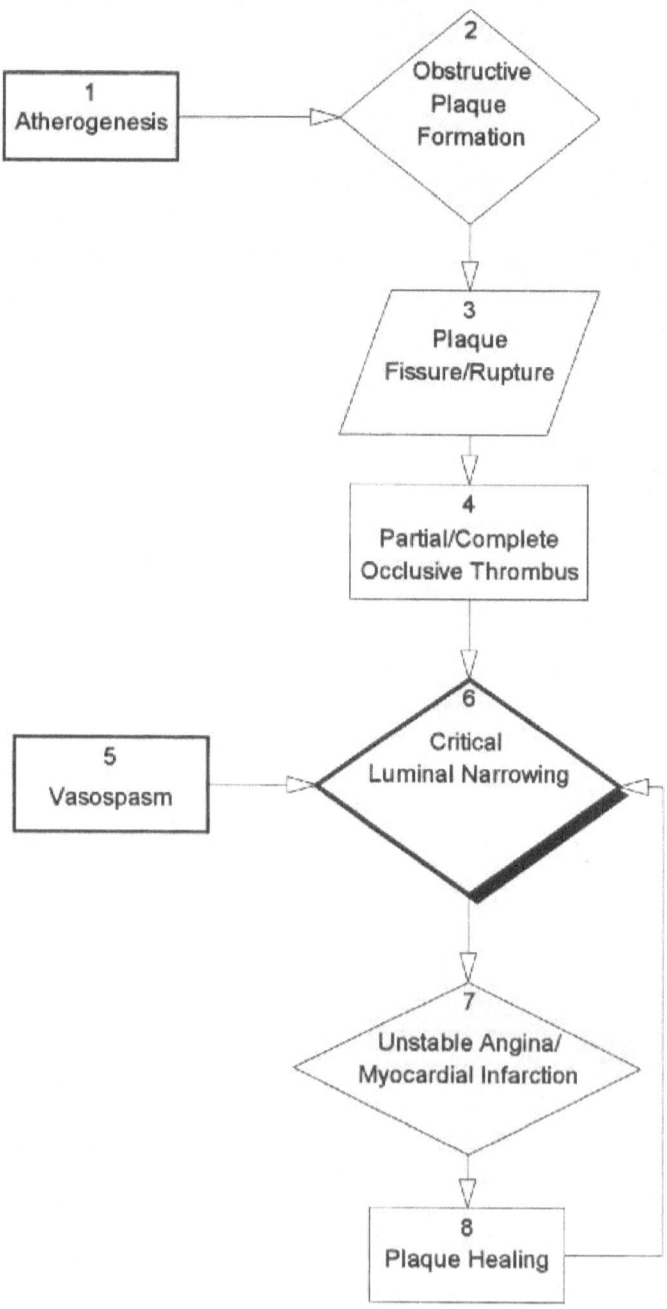

Figure 16.61. Flow chart of the pathogenesis of critical luminal narrowing in CAD.

Diameter	Absolute Area	Relative Area (Percentage)
1	0.79	100
0.9	0.64	81
0.8	0.5	64
0.7	0.38	49
0.6	0.28	36
0.5	0.2	25
0.4	0.12	16
0.35	0.1	12
0.3	0.07	9
0.25	0.05	6
0.2	0.03	4
0.1	0.01	1

Table 16.2. Relationship of arterial diameter to the absolute and relative area from a baseline of unity

This arbitrary assignment of a critical stenotic area is of course a measure of the severity of the atherosclerotic process and the potential for acute thrombogenic complication. The same critical area, however, is not necessarily the future or actual site of the thrombus formation.

Having arbitrarily imposed an absolute pathological binary standard for CAD, it is necessary to translate the anatomical criteria to an equivalent gold standard in the patient population. It seems logical to assume that the diameter of the vessel visualized on angiography corresponds to the diameter of a concentric stenotic area noted on pathological section. What is at the variance is the reference diameter with which the observed diameter is compared in order to compute the percent reduction in area, in other words, the reference value assigned to the original diameter prior to the advent of the stenotic process. This reference value may differ substantially in the two measurements. In pathology, the internal elastic membrane defines the diameter of the original cross-sectional area; and in angiography, the normal diameter is derived from what appears as a normal nonstenotic segment, which may or may not correspond to the original anatomical cross-sectional area. With this in mind, the percent reduction in the area may differ between the anatomy and the angiography, irrespective of the fact that the observed stenotic diameter is the same in both cases.

Nevertheless, despite the noted discrepancy, the diameter of the stenotic vessel and the percent reduction in the cross-sectional area angiographically calculated is accepted as the gold standard in the quantitative analysis of obstructive coronary disease.

It is important to remember that the dividing line between CAD and freedom from CAD is arbitrarily imposed both physiologically and anatomically in order to divide a continuous spectrum into two mutually exclusive and exhaustive categories of hemodynamically significant and hemodynamically insignificant CAD.

Once a gold standard is postulated, imperfect as it may be, the sensitivity and specificity of any given test may be computed for any given cutoff point. In one early study,[1] 1,465 male symptomatic patients were stress tested. The exercise test was considered positive when there was ≥ 1 mm of ST segment depression for at least 0.08 second, as compared with the resting baseline value. Note that the protocol of this study assigned a negative result to any value below the cutoff point of 1 mm. In a similar fashion, clinically important CAD was defined as ≥ 70 percent narrowing of the diameter of at least one major vessel. By this criterion of the gold standard, 1,023 were considered positive for CAD and the balance 442 were defined as free from CAD (Table 16.4).

		Coronary Artery Disease			
		Prevalence $P(D^+) =$	1-Prevalence $P(D^-) =$	Sample universe $P(U) = 1$	
		Disease present 1,023	Disease absent 442	Sample universe 1,465	
Stress test	Positive test, T^+ Abnormal test	True positive 815	False positive 115	T^+ row total 930	Predictive value of positive test $PV[-] = \dfrac{TN}{TN + FN} = \dfrac{222}{222 + 9} = 96\%$
	Negative test, T^- Normal test	False negative 208	True negative 327	T^- row total 535	Predictive value of negative test $PV[-] = \dfrac{327}{208 + 327} = 61\%$
		D^+ column total = 1,023	D^- column total = 442	U total	
		Sensitivity $\dfrac{815}{815 + 208} = 80\%$	Specificity $\dfrac{327}{115 + 327} = 74\%$		

Table 16.3. Derivation of sensitivity and specificity for a defined cutoff point using a predetermined gold standard criterion to determine the prevalence of the disease in the sample population

In this case, the sensitivity and the specificity of the test in question were calculated given the exact prevalence or prior probability of CAD angiographically documented. The stress test results were then assigned to the respective cells as determined by the conjoint result of ST segment response and the angiographically calculated arterial narrowing. Once in place, the calculation of sensitivity and specificity for this particular test is reduced to a simple ratio. The process of establishing the sensitivity and specificity of any one test is a challenge that needs to consider all factors that may inject an element of bias in the selection of subjects, the choice of the gold standard, the assignment of cutoff points, and the interpretation of the tests. Note that in this particular study, all subjects were symptomatic (chest pain), so that the generic results of the test may not be applicable at large.

16.2 The Ischemic Response: Physiologic Background

Isotonic exercise stress test is designed to increase myocardial oxygen demand. The increase in cardiac output associated with increase in heart rate and blood pressure requires a commensurate increase in myocardial oxygen consumption (MVO_2) provided by proportionate increase in coronary blood flow. The supply-demand ratio remains constant despite the altered factors,

$$\frac{\text{Epicardial (coronary blood flow)}}{\text{Myocardial oxygen consumption}} = \frac{\uparrow \text{Supply}}{\uparrow \text{Demand}} = 1$$

Fick formula modification: Flow $\times$ O_2 extraction = O_2 consumption.

$$\frac{\text{Flow} \times \text{Extraction (Supply)}}{O_2 \text{ Consumption (Demand)}} = \frac{\text{mL / min} \times \text{mL } O_2 / 100 \text{ mL blood}}{\text{mL } O_2 / \text{min}} = 100\%$$

In atherosclerotic CAD, as defined earlier, the increased demand is not compensated for by increase in supply, thus driving the ratio to less than unity,

$$\frac{\text{Supply}}{\uparrow \text{Demand}} = <1$$

The failure of the supply to meet the demand results in myocardial ischemia. Note that a decrease in the ratio could be equally obtained by reduction in epicardial coronary blood flow, as follows:

$$\frac{\text{Epicardial (coronary blood flow)}}{\text{Myocardial oxygen consumption}} = \frac{\downarrow \text{Supply}}{\text{Demand}} = < 1$$

The resultant transmural myocardial ischemia is to be differentiated from the subendocardial ischemia generally associated with increase in demand. The supply side ischemic response is associated with coronary artery spasm in the absence of significant obstructive CAD and is therefore insensitive to exercise stress provocation. In this case, only ergonovine challenge test is capable of provoking coronary artery spasm.

In the presence of left ventricular hypertrophy, the increase in demand may overwhelm a normally increase in supply to precipitate an ischemic response,

$$\frac{\uparrow \text{Supply}}{\uparrow\uparrow \text{Demand}} = < 1$$

The response in this instance confounds the purpose of the test, which targets obstructive CAD. Other factors that need to be excluded if the test is to remain specific for CAD include drug treatment, Mitral Valve Prolapse (MVP), Left bundle branch block (LBBB), and Wolf Parkinson White (WPW).

16.3 The Diagnostic Impact of the Predictive Value: Exercise Stress Test in Perspective

The predictive value (PV) stands as a shorthand symbol for Bayes' formula. Given its various mathematical formats and verbal expressions (posterior probability, predictive accuracy, predictive value, etc.), it would seem inappropriate to suggest that these shorthand symbols or expressions do not convey the centrality of the concept in the diagnostic process. Devoid of its symbolic jargon, PV is in effect a measure of the weighted diagnosis into which all the historical, physical, and laboratory data have been factored. This may be seen as an overstatement, which on casual examination may not seem to be justified unless one notes that the three variables that enter into its composition, namely, prior probability or prevalence, sensitivity, and specificity, are in effect quantitative assessment of the historical data, the physical examination, and the available lab data.

In a sense, PV is a measure of the final diagnosis arrived at taking into consideration all the clinical data. The prevalence is in effect the tentative diagnosis assigned to the case, taking into consideration the demographics, the signs and symptoms, and the results of the physical exam. The sensitivity and the specificity of the test in question are a measure of the accuracy of the given test in correctly identifying a given tentative diagnosis. All three parameters when expressed by Bayes' relation become a measure of the validity of the tentative diagnosis and as such may be considered as the arbiter of the diagnosis.

The following three examples represent a variation on a common chief complaint, namely, chest pain, where the prior probability of CAD assigned in each case is a reflection of the clinical judgment of the attending physician while the sensitivity and the specificity used will be those derived earlier in the study of symptomatic patients.

Consider the first case (Case 16.1), a fifty-six-year-old executive, nonsmoker, complaining of vague chest pains, at times related to stress. High Density Lipoprotein (HDL) is under 35 mg/DL. In view of the atypical presentation and the associated demographics, the prior probability in this case is estimated at 50 percent. Clinicians may differ as to the exact percentage assigned; however, a range of 40 to 60 percent seems appropriate given the clinical data.

A positive test result yields a predictive value of 75 percent. The clinical implication is that 75 percent of those presenting with an equivalent pattern turn out to be truly positive, that is, harboring an obstructive coronary lesion equal or greater than the minimum criterion set by the test gold standard.

The patient may or may not turn out to be truly positive on further definitive examination; however, his chance of being truly positive is 3:4, and the odds for his harboring the disease is 3:1.

The chance of his having the disease now is quite substantive, particularly when compared with the initial tentative diagnosis of 50 percent postulated in favor of the disease, which translated into 25 percent gain in certainty. A negative test result, on the other hand, will boost his chance of not having the disease to 79 percent or almost four out of five, and the odds against having the disease is now reduced to 1:4.

In the first instance, the tentative diagnosis has been substantially reinforced given the positive result; whereas in the second instance, a serious doubt is now entertained given the negative result.

The second case to be considered is that of a sixty-year-old surgeon (Case 16.2) presenting with a history of classical anginal pain associated with multiple risk factors. A prior probability of 0.9 was assigned prior to the performance of the test. This is an extremely high probability that in the opinion of the physician, the patient does suffer from CAD. In fact, given such a high probability, the indication for a simple stress test may be questionable and a more definitive approach is warranted. Nevertheless, following a prescribed routine, the test was performed, resulting in a predictive value for the positive result of 97 percent, an increase in certainty of mere 7 percent that in reality did not affect the basic tentative diagnosis. In the unlikely event that the test did turn out to be negative, the predictive value of 29 percent seems to suggest that his chance of not harboring the disease is one in three, which did not dispel the initial clinical impression. On balance, the tentative diagnosis remains unchallenged, and nothing short of a definitive approach is likely to affect the initial diagnosis.

The third case to be considered is that of young woman with no specific risk factors complaining of vague chest discomfort (Case 16.3). A prior probability for CAD of 0.1 was assigned. This case represents the counterpart of the second case where the prior probability is now low enough to cast serious doubt on the tentative diagnosis. The predictive value of a positive test is 26 percent. Note that the predictive value of the complement is computed as follows: $1 - PV[+] = P(D^- \mid T^+) = 74$ percent, which is another way of saying that the odds in favor of its being false positive 74:26 or approximately 3:1. The predictive value of a negative result, on the other hand, is given at 97 percent, which is certainly high enough to rule out the remote possibility of CAD. In the negative case, the rule out gain of 7 percent is marginal and has little bearing on our initial estimate of the absence of disease. The rule in gain of 15 percent is similarly not impressive enough to change our initial estimate of the presence of disease.

Of the three case, the test result is most valuable in support or rejection of a tentative diagnosis when the initial or prior estimate of the probability of disease is essentially a toss-up, admitting in effect the lack of evidence in support of either proposition.[16]

---

[16] D. A. Weiner et al., "Exercise Stress Testing: Correlations among History of Angina, ST-Segment Response and Prevalence of Coronary-Artery Disease in the Coronary Artery Surgery Study (CASS)," *New England Journal of Medicine* 301 (1979): 230-235.

		Coronary Artery Disease			
		Prevalence $P(D^+) = 0.5$	$1 -$ Prevalence $P(D^-) = 0.5$	Sample universe $P(U) = 1$	
		Disease present 500	Disease absent 500	Sample universe 1,000	
Stress test	Positive test, T^+ Abnormal test	True positive $n(D^+) \times$ Sens $0.8 \times 500 = 400$	False positive $n(D^-) - n(TN)$ $500 - 370 = 130$	T^+ row total 530	Predictive value of positive test 400 / 530 = 75 percent Rule in gain = ↑25 percent
	Negative test, T^- Normal test	False negative $n(D^+) \times n(TP)$ $500 - 400 = 100$	True negative $n(D^-) \times SP$ $0.74 \times 500 = 370$	T^- row total 470	Predictive value of negative test 370 / 470 = 79 percent Rule out gain = ↑29 percent
		D^+ column total = 500	D^- column total 500	U total	
		Sensitivity = 0.80	Specificity = 0.74		

Case 16.1. Fifty-six-year-old CEO complaining of vague chest pain, at times related to stress. HDL less than 35 mg/DL

		Coronary Artery Disease			
		Prevalence $P(D^+) = 0.90$	1-Prevalence $P(D^-) = 0.10$	Sample universe $P(D^+) + P(D^-) = P(U) = 1$	
		Disease present $n(D^+) = P(D^+) \times n(U)$ $0.9 \times 1,000 = 900$	Disease absent $n(D^-) = P(D^-) \times n(U)$ $0.1 \times 1,000 = 100$	Sample universe $n(U) = n(D^+) + n(D^-)$ 1,000	
Stress test	Positive test, T^+ Abnormal test	True positive 720	False positive 26	T^+ row total 746	Predictive value of positive test $PV[+] = \dfrac{720}{746} = 97\%$
	Negative test, T^- Normal test	False negative 180	True negative 74	T^- row total 254	Predictive value of negative test $PV[-] = \dfrac{74}{254} = 29\%$
		D^+ column total $= 900$	D^- column total $= 100$	U total	
		Sensitivity = 0.80	Specificity = 0.74		

Case 16-2. A sixty-year-old surgeon with a history of classical angina associated with multiple risk factors

		Coronary Artery Disease			
		Prevalence $P(D^+) = 0.10$	1-Prevalence $P(D^-) = 0.90$	Sample universe $P(D^+) + P(D^-)$ $= P(U) = 1$	
		Disease present	Disease absent	Sample universe	
		$0.1 \times 1{,}000 =$ 100	$0.9 \times 1{,}000$ $= 900$	1,000	
Stress test	Positive test, T$^+$	True positive	False positive	T$^+$ row total	Predictive value of positive test
	Abnormal test	$0.8 \times 100 = 80$	$0.26 \times 900 =$ 230	$80 + 230 =$ 310	$PV[+] = \dfrac{80}{80 + 230} = 26\%$ Rule in gain $= 26 - 10$ $= 16$ percent
	Negative test, T−	False negative	True negative	T$^-$ row total	Predictive value of negative test
	Normal test	$0.2 \times 100 = 20$	$0.74 \times 900 =$ 670	$20 + 670 =$ 690	$PV[+] = \dfrac{80}{80 + 230} = 26\%$ Rule out gain $= 97 - 90$ $= 7$ percent
		D$^+$ column total = 100	D$^-$ column total = 900	U total	
		Sensitivity = 0.80	Specificity = 0.74		

Case 16.3. Young woman; no risk factors; vague atypical chest discomfort

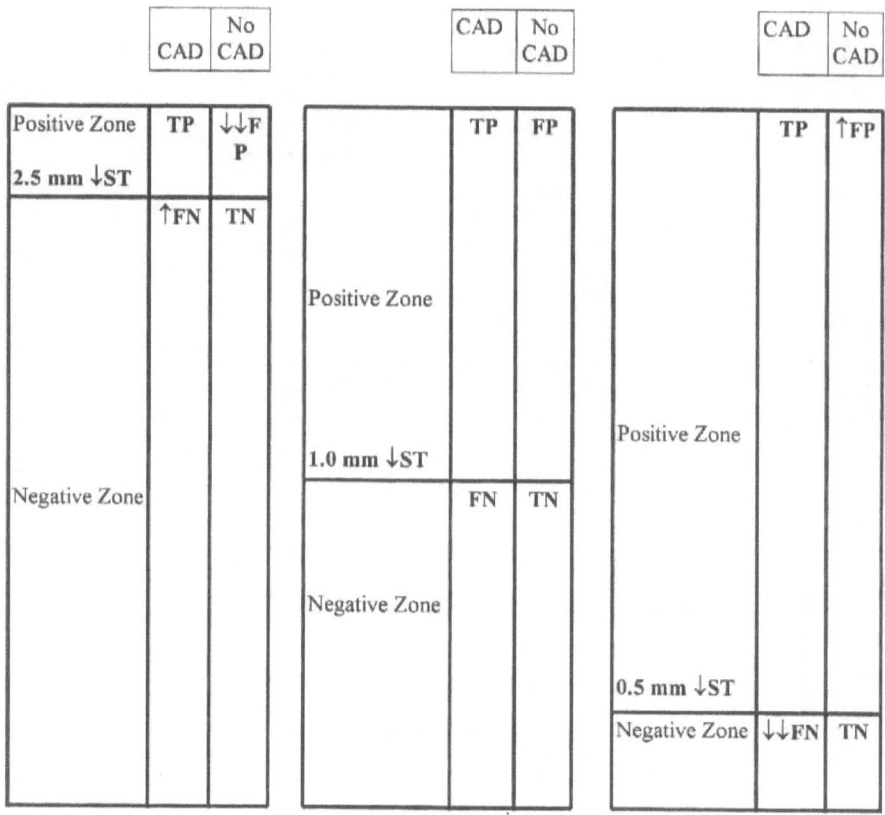

Table 16.1. The effect of altering the cutoff level of ↓ST segment on the sensitivity and specificity of the stress test, as manifested by the change in the relative magnitude of TP and FP with respect to FN and TN

Cutoff set high (strict) ↓↓FP = ↑Specificity T⁺ ⇒ rules in CAD	Cutoff set intermediate Optimal	Cutoff set low (loose) ↓↓FN = ↑Sensitivity T⁻ ⇒ Rules out CAD

Chapter 17

Syphilis and Lyme Disease: Diagnostic Strategy

The parallel evolution and similarities between the natural history of syphilis and Lyme disease underline the parallel immune response to the two members of the Spirochaetaceae family: *Borrelia burgdorferi* and *Treponema pallidum* (Table 17.1).

	Syphilis		Lyme Disease
Incubation period	Three weeks (average)	Incubation period	Three to thirty-two days
Primary	Chancre + regional lymphadenopathy	Stage I	Erythema migrans + lymphadenopathy
Secondary	Three to four weeks (average) after appearance of chancre Eight weeks after exposure Flulike symptoms Generalized lymphadenopathy + cutaneous lesions ± liver, kidney, myocardium, nervous system	Stage II	Days after erythema migrans Days or weeks after inoculation Flulike symptoms Regional or generalized annular lesion ± liver, kidney, myocardium, meninges, cranial or peripheral nerves
Latent	Years	Latent	Months-years
Tertiary	Benign Cardiovascular Neurological Asymptomatic Meningovascular Parenchymal Tabes	Stage III	Arthritis, chronic Late skin manifestation Neurological Asymptomatic Chronic encephalomyelitis Dementia Ataxia

Table 17.1. Parallel evolution of the natural history of syphilis and Lyme disease

17.1 Targeting a Test Order

In general, a test is ordered with one of two primary objectives:

1. As a screening tool in an asymptomatic person where the possibility of a latency phase in the disease process hides the incipient progress of the disease, or to detect early structural, physiological, or biochemical changes that may herald or precede the development of the overt disease in the asymptomatic patient

2. As a diagnostic tool in the symptomatic patient to confirm a tentative diagnosis based on the available evidence at hand

It is essential to keep in mind that each of the above-mentioned two objectives differ with regard to the prior assumption regarding the disease in question as well as the required level of predictive accuracy needed to confirm or deny the tentative diagnosis put forward (Table 17.2).

In the screening mode, it is implicitly assumed that the prevalence of the silent abnormalities being sought, given an asymptomatic individual, is at the lower end of the prevalence range. The sensitivity of the screening test, however, needs to be high enough so as to snare the maximum number of truly positive patients, thus reducing the false-negative count to the bare minimum. As noted in Table 17.2, the double effect of decreased prevalence ($\downarrow$Prev) and increased sensitivity ($\uparrow$Sens), resulting in decreased false-negative count ($\downarrow$FN), will ensure a very high predictive value of a negative test even at moderate sensitivity, which is another way of saying that a negative test guarantees the absence of occult disease or incipient abnormality.

In the diagnostic mode, it is implicitly assumed that the prevalence of disease being entertained in the differential diagnosis in the symptomatic patient is in the upper range of prevalence. In a sense, the preassumed prevalence is a reflection of the belief in the proposed tentative diagnosis given the data at hand. To be sure, in the diagnostic mode, the clinical perception of the disease being tested is reflected in the weight assigned to the prevalence parameter. In probabilistic terms, it is the prior probability assigned to the disease in question. In the limit, a classic history, a pathognomonic sign or symptom, ensures the highest possible prevalence (prior probability).

In the diagnostic mode, a high specificity is required to ensure the minimal number of false positives. As noted in Table 17.2, the combined effect of increased prevalence ($\uparrow$Prev) and increased specificity ($\uparrow$Sp), resulting in decreased false-positives count ($\downarrow$FP), will guarantee a very high predictive value of a positive test required for confirming the tentative diagnosis, which is another way of saying that a positive test confirms the prior diagnosis based on the then available clinical data.

17.2 Testing for Syphilis and Lyme disease

The Venereal Disease Research Laboratory (VDRL) flocculation test is probably the most widely used serological screening test. The test is one of several modifications of flocculation reaction for the detection of reagin by direct mixture of syphilitic sera with cardiolipin antigen. The reagin-type antibodies are not specific antibodies against the spirochete itself, rather the reagin-type antibodies (Against cardiolipin) are the indirect response to the treponema infection.

The sensitivity of VDRL is a function of the disease stage in which it is ordered. Because of the lag period involved in the evolution of the antibodies to the spirochete, the sensitivity during the primary stage is often less than 80 percent (70-80 percent). The sensitivity during the secondary stage, however, approaches 100 percent. For screening purposes in the asymptomatic patient, which include patients in the latent phase as well as patients in the asymptomatic tertiary stage, VDRL sensitivity is given at 86 percent with a specificity of 97 percent.

A negative result rules out syphilis with absolute certainty. A positive result pauses the quintessential dilemma in diagnostic testing. At the assumed prevalence level of one per thousand and a specificity approaching the upper limit, the PV[+] is just 3 percent (Table 17.3), reflecting the unavoidable and inordinate number of false positives associated with the test.

		Any Given Disease			
		Prevalence $P(D^+)$ $n(D^+) = P(D^+) \times n(U)$	$1 -$ Prevalence $1 - P(D^+)$ $n(D^-) = n(U) - n(D^+)$	Sample universe $P(U) = 1$	
Any test	Positive test, T$^+$ Abnormal	True positive $n(D^+) \times$ Sens	False positive $n(D^-) \times 1(1 - Sp)$	T$^+$ row total	$P(D^+ \mid T^+) =$ PV[+] TP / TP + FP
	Negative test T- Normal test	False negative $=$ $n(D^+) \times (1 - Sens)$	True negative $n(D^-) \times Sp$	T$^-$ row total	$P(D^- \mid T^-) =$ PV[−] TN / TN + FN
		D$^+$ column total	D$^-$ column total	U total	
		Sensitivity TP / TP + FN	Specificity TN / TN + FP		

Corollaries	Corollaries
$\uparrow$TP = $\uparrow$Sens $\times$ $\uparrow$Prev	$\uparrow$TN = $\uparrow$Sp $\times$ $\uparrow(1 - \downarrow$Prev)
TP is a function of sensitivity and prevalence.	TN is a function of specificity and prevalence.
$\uparrow$FN = Prev $- \uparrow$TP	$\downarrow$ FP = $(1 - $Prev) $- \uparrow$TN
For a given prevalence, FN is inversely proportional to TP, or	For a given prevalence, FP is inversely proportional to TN, or
$\downarrow$FN = $\downarrow(1 - \uparrow$ Sens) $\times \downarrow$Prev	$\bullet\downarrow$ FP = $\downarrow(1 - \uparrow$Sp) $\times \downarrow(1 - \uparrow$Prev)
FN is inversely proportional to sensitivity and directly proportional to prevalence.	FP is inversely proportional to specificity and prevalence.
Therefore, the higher the sensitivity, the smaller the FN. On the other hand, the lower the prevalence, the smaller the FN. Because $\uparrow$PV = [−] = TN / TN + $\downarrow$FN, the predictive value of a negative test approaches 100 percent and $(1 - $PV[−]) approaches 0 as FN approaches 0.	Therefore, the higher the specificity, the smaller the FP. On the other hand, the higher the prevalence, the smaller the FP. Because $\uparrow$PV[+] = TP / TP + $\downarrow$FP, the predictive value of a positive test approaches 100 percent and $(1 - $PV[+]) approaches 0 as FP approaches 0.
$\therefore$ A low prevalence and a high sensitivity imply a PV[−] approaching 100 percent.	$\therefore$ A high prevalence and a high specificity imply a PV[+] approaching 100 percent.
In effect, high sensitivity and low prevalence guarantee the highest predictive value for a negative test, which is another way of saying that the negative result rules out the disease in question.	In effect, high specificity and high prevalence guarantees the highest predictive value for a positive test, which is another way of saying that the positive result rules in the disease in question.

Table 17.2. Correlation of the required level of predictive value of positive or negative result with prevalence, sensitivity, and specificity as a marker for screening or diagnosis.

However, despite the fact that all 97 percent of those tested positive are in fact false positive and only 3 percent are presumed to be truly positive, the fact remains that for the persons tested, even this minor uncertainty needs to be verified and correctly assigned.

This is another way of saying that the patient in question may or may not be truly positive. In fact, the chance of his being truly positive is one in thirty-three, whereas the chance of his being false positive, that is, free of infection but branded as positive, is thrity-two of thirty-three or 97 percent.

		Syphilis			
		Prevalence $P(D^+) = 0.001$	1 – Prevalence $1 - P(D^+) = 0.999$	Sample universe	
VDRL	Positive test, T$^+$	True positive	False positive	T$^+$ row total	$P(D^+ \mid T^+)$ $P(D - \mid T^+)$
	Abnormal test	0.86	29.97	30.83	PV[+] = 0.028 = 3 percent ↔ 1 – PV[+] = 97 percent
	Negative test, T$^-$	False negative	True negative	T$^-$ row total 969.17	$P(D^+ \mid T^-)$ $P(D - \mid T^-)$
	Normal test	0.14	969.03		PV[–] = 0.01 percent ↔ PV[–] = 99.99 percent
		D$^+$ column total = 1	D$^-$ column total = 999	U total = 1,000	
		Sensitivity = 0.86	Specificity = 0.97		

Table 17.3. Predictive value of a positive and negative VDRL given a prevalence of 0.001 (1 per 1,000)

The diagnostic strategy, given a seropositive VDRL and a very low predictive value for the positive test result, is to proceed to the definitive test based on spirochete type antigen as used in the fluorescent treponemal antibody absorption test (FTA-ABS). In this test, antibodies in the serum will combine with the spirochete and then will be made visible by attaching the complex to an antihuman gamma globulin tagged with a dye and viewed under a fluorescent microscope (Table 17.4).

		Syphilis				
		Prevalence $P(D^+) = 0.03$	1 – Prevalence $1 - P(D^+) = 0.97$	Sample universe		
FTA-ABS	Positive test, T^+	True positive	False positive	T^+ row total	$P(D^+ \mid T^+)$ $P(D - \mid T^+)$	
	Abnormal test	0.85	0.3	1.15	PV[+] = 73.9 percent = ↔ 1 – PV[+] =26.1 percent	
	Negative test, T^-	False negative	True negative	T^- row total	$P(D^+ \mid T^-)$ $P(D - \mid T -)$	
	NORMAL TEST	=0.01	=29.67	=29.68	1 – PV[–] = 99.97 percent ↔ PV[–] =0.03 percent	
		D^+ column total = 0.86	D^- column total = 29.97	U total = 30.83		
		Sensitivity = 0.99	Specificity = 0.99			

Table 17.4. Predictive value of positive and negative FTA-ABS performed following a positive VDRL. Note the prevalence in this case is assumed to be the PV[+] of the reported VDRL of 3 percent or 0.03.

Lyme disease, like syphilis, tends to follow a pattern characterized by stages exhibiting different clinical manifestations. Unlike the VDRL, the serological testing for Lyme disease evaluates the actual antibody titer to *B. burgdorferi* in the form of sonicated whole spirochetes as the antigen using the classic ELISA.

Putting aside for the moment the lack of standardization among the different laboratories and cross-reactivity of IgM to other diseases including syphilitic and other autoimmune disorders, the slow progression of seropositivity following inoculation accounts for the reported 40 percent sensitivity (and 94 percent specificity) of IgM ELISA in the early phase associated erythema migrans.

Further complicating the picture is the adverse effect of early antibiotic intervention on the normal development of antibody response often associated with what might be called *arrested antibody reaction*, which results in further significant loss of sensitivity. The sensitivity of IgG ELISA in the following weeks normally increases to 89 percent while the specificity drops to 72 percent.

Given that 5 to 10 percent of infected patients are asymptomatic, IgM response generally peaks between three and six weeks and then gradually declines. The IgG response lags the IgM response and generally increases to peak levels during the arthritic symptoms. Therefore, a fast positive titer after treatment is not a reflection of activity or treatment failure. A negative ELISA early in the course of the disease does not rule out the disease.

		Lyme Disease			
		Prevalence $P(D^+)$ 23 percent = 0.23	1 – Prevalence $1 - P(D^+) = 77$ percent = 0.77	Sample universe	
IgG ELISA	Positive test, T$^+$	True positive	False positive	T$^+$ row total	PV[+] = 49 percent
	Abnormal	20.47	21.56	42.03	1 – PV[+] =
	Negative test, T$^-$	False negative	True negative	T$^-$ row total	1 – PV[–] =
	Normal test	2.53	55.44	57.97	PV[–] = 96 percent
		D$^+$ column total = 23	D$^-$ column total = 77	U total = 100	
		Sensitivity = 0.89	Specificity = 0.72		

Table 17.5. Predictive value of a positive or negative ELISA given a prevalence of 0.23

Extrapolating from published data regarding the overdiagnosis of Lyme disease in the symptomatic population given a sensitivity of 89 percent and a specificity of 72 percent for the IgG ELISA after the first weeks of infection, it is evident that even in the presence of relatively high prevalence or assumed prior probability for Lyme disease, a negative result rules out latent, asymptomatic, or active infection. As noted in Table 17.5, despite a high degree of prior probability of 23 percent, the predictive value of a negative test is 96 percent.

This result is predicated on the proficiency of the laboratory performing the ELISA. The predictive value of the positive result even at this value of prior probability is still 49 percent, implying a significant number of false positives. By definition, false positive has been designated as positivity in the absence of disease. In borreliosis as well as in treponemiasis, a positive test may be a reflection of seropositivity in the absence of active infection, which may prevail after successful treatment or seropositivity in the absence of infection passive or active and solely related to cross-reactivity with nonrelated antibodies.

		Lyme Disease			
		Prevalence $P(D^+)$ 49 percent = 0.49	1 − Prevalence $1 − P(D_-^+) = 51$ percent = 0.51	Sample universe	
Western blot	Positive test, T^+	True positive	False positive	T^+ row total	PV[+] = 94 percent
	Abnormal	16.99	1.08	18.07	1 − PV[+] =
	Negative test, T^-	False negative	True negative	T^- row total	1 − PV[−] = 14 percent
	Normal test	3.47	20.48	23.96	PV[−] = 86 percent
		D^+ column total = 20.47	D^- column total = 21.56	U total = 42.03	
		Sensitivity = 0.83	Specificity = 0.95		

Table 17.6. Predictive value of positive or negative Western blot performed following a positive ELISA. Note the prevalence in this case is assumed to be the PV[+] of the reported ELISA of 49 percent

As in the case of FTA-ABS in the definitive diagnosis of syphilis, Western blot is used not for screening but to eliminate the false positives associated with cross reacting antibodies in the absence of true seropositivity. The differentiation between seropositivity associated with active infection and that prevailing after successful treatment can only be resolved through clinical expertise (Table 17.6).

Part IV

Statistical Inference

Chapter 18A

The Discrete Random Variable Probability Distribution[17]
Probability Mass Function
(Probability Distribution and Function of Discrete Random Variables)

This chapter and the following two chapters focus on the degree of conformity (or lack of it) that consigns the random variable to a particular level of pattern of differential occurrences. Simply stated, the question addressed is whether the occurrence of events is random and haphazard or conceals an innate order.

The nature and parameters of such an emerging pattern that might modify or influence the probability of occurrence of the random variable constitute in an indirect way the only link between probability and inferential statistics that would allow a glimpse into the contents of the black box, the classic euphemism for the population at large.

This chapter introduces the reader to the landmark merger between random events (random variables), organized and tabulated in terms of the frequency of their occurrence (descriptive statistics) and all the important concepts of probability, which made up the initial half of this monograph. The aim of the merger is to introduce a quantifiable measure to the chance occurrence of the random events, thus allowing the observer to predict, but with limited certainty, the outcome of the chance events.

---

[17] The terms used in connection with the probability distribution of random variables lack a uniformity of standard usage. The term often used for the probability distribution is *distribution function*. However, because the subject of the three chapters deals with the probability distribution of random variables, discrete, binomial, continuous, and normal, a modified title was used for this chapter to underline the inherent connection and uniformity of subject matter. The use of the probability mass function and probability density function seems to be the standard terminology in recent literature.

Given a meager sample of the black box contents, our only clue is to relate the sample at hand to the probability of its occurrence if indeed there is a pattern that categorize the probability of its occurrence. In other words, if there is a method or a pattern by which events, assumed to be random, tend to occur, then deciphering the code should provide the necessary intelligence to arrive at a reasonable estimate of the contents.

The subject is thus an introduction to inferential statistics, which in effect is the complement of the probability theory. In probability, we have been able to deduce the likelihood of a specific event (white and red balls), given the structure and composition of the sample space (population) from which the event (sample) is derived. In inferential statistics, we are in effect faced with the specific outcome (sample). The inference in this case relates to the structure and composition of the sample space (population), which unlike the probability case, is unknown.

The three chapters may be viewed as a bridge between the deductive probability expounded earlier and the inferential statistics to be explained later. It may be worth recalling that Bayes' attempt at inductive reasoning was a step in the right direction, although short of desired target. His use of prior probability to modify the posterior probability was certainly a masterful stroke of inferential technique. In Bayes' technique, we are given an initial estimate of the contents of the black box; and then when confronted with a random sample, we are in effect given a second a posteriori chance to modify the original estimate.

In inferential statistics, on the other hand, armed with a random sample drawn out of an unknown population, inference concerning the total population can only be applied if and only if the probability of the occurrence of the given sample is related in some way to a pattern that dictates the probability of the occurrence of samples of a given composition.

18A.1 The Conversion of Raw Data into Empirical Frequency Distribution

Distribution implies, as noted earlier, the allocation or apportioning of measurable, quantifiable, or otherwise definable units to individuals or items comprising a set or a subset. The process involves the assignment of a unique numerical value to the members or components of the group or sample, for example, AST score to a student, weight in ounces to a newborn, serum cholesterol level (mg/100 mL) to a diabetic patient, resting heart rate (bpm) to an athlete, age to hospitalization, annual income to a family, volume in cubic centimeters to a bottle, number of papers to an author, and waiting time in minutes to an ambulance arrival.

The totality of the unordered, discrete values thus collected constitute the raw data. The extraction of relevant or pertinent information from the mass of raw data requires the application of a shuffling process designed to organize and summarize the numerical values. Note that the process involved in the reorganization does not yield any new information that is not inherently present in the raw data. What is being achieved is a mode of presentation amenable to deductive reasoning.

The initial step is to process the unordered raw data into an ordered array of measurements (variables) in either ascending or descending order in exact numerical sequence. The array provides the simplest distribution mode, where the range spread between maximum and minimum is clearly discernible.

The next step is to tally the number (frequency) with which each measured value or score occurred, that is, to count the number of members or items exhibiting the same value or score.

How many students scored the same number on the AST? How many patients exhibited the same cholesterol level?

The graphic representation of the same ordered array takes the form of a line chart, in which the horizontal scale delineates the individual numerical values or scores and the vertical scale denotes the frequency f corresponding to the tally marks.

Because data can be voluminous, they need to be arranged or grouped to reduce volume, graphed for display, and finally expressed in measures that describe central tendencies and variability. The most common method of condensing data is to group them into classes. This may be done directly from the unordered data list or the ordered array. The usual technique is to prepare a tally sheet for recording the number of items in each class and then transfer the information to a frequency distribution showing the classes and number of items in each class.

The process of frequency distribution may thus be described as the method by which a wide range of measurements is divided into several narrow nonoverlapping contiguous ranges or intervals and the subsequent assignment of each measurement to one and only one of the defined intervals.

Because the sum of the frequency assignment associated with all the class intervals cover the whole range of measurements, the full range of the frequency assignment constitutes the frequency distribution, whereas the resultant number of measurements that fall into a given range or interval constitutes the absolute class frequency of such measurements.

When the distribution is qualified by characterizing it as frequency distribution, the discrete values are bunched into classes, which then are tabled or graphed.

Thus, a frequency table lists categories of scores along with their corresponding frequencies. The frequency for a particular category or class is the number of original scores that fall into that class.

Finally, a histogram is constructed to represent a set of scores after having completed a frequency table. The standard format for a histogram usually involves a vertical scale that delineates frequencies and a horizontal scale that delineates values of the data being presented.

18A.2 The Transformation of Empirical Frequency Distribution

The term frequency distribution is generic in context in the sense that the pattern of the resulting histogram can assume any regular or irregular configuration or shape (e.g., unequal heights interspersed with vacant intervals) covering the range of all the values. The dispersion of the rectangles along the x axis need not conform to any particular pattern or design.

The line chart and the histogram are designed to represent discrete RV, as individual in the case of the line chart and as grouped, classed, or categorized subsets of the total in the case of the histogram. The only restriction is that the sum of the relative frequencies adds up to $1 = 100$ percent.

Thus, the distribution that results from organizing the raw data is empirical and does not necessarily conform to any particular model or mold. It is simply a technique for displaying and summarizing raw data, starting with an ordered array and ending with a histogram.

A frequency distribution thus tabulated from the sample raw data is called an empirical distribution to denote actually observed and measured data rather than theoretically derived values.

The distribution that occupies center stage in statistics, however, is one that conforms to specific recognizable pattern such that the midpoint of the rectangles or the tip of the lines in a line chart follows or conforms to a smooth transition between the classes of the range, in effect outlining a specific curve.

The empirical frequency distribution now becomes a theoretical frequency distribution that is, a theoretical distribution function that conforms to a predefined pattern in the case of a discrete random variable or a smooth curve that can be plotted as a function of a given formula. The term function implies that the distribution follows in exact and perfect order the contour of the graph dictated by the function. What started as a "random collection of data or measurement" is now constrained to follow the outline of a function, just the as the area of the square is a function of its side length.

Despite their separate derivation, it is the confluence between the theoretical and the empirical frequency distributions that forms the backbone of inferential statistics. The crucial connection is the often observed subtle transition from the empirical to the theoretical pattern of distribution that characterizes multiple phenomena in nature. What is even more intriguing is the existence of several theoretical distribution patterns that are custom tailored to specific situations.

The concept of distribution, however, as noted earlier, is more complex. When the empirical distribution assumes or approaches the form of a theoretical distribution, it acquires the properties of the function, which makes it amenable to mathematical manipulation and ultimately to inferential prediction.

The interesting aspect of this transformation is the notion that a random phenomenon may under certain circumstances loosen its randomness and behave in accordance with the rules imposed by a given function.

In practice, strict compliance with the rules required by the function is the exception rather the rule. Nevertheless, if the rules imposed by the function are followed, the random phenomenon approaches the mathematical counterpart with greater and greater fidelity.

The philosophical question as to why such haphazard occurrences or measurements assume a rigorous mold or model is a question to be reflected upon in search for an answer.

On the practical level, certain phenomena in nature assume a particular distribution pattern, either in discrete or in continuous form, peculiar to the phenomenon in question, making it possible to judge the probability of its occurrence under a specific set of circumstances.

The subtle transition from the empirical to the theoretical and the implication derived is best illustrated by the following example:

Example 1. The simplest display of such a distribution takes the form of a table. Table 18A.1, columns 1 and 2, depicts the frequency distribution of the heights (a continuous quantitative variable) of eighty students into six contiguous and mutually exclusive class intervals 4 inches wide, covering the range of 58-82 inches noted in the random sample of eighty students whose heights were individually measured and classified.

The corresponding graphic display of such a distribution takes the form of a frequency histogram, where each of the resultant absolute class frequencies is represented by the area (not the height) of a rectangle (Figure 18A.1).

Such being the case, the area of the rectangle becomes a function of the width of its base as well as the height of its vertical side. By deliberately dividing the range into equal class intervals, the base of the rectangles may be considered to be equivalent to a unit interval, thus making the height of the rectangle numerically equal to the absolute frequency density for the given class. Density, as you may recall, refers to mass per unit volume. In the context of population, density refers to the number of people per unit area (contrast the population density of a block in mid town with an equivalent block in the suburbs). The perusal of the histogram makes it obvious that twenty-four students' heights packed into one unit interval represent a denser distribution than the four students occupying the initial or the last interval. Thus, the ratio of the rectangle area to its base becomes the frequency density of the particular class in question (Figure 18A.2). Alternatively, the product of the frequency density and the interval unit yields the column area, the equivalent of the absolute number in the unit interval (Figure 18A.3).

Class Interval	Frequency	Relative Frequency	Relative Frequency Density
Student's height in inches	Number of students per class	Frequency per class / Σf_i	Relative Frequency / class width of 4
58-62	4	0.05	0.01
62-66	16	0.2	0.05
66-70	24	0.3	0.07
70-74	20	0.25	0.06
74-78	12	0.15	0.04
78-82	4	0.05	0.01
	$\Sigma f_{i=80}$	Σ relative $f_i = 1$	Σ frequency density $= 0.25$
		Total area of all rectangles $= 4 \times 1$	Total area of all rectangles $= 1$

I.

Table 18A.1. Frequency, relative frequency, and relative frequency density of heights in a sample of eighty students

Class Interval	Class Frequency	Relative Frequency	Relative Frequency Density
Height in inches	Number of students in class		
58-66	4	0.05	0.01
62-74	60	0.75	0.18
74-82	16	0.2	0.05
	$\Sigma f_{i=80}$	Σ relative $f_i = 1$	Σ frequency density $= 0.25$
		Total area of all rectangles $= 4 \times 1$	Total area of all rectangles $= 1$

Table 18A.2. Frequency, relative frequency, and relative frequency density of heights in a sample of eighty students

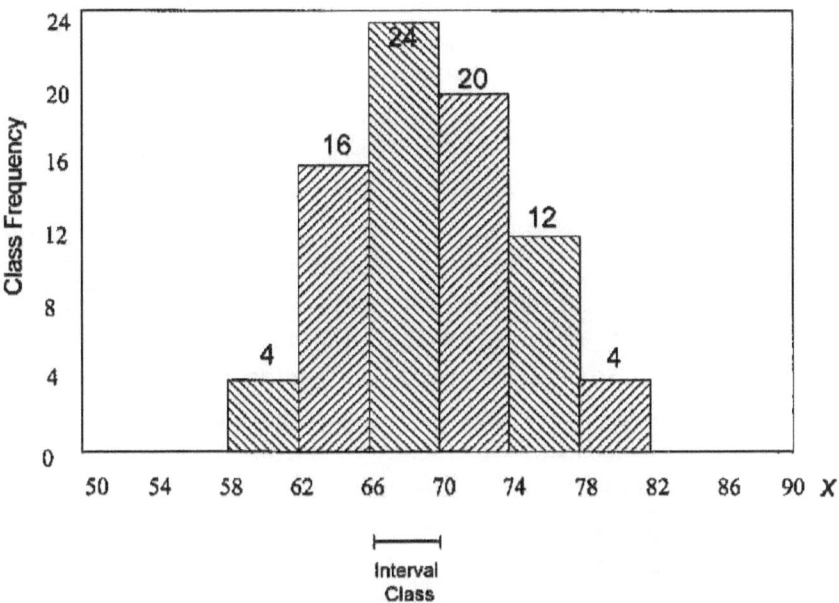

Figure 18A.1. Histogram of the frequency distribution of heights in a random sample of eighty freshmen. Because the width of each rectangle is equivalent to one unit interval, the height of the rectangle is numerically the same as the area of the rectangle, corresponding to the number of students in each of the 4-inch intervals (category and class).

The process of distribution may be equally conducted by determining the relative frequency (fraction or percentage of measurements out of the total number) that fall within a particular class interval rather than the absolute number of measurements as done in the quantitative distribution noted previously.

Because the sum of the relative frequency assignment associated with all the class intervals covers the whole range of measurements, the full range of the relative frequency assignment constitutes the relative frequency distribution, whereas the resultant fraction or percentage of measurements that fall into a given range or interval constitute the relative class frequency of such measurements (Figure 18A.2).

The neat correspondence of height and area breaks down when the base of the rectangle exceeds the unit interval. This is evident in the distribution of the sample of students' heights into three classes of different widths in response to a biometrics survey (Table 18A.2).

In the corresponding histogram (Figure 18A.6), the area of the respective rectangle is similarly drawn to represent the absolute numerical frequency of the class. In this case, however, the class width is not equivalent to the unit interval, so that the frequency, that is, the height of the corresponding rectangle, is reduced to accommodate the increased width associated with a given area. Accordingly, sixty students range in height between 62 and 74 inches, so that the absolute frequency of the extended class becomes 60 / 3 = 20 per unit interval. The frequency is reduced to reflect the fact that three contiguous unequal classes are merged into one. The same logic extends to the relative frequency distribution when the class width is not uniform. As can be seen in Histograms 18-5 and 18-6, the area being made equivalent to fraction or the percentage of the total classified within the specific range.

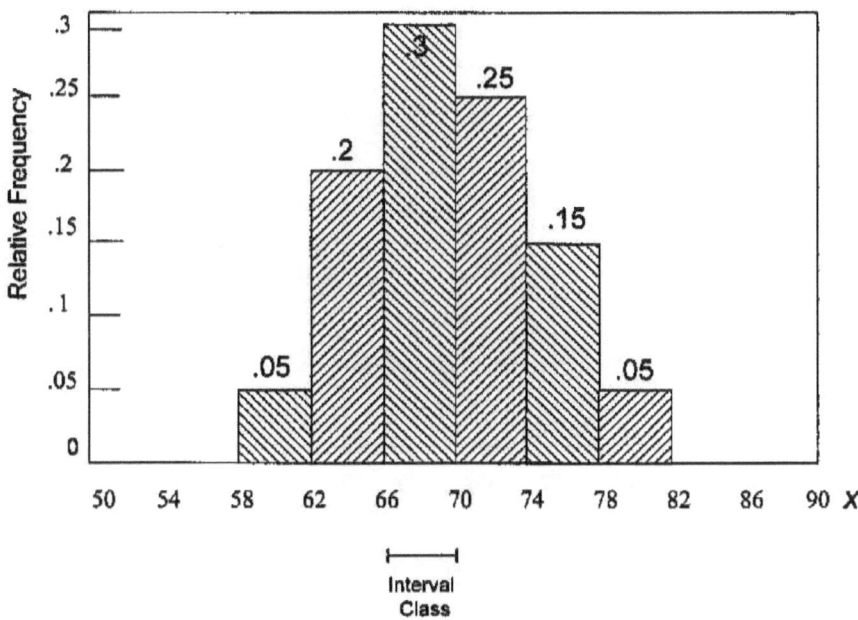

Figure 18A.2. Histogram of the relative frequency distribution of the same random sample of eighty freshmen. Note that the height of the rectangle rather than the area that corresponds to the class relative probability because the base of each rectangle is four units instead of one. Accordingly, the total area is four times the sum of the normal probability distribution of one.

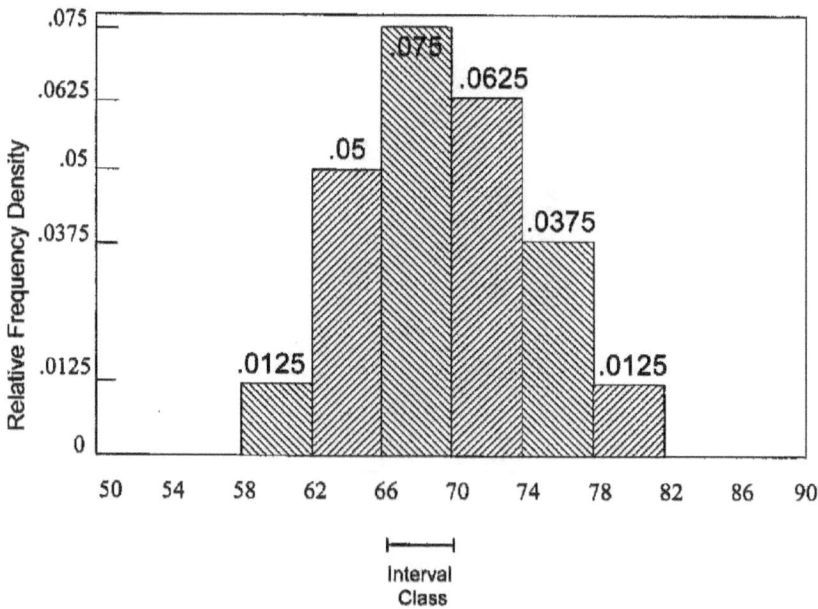

Figure 18A.3. Histogram of the relative frequency density distribution of the same random sample of eighty freshmen. In this format, the area of each rectangle corresponds to the fraction (percentage) of students in each of the class intervals set at 4-inch difference in height. The area of each rectangle thus represents the percent of the total in each category. The total are being the sum of the percentages, that is, the sum of all probabilities or 100 percent. The histogram in this case, that is, the area involved if a curve was to connect the midpoint of each rectangle, is an exact visual representation of the probability distribution among the random variable x, representing the height of the students.

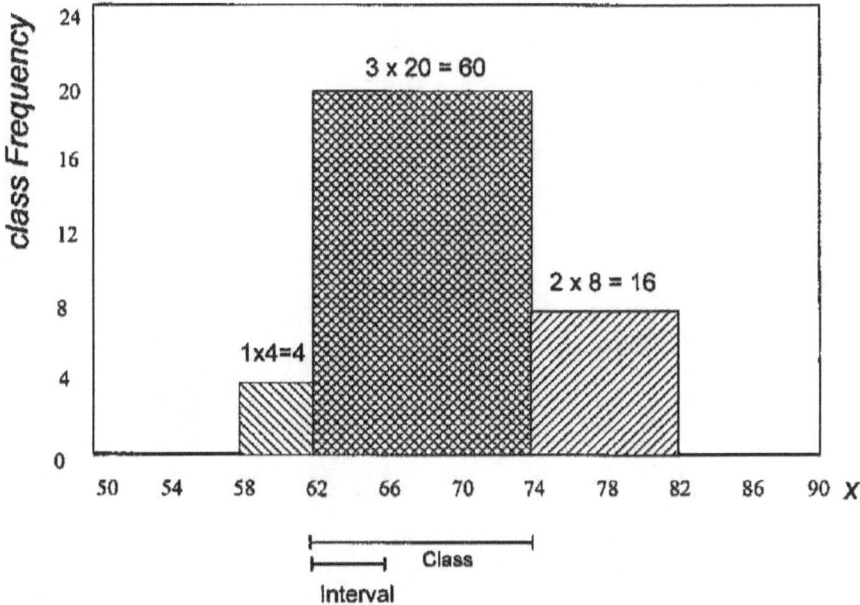

Figure 18A.4. Histogram of the frequency distribution of heights in the same random sample of eighty students. In this case, however, because the base width of the middle and last rectangles is a multiple of the unit interval of 4 inches, the height of the middle rectangle is adjusted to reflect its density $(60 / 3 = 20)$. Similar adjustment is made in the height of the last rectangle $(16 / 2 = 8)$.

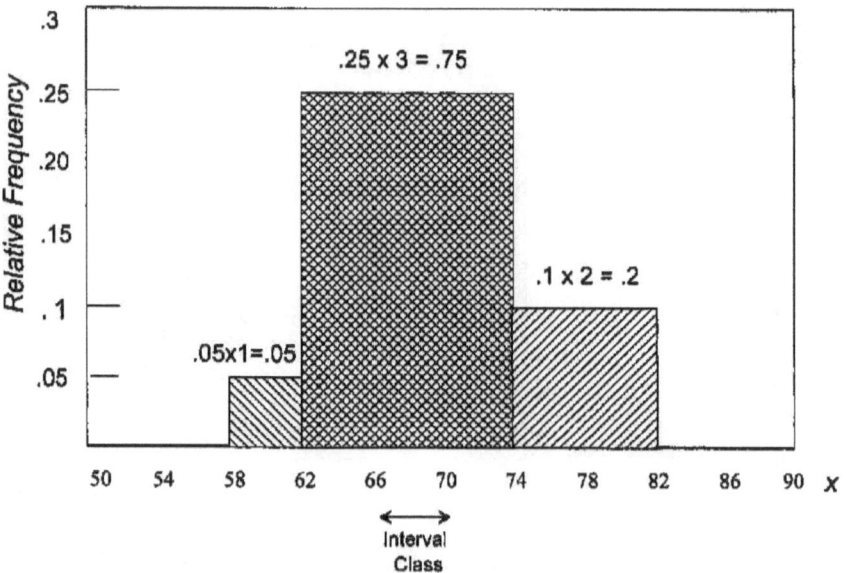

Figure 18A.5. Histogram of the relative frequency distribution of heights in the same random sample of eighty students. Note that the relative frequency of each class needs to be adjusted to reflect the width of the class interval.

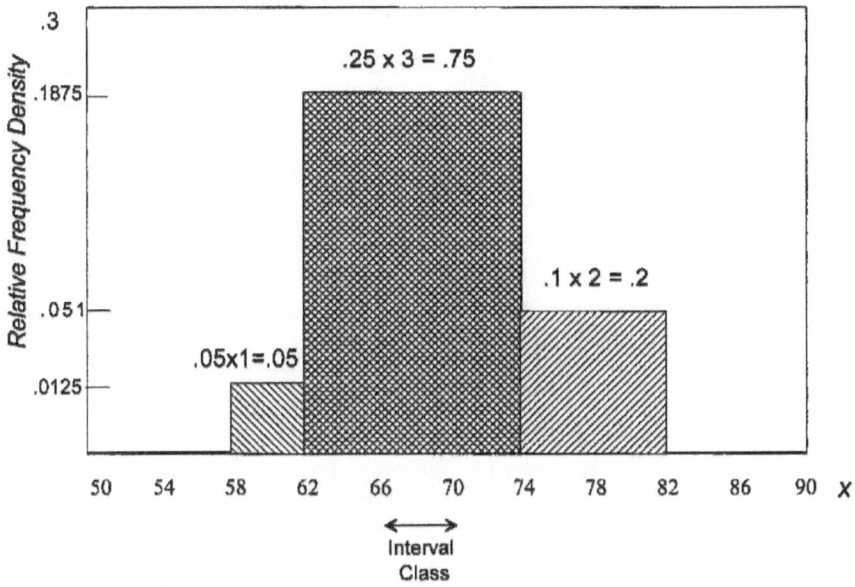

Figure 18A.6. Histogram of the relative frequency density of heights in the same random sample of eight students. Here again, the area of each rectangle corresponds to the fraction (percent) of the students out of the total. The total area of the three rectangles, being the sum of the percentages, is 100 percent. In this case, however, because the base width of middle and last rectangles is a multiple of the unit interval of 4 inches, the height of the middle rectangle is adjusted to reflect its relative density (0.75 / 3 = 0.25). Similar adjustment is made in the height of the last rectangle (0.2 / 2 = 0.1).

18A.3 The Concept of Function as an Operation

In the so-called dynamic approach, f is regarded as an operator to which when the appropriate number, x, is fed, f produces the required number $f(x)$.

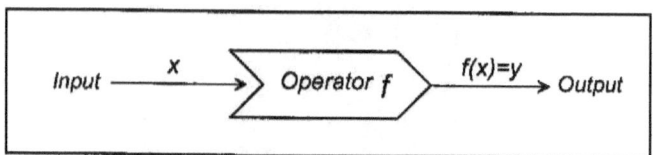

Thus, to each x, there corresponds exactly one y, which is called the *function of x* and is denoted by $f(x)$, so that $y = f(x)$. In this view, f is a law or rule by means of which $f(x)$ can be calculated when x is given. This operational viewpoint is the familiar modality presented in traditional texts.

18A.3.1 The Concept of Function as a Set of Ordered Pairs $(x, f(x))$

From this point of view, f may be regarded as a set of ordered pairs $(x, f(x))$ in which x is the first element while the function $f(x)$ is the second.

Arbitrary sets of ordered pairs are formally called *relations*. A function, then, is a particular kind of relation. A function is defined to be a set of ordered pairs such that no two ordered pairs have the same first coordinate and different second coordinates.

To illustrate the difference between a relation and a function, consider the following three sets:

$$f = \{(2,1), (3,2), (4,3)\}$$
$$f = \{(2,1), (3,2), (4,1)\}$$

$$f \neq \{(2,1), (3,0), (2,4)\}$$

The first two sets are functions (the second set has 1 as a second coordinate of two different pairs, which is still within the pairing rule), but the third set is not a function because (2,1) and (2,4) are ordered pairs with the same first coordinate and different second coordinates.

18A.3.2 Linear Ordering of Real Numbers[18]

With each real number x from the set of real numbers R, we associate a point on a line as in Figure 1.12. The line is called the *real line* or the *x axis*, and the point associated with zero is called the *origin O*. If x is positive, the point associated with x lies to the right of the origin. If x is negative, the point lies to the left of the origin. By this procedure, we are assigning a unique real number to correspond to each point in 1 − space, so that as a consequence, there corresponds to each real number a unique point on the line. This correspondence between the real number line (x axis of 1 − space) and the set of real numbers (R) is a one-to-one correspondence, such that to each number, there corresponds exactly one point and to each point there corresponds exactly one number.

---

[18] Natural numbers = counting numbers = positive integers

$$1, 2, 3, 4, \ldots$$

Integers = positive integers + 0 + negative integers

$$\ldots, -4, -3, -2, -1, 0, 1, 2, 3, 4, \ldots$$

Rational numbers = integers + set of all fraction p/q. Expressed as a decimal that either terminates or else repeats in regular cycles forever.
Real numbers = rational numbers + irrational numbers (nonterminating or nonrepeating) (all numbers that have decimal representation).
These positive and negative real numbers, together with 0, which is neither positive nor negative, constitute the set of real numbers, R, or the real-number system.

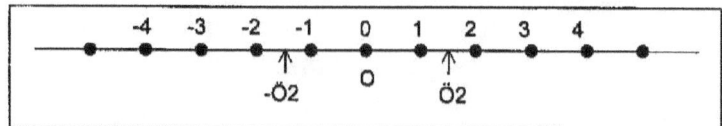

18A.3.3 Cartesian Placement of Ordered Pairs of Real Numbers

If R represents the set of real numbers, then $R \times R$ is the set of all ordered pairs of real numbers. Just as each point on a line corresponds to one and only one real number, hence every point in the plane defined by a Cartesian or rectangular coordinate system can be made to correspond to one and only one ordered pair of real numbers. Thus, point P is located by specifying the ordered pair (x, y) of real numbers, where x is the x projection of P and y is the y projection of P. In this way, a one-to-one correspondence between the set of points in a plane and the set $R \times R$ is established. The order in the pair of (x, y) is essential for the exact positioning of a given point because $(1, 2)$ and $(2, 1)$ are obviously two different points.

Thus, in accordance with the definition of function noted above, set $f = \{(1,2), (2,2), (3,4), (4,3)\}$ in Figure 18A.7 represents a function of four ordered pairs, whereas set $f \neq \{(1,2), (1,3), (3,4), (4,3)\}$ in Figure 18A.8 is not a function.

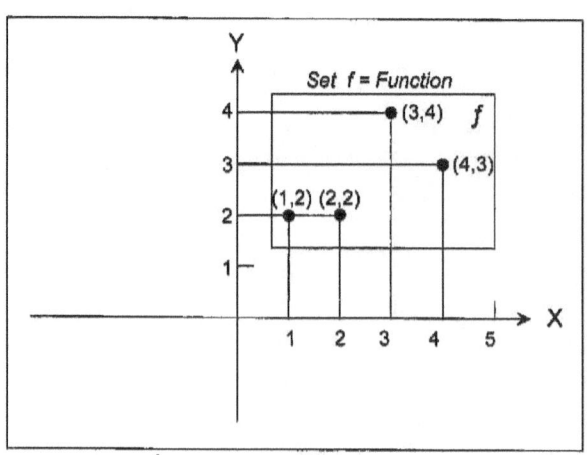

Figure 18A.7. Chart of set $f = \{(1,2), (2,2), (3,4), (4,3)\}$

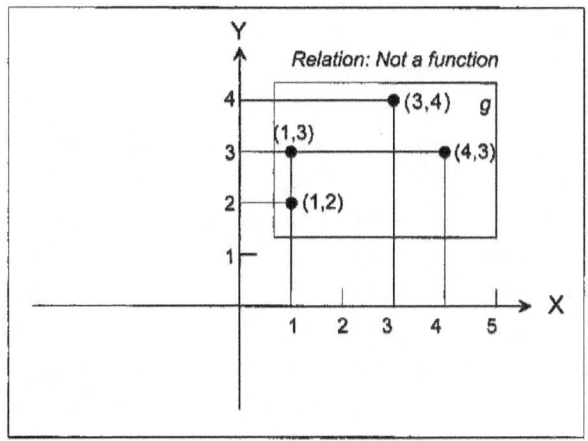

Figure 18A.8. Chart of set $f \neq \{(1,2), (1,3), (3,4), (4,3)\}$

The set of all the first components of a function f is called the *domain of f* and is denoted by D. Similarly, the set of all the second components of f is called the *range of f* and is denoted by R.

Given $f = \{(1,2), (2,2), (3,4), (4,3)\}$ as in Figure 18A.7,

$$D = \{1, 2, 3, 4\}$$
$$\text{and}$$
$$R = \{2, 2, 3, 4\} = \{2, 3, 4\}.$$

Thus, to each x in the domain, there corresponds exactly one y in the range, which is called the *function of x* and is denoted by $f(x)$ so that $y = f(x)$. Thus, the symbol $f(x)$ denotes the second component of that ordered pair in which x is the first component. In other words, if x is in the domain of f, then $f(x)$ denotes the image of x in the range.

The function defined earlier as a set of ordered pairs may be viewed as a correspondence between set x of elements, called the domain of the function, and another set y of different elements, called the range of the function, such that to each element of the domain, there corresponds one and only one element of the range; and to each element of the range, there corresponds at least one element of the domain.

Stated differently, function *f* from *x* into *y* is the set of all ordered pairs (*x,y*) in which each *x* is the first element in one and only one ordered pair of the function.

Example 2. The area, *y*, of a square is uniquely determined when the length, *x*, of an edge is given because to each positive value of *x*, there corresponds one and only one value of *y*. The formula $y = f(x) = x^2$ is the rule of correspondence between the domain, which is the set of all positive real numbers *x* (i.e., the length of the edge of the square), and the range, which is the set of all positive real numbers *y* (i.e., the area of the square corresponding to the given length of the edge). Note that for each positive value of *x* (the domain), there corresponds one and only one value of $y = f(x) = x^2$ (the range). It is the correspondence between the set of all positive values of *x* and the set of values of *y* dictated by the rule that constitute the function in this case. Note that length is measured using an interval scale, such that length of the edge may assume any positive real number (all numbers that have decimal representation) and thus can be considered to be a continuous domain. By the same token, the range may likewise result in a continuous positive real number. The correspondence in this case is thus between a continuous domain and a continuous range.

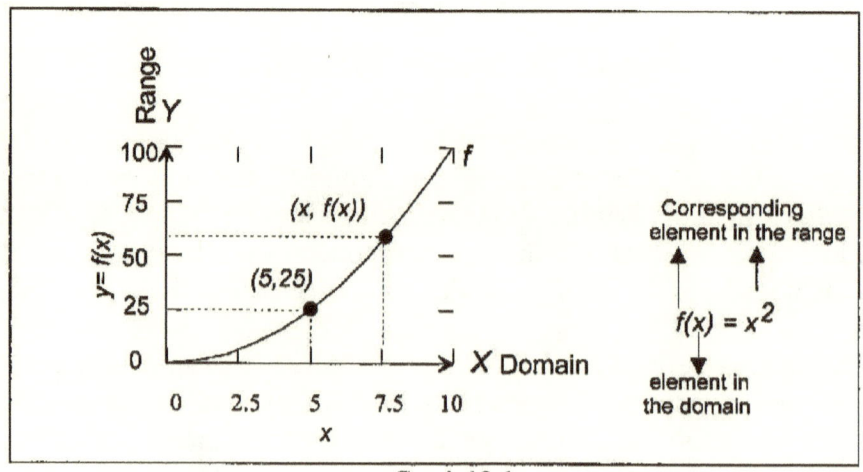

Figure 18A.9. Correspondence between continuous domain and continuous range

Thus, given $f(x) = x^2$, we can think of f as being the operator that converts x into x^2 when $x > 0$ or as being the set of ordered pairs (x, x^2) for which $x > 0$.

In the first instance, when an element x of the domain is selected and fed into the black box, the x is called an *input* and the black box is supposed to produce an *output*, which is an element y of a set R, which is called a range.

Alternatively, in the second instance, f may be regarded as a **set** of ordered pairs $(x, f(x))$, in which x of the domain is the first element while the function $f(x)$ is the second element.

A function then involves three things: a set of elements called the domain of the function, a set of elements called the range of the function, and a rule of correspondence, which enables us to determine precisely which element of the range corresponds to each element of the domain.

Once it is clearly understood that when a function exists the function is the correspondence, it will often be convenient to refer to the typical element of the range as a function of the typical element of the domain. $f(x)$ is thus a short way of writing the phrase "the value of the function f for the number x" or more briefly, "f of x." Implicit to these notations is the subtle concept of correspondence, whereby x stands for any one value in the domain and $f(x)$ stands for the corresponding value of the range.

Thus, we can say that the "the area of a square is a function of the length of an edge of the square" and the "the sum of the face values of a pair of rolled dice is a function of the elements (simple events) of the sample space which in turn is composed of all the possible ordered pairs." It is customary to refer to the typical element of the domain as the independent variable and the typical element of the range as the dependent variable.

18A.4 The Random Variable

This chapter introduces the reader to the concept of the random variable, the leitmotiv of modern probability. The framework within which the concept is based is related to the previously discussed models of probability (the equally likely outcome or the relative frequency interpretation models) as well as to the concept of the function detailed earlier.

To return to the ubiquitous sample space of all ordered pair resulting from the roll of a pair of dice (Table 4.2.), the familiar sample space defined as SS = {(1,6), (1,5), . . . , (6,6)} contains thirty-six elements of ordered pairs or simple events (Table 4.3). Let E_2, E_3, . . . , E_{12} denote the event composed of the sum of the face values of the ordered pairs such that the compound events are subsets of the sample space, for example, E_3 = {(1, 2), (2, 1)} or E_5 = {(1, 4), (2, 3), (3, 2), (4, 1)}, whereas the event E_{12} = {(6, 6)} is a simple event, being restricted to a single ordered pair (column 1 of Table 4.4).

Let X denote the functions $X(E_2)$, $X(E_3)$, . . . , $X(E_{12})$, whose domain is the set of events, E_2, E_3, . . . , E_{12}, of the sample space and its range is the numerical set of the eleven corresponding values of the derived functions, $X(E_2) = 2$, $X(E_3) = 3$, . . . , $X(E_{12}) = 12$.

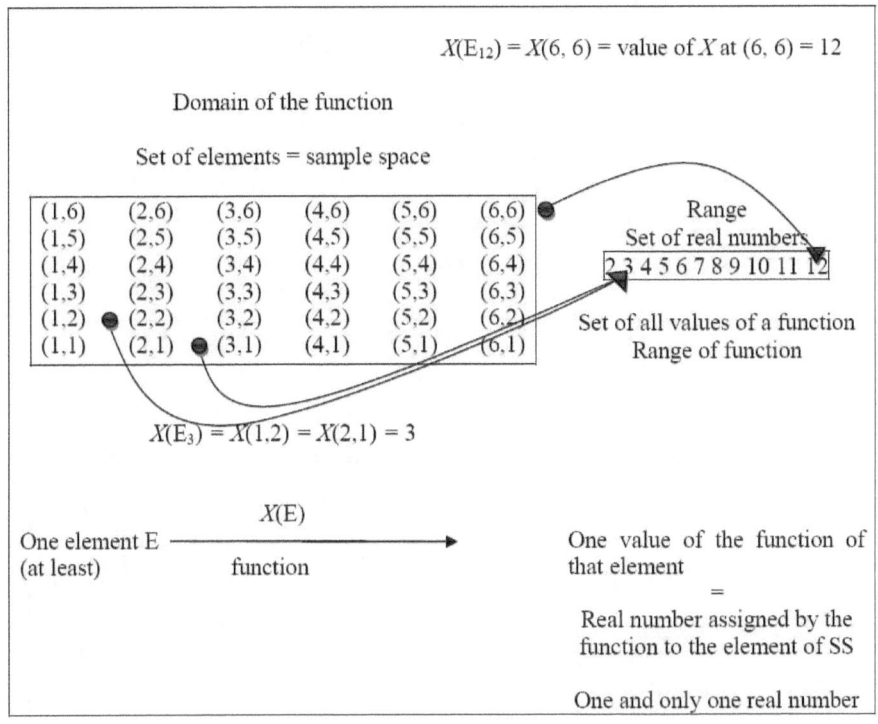

Figure 18A.10. Diagram of the interplay of Domain Vs. R

Each ordered pair of SS has associated with it exactly one element of the range; however, the same value of X may be derived from more than one outcome. For example, $X(E_3) = 3$, if E is any one of the two elements of the event $\{(1,2), (2,1)\}$.

A given input element always leads to exactly one output number, but the same output number may be obtained from more than one input element.

Notice that in example 2, the correspondence was one-to-one because there corresponded one and only one element of the other set to each element of either set. But in this case, the correspondence is not always one-to-one; in here, each element in the range corresponds to one or more than one element of the domain. But despite this, the correspondence is a function whose domain is the set composed of thirty-six elements (simple events) and whose range is the set composed of 11 events because to each element of the domain, there corresponds one and only one element of the range; and to each element of the range, there corresponds at least one element of the domain.

Return to the tossing of three coins (quarter, penny, and dime). The resulting sequence of heads (Washington, Lincoln, and Roosevelt) and tails makes up the sample space of the experiment.

$$S = \{HHH, HHT, HTH, THH, HTT, THT, TTH, TTT\}.$$

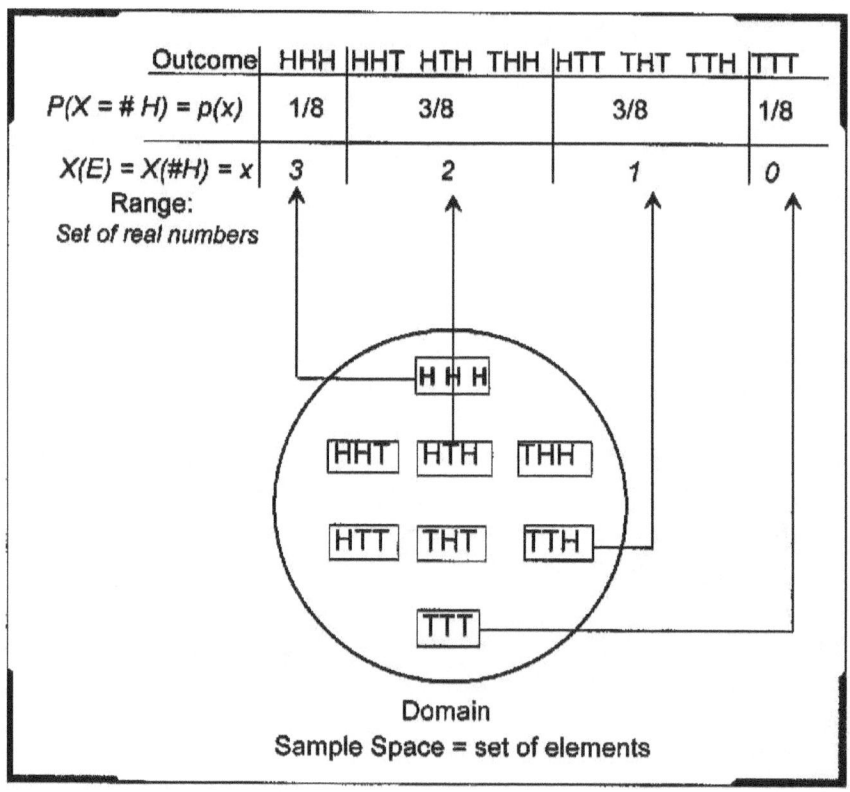

Figure 18A.11. Flow chart of the random variable defined in terms of the number of heads associated with the experiment of tossing three coins

Denote the events corresponding to the number of heads on any given outcome by E_n. Let X be the function whose domain is the set of events (subsets), E_1, E_2, E_3, and E_0 of the resulting events, simple or compound, and its range the set of four numerical corresponding values, then

$$E_3 = \{(HHH)\} \text{ and } X(E_3) = X(HHH) = 3$$

$$E_2 = \{(HHT), (HTH), (THH)\} \text{ and } X(E_2) = X(HHT) = X(HTH) = X(THH) = 2$$

$$E_1 = \{(HTT), (THT), (TTH)\} \text{ and } X(E_1) = X(HTT) = X(THT) = X(TTH) = 1$$

$$E_0 = \{(TTT)\} \text{ and } X(E_0) = X(TTT) = 0$$

Note once again the correspondence between the domain of X (number of simple events in the original sample space) and its range, the set of numbers generated by the corresponding function (number of heads in a given outcome). Here, as in the dice example, to each element of the domain, there corresponds one and only one element of the range, $X(E_2) = 2$; whereas to any one element of the range, there corresponds at least one element of the domain.

Consider the trite experiment of observing the result of tossing a single die. The set of possible outcomes assumes one of six equally likely, disjoint, and mutually exclusive values: $S = \{1, 2, 3, 4, 5, 6\}$. If X is made to denote the function of any one element of the sample space, then $X(E) = X(1) = 1$ and $X(E) = X(6) = 6$, etc. In this case, the outcome of the experiment is identical with the value of the function, so that $X(E) = E$, the identity function.

The common theme in the above three examples is the assignment of a numerical value to each outcome in S. The perusal of the three examples and the associated flow charts should be enough to convince the reader that X is essentially a function whose domain is the set of outcomes while its range is a subset of real numbers. The notation $X(E) = x$ means that X as a function of the outcome E is equal to x, a real number, the value of $X(E)$.

The reader may have surmised that X in the context detailed previously is the sought after **random variable** under discussion. Recall that prior to the performance of an experiment, the unknown although anticipated outcome is designated as a random variable, underlying the fact that the RV may assume any one value depending on the actual outcome of the experiment. Thus, the RV X is a generic symbol that stands for the potential value x that will obtain on the performance of the experiment. Which is another way of saying that when materialized, the RV represented by the capital X takes the value of the lower case x, which is any number represented by x.

Because the random variable is a numerical quantity, whose value is defined for each outcome of the experiment and thus indirectly with each element of the sample space corresponding to the resulting outcome, it may be represented by a table that lists the elements of a finite sample space and the corresponding number the random variable assumes with each outcome (Figures 18A.10 and 18A.11).

Furthermore, because the outcome of any one experiment is unpredictable beforehand, it must, however, correspond to the particular numerical value associated with the particular outcome and ultimately with the corresponding element of the sample space. For the event of two heads outcome, the random variable $X(E_2) = X(HHT) = X(HTH) = X(THH) = 2$.

The random variable is in effect a function denoted by X (rather than f), whose domain is the set of elements in a sample space and whose range is a set of real numbers. In accordance with the accepted notation of a function, $X(E) = x$ stands for the value of the function X at every event E of the sample space. Stated differently, $X(E)$ is the value of the function X corresponding to all possible events that can be derived from the simple events of the sample space in accordance with the defined rule. The notation stipulates that capital X stands for the random variable, whereas the lower case x denotes the particular value of a random variable. The analogous use of notation for the standard function, f, and the random variable, X, further emphasizes the functional nature of the random variable

Random variable	$X(E) = x$
Function	$f(x) = y$

This roundabout way of introducing the random variable is not the standard method of presentation. The following definitions are excerpted from standard texts. As can be noted, not all definitions adequately convey the functional aspect of the random variable.

Note that the set of all possible values of X, that is, the range, may be considered as another sample space in its own right, representing the numerical outcome of the function, in contrast to the sample space of the domain corresponding to all possible outcomes of the domain.

Finally, to divest the random variable from its coterie of coins and dice and to project into a real-life situation, consider the following experiments and the random variable generated by the outcome of the experiment are tabled. The application as can be seen is universally relevant to every field of endeavor.

---

1. A random variable X is a function defined over a sample space S: $\{e_1, e_2, , e_n\}$. This means that to each element e_i of S, there is a corresponding a unique real number, namely, the value of X. Thus, we may write $X(e_i) = x_i$ (Mode).

2. Let E be an experiment and S a sample space associated with the experiment. A function X assigning to every element $s \in S$, a real number, $X(s)$, is called random variable (Meyer).

3. A random variable X associated with a probability space S is a function that assigns a real number to each simple event in S (K. Smith).

4. A random variable is a rule that assigns a number to each outcome of a chance experiment. More precisely, a random variable is a function with domain given by the set of outcomes of a chance experiment and range contained in the set of real numbers (Tan).

5. A random variable is a rule that assigns a numerical value to each outcome *of* an experiment (Anton). For a given sample space S of some experiment, a random variable is any rule that associates a number with each outcome in S.

   The notation $X(s) = x$ means that x is the number associated with the outcome s by the RV X, so x is called the value of the variable associated with s (Devore).

6. A random variable is a function or rule that assigns a number to each possible outcome in a sample space (Hildebrand).

7. Any quantitative variable the numerical value of which is determined by a random experiment and thus by chance is called a random variable. The variable's name (such as "heads" when tossing a coin) is designated by X; any one of its possible values (such as "two heads" in five tosses) is symbolized by x (Kohler).

Random Experiment	Discrete Random Variable
Count the number of correct answers on a twenty-question exam	The number of correct answers on exam
Count the nightly number of patients attending the ER between 12 midnight and 8:00 a.m. for thirty days	The number of nightly attendance at the ER for thirty nights
Random Experiment	**Continuous Random Variable**
Record the life of an alkaline battery pack	The number of hours a battery pack lasts
Record the weight of a newborn term baby in ounces	The actual weight of a newborn in ounces
Check the time it takes for a drug to take effect	The number of hours and minutes
Measure the height (in inches) of a male college freshman	The height in inches of a freshman
Determine serum blood total cholesterol level in a diabetic patients	Level of serum blood cholesterol in mg/dL
Measure the systolic blood pressure	Level of systolic blood pressure in mm Hg.

Table 18A.3. Variables defined in random experiments

18A.5 The Probability Mass Function: The Probability Distribution Function for Discrete Random Variable

Consider, hopefully for the last time, the experiment of tossing a single die. Given a discrete random variable, X, defined on sample space $S = \{1, 2, 3, 4, 5, 6\}$, and whose range consist of a number of values 1, 2, . . . , 6, then the probability of the outcome assuming any one value of the simple events of the set $\{1\}$, $\{2\}$, $\{3\}$, $\{4\}$, $\{5\}$, and $\{6\}$ is expressed as follows:

$$P(X = 1) = \frac{1}{6}; \quad P(X = 2) = \frac{1}{6}; \ldots; \quad P(X = 6) = \frac{1}{6}$$

Note that the functional aspect of the random variable has been suppressed in this notation, which could be expanded to read

$$P(X(E) = 1) = P(X = 1) = P(\text{the event that } X = 1) = \text{Probability function of } X = p(x) = \frac{1}{6}.$$

What is being implied in this abbreviated notation is as follows:

1. The event in the sample space defined by the random variable $X(E) = 1$ occurs with a probability of 1/6 or what amounts to the same thing that the probability of the value of the random variable (function) of the event occurs with a probability of 1/6.
2. Consider once more the experiment of tossing two dice. The sample space in this case is the Cartesian product $n(S) \times n(S) = 6 \times 6 = 36$ equally likely outcomes:

$$S = \{(1, 1), (1, 2), \cdots, (6, 5), (6, 6)\}.$$

If X is to represent the outcome of any one toss, then

$$X = (1, 1); X = (1, 2); \ldots; X = (6, 5); X = (6, 6).$$

In this case, the probability of X assuming the value corresponding to the sum of any one ordered pair is expressed as follows, given that the elements of the sample space are equiprobable:

$$P(X(1,1)) = \frac{1}{36}; \; P(X(1,2)) = \frac{1}{36}; \; P(X(6,5)) = \frac{1}{36}; \; P(X(6,6)) = \frac{1}{36}$$

3. The event that the sum of the face numbers of the two dice is 5 is

$$E_5 = \{(1, 4), (2, 3), (3, 2), (4, 1)\}.$$

If X is assigned to the outcome of any ordered pair whose sum equals 5, then

$$X(1,4) = 5; \; X(2,3) = 5; \; X(3,2) = 5; \; X(4,1) = 5.$$

The probability of X displaying any one pair of the subset of E_5 is

$$P(X(1,4)) = \frac{1}{36}; \; P(X(2,3)) = \frac{1}{36}; \; P(X(3,2)) = \frac{1}{36}; \; P(X(4,1)) = \frac{1}{36}$$

The probability that X assumes the sum of 5 as the outcome so as to include all the possible sums that total 5 is by the addition principle,

$$P(X = E_5) = P(X(1,4)) + P(X(2,3)) + P(X(3,2)) + P(X(4,1)) = \frac{1}{36} + \frac{1}{36} + \frac{1}{36} + \frac{1}{36} = \frac{4}{36}$$

This is the probability that the sum of the face values on the dice turns out to be 5. In other words, the new function gives the probability for every value in the range, that is, for every x value that the random variable assumes.

4. Return to the tossing of three coins. The resulting sequence of heads and tails makes up the sample space of the experiment.

$$S = \{HHH, HHT, HTH, THH, HTT, THT, TTH, TTT\}.$$

Assign X to the outcome of any one toss, then

$$X = (HHH); \ X = (HHT); \ \dots; \ X = (TTT).$$

The probability of X turning up any one outcome of the set,

$$P(X(HHH)) = \frac{1}{8}; \ P(X(HHT)) = \frac{1}{8}; \ \dots; \ P(X(TTT)) = \frac{1}{8}$$

5. Assign X the number of heads in any one outcome, then

$$X(HHH) = 3; \ X(HHT) = 2; \ \dots; \ X(TTT) = 0.$$

The probability of X displaying two heads is then the sum of the probabilities of the mutually exclusive and disjoint events.

$$P(X = 2H) = P(X(HHT)) + P(X(HTH)) + P(X(THH)) = \frac{1}{8} + \frac{1}{8} + \frac{1}{8} = \frac{3}{8}.$$

Examples 1-5	RV X	Probability function of the RV X
Example 1	$X(1) = 1$	$P(X=1) = 1/6$
Example 2	$X(1, 1) = 1$	$P(X(1, 1)) = 1/36$
Example 3	$X(1, 4) = 5$	$P(X = E_s) = 4/36$
Example 4	$X(HHH) = 1$	$P(X(HHH)) = 1/8$
Example 5	$X(HHT) = 2$	$P(X = 2H) = 3/8$
RV	$X(E) = x$	$P(X = x) = p(x)$
Function	$f(x) = y$	$P(f(x)) = p(x)$

Table 18A.4. Random Variable Vs. Probability function

We are now dealing, so to speak, with a function of a function. The original function being that of the RV, which assigns a range value to each event of the sample space. In turn, the value of the range now becomes the domain of a function that assigns probability values to each value of the range. Note that the probability function is a new function whose domain is the range of the RV (function) defined on the original sample space.

The probability function, $p(x)$, thus represents the probability at any given value in the range in which the random variable X assumes one x value, in formal notation, $P(X=x) = p(x)$, where x is the discrete value of the random variable, which is a shorthand way of stating that the probability of the outcome is the probability of the value that X will assume.

Given a discrete random variable, X, defined on sample space, and whose range consist of a number of values, then each possible outcome x is associated with a certain probability that defines its probable occurrence within the range. In other words, the probability of a given outcome in the range denoted by $p(x)$ is identical with the probability that the random variable X assumes the value x, so that

$$P(X = x) = p(x)$$

Furthermore, the probability that X assumes the value x is $P(X = x) = p(x)$, which specifies the probability of the x value on the conclusion of the experiment.

If the number of possible values of X is finite (i.e., if the range is made of a finite number of outcomes), then X is called a *discrete random variable*. In such a case, the possible values of X may be listed as $x_1, x_2, \ldots, x_n$.

If X, on the other hand, can assume any real number (i.e., all numbers that have decimal representation), then X is called a *continuous random variable*.

Note that even when the measurements are performed on a continuous interval scale that can take any value in a continuum (e.g., blood chemistry, weight, blood pressure, etc.), the values are rounded and thus converted into discrete values then plotted on a continuous axis.

Domain of the function

Set of elements = sample space

(1,6)	(2,6)	(3,6)	(4,6)	(5,6)	(6,6)◄──	Simple even which gave
(1,5)	(2,5)	(3,5)	(4,5)	(5,5)	(6,5)	rise to $X(E) = 12$
(1,4)	(2,4)	(3,4)	(4,4)	(5,4)	(6,4)	
(1,3)	(2,3)	(3,3)	(4,3)	(5,3)	(6,3)	
(1,2)●	(2,2)	(3,2)	(4,2)	(5,2)	(6,2)	
(1,1)	(2,1)●	(3,1)	(4,1)	(5,1)	(6,1)	

Compound event (subset) which gave rise to $X(E) = 3$

Figure 18A.12. Domain Vs. Simple or Compound events

It has been made abundantly clear that the probability function $p(x)$ defines the probability that the value of X assumes a given range number. In effect, the probability function is the assignment of a probability value to each of the numbers obtained in the range of the random variable, which in turn corresponds to the elements of the sample space.

In the case in which the probability of X assumes the value corresponding to the sum of any one ordered pair as in example 5, the probabilities associated with each element of the range may be computed in an analogous manner. These values are summarized in the following probability table, where each numerical x value in the range is tabulated with its corresponding probability $p(x)$ (Table 18A.5).

x	2	3	4	5	6	7	8	9	10	11	12
$p(x)$	1/36	2/36	3/36	4/36	5/36	6/36	5/36	4/36	3/36	2/36	1/36

Table 18A.5

As noted in Table 18A.5, each numerical value of x in the range is coupled with the corresponding probability function of the random variable X, $p(x)$. The resultant ordered pairs of $(x_i, p(x_i))$ constitute the probability distribution of the random variable X.

$$P(X = x) = p(x) \quad = \text{Probability associated with each value of the RV}$$
$$= \text{Probability of occurrence of each value of the range}$$

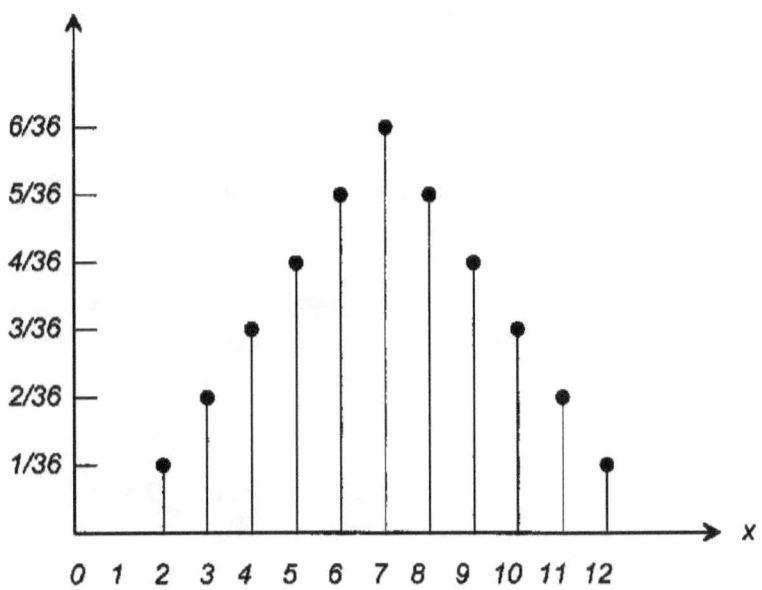

Figure 18A.13. Line chart of the $X(E) = x$ values that RV assumes at the event E; range of the discrete random variable.

The graphic counterpart to Table 18A.5 is presented in the probability Figure 18A.13. The various values of X are indicated on the horizontal x axis, and the length of the vertical line drawn from the x axis to the point with coordinates $(x,p(x))$ is the probability of the event that X has the value x.

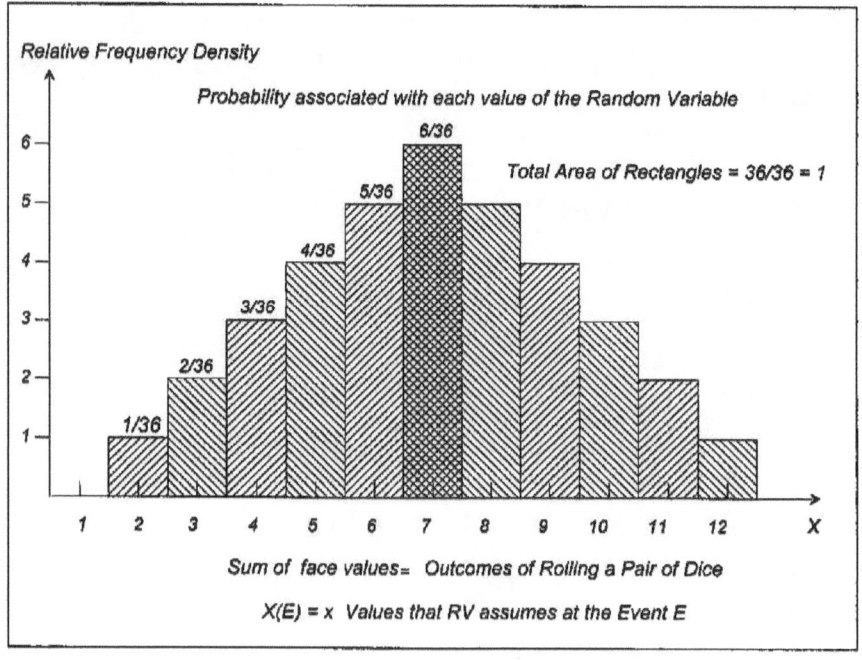

Figure 18A.14. Relative Frequency Density Vs. RV
values of the a given event

Chapter 18B

The Binomial Probability Distribution
(Probability Distribution Function of Binomial Random Variables)

18B.1 Bernoulli Random Variable

When the outcomes of a given trial or experiment are mutually exclusive (the occurrence of any one event rules out the occurrence of the other events so that joint occurrence is impossible) and independent (the occurrence of one is not affected by the occurrence of the other), the sample space is reduced to its absolute minimum of two basic mutually exclusive and complementary outcomes.

Furthermore, in a similar vein to the basic level of the binary number system where only two digits (0 and 1) are required in order to write a binary number, the Bernoulli random variable can similarly assume two and only two possible values: success p and failure q.

As previously noted, the coin is a member of a class of objects that can assume one of two mutually exclusives states of being. This class of objects, physical or conceptual, is referred to as a *Bernoulli random variable*. Accordingly, the sample space for a Bernoulli random variable may be expressed as the set {success, failure} {p, q} or, alternatively, {1, 0}.

From a practical point of view, the binomial state of a Bernoulli random variable may be applied to a wide variety of options as can be appreciated from the brief listing in the attached Table 18B.1.

Subject	State	
Binary digit	1	0
Sample space	Set	Complement
Outcome	Success	Failure
Coin	Head	Tail
Switch	On	Off
Test	Positive	Negative
Target	Hit	Miss
Statement	True	False
Answer	Yes	No
Being	Health	Disease
Birth	Boy	Girl

Table 18B.1

The practical implication, the subject of this chapter, can be readily appreciated through the simple experiment of tossing six coins and observing the outcome of heads and tails (HT) that materialize with each toss.

When the experiment is repeated over and over again, the pattern that emerges ranges from all heads to all tails and a graded mixture in between (Table 18B.2, second row).

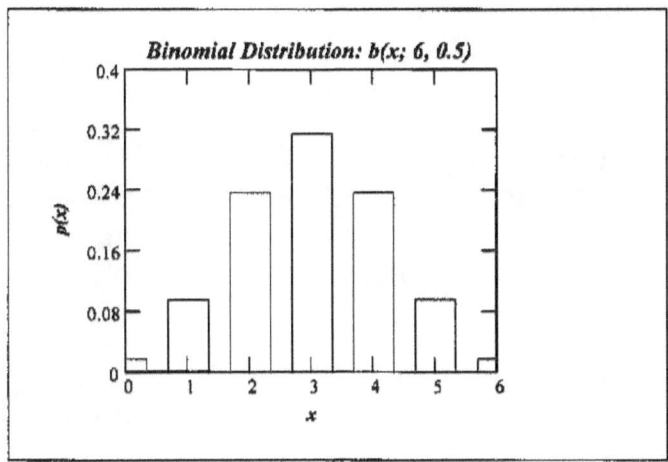

Figure 18B.1. Histogram depicting the relative frequency (probability) associated with each binomial random variable x (number of heads)

Finally, when the relative frequency (probability) of the specific outcomes resulting from repeated trials (tosses) associated with the seven possible outcomes is plotted against the random variable, depicting the number of heads for the given toss is charted, a symmetrical histogram results in which the relative frequency of the different outcomes is plotted on the y axis for each of the seven possible combinations. Thus, the coefficient of twenty associated with (H^3T^3) occurs twenty times out of possible sixty-four (20/64) combinations or equivalently 0.3125 (31.25 percent).

Additionally, because the base of each column is unity, the area of the column is essentially an exact percentage of the total. The total in this case is the sum of the areas of the seven noncontiguous columns, which adds up to 1.

$$\frac{1}{64} + \frac{6}{64} + \frac{15}{64} + \frac{20}{64} + \frac{15}{64} + \frac{6}{64} + \frac{1}{64} = \frac{64}{64} = 1$$

Note that each of the extreme columns occupies 0.0156 (1.56 percent) of the total area, consistent with the fact that all tails or all heads is a rare occurrence.

18B.2 The Binomial Random Variable

The binomial random variable is a special case of the generic discrete random variable. Its value as determined by the outcome of a random trial assumes one of two possible outcomes, usually called success, p, or failure, q. Thus, in contrast to the discrete random variable whose variable may assume multiple values, the binomial version reduces the number of variables to the absolute minimum of two, thus the name binomial.

Note that the binomial random variable X is associated with an experiment consisting of more than one trial so that its value is represented by the number of successes in n trials; thus,

$$x = \text{number of successes in } n \text{ trials.}$$

On the other hand, a binomial random variable defined as the number of successes in n trial can obviously assume any natural number from 0 to n, depending on the actual number of successes in the n trials.

18B.3 Binomial Probability Distribution: $p = q$

Suppose, as depicted in the attached Venn diagram (Figure 18B.2), that the probability of the H outcome is equal to the probability of T outcome, so that

$$P(H) = p = 0.5$$
$$P(T) = q = 0.5$$

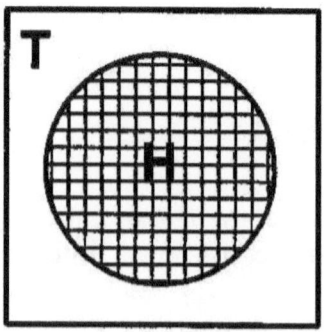

Figure 18B.2

As you may have guessed, the sample space and the outcome just describe are the theoretical models for the tossing of a single fair coin. If the number of coins tossed is more than one, say six coins, the sample space expands to sixty-four simple outcomes in order to accommodate all possible permutations with replacement that the six coins may assume on any one given toss.

To reiterate the obvious, in tossing six fair coins, 2^6 or sixty-four possible outcomes are then equally likely. Each outcome representing one particular combination (permutation) is thus associated with a probability of 1/64. The sixty-four outcomes resolve into seven possible distinct events if the number of heads, or its complement the number of tails, per toss is exclusively considered (Table 18B.2). Accordingly, the sample space, as defined for this event in terms of the number of heads (successes) per throw, is partitioned into seven corresponding subsets whose elements constitute the possible outcomes of the events. Obviously, the seven events range from all heads to no heads for any one throw. In accordance with accepted terminology, the events associated with all heads or no heads are simple events because the subset from which they originate is made up of one element only. The balances of the possible events are compound events because the subset from which they originate is made up of several elements. This is depicted in the third and fourth rows, where the frequency and the relative frequency of the outcomes are tabled, whereas the first and second row illustrates the makeup of its combination.

The frequency of occurrence of any one of the seven events on repeated tossing the six coins is shown to be identical with the corresponding binomial coefficient, third row, which in turn is the number of possible combinations obtained when six different objects are taken or combined 0, 1, 2, 3, 4, 5, and 6 at a time.

In each case, the coefficient gives the number of outcomes that make up the compound event or, alternatively, the number of elements in the corresponding subset of the sample space with which a particular combination of (x) number of heads and $(6 - x)$ number of tails appear in the sixty-four plus tosses.

Thus, the combination of four heads and two tails occur fifteen times, whereas three heads and three tails top the list of frequencies at twenty times. At the two extremes, all heads or all tails are expected to occur only once.

The finding on any one toss of the six coins, one need not be reminded, allows for one and only one combination, that is, only one outcome out of the total sixty-four possible outcomes corresponding to the sixty-four elements of the sample space is possible. What the array reads is the number of seven possible combinations (permutations to be specific) of 0, 1, 2, 3, 4, 5, and 6 heads that are expected on repeating the tossing sixty-four plus times.

This frequency of the events, or its equivalent the value of the binomial coefficient, that is, the number specifying the frequency if outcomes associated with the random variable x correspond to the number of heads in this trial. Given the frequency, the relative frequency of each of the seven coefficients is simply the ratio of the given coefficient to the sum of the coefficients as noted in the fourth row of Table 18B.2. The relative frequency may be translated into probability as a fraction or as a percentage of the total possible outcomes of 64. Thus, the probability of getting an equal number of heads and tails in the long run (i.e., sixty-four times or multiples of sixty-four times and not just a single toss) is expected to occur twenty times out of the sixty-four tosses, or 3,125 in ten thousand tosses, which is another way of saying that the combination H^4T^2 should theoretically occur fifteen times in the sixty-four throws of six balanced coins, the combination H^3T^3 should occur twenty times out of the sixty-four tosses, and the combination of all heads, H^6T^0, is expected to occur only once.

The binomial random variable, X, being considered in this case, is the number of heads on any given toss while the number assigned to it is the frequency of its occurrence on repeated trials or the equivalent theoretical expected frequency.

From the fourth row of Table 18B.2, the probability of the event with x heads, representing the probability in which the random variable X takes the specific value x, is the correct and somewhat elaborate way of defining the probability function of the number of heads, $p(x)$, for each of the possible combinations beginning with the probability function of 0, $p(0)$, for the case where the random variable X equals 0, $P(X = 0)$, that is, all tails, and ending with the probability function of 6, $p(6)$, for the case where the random variable X equals 6, $P(X = 6)$, that is, all heads. The binomial probability distribution is thus defined as the set of ordered pairs $(x, p(x))$ corresponding to all possible values of X. As noted, the numerator in each case is none other than the combination $6Cx$ of the six coins taken x at a time, equivalent to the expected frequency of occurrence of the particular event, whereas the denominator is the total number of possible outcomes of $2^6 = 64$ as noted previously.

Because the sample space is now made up of sixty-four equally likely distinct outcomes, each of which is assigned a probability of 1/64, the joint probability of the compound event could be equally derived using the addition principle for mutually exclusive events. Thus, the probability that exactly two heads turn up, E {HHTTTT, HTHTTT, TTHHTT, . . . ,}, which includes fifteen simple events or outcomes, is the sum of the probabilities of its component outcomes of simple events. Alternatively, because the number of elements in the compound event, which is a subset of the sample space, is equal to fifteen, the probability of the compound event may be expressed as follows:

$$P(\text{compound event}) = \frac{\text{No. of elements in subset}}{\text{No. of elements in sample space}} = \frac{15}{64}$$

Events	$1H^0T^6$	$6H^1T^5$	$15H^2T^4$	$20H^3T^3$	$15H^4T^2$	$6H^5T^1$	$1H^6T^0$
Binomial coefficient nCx = no. of events with x heads	$6C0 = 1$	$6C0 = 6$	$6C2 = 15$	$6C3 = 20$	$6C4 = 15$	$6C5 = 6$	$6C6 = 1$
P(event with x heads) $nCx/2^n$	$\dfrac{1}{64} = .016$	$\dfrac{6}{64} = .093$	$\dfrac{15}{64} = .23$	$\dfrac{20}{64} = .31$	$\dfrac{15}{64} = .23$	$\dfrac{6}{64} = .093$	$\dfrac{1}{64} = .016$
P(x successes in n trials) $P(X = x) =$ $p(x) = nCx \times H^xT^{n-x}$	$p(0) = \dfrac{1}{64}$	$p(1) = \dfrac{6}{64}$	$p(2) = \dfrac{15}{64}$	$p(3) = \dfrac{20}{64}$	$p(4) = \dfrac{15}{64}$	$p(5) = \dfrac{6}{64}$	$p(6) = \dfrac{1}{64}$
$E(X) = \mu_x =$ $\Sigma x \bullet p(x)$	$0 \times \dfrac{1}{64} +$	$1 \times \dfrac{6}{64} +$	$2 \times \dfrac{15}{64} +$	$3 \times \dfrac{20}{64} +$	$4 \times \dfrac{15}{64} +$	$5 \times \dfrac{6}{64} +$	$6 \times \dfrac{1}{64}$
$\dfrac{192}{64} = 3$							

Table 18B.2

In the six coins tossing experiment, the number of heads that may turn out is the RV represented by the capital letter x, which assumes its actual n value of 0 to 6 when the tossing experiment is done.

Because the number of heads reported for each of the sixty-four outcomes correspond to the random variable assigned in this case to each of the outcomes and because the probability of each of the outcomes = 1/64, the probability of the outcome for $x = 2$ is defined by the probability function that gives the probability associated with each value of the random variable as follows:

$$p(x) = P(X = x) = nCx \times \frac{1}{64} \text{ which for } x = 2, \ = 6C2 \times \frac{1}{64} = \frac{15}{64}.$$

Note that the combinations specifying x number of heads is computed from the following relation, where x denotes the number of heads and n the number of elements in the set as follows:

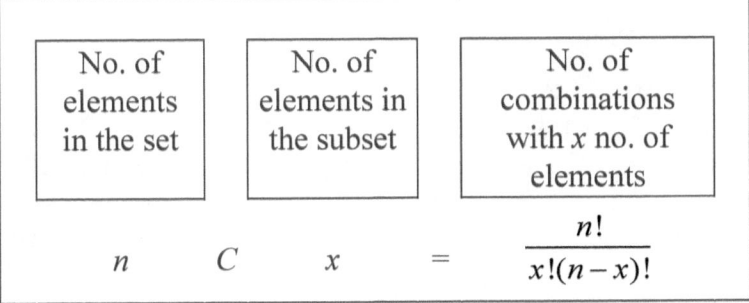

Because $nCx = nCn - x$, then if x = number of heads, $n - x$ = number of tails.

18B.4 Graphic Display of the Discrete Binomial Probability: $p = q$

The probability distribution of the random variable is to be differentiated from the individual probabilities associated with each outcome. The probability distribution for a discrete RV in contrast to the probability of any one discrete value of the random variable is an assignment of probability to each of the distinct numerical values of the RV (row 4 of Table 18B.2). The focus of interest in the distribution is the layout of all the values with particular stress on its central tendency and the dispersion of its values around its central location. For discrete random variables, the probability distribution is best appreciated in tabular form or as a line chart where the main characteristics of the distribution can be appreciated at a glance. In essence then, a distribution is characterized by two distinctive features that fully account for its form; the first may be loosely described as the measure of its central tendency or location, and the second may be equally visualized as the measure of the dispersion of the individual values around the central tendency.

In the following paragraph, the central tendency of the tossing experiment will be addressed using the standard method used for the discrete random variable, not necessarily binomial. This approach, although unorthodox, is designed to underline the common logical thread that unites all the discrete random variables. The abbreviated, shortcut approach unique to the binomial random variable will be addressed later.

18B.5 The Expected Value

The derivation of the expected value of a discrete random variable X, denoted by $E(X)$, is detailed in row 5 of Table 18B.2 and row 3 of Table 18B.3. In so many words, it is equal to the sum (Σ) of the product ($\bullet$) of the values (x) assigned to the random variable X (i.e., the number of heads, 0-6) and the corresponding probability, $p(x)$, associated with each value of x.

$$\underset{\substack{\text{Expected} \\ \text{Value}}}{E(X)} = \underset{\text{Mean}}{m_X} = \sum x \bullet P(X = x) = \underset{\text{Sum}}{\underset{\substack{\text{Weighted} \\ \text{Average}}}{\sum}} x \bullet p(x).$$

The expected value so derived is nothing more than the mean value of X, μ_x, or the expectation of X, $E(X)$, which is the weighted average of all the possible values. The weights in this case are the actual probabilities associated with each value. The expected number of heads obtained on tossing six balanced coins in the long run thus equals three heads (row 6, Table 18B.2). This number can be equally derived if one keep tossing and adding the number of heads, in which case one would expect the heads to number about 50 percent of the number of tosses. Intuitively, one would expect that in one toss of the six coins, three tails and three heads are likely to appear.

The following expression makes it clear that the expected value $E(X)$ is an alternate notation for the weighted average value $\overline{X}$ or the mean value μ_x. Moreover, the sum of the product of the random variable x and its corresponding probability $p(x)$ could similarly be derived by substituting $nCx/2^n$ for the corresponding probability $p(x)$. This is fully documented for each value of the random variable x, in the fifth row of Table 18B.2.

$$\underset{\substack{\text{Expected} \\ \text{value}}}{E(X)} = \underset{\substack{\text{Weighted} \\ \text{average}}}{\overline{X}} = \underset{\substack{\text{Mean} \\ \text{value}}}{m_X} = \underset{\text{Sum}}{\sum} \underset{\substack{x \\ \text{value}}}{} \bullet p(x) = \sum x \bullet \frac{nCx}{2^n} = \frac{192}{64} = 3$$

It is important to keep in mind the nCx actually stands for nPr in this case because we are dealing with the permutation of n objects with x and $(n - x)$ kinds (two kinds only). nCx, on the other hand, as you may recall from chapter 2, is the number of combination of x and $(n - x)$ subsets out of n distinct objects.

$$nC\,x = \frac{n!}{x!(n-x)!} = \text{Number of subsets (unordered } x\text{-tuples)}$$

$$nP\,x = \frac{n!}{x!(n-x)!} = \text{Number of permutation of n objects of two kinds (ordered } x\text{-tuples).}$$

The probability distribution of the random variable x, the number of heads on any given toss, can be fully appreciated by scrutinizing Table 18B.3 and Figure 18B.3. From both, it can be readily seen that $x = 3$ constitutes the measure of central tendency of the whole array, such that the balance of remaining values both larger and smaller are clustered around the central value.

Random variable $X = x$	$x = 0$	$x = 1$	$x = 2$	$x = 3$	$x = 4$	$x = 5$	$x = 6$
P(x successes in n trials) $P(X = x) = p(x) = nCx \times p^x q^{n-x}$	$p(0) = \dfrac{1}{64}$	$p(1) = \dfrac{6}{64}$	$p(2) = \dfrac{15}{64}$	$p(3) = \dfrac{20}{64}$	$p(4) = \dfrac{15}{64}$	$p(5) = \dfrac{6}{64}$	$p(6) = \dfrac{1}{64}$
$E(X) = \mu_x = \Sigma\, x \cdot p(x)$	$0 \times \dfrac{1}{64}$	$1 \times \dfrac{6}{64}$	$2 \times \dfrac{15}{64}$	$3 \times \dfrac{20}{64}$	$4 \times \dfrac{15}{64}$	$5 \times \dfrac{6}{64}$	$6 \times \dfrac{1}{64}$

Table 18B.3. Probability for a given RV

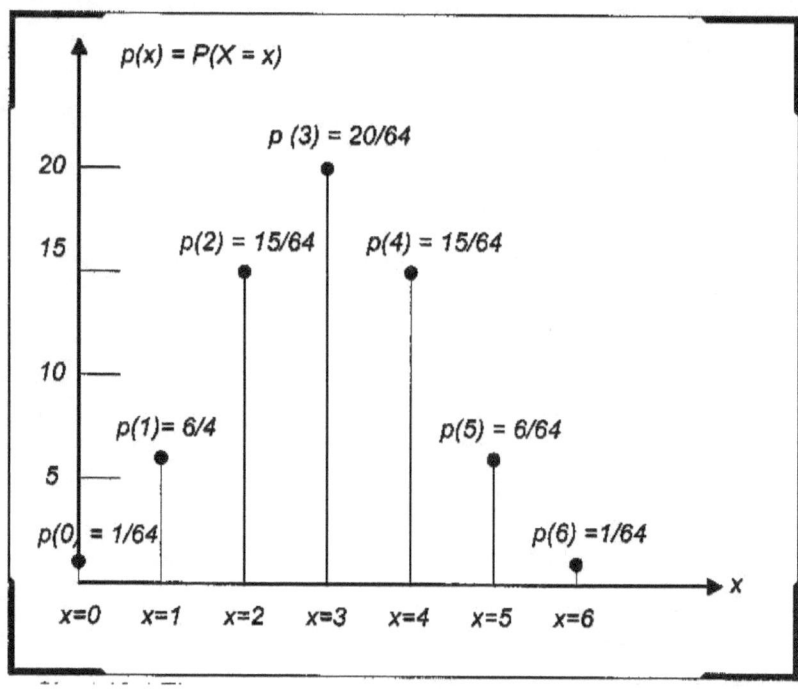

Figure 18B.3. Line chart of the probability distribution
of a binomial random variable

18B.6 Binomial Probability Distribution: $p \neq q$

The binomial population just described consisted of 50 percent heads and 50 percent tails. Thus, the derivation of the probability function (distribution function) of the binomial random variable was based on the assumption of equally probabilities for the two mutually exclusive states. Unlike the current example where $p = q = 1/2$, this is not the norm in most practical applications.

In statistical language, the proportion of one state is designated as p, and the proportion of the other state is designated as q. Obviously, the sum of the two states adds up to 1 or 100 percent so that given p, the other state q is readily derived from the balance, that is, $q = 1 - p$.

A binomial population, however, composed of two mutually exclusive categories need not be equally probable as in the coin case. When the two states in the binomial population are not of equal proportion, that is, $p \neq q \neq 0.5$, the problem must consider the probabilities associated with each of the states.

Consider, for example, the probability of rolling exactly two sixes in three rolls of a die. Because each of the three rolls will result in either six (success) or a nonsix (failure), the sample space can be reduced to a basic binomial configuration. Because three rolls is the equivalent of three trials, the number of possible outcomes equals $2 \times 2 \times 2 \times = 2^3 = 8$, as per the formula for permutation with replacement or its equivalent the multiplication rule, namely,

$$\{SSS, SSF, SFS, FSS, SFF, FSF, FFS, FFF\}$$

These outcomes are allocated to four subsets as noted in Table 18B.4.

$nCx = 3C0 = 1$	$nCx = 3C1 = 3$	$nCx = 3C2 = 3$	$nCx = 3C3 = 1$
$1 \times p^x q^{n-x}$	$3 \times p^x q^{n-x}$	$3 \times p^x q^{n-x}$	$1 \times p^x q^{n-x}$
$1 \times p^0 q^3$	$1 \times p^1 q^2$	$1 \times p^2 q^1$	$1 \times p^3 q^0$
$1 \times \left(\dfrac{1}{6}\right)^0 \left(\dfrac{5}{6}\right)^3 = \dfrac{125}{216} = .58$	$3 \times \left(\dfrac{1}{6}\right)^1 \left(\dfrac{5}{6}\right)^2 = .35$	$3 \times \left(\dfrac{1}{6}\right)^2 \left(\dfrac{5}{6}\right)^1 = \dfrac{5}{216} = .07$	$1 \times \left(\dfrac{1}{6}\right)^3 \left(\dfrac{5}{6}\right)^0 = \dfrac{1}{216} = .004$

Table 18B.4. Probability Distribution in Tabular form

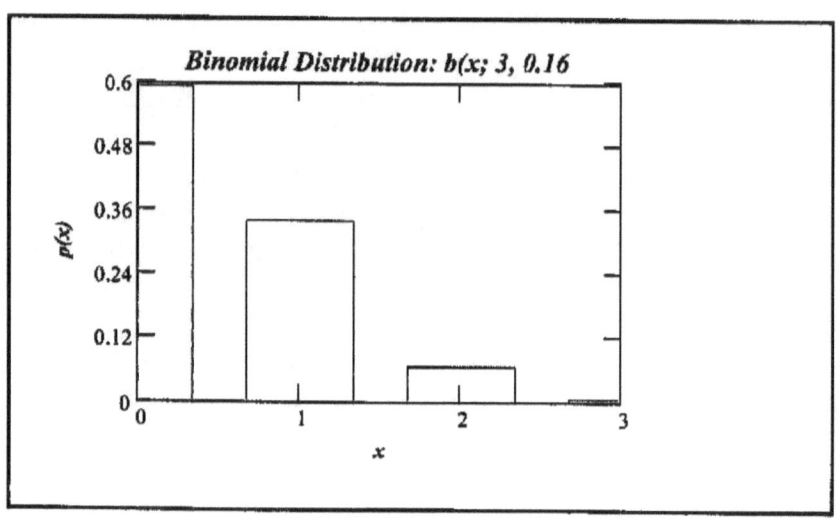

Figure 18B.4. Probability Distribution in Histogram form

The corresponding histogram in this case is unsymmetrical with the probability of failure comprising 58 percent of the total area, while column 4 occupies less than half percent of the total area (0.004 percent).

Table 18B.5 lists the eight possible permutations of Ss and Fs representing the eight possible outcomes. The probability of each outcome is computed by the multiplication of the corresponding probability associated with S and F because the outcomes are mutually exclusive and independent.

The last column lists the number of successes associated with each trial. From Table 18B.5, it can be observed that

P(exactly two sixes in three rolls) = P(SSF or SFS or FSS); second to fourth row inclusive.

And from Table 18B.6, the probability associated with two successes in three trials is given, such that

$$P(SSF \text{ or } SFS \text{ or } FSS) = P(SSF) + P(SFS) + P(FSS) = 15/216 \cong 0.069; \text{ third row.}$$

However, because each of the three outcomes is equally likely, associated with a probability of 5/216, the probability of the compound event of two sixes in three rolls may be derived by multiplying the probability of one of the outcomes by the number of elements in the subset; thus,

$$P(\text{SSF or SFS or FSS}) = 3 \times 5/216 = 15/216$$

Outcome	Probability of Outcome						No. of Successes
SSS	$P(SSS) =$	$P(S) \bullet P(S) \bullet P(S) =$	p^3	$(1/6)^3$	$= 1/216$	3
SSF	$P(SSF) =$	$P(S) \bullet P(S) \bullet P(F) =$	$p^2 q$	$(1/6)^2 \times (5/6)$	$= 5/216$	2
SFS	$P(SFS) =$	$P(S) \bullet P(F) \bullet P(S) =$	$p^2 q$	$(1/6)^2 \times (5/6)$	$= 5/216$	2
FSS	$P(FSS) =$	$P(F) \bullet P(S) \bullet P(S) =$	$p^2 q$	$(1/6)^2 \times (5/6)$	$= 5/216$	2
SFF	$P(SFF) =$	$P(S) \bullet P(F) \bullet P(F) =$	pq^2	$(1/6) \times (5/6)^2$	$= 25/216$	1
FSF	$P(FSF) =$	$P(F) \bullet P(S) \bullet P(F) =$	pq^2	$(1/6) \times (5/6)^2$	$= 25/216$	1
FFS	$P(FFS) =$	$P(F) \bullet P(F) \bullet P(S) =$	pq^2	$(1/6) \times (5/6)^2$	$= 25/216$	1
FFF	$P(FFF) =$	$P(F) \bullet P(F) \bullet P(F) =$	q^3	$(5/6)^2$	$= 125/216$	0

Table 18B.5. The Probability of a given outcome

Hence, the probability of x successes out of three trials is the sum of the probabilities associated with the particular number of successes, that is, 0, 1, 2, and 3. These probabilities are tabulated separately in Table 18B.7

No. of Successes	Probability of x Successes in Three Trials $p(x)$		Probability of (No. of successes) $p(x)$
0	$P(0) = P(FFF) =$	q^3	$= 125/216$
1	$P(1) = P(SFF) + P(FSF) + P(FFS) =$	$3pq^2$	$= 75/216$
2	$P(2) = P(SSF) + P(SFS) + P(FSS) =$	$3p^2 q$	$= 15/216$
3	$P(3) = P(SSS) =$	p^3	$= 1/216$

Table 18B.6. Probability of a given number of Success

The probability of rolling exactly two sixes in five rolls instead of three can be equally stated in terms of S and F as the probability of rolling two Ss and three Fs in any sequence in five trials. We are here dealing with the permutation of two distinct objects two Ss and three Fs or, alternatively, what amounts to numerically equivalent result, the combination of five items taken two at a time. Thus,

$5P2, 3 = 5C2 = 10$ possible permutation of the two Ss and three Fs.

Now the probability of rolling any one permutation, that is, two Ss and thee Fs in any order is

$$(1/6)^2 \times (5/6)^{5-2=3} = 125/7,776.$$

For the ten possible permutations, the probability is ten times the probability for one permutation; that is,

$$10 \times (1/6)^2 \times (5/6)^{5-2=3} = 1,250/7,776 \approx 0.161.$$

In the above-noted experiment as in most binomial experiments, it is the total number of Ss that is of interest. Thus, given a binomial experiment consisting of n trials, the binomial random variable X associated with this experiment is defined as
$X =$ the number of Ss among n trials.

As frequently noted, the probability distribution of a discrete random variable is defined for every number x by the following relation:

$$p(x) = P(X = x),$$

which is a shorthand way of saying that for every possible value x of the random variable, the probability $p(x)$ specifies the value obtained when the experiment is performed. The probability distribution of X is therefore a comprehensive tabulation of all the values of X along with their corresponding probabilities. Because the probability distribution of a binomial random variable X depends on the two parameters n and p, the distribution may be denoted by another shorthand abbreviation.

18B.7 Probability Distribution: $b(x;n,p)$

In this special case, in which the outcomes and probabilities for a binomial experiment with three trials are tabulated, the probability of x successes in three trials is given by the following expression:

$$P(X = 2) = p(2) = P(SSF) + P(SFS) + P(FSS) = 3C2 \times p^2 \times (1-p)^{3-2}$$

Because the number of outcomes with $x = 2$ is 3 and each of the three has probability $p^2 (1-p)^1$, the probability distribution of the random variable X depends on the two parameters $n(3)$ and p, the binomial relation can be depicted as a function of its given parameters

$$\boxed{3C2 = 3} \qquad \boxed{p^2(1-p) = \left(\frac{1}{6}\right)^2 \times \frac{5}{6}}$$

$b(2; 3, p) = $ (no. of outcomes with $X = 2$) $\times$ {probability of any outcome with $X = 2$}.

In general,

$$\boxed{nCx} \qquad \boxed{p^x \times (1-p)^{n=x}}$$

$b(x; n, p) = $ (no. of n trials consisting of x successes} $\times$ {probability of any sequence}.

The first factor is the number of ways of choosing x of the n trials to be Ss, that is, the number of combinations of size x that can be constructed from n distinct objects (trials or sequences here). Because the ordering of Ss and Fs is not important, the second factor above is $p^x(1-p)^{n-x}$.

$$b(x; n,p) = nCx \times p^x \times q^{n-x} \quad x = 0, 1, \ldots, n.$$

Any random experiment that satisfies the conditions observed in the tossing of a coins or the rolling of a die must exhibit the following features in order to qualify as a binomial experiment:

1. The experiment consists of a fixed number of trials, n.
2. The n trials are independent and repeated under identical conditions.

3. Each trial ends up with one of two complementary outcomes, designated by S for success and F for failure.
4. The probability of success remains constant throughout the experiment. Because the probability of failure is the complement of success, $q = 1 - p$.

Because the main objective of the binomial experiment is to find the probability of x successes out of n trials (two sixes in five rolls of a die, three heads in a six-coin toss), the following are the necessary data that must be considered in the calculation:

☑ n = number of repeated trials; equivalent to the size of the sample
☑ p = probability of one state, ranging from 0 to 1, usually designated as success, however, without the implication of the inherent meaning of the word
☑ $1 - p = q$ = probability of the other state, the complement of p, usually designated as failure, again without the attribute of the word
☑ x = number of successes in n trials (0 to 6 for the number of heads in the six coins tossing experiment, number of sixes in five rolls of a die)
☑ $n - x$ = number of failures in n trials

The formula that emerges from the correct compliance with the salient features of the binomial experiment and the correct interpretation of the variables assumes the following expression:

$$P(X = x) = p \binom{\text{Success in } n \text{ trials}}{x} = nCx\, p^x q^{n-x} = \frac{n!}{x!(n-x)!} p^x q^{n-x} \text{ for } x = 0, 1, 2, \ldots, n.$$

Using the simple binomial expansion, it is now possible to derive a formula (a rule) that would give the probability of a discrete random variable in a binomial population of two different proportions (not necessarily 50-50 percent) in conjunction with any number of trials (number of coins). Thus, in the case of the six coins, by applying the binomial expansion, the probabilities associated with each random variable can be readily derived by appropriate substitution in the above expression

Where $n = 6 =$ number coins
$p = q = 1 - p = 1/2$

$$P(X = 0) = P(0H, 6T) = p(0) = nC \, x \, p^x q^{n-x} = \frac{6!}{6!0!} \times \left(\frac{1}{2}\right)^6 \left(\frac{1}{2}\right)^0 = 1\left(\frac{1}{2}\right)^6 = \frac{1}{64}$$

$$P(X = 1) = P(1H, 5T) = p(1) = nC \, x \, p^x q^{n-x} = \frac{6!}{5!1!} \times \left(\frac{1}{2}\right)^5 \left(\frac{1}{2}\right)^1 = 6\left(\frac{1}{2}\right)^6 = \frac{6}{64}$$

$$P(X = 2) = P(2H, 4T) = p(2) = nC \, x \, p^x q^{n-x} = \frac{6!}{4!2!} \times \left(\frac{1}{2}\right)^4 \left(\frac{1}{2}\right)^2 = 15\left(\frac{1}{2}\right)^6 = \frac{15}{64}$$

$$P(X = 3) = P(3H, 3T) = p(3) = nC \, x \, p^x q^{n-x} = \frac{6!}{3!3!} \times \left(\frac{1}{2}\right)^3 \left(\frac{1}{2}\right)^3 = 20\left(\frac{1}{2}\right)^6 = \frac{20}{64}$$

$$P(X = 4) = P(4H, 3T) = p(4) = nC \, x \, p^x q^{n-x} = \frac{6!}{2!4!} \times \left(\frac{1}{2}\right)^2 \left(\frac{1}{2}\right)^4 = 15\left(\frac{1}{2}\right)^6 = \frac{15}{64}$$

$$P(X = 5) = P(5H, 3T) = p(5) = nC \, x \, p^x q^{n-x} = \frac{6!}{1!5!} \times \left(\frac{1}{2}\right)^1 \left(\frac{1}{2}\right)^5 = 6\left(\frac{1}{2}\right)^6 = \frac{6}{64}$$

$$P(X = 6) = P(6H, 3T) = p(6) = nC \, x \, p^x q^{n-x} = \frac{6!}{0!6!} \times \left(\frac{1}{2}\right)^0 \left(\frac{1}{2}\right)^6 = 1\left(\frac{1}{2}\right)^6 = \frac{1}{64}$$

The initial expression could be further expanded into a binomial generic format by applying the following modified equivalent notation:

$$P\left(\frac{x}{n}\right) = P\left(\frac{\overset{\text{No. of successes}}{x}}{\underset{\substack{\text{No. of trials}\\\text{Sample size}}}{n}}\right) = \frac{\overset{\substack{\text{No. of trials}\\\text{Sample size}}}{n!}}{\underset{\substack{\text{No. of successes No. of failures}}}{x!\;(n-x)!}} \times \left(\underset{\substack{\text{Probability of}\\\text{success}}}{p}\right)^{\overset{\text{No. of successes}}{x}} \times \left(\underset{\substack{\text{Prob. of}\\\text{failure}}}{q}\right)^{\overset{\text{No. of failures}}{n-x}}$$

Note once more that x replaces r in the classic combination formula, nCr. In the previously mentioned expression, x the number of successes in n trials is the numerical equivalent of r distinct objects taken from n distinct objects at a time. This equivalence need not obscure the fact that the value represents the permutation of two distinguishable objects of x and $n - x$.

$$\frac{\overset{\substack{\text{No. of trials}}}{n!}}{\underset{\substack{\text{No. of successes No. of failures}}}{x!\;(n-x)!}} = nP\,x \;=\; \text{No. of Permutations of } n \text{ objects with } x \text{ and } (n - x) \text{ kinds (2 kinds).}$$

The previously mentioned coefficient is obviously a function of the number of successes and thus would vary from 0 to n for any given trial (from zero heads to six heads in the previously mentioned trial).

The previously mentioned relation is now applicable to any discrete binomial variable in which p defines the probability of success (which is equivalent to the designated proportion in sample size) and q or $1 - p$ defines the probability of failure (which is equivalent to the designated balance of the proportion in the sample size).

18B.8 Finite versus Continuous Probability Distribution

In the preceding chapter, where the random variable assumed finite discrete values, the outline of the probability distribution was finite, noted to be symmetrical about a central axis for $p = q = 0.5$ and asymmetrical for $p \neq q$. An intriguing and unexpected aspect of the emergent outline could be seen to evolve as the value of the exponent n tends to increase. As $n = 10$, for $p = q = 0.5$, the line joining the midpoint of the discrete columns approaches the familiar characteristic of the normal curve (normal probability density function). At $n = 20$, the pattern of the normal curve appears to be more plausible.

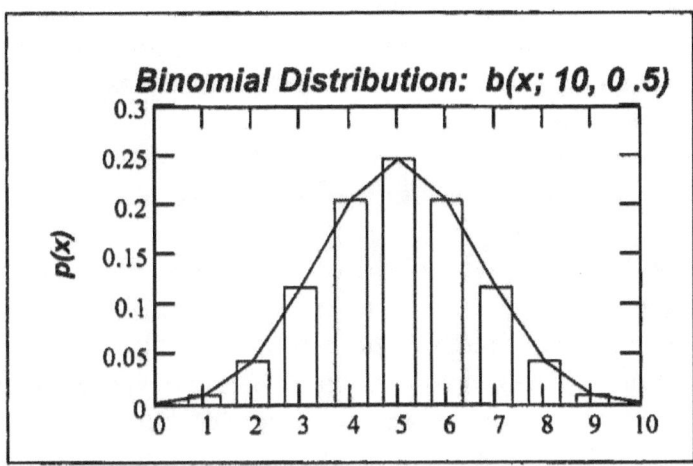

Figure 18B.5. Finite Discrete values of Binomial Distribution
approaching The Normal Distribution

This actual evolution of the contour holds equally well for $p \neq q$ if n
is further increased from its corresponding value for $p = q$.

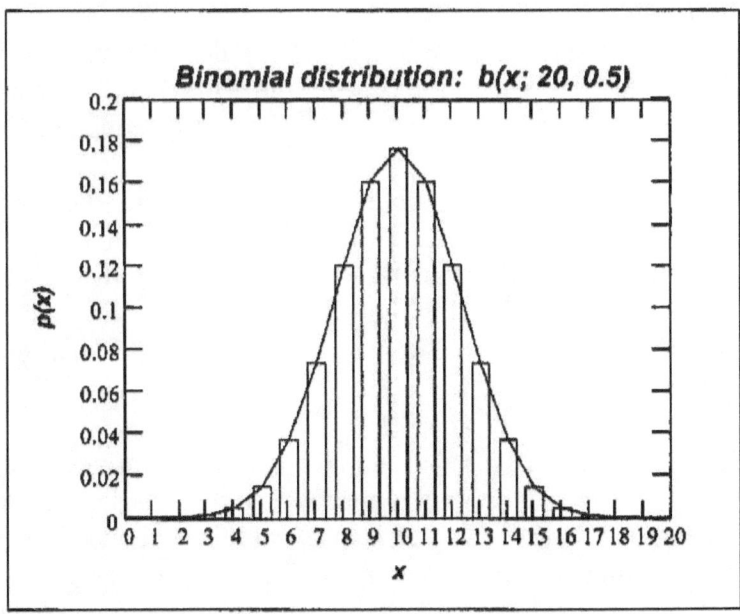

Figure 18B.6. Finite smaller Discrete values of Binomial Distribution
Further approaching The Normal Distribution

The practical implication is that a finite probability distribution of discrete random variables may be treated (with minimal correction) as a continuous probability distribution normally associated with a contiguous random variable.

18B.9 The Binomial Probability Distribution

The probability associated with the random variable is, in essence, a measure of the likelihood of its occurrence. In other words, one can assume in view of the high probability that the event in question is of common occurrence and is therefore to be expected or in view of the probability, and one may assume that the likelihood of its occurrence is remote and thus dismisses the chance occurrence. In other words, decide whether the event is common or otherwise rare and draw the appropriate conclusion from the derived fact.

In the case of the six coins, the number of heads obtained, however, varies about a mean of $n/2$ heads, or three heads. Thus, the frequency distribution of outcomes would in reality cluster around the mean of $n/2$. This can be observed from the central column of Tables 18B.2 and 18B.3, where the frequency of twenty is bordered on either side by symmetrically declining values. The graphic counterpart is noted from Figure 18B.3 in which the central line corresponding to $x = 3$ is bordered on each side by symmetrically declining frequencies.

The tight spread of the possible outcomes around the mean of three heads is readily verified by noting that fifty of the possible sixty-four outcomes are clustered between two and four heads, which is another way of saying that the probability of an outcome of two to four heads makes up 50/64 or 78 percent of the total number of possible outcomes.

The degree or extent of spread around the mean, the variance, denoted by $V(X)$ or σ^2, is the second key concept that characterizes the layout of the outcomes of a given experiment or sample. The weighted mean or expected value is a measure of the central tendency or location around which the values tend to cluster, whereas the variance or its square root, the standard deviation, measures the dispersion or variability of the spread around the mean.

The concept underlying the measurement of dispersion is made unnecessarily complicated considering the computation effort involved in arriving at a number that is essentially a measure of the spread or dispersion of the values around the central mean. The problem would have been readily resolved and intuitively appreciated if the corresponding distance of each variable from the central mean $(x - \mu)$ on both sides is added and averaged. Unfortunately, the result of such an average, its expected value, $E(X - \mu)$, would have been zero, considering that negative values are being added to positive values.

Now comes the problem of how to circumvent this difficulty. Of the many approaches proposed, the one solution that addresses the objectionable negative number is by simply squaring the deviated distance on both sides, $(X - \mu)^2$. Once this solution is accepted, the variance, the measure of dispersion, is the average or expected value of the squared deviated distance, $E(X - \mu)^2$.

What appears as reasonable and simple solution turns out to be a rather tedious task of computation. Once this solution is accepted, the measure of dispersion then becomes the sum (Σ) of the product $(\bullet)$ of the square of the distance of each value of the random variable X, from the central mean $(x - \mu)^2$ and the associated weight of probability of the same variable $p(x)$. The formula now takes the following format:

$$\underset{\text{Variance}}{V(X)} = \left(\underset{\substack{\text{Standard} \\ \text{deviation}}}{\sigma} \right)^2 = E \left(\underset{\text{Distance}}{x - \mu} \right)^2 = \underset{\text{Sum}}{\sum} (x - \mu)^2 \bullet p(x) \; \underset{\text{random variable } X.}{= \text{the variance of}}$$

Note that the result is still artificially squared as a consequence of the attempt to eliminate the negative values of the deviated distances. The obvious solution is to retrieve the original values by square rooting the variance. The result is the classical standard deviation, the second key measure desired for the complete characterization of the layout of any given distribution

$$\sqrt{V(X)} = \sigma^2 \sum (x - \mu)^2 \bullet p(x) = \sigma = \text{Standard deviation}$$

The process involves a sequence of squaring, multiplications, and additions. The difficulty is partially alleviated by the algebraic manipulation of the above formula to yield what is dubbed as a shortcut formula; thus,

$$V(X) = \sigma^2 = E(x - \mu)^2 = \Sigma(x - \mu)^2 \bullet p(x) = \Sigma \, x^2 \bullet p(x) - (\mu)^2 = E(X^2) - [E(X)]^2.$$

As per the last expression in the previously mentioned formula, we are required to square each x, multiply it by its probability $p(x)$, and then sum (Σ) the total, rows 2, 3, and 4, of Table 18B.6. From the total thus obtained, subtract the square of the mean, μ, and the result is the weighted average or expected value of the square of the deviated distances from the actual mean of the distribution, row 6. To get to the real measure of dispersion, a square root of the variance yields the standard deviation, row 7. The process is detailed in the following table for the experiment of six coins.

Random variable $X = x$	0	1	2	3	4	5	6
x^2	0	1	4	9	16	25	36
$p(x)$	1/64	6/64	15/64	20/64	15/64	6/64	1/64
$E(X^2) = \Sigma x^2 \bullet p(x) = 10.5$	$0 \times 1/64$	$1 \times 6/64$	$4 \times 15/64$	$9 \times 20/64$	$16 \times 15/64$	$25 \times 6/64$	$36 \times 1/64$
$E(X) = \mu = \Sigma x \bullet p(x) = 3$	$0 \times 1/64$	$0 \times 1/64$	$2 \times 15/64$	$3 \times 20/64$	$4 \times 15/64$	$5 \times 6/64$	$36 \times 1/64$
$V(X) = \sigma^2 = \Sigma x^2 \bullet p(x) - (\mu)^2 = E(X^2) - [E(X)]^2 = 10.5 - 3^2 = 10.5 - 9 = 1.5 = \text{variance}$							
$\sqrt{V(X)} = s = \sqrt{1.5} = 1.224 = \text{Standard deviation}$							

Table 18B.7. Variance and Standard Deviation of the RV X=x

In practical work, however, this is highly inefficient procedure because it can be shown that for a binomial random variable.

In practice, as alluded to earlier, the generic procedures for deriving the expected value $E(X)$ and standard deviation $\sigma(X)$ of any discrete random variable, including the binomial, can be drastically revised and reduced in special case of the discrete binomial random variable.

For the expected value, given the key parameters of the binomial distribution of n, the number of trials, and p, the probability of success and assuming that the condition noted earlier are met, then

$$\underset{\substack{\text{Expected}\\\text{Value}}}{E(X)} = \underset{\substack{\text{Number of}\\\text{trials}}}{n} \times \underset{\substack{\text{Probability}\\\text{of success}}}{p}$$

The procedure is reduced to the simple multiplication of the number of trials by the probability of success, assumed to be constant for each trial.

Applying this new formula to the tossing experiment of six coins, which is the equivalent of tossing one coin six times or six trials, and assuming that we are tossing a fair coin whose probability p of success = 1/2, then the expectation of the number of heads $E(X) = 6 \times 1/2 = 3$. Intuitively, the equation is simply a shorthand statement of the fact that given n trials, in which the probability of success is constant and the same for each trial, then the number of successes is simply the product of the two factors.

Consider now the standard deviation of a binomial random variable. As in the case of the expected value, the derivation and the rather tedious computation were necessary in order to highlight the key idea of the standard deviation as applied to any discrete random variable. However, in the special case of the binomial distribution, the expression collapses to the following:

$$\underset{\text{Variance}}{V(X)} = \underset{\substack{\text{Number of}\\\text{trials}}}{n} \times \underset{\substack{\text{Number}\\\text{of successes}}}{p} \times \underset{\substack{\text{Number}\\\text{of failures}}}{(-p)} = npq$$

and

$$\boxed{\begin{array}{l} \text{Standard} \\ \text{deviation} \\ \mathsf{s}\,(X) = \sqrt{npq} \end{array}}$$

Thus, the process is reduced to the simple multiplication of the key parameters of success, failure, and number of trials, followed by the square root to arrive at the standard deviation. In the case of the six coins,

$$\boxed{\mathsf{s}\,(X) = \sqrt{npq} = \sqrt{6 \times \frac{1}{2} \times \frac{1}{2}} = \sqrt{\frac{3}{2}} = \sqrt{1.5} = 1.224}$$

18B.10 Clinical Application of the Binomial Distribution

To put the concept of the discrete random variable in a binomial setting in its proper perspective, it might be helpful to translate the coin tossing and die rolling exercises into more realistic scenarios.

18B.11 Malignant Viral Infection

A highly contagious viral infection with 50 percent spontaneous recovery was taking its toll in a closed community. A new antiviral cocktail was administered to ten patients selected at random. The medical staff was delighted to note that eight of the selected patients recovered. The epidemiology department was consulted as the significance of the trial result.

The question that needs to be addressed in statistical terms is the probability of eight or more cures out of ten randomly selected treated patients.

Note that in this case, the spontaneous recovery is 50 percent, that is, $p = q = 0.5$; accordingly,

$$p(x) = nCx \times p^x q^{n-x} = 10Cx \times (0.5)^x \times (0.5)^{10-x} = 10Cx \times (0.5)^{10}.$$

Note that when $p = q$, multiplying the exponent $10 - x$ by its complement reduces the two exponents to the single numerical exponent.

The probability of eight or more cures out of ten is simply the sum of the individual probability associate with eight out of ten, nine out of ten, and ten out of ten.

$10C8 \times (0.5)^{10} + 10C9 \times (0.5)^{10} + 10C10 \times (0.5)^{10} = 45 \times (\frac{1}{2})^{10} + 10 \times (\frac{1}{2})^{10} + 1 \times (\frac{1}{2})^{10} = 0.055$.

The perusal of Figure 18B.5 assigns this probability to the area of the last three columns on the right as the exact percentage out of the total area of one occupied by the full histogram.

The probability of eight or more cures out of ten is 5.5 percent. Can we then conclude that such an outcome is just pure chance that could have occurred anyway without treatment, that is, a 5.5 percent chance this large or larger could have occurred through random coincidence?

As you are well aware from the ubiquitous use of the p value in all clinical trials, the cutoff point is usually and arbitrarily place at the 5 percent lever (0.05), which may be translated as the dividing line between significant and nonsignificant. In our case, the probability is just over the borderline, which renders the result nonsignificant, in the sense that such an outcome could occur through mere chance without intervention. Stated differently, the chance occurrence on tossing ten coins and getting eight, nine, or ten heads on any one toss is not beyond expectation. Note that if nine of ten patients recovered as a result of the intervention, the probability of such a recovery rate would be as follows:

$10C9 \times (0.5)^{10} + 10C10 \times (0.5)^{10} = 10 \times (\frac{1}{2})^{10} + 1 \times (\frac{1}{2})^{10} = 11/1,024 = 0.010$ (1 percent).

This probability is assigned to the last two columns on the right comprising 1 percent of the total area. Such an occurrence is as rare as getting nine of ten heads on any one toss. The result of such an outcome would be significant, corroborating the effectiveness of the new therapeutic modality.

18B.12 New Antibiotic

Consider the response of a set of four patients with *Mycoplasma pneumoniae* specifically selected to be similar in all biological traits (age, sex, ethnic background, personal history, and family history) to a new antibiotic drug presumed to be more effective in eradicating the organism from the respiratory tract (cure) than the standard current treatment in which a carrier state persists in 50 percent of the cases. The analogy of this trial to the tossing experiment of four fair coins bears a closer scrutiny.

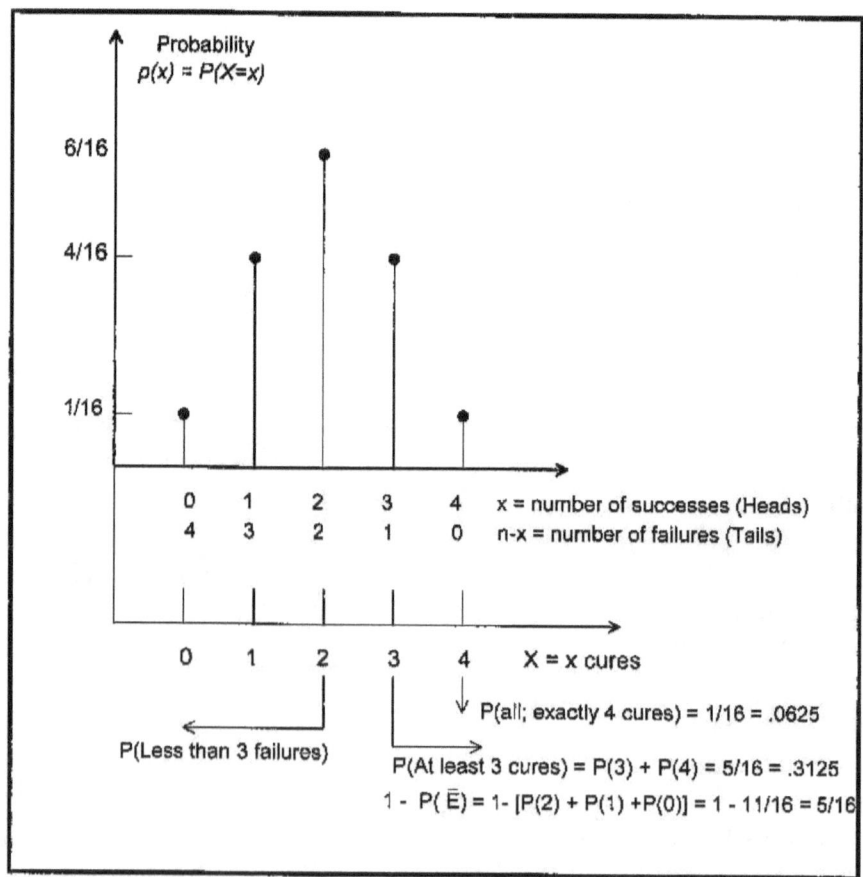

Figure 18B.7. Analogy of Treatment response to a tossing experiment

Strictly speaking, a random experiment that satisfies the conditions observed in the tossing of a coin must exhibit the following features in order to qualify as a binomial experiment:

1. Each trial ends up with one of two complementary outcomes, success or failure.
2. The n trials are independent.
3. The n trials are repeated under identical conditions.
4. The probability of success remains constant throughout the experiment.

Conditions 1 and 2 are applicable in the context of the clinical trial because the response of any given patient (the outcome of the Rx) is independent of any other patient. Conditions 3 and 4, however, cannot be strictly met under the conditions of a clinical trial. The response of the individual patients across the board to the standard Rx cannot be strictly considered 50 percent, although the selection process was designed to eliminate biologic traits that may influence the odds in favor or against.

Within the constraints noted previously, the trial may qualify as a binomial experiment analogous to the tossing of four coins. The response of the four patients to the new antibiotic resulted in a cure in all of them. The results appear promising as to the merit of the new treatment compared with the standard. The question that needs to be addressed in order to put the results in the context of the old experience is to inquire as to the probability of four successive cures under the standard treatment.

Because a 50 percent cure rate implies a binomial probability distribution equivalent to tossing four coins, four consecutive cures may be considered equivalent to the outcome of four heads on a given tossing trial (Figure 18B.7).

$$P(X = 4) = P(\text{Exactly 4 cures}) = 4C4 \bullet \left(\frac{1}{2}\right)^4 \times \left(\frac{1}{2}\right)^0 = \frac{1}{16} = .0625$$

The probability of four heads is rather rare, resulting in a probability of $1/16 = 0.06256$, accounting for one success (four heads) in sixteen trials = or roughly six successes in one hundred trials, which is another way of concluding that four consecutive successes are a rare occurrence under the old Rx. The probability is small but not out of the ordinary. The best that can be said is that a trial involving a larger sample is indicated.

A new trial involving six new patients was conducted, which resulted in six consecutive cures.

$$P(X = 6) = 6C6 \times \left(\frac{1}{2}\right)^6 \times \left(\frac{1}{2}\right)^0 = \frac{1}{64} = .016$$

The probability of six cures under the standard Rx, as noted in Line Chart 18-1, which is Figure 18B-3, is $1/64 = 0.016$. The probability of such an event (six consecutive cures) under the standard Rx (once in sixty-four trials or sixteen times in a thousand trial) may be considered so rare that one may be forced to conclude that its occurrence under the standard treatment cannot be realistically considered except as a remote possibility. A more logical deduction is to conclude that the new treatment is indeed superior to the standard cure rate of 50 percent.

On the other hand, if the initial trial ended with at least three cures (which translates into three or four cures in this case), the probability of such an outcome requires the addition of the respective probabilities, as derived in the following expression:

$$P(\text{At least 3 cures}) = P(\text{exactly 3 cures}) + P(\text{exactly 4 cures}) = \frac{4}{16} + \frac{1}{16} = \frac{5}{16} = 0.312.$$

The same result is obtained by subtracting the complement of at least three cures, namely, less than three cures from the probability of one; thus,

$$P(\text{Less than 3 cures}) = 1 - [P(2) + P(1) + P(0)] = 1 - \frac{11}{16} = \frac{5}{16} = 0.312.$$

The probability of such an outcome (slightly more than thirty-one successes in one hundred trials of the same sample size of four) under the standard regimen is common enough as to discredit any claim of superior effectiveness of the new drug.

Unlike the previous example where $p = q = 1/2$, the norm in most practical applications is $p \neq q$, in which the inequality between success and failure prevails. In order to put the binomial probability distribution in perspective, the following examples illustrate its universal mode of application.

18B.13 Heart Transplant Program

The probability that a heart transplant performed at the medical center is successful (i.e., the patient survives a year or more after undergoing such an operation) is 0.85. Of six patients who have recently undergone such an operation, what is the probability that a year from now

    a. none of the heart recipients will be alive?
    b. exactly three will be alive?
    c. at least three will be alive?
    d. all will be alive?

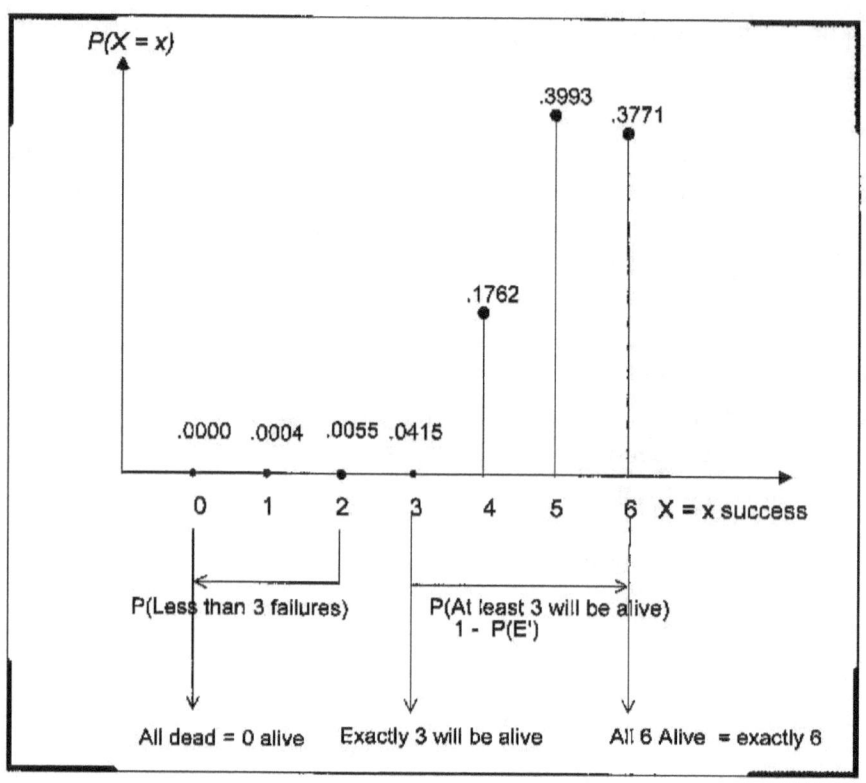

Figure 18B.8. Probability of success or
failure in Heart Transplant Program

Here, $n = 6$, $p = 0.85$, and $q = 0.15$. Let X denote the number of five years of survival. Then,

a. the probability that no heart recipients will be alive after five years is given by
$$P(X = 0) = 6C0 \times (0.85)^0 \times (0.15)^6 = 1 \times (1) \times (0.15)^6$$
$$= 0.0000$$

b. the probability that exactly three will be alive after five years is given by
$$P(X = 3) = 6C3 \times (0.85)^3 \times (0.15)^3 = 20 \times (0.85)^3 \times (0.15)^3$$
$$= 0.0415$$

c. the probability that at least three will be alive after five years is given by

$$P(X = 3) + P(X = 4) + P(X = 5) + P(X = 6)$$

$6C3 \times (0.85)^3 \times (0.15)^3 + 6C4 \times (0.85)^4 \times (0.15)^2 + 6C5 \times (0.85)^5 \times (0.15)^1 + 6C6 \times (0.85)^6 \times (0.15)^0$

$20 \times (0.85)^3 \times (0.15)^3 + 15 \times (0.85)^4 \times (0.15)^2 + 6 \times (0.85)^5 \times (0.15)^1 + 1 \times (0.85)^6 \times (0.15)^0$

$0.0415 + 0.1762 + 0.3993 + 0.3771 = 0.9941$

d. the probability that all will be alive after 5 years is given by

$$P(X = 6) = 6C6 \times (0.85)^6 \times (0.15)^0 = 1 \times (0.85)^6 \times (1) = 0.3771$$

18B.14 Public Health Problem

The relevance of binomial probability in epidemiology and public health is illustrated by the following simulated example.

The prevalence of an infectious disease in a particular area has been estimated at 0.1 of the resident population. Of the six newly admitted cases to the county hospital, three were proven to harbor the infection. The public health authorities suspect a rise in the prevalence. Can this premise be proven?

Assume for the moment that there is no change in the prevalence of the disease. Under this assumption, the probability of disease, $p = 0.1$, remains unchanged at 10 percent.

The sample size n is the number of admissions, three of which were infected. The probability that this sample is representative of the status quo, that is, no change in prevalence, may be computed, using the binomial equation, as follows, where $p = 0.1 =$ probability of infection, $q = 0.9 =$ probability of health:

Probability of three infected cases in six $= 6C3 \times (0.1)^3(0.9)^3 = 0.015.$

The probability of 0.015 implies that three consecutive cases out of six may be encountered fifteen times in 1,000 admissions or just about once in a one hundred admissions of similar proportions to the current one. What is being asserted is the rarity of such an occurrence, namely, the consecutive admission of three identical cases. Such being the case, the small probability (15 in 1,000) that the three consecutive cases are just a chance occurrence cannot be sustained. In effect, asserting that a change in prevalence of the disease is indeed probable and needs to be seriously considered.

Note that if only two of the newly admitted cases were to prove positive, the probability of such an event would be as follows:

Probability of two infected cases in six = $6C2 \times (0.1)^2(0.9)^4 = 0.098$.

By comparison with the previous probability of fifteen per thousand, the probability in this instance increases to 98 of 1,000 similar admission, roughly 10 percent of similar admission. A probability of this magnitude cannot be considered rare, which is another way of saying that such an occurrence could be ascribed to chance factors. The conclusion in this instance is the opposite of the previous conclusion in that a 10 percent probability does not support the thesis of increased prevalence of the disease in the community.

18B.15 Critical Care Technique

The fellow in the pulmonary intensive care unit is fairly well experienced in drawing arterial blood samples for gas analysis. The probability of a single try arterial puncture in his experience is 0.8.

What is the probability that in four different attempts, the fourth puncture will miss the artery?

Note that the probability associated with each attempt is independent of each other (the outcome of one trial has nothing to do with the outcome of the other trial) so that the probability of a series of attempts is equal to the product of their respective probabilities, which in this case is calculated as follows:

$0.8 \times 0.8 \times 0.8 \times 0.2(1-0.8) = 0.1024$ = probability of a miss on the fourth scheduled puncture.

What is the probability that in four different attempts, exactly two will miss the artery?

The probability of exactly two misses may be realized following two successes so that the probability of this particular sequence may be calculated as follows:

$0.8 \times 0.8 \times 0.2 \times 0.2 = 0.0256 =$ probability of two successful punctures and two failed attempts.

The same probability is obtained by postulating a different sequence, such as

$0.8 \times 0.2 \times 0.8 \times 0.2 = 0.0256$

The probability of exactly two misses must consider all the possible sequences of two successes and two misses, resulting from the permutation of four attempts of two kinds, successful and failed, or what amount to the same thing the number of ways in which two out of four attempts may be chosen,

$$4P2,2 = 4C2 = \frac{4!}{2!2!} = 6$$

Because each of the sequences is mutually exclusive, the probability of obtaining two misses through the first sequence or the second sequence or . . . , is the sum of the probabilities of the individual sequences, as follows:

$0.0256 + 0.0256 + \ldots = 0.0256 \times 6 = 0.1536 =$ probability of missing two punctures out of four attempts.

Alternatively, the problem is a binomial example because it involves a hit and miss situation in which $p = 0.8$ and $q = 0.2$, respectively. Thus,

P(exactly two misses in four trials) = $nCxP^xq^{n-x}$ = $4C2 \times (0.8)^2 \times (0.2)^2$ = 0.1536.

18B.16 Critical Care Procedures Proficiency

An intern, a resident, and a pulmonary fellow were to alternate in drawing arterial blood sample from a critical pulmonary patient. The probability of the intern accessing the artery on first try is 0.4, that of the resident is 0.6, and that of the fellow is 0.8.

What is the probability that one of them will fail to access the artery?

In this case, as in the former example, the probability of each sequence in the rotation schedule must be added in order to assess the probability of one failure, shown as follows:

0.4 (Intern) × 0.6 (Resident) × 0.2 (Fellow) = 0.0480
0.4 (Intern) × 0.4 (Resident) × 0.8 (Fellow) = 0.1280
0.6 (Intern) × 0.6 (Resident) × 0.8 (Fellow) = 0.2880

Note that the probability of a miss in which the fellow failed (first round) is much smaller than the probability in which the intern failed (third round). Taking into consideration all the rounds, the probability of a miss in the first, second, or third round is equal to the sum of the probabilities of each round because the sequence in each round is mutually exclusive from that of the next round.

0.0480 + 0.1280 + 0.2880 = 0.4640 = probability of one failure in the rotating schedule.

18B.17 Monitoring System Failure

The cardiac monitoring system of the ICCU, made of three mutually exclusive and independent units, was inspected recently and found to be in working order. Of the three major components of the system, the probability of connection failure (wiring disruption, transducer blockage, misplacement of electrode or loss of contact, etc.) was rated at 0.1. The probability of transducer and microprocessor failures were rated at 0.01 and 0.001, respectively. The need to evaluate the probability of system failure, given the individual unit failure probabilities, is relevant to the management protocol of the unit.

The probability of the faultless operations of the individual units may be calculated as follows:

$1 - 0.1 = 0.9000$ = probability of success (faultless operation) of the connection system.
$1 - 0.01 = 0.9900$ = probability of success (faultless operation) of the transducer.
$1 - 0.001 = 0.9990$ = probability of success (faultless operation) of the microprocessor.

The probability of failure of any one component is thus calculated as follows:

$0.1 \times 0.9900 \times 0.9990 = 0.0989$ probability of system failure due to first unit failure.
$0.01 \times 0.9000 \times 0.9990 = 0.0089$ probability of system failure due to second unit failure.
$0.001 \times 0.9900 \times 0.9000 = 0.0009$ probability of system failure due to third unit failure.

The probability of failure of at least one component is thus calculated as follows:

$1 - 0.9000 \times 0.9900 \times 0.9990 = 1 - 0.8901 = 0.1099 \cong 11$ percent.

Note that despite the low probability attached to each component of the system, the overall probability of failure remains unacceptably high.

Note that the probability of a miss in which the fellow failed (first round) is much smaller than the probability in which the intern failed (third round).

Taking into consideration all the rounds, the probability of a miss in the first or the second or the third round is equal to the sum of the probabilities of each round because the sequence in each round is mutually exclusive from that of the next round.

18B.18 Frequency of Procedures

Suppose that 65 percent of all patients at central hospital get a routine ECG on admission, whereas only 25 percent are further evaluated using a Doppler echocardiography study. However, in 40 percent of the patients, a Doppler echocardiography study is performed without a concurrent ECG.

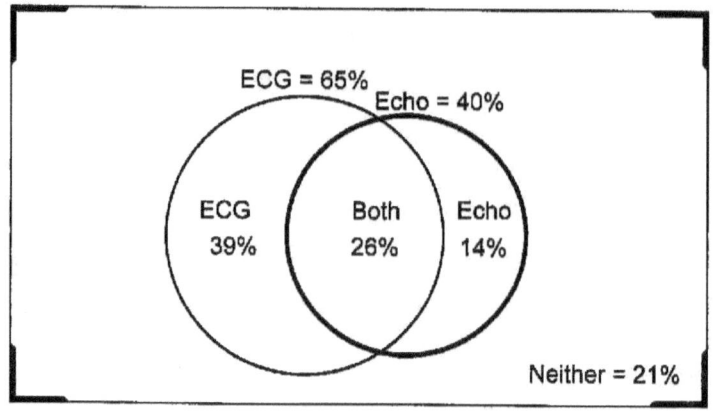

Figure 18B.9. Frequency of Procedures in Venn Diagram

Note the specific usage of the words "or" and "and" in the context of probability as distinct from its grammatical usage. Assuming independence, that is, the performance of ECG is independent from the performance of echocardiography, the following questionable propositions were derived:

1. What is the percentage of patients that that will undergo an ECG and an echocardiography? (panel 5, Figure 5.8b)

$$\text{ECG} \cap \text{echocardiography} = 0.65 \times 0.40 = 0.26$$

2. What is the percentage of patients that that will undergo either an ECG or an echocardiography? (panel 8)

$$\text{ECG} \cup \text{echocardiography} = 0.65 + 0.40 - 0.26$$
$$= 0.79 = 79 \text{ percent (inclusive or)}$$

3. What is the percentage of patients that will receive neither an ECG nor an echocardiography? (panel 12)

$$100 - 79 = 21 \text{ percent}$$

4. What is the percentage of patients that will receive neither an ECG nor an echocardiography? (panel 9)

$$100 - 26 = 74 \text{ percent}$$

5. What is the percentage that will undergo an echocardiography and not an ECG? (panel 7)

Echocardiography $\cap$ not (ECG) $= 0.40 \times 0.35 = 0.14 = 14$ percent

6. What is the percentage that will undergo an echocardiography or not an ECG? (pane 11)

$$\text{Echocardiography} \cup \text{not (ECG)} =$$
$$(0.4 + 0.35) - 0.14 = 0.61 = 61 \text{ percent}$$

7. What is the percentage of those having an echocardiography who will also get an ECG?

$$26 / 40 = 65 \text{ percent}$$

	Echocardiography	No Echocardiography	Total
ECG	0.26	0.39	0.65
No ECG	0.14	0.21	0.35
Total	0.4	0.6	1

Table 18B.8. Frequency of Procedures in Tabular form

18B.19 Question of Life Expectancy

Mr. and Mrs. Smith are both sixty-five years of age. Based on actuarial tables, the probability that Mr. and Mrs. Smith will celebrate their seventy-fifth birthday is 0.6 and 0.7, respectively. Given that the life expectancy of either spouse is independently determined, consider the following:

1. The probability that both will be alive in ten years

$P(A$ and $B) = P(A \cap B) = P(A) \times P(B) = 0.6 \times 0.7 = .42$ (panel 5, Figure 5.6b)

2. The probability that neither will be alive in ten years

$P[(\text{not } A)$ and $(\text{not } B)] = P(A' \cap B') = P(A') \times P(B') = 0.4 \times 0.3 = 0.12$ (panel 12)

3. The probability that only one will be alive

$P[A$ and $(\text{not } B)] + P[(\text{not } A)$ and $B] = (0.6 \times 0.3) + (0.4 \times 0.7) = 0.46$ (panels 6 and 7)

4. The probability that neither A nor B will be alive

$P(\overline{A} \cup \overline{B}) = P(\overline{A \cap B}) = P(\overline{.42}) = 1 - .42 = .58$ (panel 9)

	A	$\overline{A}$	Total
B	0.42	0.28	0.7
$\overline{B}$	0.18	0.12	0.3
Total	0.6	0.4	1

Table 18B.9. Life Expectancy Probability in Tabular form

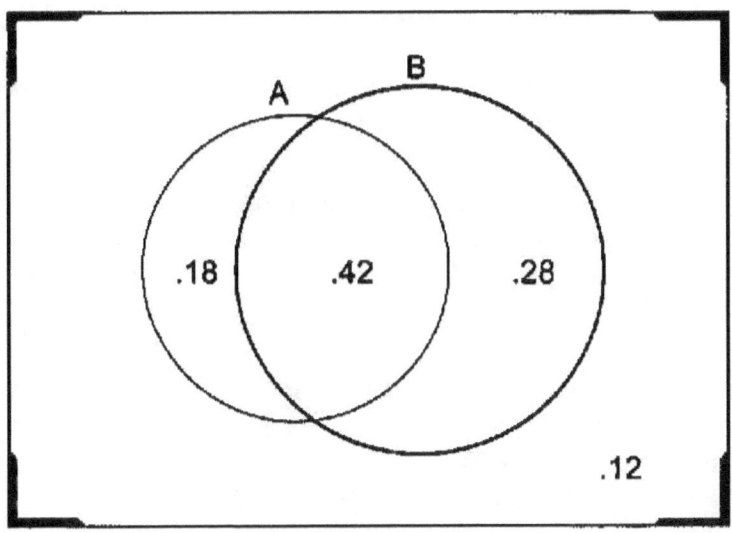

Figure 18B.10. Life Expectancy Probability in Venn diagram

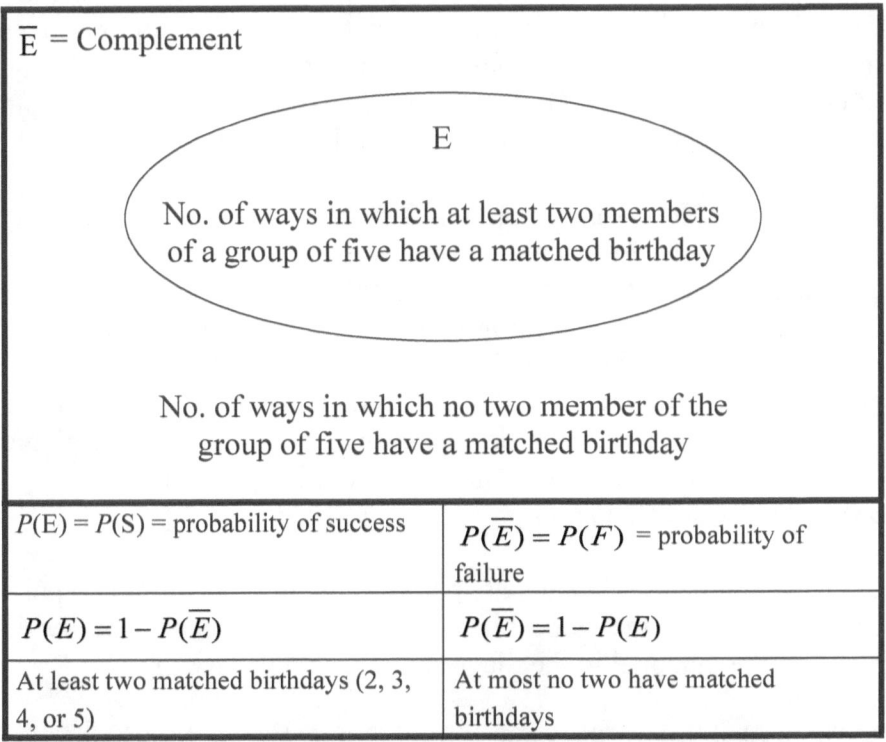

$\overline{E}$ = Complement	
$P(E) = P(S)$ = probability of success	$P(\overline{E}) = P(F)$ = probability of failure
$P(E) = 1 - P(\overline{E})$	$P(\overline{E}) = 1 - P(E)$
At least two matched birthdays (2, 3, 4, or 5)	At most no two have matched birthdays

Table 18B.10. The Birth day Problem in Venn and Tabular format

18B.20 The Birthday Problem

The birthday problem is ubiquitous to all elementary texts. Its almost universal inclusion seems to derive in part from its inherent fascination to any assembled group of people concerning a cherished personal date. Its inclusion in this monograph, aside from its entertaining appeal, is related to the fact that the problem illustrates two counting principles and three probability rules, often submerged in the outline of the solution.

Consider a waiting room with five patients. The question raised by the birthday problem can be simply stated as follows: What is the probability that at least two randomly selected persons of the five persons in the room have the same birthday?

To put the problem in perspective, consider two Martians living in a planetary distant moon where the year is made up of six planetary days. The question for the two Martians would be rephrased as follows: What is the probability that the two Martians share the same birth date, that is, $(1, 1), (2, 2), \ldots, (6, 6)$ as per the Martian calendar? The perusal of Figure 4.2 should convince the reader that

1. There are thirty-six ordered pairs of possible dates that may correspond to the birth date of the two Martians. In other words, the sample space that covers all possible pairs of dates is simply the permutation with repetition of the six calendar dates, that is, n^r = 6^2 = 36 ordered pairs of dates. Alternatively, the multiplication principle may be used to derive the number of elements in the sample space because each day of the calendar year can be paired with six different days, resulting in a sample space of $6 \times 6 = 36$ ordered pairs of calendar days.

2. The number of matched pairs, that is, the number pairs corresponding to the same birth date, is readily seen to be six in number (the diagonal in the diagrammatic sample space).

3. The probability of the same birth date for the two Martians is the ratio of the number of matched pairs to the total number of ordered pairs, both matched and unmatched, in the sample space. Thus,

$$\frac{\text{Number of matched pairs}}{\text{Total number of ordered pairs in the sample space}} = \frac{6}{36} = \frac{1}{6}$$

Consider now three Martians and rephrase the question as follows: What is the probability that at least two of them share the same birth date?

1. The increase in the number of Martians to three adds a third dimension to the sample space. In other words, the elements of the sample space are now made of ordered triplets corresponding to all the possible permutation of size 3 taken from the set of six elements with repetition. The sample space is now made up of 6^3 = 6 × 6 × 6 = 216 ordered triplets that correspond to all possible birth dates of the three Martians.
2. Note that the quantifying number of at least implies in statistical parlance, two or all three Martians as having the same date, which translates into the count of all triplets exhibiting a matched pair, for example, (2, 2, 6) as well as the "flush" triplets, for example, (3, 3, 3), that is, all three having the same date. The problem thus posed may be approached either directly or indirectly.

18B.20.1 Direct Approach

This approach requires the direct count of all the flush and matched pairs triplets. The number of flush triplets remains unchanged because each matched pair can become flush triplets in one way. The number of matched pairs triplets, however, equals 90 (60 + 30 by direct count using Figure 4.2 as a guideline[19]). A total of ninety-six flush and matched pair triplets are counted in the sample space of 216 triplets.

---

[19] Each ordered pair in the triangles of the diagram generates two paired triplets when crossed with third calendar year (30 × 2), whereas each matched pair in the diagonal generates five additional paired triplets (6 × 5).

Thus, the probability that at least two Martians (i.e., two or three) share the same birth date is as follows:

$$\frac{\text{Number of ways three Martians can have at least two matched birthdates}}{\text{Total number of ways that three martians can have birthdates}} = \frac{96}{216} = \frac{4}{9} = 0.44$$

In this case, there is a 44 percent chance for two of the Martians to have the same birth date, compared with 1/6 or 16 percent chance for just two of them as in the first case.

18B.20.2 Indirect Approach

The approach is an exclusionary process aimed at simplifying the unmanageable numbers when the number of candidates exceeds three.

1. As in the direct approach, the total number of all possible triplets that make up the sample space under consideration is calculated. The process involved is permutation with repetition, taking into consideration the size and the number of elements involved.
2. The number of triplets made up of three distinct, unmatched numbers, for example, (2, 3, 5), is counted. This number accounts for all three Martians with no birth date in common. The process in this case involved permutation without repetition so that the number of such triplets of dates is the number of days in the calendar year taken three at time or $6P3 = 120$. The same result is obtained by the direct use of the multiplication principle so that $6 \times 5 \times 4 = 120$.
3. The probability that none of the three Martians share the same date is derived as follows:

$$\frac{\text{Number of ways three Martians can have unmatched birthdates}}{\text{Total number of ways that three Martians can have birthdates}} = \frac{120}{216} = \frac{5}{9} = 0.55.$$

4. To arrive at the probability required as the answer to the posed question, the complement law of probability is invoked; thus,

$\boxed{1-\dfrac{5}{9}=\dfrac{4}{9}}$ the probability that at least two Martians (i.e., two or three) share the same birth date.

Returning to our lonely planet, consider the probability of a shared birth date for just two persons. Obviously, for any one person, the possibilities of one's birthday are 365 corresponding to the number of days in a year. For any two persons, the sample space, just as in the case of the two dice, is now made up of $365^2 = 365 \times 365 = 133,225$ ordered pairs corresponding to all possible matching and unmatching birth dates, out of which the number of matched pairs in the diagonal is counted at 365 matched pairs [e.g. (12, 12), . . . , (64, 64), . . . , (263, 263), . . . , (365, 365)].

The probability of any two people sharing the same birth date may thus be directly derived as follows:

$$\frac{\text{Number of matched pairs}}{\text{Total number of ordered pairs (matched and unmatched) in the sample space}} = \frac{365}{133225} = \frac{1}{365}$$

For two people, the probability of sharing the same birth date amounts $1/365 = 0.003$, just three times among a thousand pairs.

Finally, to respond to the initial question as to the probability that at least two of the five persons in the waiting room share the same birth date, the indirect approach is the only practical method given the astronomical counts. Nonetheless, the basic premises and principles remain unchanged and equally applicable.

To begin with, the sample space is made up of quintuplets as the unit element corresponding to the permutation with repetition of 365 distinct items (days),

$$\boxed{n^r = 365^5 = 365 \times 365 \times 365 \times 365 \times 365.}$$

This total number, however, includes both matched and unmatched quintuples, only a fraction of which is matched.

Yet the focus of the problem is to count by any means possible the number of matched quintuples that qualify as the shared common date for at least two members of the five, a fraction of the sample space of matched and unmatched quintuples.

The number of matched quintuplets, which include those exhibiting a matched pair, a matched triple, a matched quadruple, or a matched quintuple, needs to be calculated. This number of course excludes all quintuples having five distinct and mismatched numbers. In this case, however, the direct approach through the classical technique of counting, detailed in chapter 2, is not possible given the astronomical number generated by the sample space of quintuples, the counting methods. We are thus forced to use the indirect method in which the number of distinct mismatched quintuplets is counted.

To implement this approach, one needs to consider that the first-person birth date can be selected in 365 ways whereas the second-person birth date can only be assigned to 364 days because the mismatch requires that the second person cannot have the same birthday as the first. Similarly, for the third person, only 363 days are left open. Thus, the total number of ways that five persons can have their birthday mismatched is by the multiplication rule, the product of the individual assignments; thus,

Total number of ways of mismatching five birthdays = 365 × 364 × 363 × 362 × 361.

The same result could be equally derived through the permutation without repetition of a set of 365 taken five at a time, which gives the number of distinct mismatched quintuplets that excludes all matched pairs, triplets, quadruplets, and quintuplets,

$$365P5 = 365 \times 364 \times 363 \times 362 \times 361.$$

Because each quintuplet in the sample space is equally likely, we are now in a position to calculate the probability that no two people of the five present share the same birth date; thus,

$$P(5\,\text{mismatched birthdates}) = P(\overline{E}) = \frac{\text{Number of mismatched quintuples}}{\text{Total number quintuples}}$$

$$= \frac{365P5}{365^5} = \frac{365\times364\times363\times362\times361}{365\times365\times365\times365\times365} = 0.973$$

P(no two people in the five share the same birth date) $= P$ (five distinct and mismatched birth dates).

The probability of interest is of course the complement of the above probability, that is, the probability of matched birth dates; thus,

$$P(\text{at least two people have the same birthdate}) = p(E) = 1 - \frac{365P5}{365^5} = 1 - 0.973 = 0.027$$

Thus, the probability of having at least two people share the same birth date is an insignificant 2.7 percent. The popularity and the fascination with the problem derive from the fact that given a waiting room with twenty-three patients, the probability at least two of them share the same birth date is now a respectable figure of 0.507, slightly more than a 50 percent chance.

18B.21 Terminology in Probability

In the formulation of problems related to probability, the phrasing of the question may confront the reader with a set of adverbs designed to modify or quantify the number of successes or failures encountered in a given series of trials. In addition, the complementary nature of the binary states allows the automatic reversal of the question in terms of either success or failure in order to circumvent cumbersome calculation.

The following examples will address the points noted previously. In the first example, the use of adverbs to designate a cutoff point will be illustrated. In the second example, the interchange in the formulation of binomial probability through success and its complement, failure, will be shown.

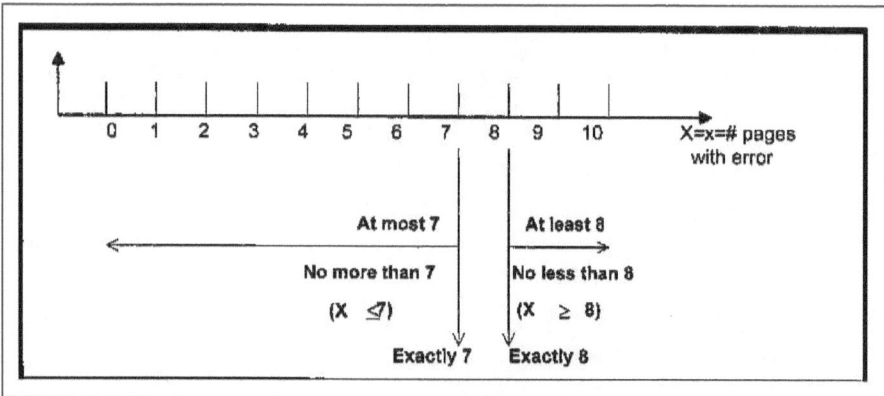

At most seven of ten pages have errors	At least eight of ten pages have errors
= No more than seven have errors	= No less than eight have errors
= Less than eight have errors	= More than eight have errors
= 0, 1, 2, 3, 4, 5, 6, or 7 pages have errors	= 8, 9, or 10 pages have errors
P(At most 7) = 1 − P(At least 8)	P(At least 8) = 1 − P(At most 7)
P(No more than 7) = 1 − P(No less than 8)	P(No less than 8) = 1 − P(No more than 7)

Table 18B.11. The Graphic Equivalent of Probability Terminology

18B.22 Probability of Error

A typist makes on the average four errors in every tenth typed page. If ten pages are typed, what is the probability that

a. Exactly seven pages have error?
b. None has an error?
c. No more than seven pages have errors?

p = probability of one state = P(making an error) = 4/10 = 0.4.
n = number of repeated trials = number of typed pages.
x = Number of success in n trials = number of pages containing errors.

a. P(exactly seven) = $10C7 \times (0.4)^7 \times (0.6)^3 = 120 \times (0.4)^7 \times (0.6)^3$
   = 0.0415
b. P(exactly 0) = $10C0 \times (0.4)^0 \times (0.4)^0 \times (0.6)^{10} = 1 \times (0.4)^0 \times (0.6)^{10}$
   = 0.0060
c. P(no more than 7) = $1 - P$(no less than 8) = $1 - [P(8) + P(9) + P(10)]$
   $10C8 \times (0.4)^8 \times (0.6)^2 + 10C9 \times (0.4)^9 \times (0.6)^1 + 10C10 \times (0.4)^{10} \times (0.6)^0$
   $[1 - (0.0113 + 0.0016 + 0.0001)] = (1 - 0.0130) = 0.9870$

The three adverbs associated with number of pages with error subdivide the total number of pages, n, into two arbitrary segments whose probability is made up of the sum of the individual probabilities of its components. Accordingly, at least three pages with error directs the question to the probability of error in the eighth, ninth, and tenth pages inclusive, whereas its complement, at most, takes into account the errors involved in the first seven pages as well as the probability of 0 error.

Finally, the probability of at most seven may prove too cumbersome to calculate involving the sum of eight separate probabilities, and because the total probability of error cannot exceed 1, the result may be equally obtained by subtracting the probability of at least 3 from 1. In contrast, the probability of an exact number of pages involves simply the direct application of the binomial formula for the specified number.

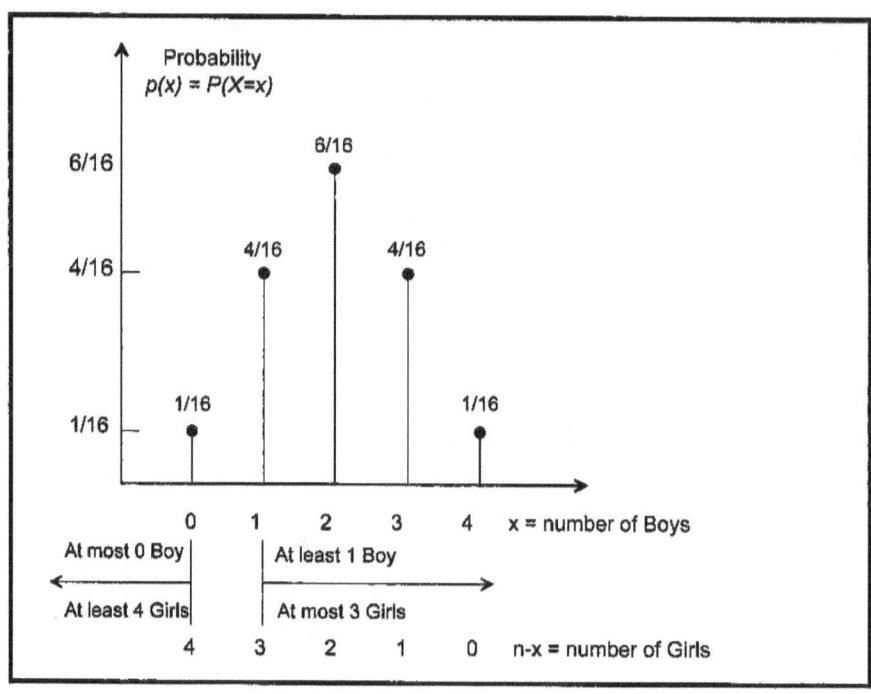

Figure 18B.11. The Probability of Gender

An interesting facet of this juxtaposition is that the probability of "at least one success" is the equivalent of "1 − at most 0 success," which in turn is identical to "1 − at least n failures." Thus, for a woman who has four children, the probability of at least one boy translates as follows:

$$P(\text{At least one boy}) = P(1 - P(0 \text{ boy})) = 1 - (4C0 \times p^0 q^4) = 1 - (1 \times 1 \times \frac{1}{16}) = \frac{15}{16}.$$

Alternatively,

$$P(\text{At least one boy}) = P(1 - P(0 \text{ boy})) = 1 - (\text{At least four girls}) = 1 - \frac{1}{16} = \frac{15}{16}.$$

18B.22.1 Probability of Success and Failure

A return visit to the probability distribution associated with the tossing of six coins, detailed in Figure 18B.3 and reproduced in a concise form in the following Table, offers a detailed version of the terminology often associated with the formulation of probability questions.

Table 18B.12 lists the probability in terms of success and failure, rows 1 and 2. In addition, the probability of success is restated both in terms of the event and its complement for the total sample space. The same applies for the probability of failure.

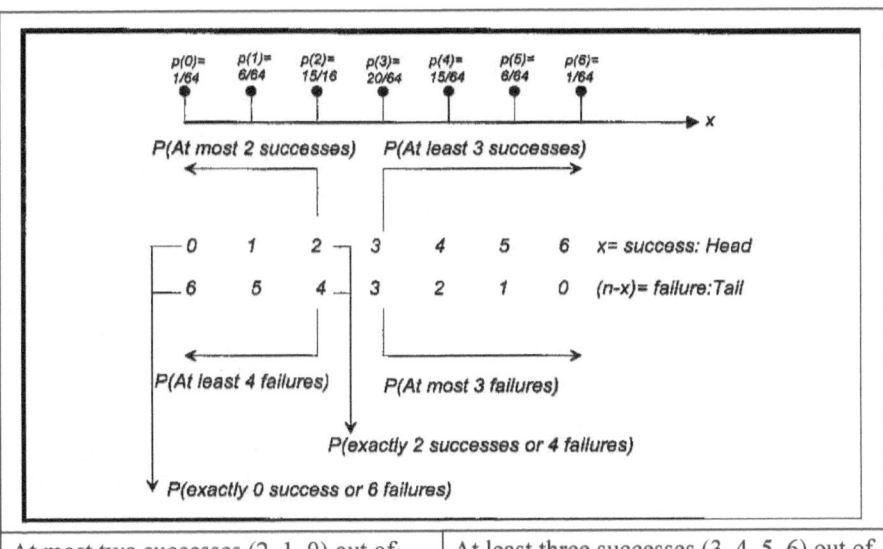

At most two successes (2, 1, 0) out of six trials	At least three successes (3, 4, 5, 6) out of six trials
Two or less successes	$P(x \geq 3)$
Not more than two successes $P(x \leq 2)$	Three or more successes $P(x \geq 3) = P(x = 3 \text{ or } x = 4 \text{ or } x = 5 \text{ or } x = 6) = P(3) + P(4) + P(5) + P(6)$
	Not less than three successes $P(x \geq 3)$

At least four failures (4, 5, 6) out of six trials $P(n - x \geq 4)$ Four or more failures $P(n - x \geq 4) = P(n - x = 4$ or $n - x = 5$ or $n - x = 6) = P(4) + P(5) + P(6)$ Not less than four failures $P(n - x \geq 4)$	At most three failures (3, 2, 1, 0) out of six trials Three or less failures Not more than three failures $P(n - x \leq 3)$
At least four failures $= 1 -$ at most three failures $P(\text{at least } 4) = 1 - P(\text{at most } 3)$ $P(n - x \geq 4) = 1 - P(n - x \leq 3)$	At least three successes $= 1 -$ at most two successes $P(\text{at least } 3) = 1 - P(\text{at most } 2)$ $P(x \geq 3) = 1 - P(x \leq 2)$
$P(\text{at least } 1 \text{ (F)}) = 1 - \Pr(\text{at most } 0 \text{ (F)})$ $= 1 - P(\text{at least } 6 \text{ (S)})$ $P(n - x \geq 1) = 1 - P(n - x \leq 0) = 1 - P(x \geq 6)$	$P(\text{at least } 1 \text{ (S)}) = 1 - \Pr(\text{at most } 0 \text{ (S)}) = 1 - P \text{ (at least } 6 \text{ (F)})$ $P(x \geq 1) = 1 - P(x \leq 0) = 1 - P(n - x \geq 6)$
More than three successes (4, 5, 6); $P(x > 3)$ Less than three successes (2, 1, 0); $P(x < 3)$;	More than four failures (4, 5, 6); $P(x > 4)$ Less than four failures (3,2,1,0); $P(x < 4)$

Table 18B.12. Probability Distribution associated with the tossing of 6 coins
The complement of at least one is exactly zero.

At most $(x - 1)$ successes out of n trials. $(x - 1), (x - 2), \ldots, 0$	AT least x successes out of n trials $x, (x + 1), (x + 2), \ldots, n$
At least $(n - x)$ failures out of n trials $(n - x), (n - x - + 2),$ $(n - x + 2), \ldots, n$	At most x failures out of n trials $(x - 1), (x - 2) \ldots, 0$
Binomial partition of the sample space of n trials into at least x successes and its complement $(x - 1)$ or at least $(n - x)$ failures and its complement $(x - 1)$. Note that "at most $(x - 1)$ success" is numerically equivalent to "at least $(x - x)$ failure."	
$n =$ number of trials, experiments, cases	
$x =$ Number of successes in n trials	$n - x =$ number of failures in n trials
$p = P(\text{success in one trial, experiment, case})$	$q = P(\text{failure in one trial, experiment, case})$

$p = 1 - q$	$q = 1 - p$
$p(x) = P(x$ successes in n trials$)$	$p(n - x) = P((n - x)$ failures in n trials$)$
$P(x) = nCx \times p^x \times q^{n-x}$	$P(n - x) = nC(n - x) \times p^x \times q^{n-x}$
$b(x; n, p)$	$b[(n - x); n, (1 - p)]$

Table 18B.13. Partition of the Sample Space into 4
complementary compartments

These considerations are summarized in Table 18B.3, where the sample space of n trials or sequences is partitioned into four designated compartments. Taken horizontally, they constitute complements of each other. Taken vertically, they are equivalent in terms of their complementary elements of success and failure.

A drug firm administers a new drug to twenty people with a certain disease. If the probability is 0.15 that the drug will cure each person of the disease, and if the result for one person is independent of that of another person, what is the probability that three or more of the twenty people will be cured? The probability that X is greater than or equal to 3 ($\geq$) equals 1 minus the probability that X is less than or equal to 2 ($\leq$). Thus, the probability that X is greater than or equal to 3 is $1 - 0.4049$, or 5,951. In other words, the probability that three or more people will be cured is approximately 0.60.

Coefficient=
frequency=
$nCx \times H^x T^{n-x}$; x = No. successes (heads) in n trials
No. events with x heads

$P($event with x number of heads$) = P(X = x) = p(x) = \dfrac{nCx}{2^n}$.
No. elements in sample space

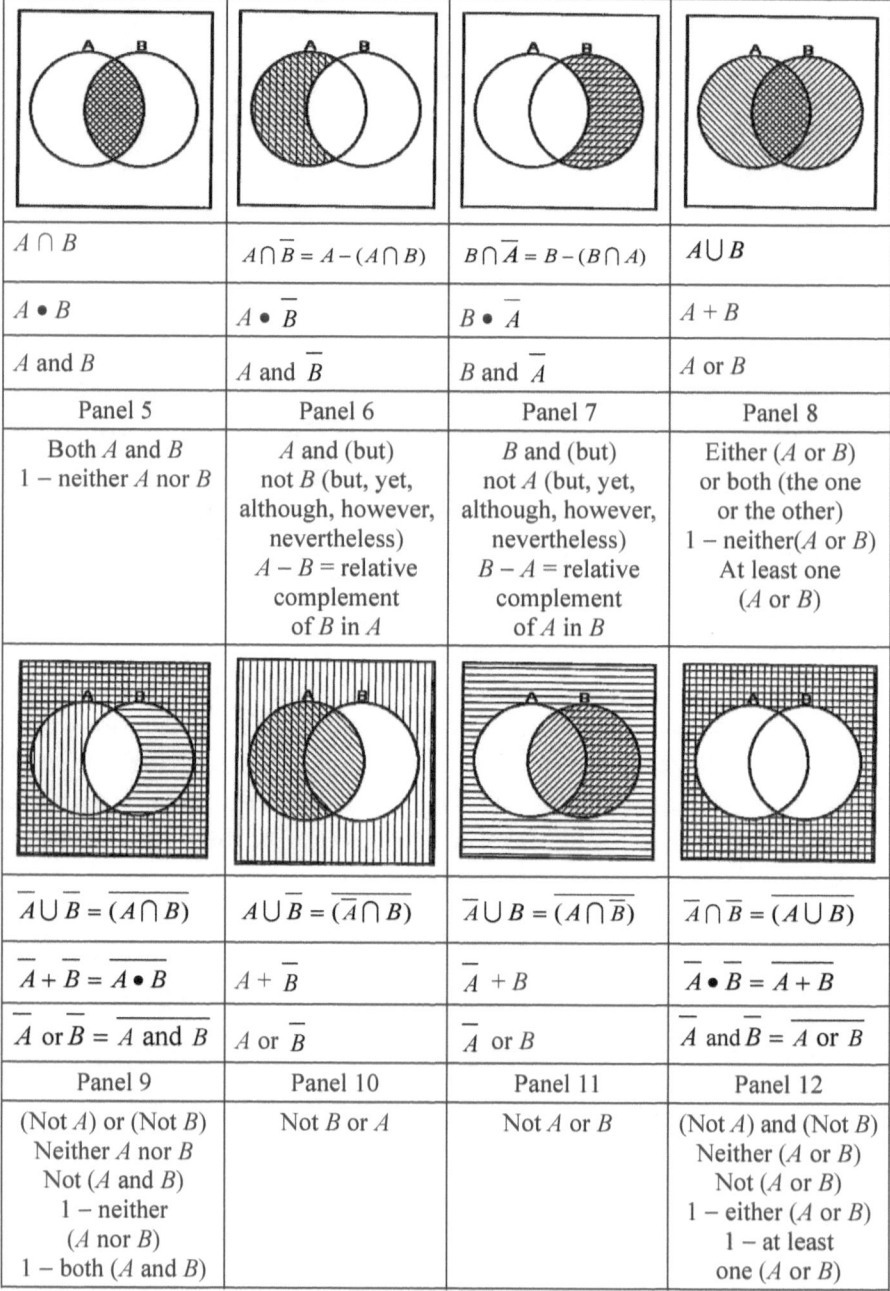

$A \cap B$	$A \cap \overline{B} = A - (A \cap B)$	$B \cap \overline{A} = B - (B \cap A)$	$A \cup B$
$A \bullet B$	$A \bullet \overline{B}$	$B \bullet \overline{A}$	$A + B$
A and B	A and $\overline{B}$	B and $\overline{A}$	A or B
Panel 5	Panel 6	Panel 7	Panel 8
Both A and B 1 − neither A nor B	A and (but) not B (but, yet, although, however, nevertheless) $A - B$ = relative complement of B in A	B and (but) not A (but, yet, although, however, nevertheless) $B - A$ = relative complement of A in B	Either (A or B) or both (the one or the other) 1 − neither(A or B) At least one (A or B)

$\overline{A} \cup \overline{B} = \overline{(A \cap B)}$	$A \cup \overline{B} = \overline{(\overline{A} \cap B)}$	$\overline{A} \cup B = \overline{(A \cap \overline{B})}$	$\overline{A} \cap \overline{B} = \overline{(A \cup B)}$
$\overline{A + B} = \overline{A} \bullet \overline{B}$	$A + \overline{B}$	$\overline{A} + B$	$\overline{A \bullet B} = \overline{A} + \overline{B}$
$\overline{A}$ or $\overline{B} = \overline{A \text{ and } B}$	A or $\overline{B}$	$\overline{A}$ or B	$\overline{A}$ and $\overline{B} = \overline{A \text{ or } B}$
Panel 9	Panel 10	Panel 11	Panel 12
(Not A) or (Not B) Neither A nor B Not (A and B) 1 − neither (A nor B) 1 − both (A and B)	Not B or A	Not A or B	(Not A) and (Not B) Neither (A or B) Not (A or B) 1 − either (A or B) 1 − at least one (A or B)

Figure 5.8b. Basic set operations in Venn diagrams, symbols, and words

Chapter 18C

The Continuous Probability Distribution
Probability Density Function
(Probability Distribution Function for Continuous Random Variables)

In chapters 18A and 18B, the probability distribution of discrete random variables whose measurements are obtained through a counting process limited to the set of integer was explained and illustrated. In this chapter, the probability distribution of a continuous random variable, whose measurements may assume any value along a continuum limited only by the degree of accuracy of the measuring instrument, is considered. This include measurements of weight, blood pressure, temperature, and serum cholesterol levels, each of which can be calibrated and refined to an arbitrary number of decimal places.

18C.1 Probability Density Function (PDF)

When the range, x, of the random variable X assumes an infinite number of values (i.e., all points in the interval between 0 and 6 inclusive representing real numbers), the previous definition of the discrete random variable becomes untenable because we are dealing here with a continuum of an infinite possible values. Accordingly,

$P(X = 1) = p(1) =$ probability of the discrete random variable at 1,

is not applicable in the case of a continuous random variable because the probability in such a case is paradoxically equal zero (Figure 18C.1).

$P(X = 1) = p(1) =$ probability of the continuous random variable at $1 = 0$

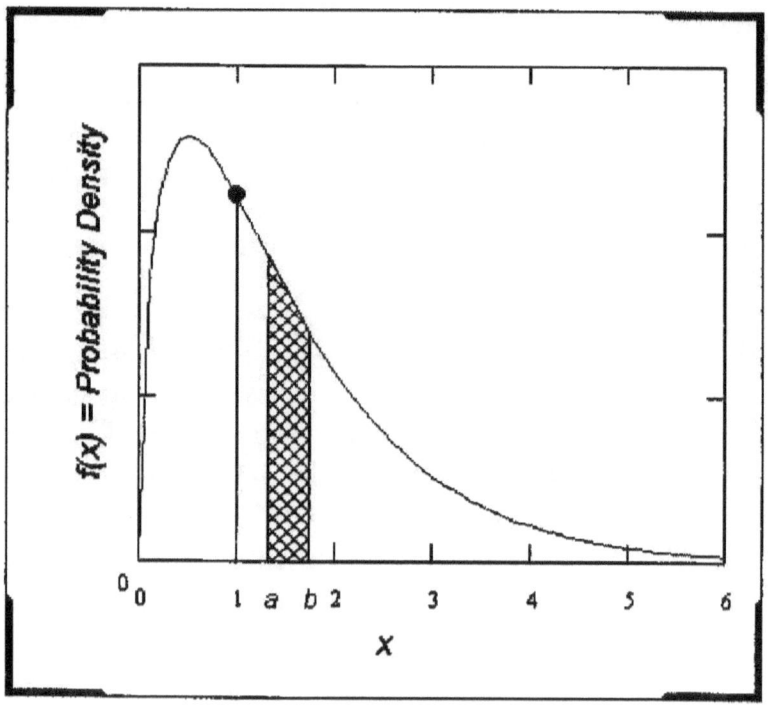

Figure 18C.1. Graph of the PDF.

The rationale behind this assertion requires a moment of reflection to realize that it is impossible to construct a probability distribution table (as was done for the discrete case) for every point on a given segment of the x axis because the number of such points is literally uncountable. The line of the x axis itself (as noted in the Concept of function in Chapter 18A) is made of dimensionless array of points, each of which is of zero length that, nevertheless, when linearly arrayed, translates into the line itself. Such being the case, the dimensionless point (i.e., of zero length) cannot possibly be associated with a measurable probability, in effect a zero probability at any given point. Thus, the probability distribution of a continuous random variable over its discrete point values is meaningless. In other words, the assignment of probability to a given point on the x axis breaks down when applied to the continuous random variable because the probability for a given value of a continuous random variable is identically zero.

The relationship of the discrete probability distribution to the continuous is best illustrated by focusing on the transitional aspect of their respective distribution. Consider once again Figure 18A.3 of chapter 18A, where the relative frequency density distribution of heights in a sample of eighty students is displayed. Note once more that the base width of each rectangle is made to equal one unit interval. The area of each rectangle thus represents the percent of the total in each category, the total area being the sum of the percentages, that is, the sum of all probabilities or 100 percent.

Thus, approaching the distribution from the discrete point of view, one begins by dividing the whole range of values of random variable X into certain intervals (categories), as demonstrated in the previous example. By calculating how many values of the random variable X are put into each category and by dividing by the total number of measurements made in order to derive the relative frequency and relative frequency density of the interval, the proportion of all students' heights within a given range and the probability that any one student's height, randomly chosen, will fall within the given range are readily noted in Figure 18C.2.

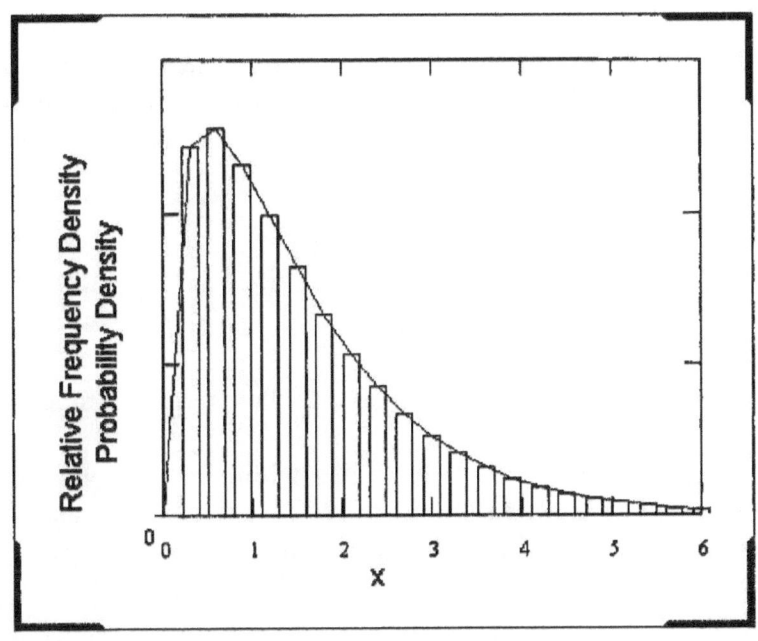

Figure 18C.2. Graph of the PDF.

If the class interval is reduced to, say, one-quarter of an inch, the columns would get narrower and sixteen times more numerous. With an increasing number of measurements, the intervals become narrower and narrower, and the step form of the histogram becomes smoother. A line along their tops would approach the smooth frequency curve that describes the probability distribution of a continuous random variable X, in which the discrete probability function, $p(x_j)$, is now replaced by the probability density function (PDF), $f(x)$ (Figure 18C.2). Along the y axis, the probability density will replace the relative frequency density.

In mechanical terms, the notion of density translates into mass per unit volume. In probabilistic terms, because the total area enclosed by the curve represents the total probability of 1 or 100 percent, a given probability demarcates a segment of the total area. Accordingly, the size of any segment thus demarcated depends on its location with respect to the central axis as dictated by its z boundaries, such that the area cutoff by the z range varies from minimum tail segment to a maximum centrally located segment.

In essence, the analogy may be stated in equivalent terms as follows:

A given probability as defined by its equivalent segmental area is a function of the z range location with respect to the central axis as noted from the probability of a z range of 1 twice removed from the central axis compared with z range once removed,

$$P(1 \leq z \leq 2) = P(0.4772 - 0.3414) = 0.1359,$$

$$P(2 \leq z \leq 3) = P(0.4987 - 0.4772) = 0.0215.$$

The curve thus reflects the probability density per unit z range.

Clearly, the probability that RV X lies within the interval (a, b) is the equivalent of the area bounded by this interval, just as the area bounded by the rectangle in the histogram. In technical terms, if we denote the PDF by $f(x)$, the probability that RV X fits into interval (a, b) will be expressed by the definite integral:

$$P(a \leq X \leq b) = \int_a^b f(x)dx$$

In this case, it is only when the function is integrated between two limits does it yield a probability. The definition may be extended to include cases where a, b, or both may become infinite.

18C.2 The Normal Distribution as an Approximation of the Binomial Distribution

The probability distribution of a binomial random variable x (number of successes in n trials) depends on the two parameter of n (number of repeated trials) and p (the probability of one state success). Because the widths of the rectangles in the histogram of a binomial distribution are equal to unity, the areas of the rectangles are equal in magnitude to their altitudes and, consequently, as measures of the relative frequencies (probabilities) of the classes.

The outline of the distribution and the changes it undergoes with different sample sizes is frequently an important parameter. In Figure 18C.3, where n (the number of independent trials, e.g., tossing a loaded penny ten times) and $p = 0.8$ (the probability of success), the distribution of x (the number of successes) is skewed with a long left tail. Its mirror image with long right tail is obtained when $p = 0.2$. A maximal probability of 0.302 was recorded in both instances for $x = 8$ and $x = 2$, respectively.

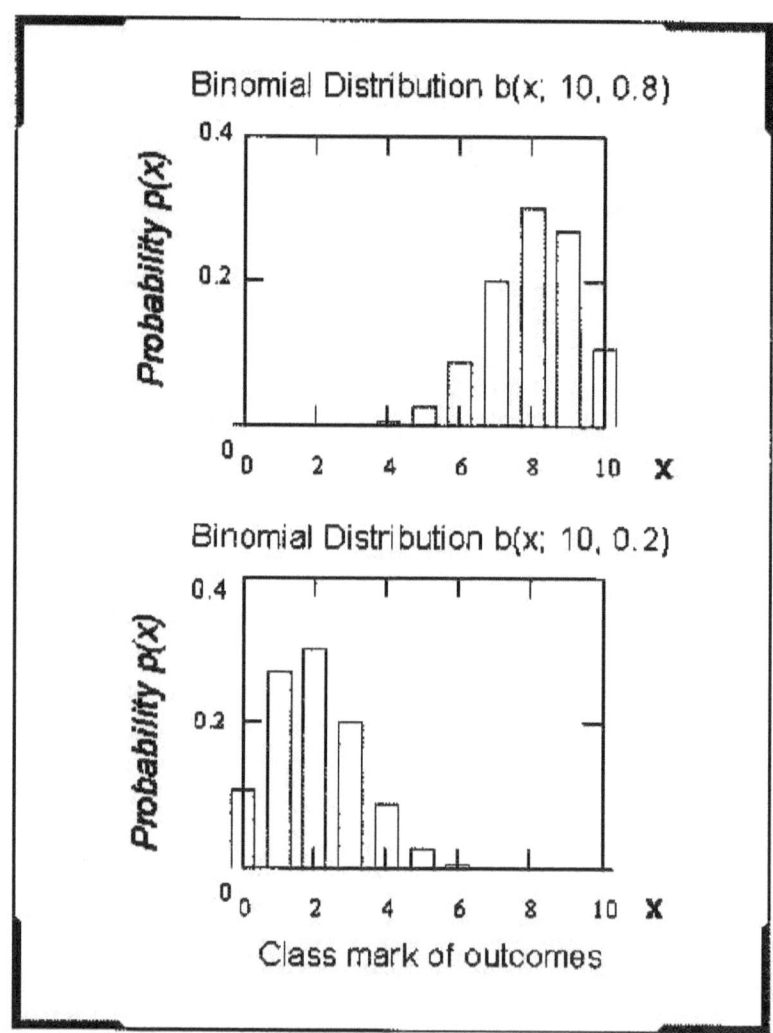

Figure 18C.3. Skewed Probability Distribution

By contrast, the distribution is perfectly symmetrical when the probability $p = 0.5$ (Figure 18C.4). Of equal importance is the fact that the outline of the probability distribution is similarly influenced by the sample size, n, the number of trials. As the sample size increases, the outline of the distribution assumes a symmetrical outline irrespective of the associated p value.

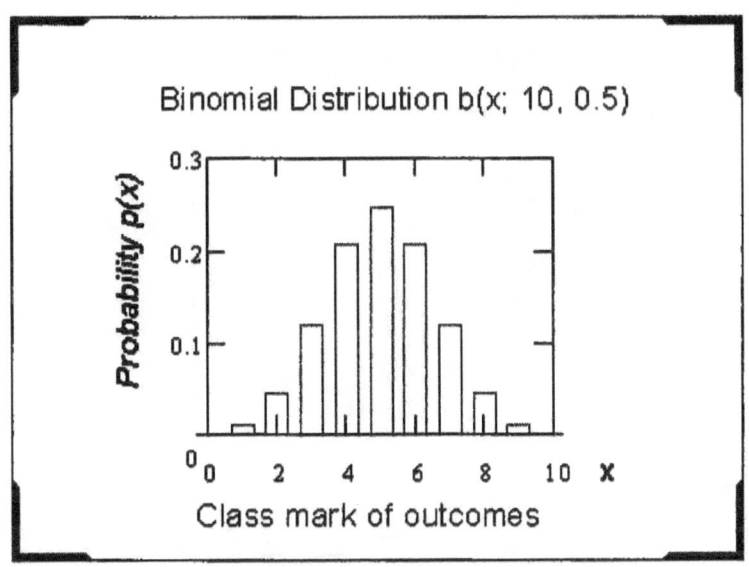

Figure 18C.4. Discrete Binomial Distribution

When $p = 0.5$ and the number of independent trials is more than 10, say $n = 20$, the histogram will begin to assume a familiar shape approaching a bell-shaped configuration.

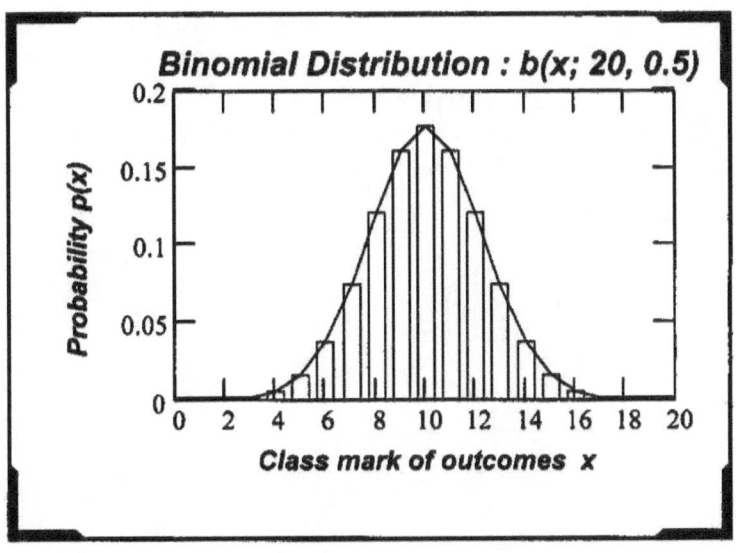

Figure 18C.5. Binomial Distribution approaching Normal Distribution

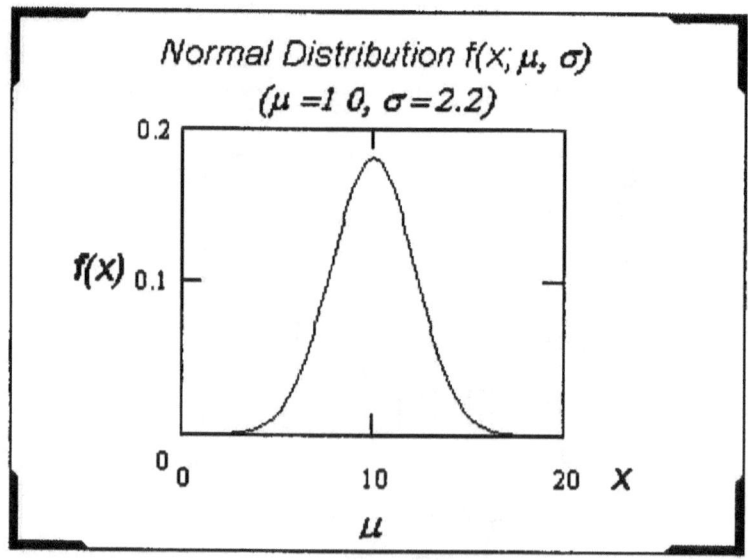

Figure 18C.6. The Normal Distribution

When $p = 0.5$ and the number of independent trials is large, say $n = 1,000$, the histogram will have the same general shape as Figure 18C.5. The histogram is not a smooth curve. In actual fact, what appears to be a smooth curve is in reality segmental made up of the connecting short lines spanning the centers of the sequential rectangles. In the limit, however, as the number of trials, n, increases indefinitely, it can be proven that the emerging curve is truly continuous and what is even more important it assumes the exact shape of the normal bell-shaped curve that is the subject of the next chapter (Figure 18C.6).

Chapter 19A

The Normal Probability Distribution
Normal Probability Density Function

19A.1 The Normal Distribution

Experimental results always involve errors. Two types of common errors may be observed in a given experiment: systematic errors and random errors. The systematic errors are due to definite causes that can be either removed or corrected (e.g., errors caused by an irregularity of the scale of an instrument or by external conditions of an experiment). The random errors are usually due to a large number of independently acting random factors, each of which has a negligible small influence on the process as a whole.

The random error x can assume arbitrary values; it is therefore a continuous random variable characterized by its probability distribution. Consider the pharmaceutical manufacturing of a given drug in capsular form. Irrespective of the control processes installed, the dosage per capsule is never as specified. The weight of each capsule will deviate from the specified weight by a measurable margin given a finely calibrated scale. The contributing factors involved are cumulative in their final effect on the actual dosage and may include such subtle and undetected physical as well as human factors acting independently of each other.

If a very large number of such measurements are made, so that the class interval of the histogram can he made smaller and smaller, say ± 0.1 mg for a 1,000-mg capsule (e.g., 999.8; 999.9; 1,000; 1,000.1; and 1,000.2) a smooth curve will come to approximate the shape of the observed distribution of weights. The resulting normal curve reflects the relative frequency with which the different capsular weights are expected to occur.

The distribution of the random errors is the practical analog of a binomial distribution when the number of trials reaches infinity, resulting in a smooth normal curve, which is how, historically, the distribution was discovered.

These errors cannot be completely excluded; only mean corrections can be introduced. Thus, familiarity with the laws governing the random errors becomes necessary, which is how, historically, the normal distribution was related to the distribution of errors of measurements.

19A.2 The Normal Probability Density Function: The Normal Curve

The normal distribution as defined by the normal probability density function (PDF) is the simplest and, in most cases, the best approximation to reality, among several theoretical distribution of continuous random variables.

The anatomy of the normal density curve is fundamental to the understanding and manipulation of statistical data. The gross perusal of the curve reveals the following salient features:

- The total area under the density curve is equal to 1 or 100 percent.
- The density curve is symmetrical with respect to a central axis, so that the area is equally divided between the left and the right half, 0.5 or 50 percent of the total for each half.
- At a certain point along the slope of the curve, termed the inflection point, the contour of the curve changes from down pointing concavity (inverted cup) to up pointing concavity.
- The wings of the curve extend to infinity, which is another way of saying that the wings, never touch the x axis, such that an infinitesimal space exists between them no matter how far extended into space.

At the microscopic level, in an elementary discussion such as this, it would seem out of place to indulge in the analysis of what appears at first sight a formidable mathematical expression for a normal curve. A closer look would in fact strip the expression of its mystique and would allow the reader to use the curve as the basic graphic tool of statistical inference in an analogous fashion to the use of the Venn diagrams in the graphic portrayal of probability relations. In essence, the formula simply provides a quantitative measure that defines and refines the above-noted gross anatomical aspects of the curve.

The normal density curve is represented by the following equation and corresponding graph (Figure 19A.1).

$$y = f(x) = \frac{1}{\sigma} \times \frac{1}{\sqrt{2\pi}} \times e^{-\frac{1}{2}\left(\frac{x-\mu}{\sigma}\right)^2} \quad \text{where } \mu \neq 0, \sigma \neq 0, \text{ and } -\infty < x < +\infty.$$

The equation is the formal expression of the PDF, in which y being the function of x, symbolized as $f(x)$, implies that for every value of x on the right side of the equation, which graphically translates into a point on the x axis, a corresponding value of y or $f(x)$ is obtained, which translates into a point on the curve, the height of which (i.e., its frequency density) is a function of the corresponding particular value of the random variable x. In addition, the equation is characterized by its two parameters, μ and σ, which, together with the random variable X, make up the exponent or power of the constant e.

To emphasize the role of the exponent in the expression, it is separately detailed in the following relation. As can be seen, μ, the arithmetic mean, determines the location of the central axis of the curve, whereas σ, the standard deviation, determines the spread or dispersion (plumb or slim) of the data around the mean (Figure 19A.2),

$$-\frac{1}{2}\left(\frac{\overset{\text{Random variable}}{x} - \overset{\text{Arithmetic mean}}{\mu}}{\underset{\text{Standard deviation}}{\sigma}}\right)^2$$

Finally, the expression contains two constants: π of course is the familiar constant ($\pi = 3.1416 \ldots$) and e is the base of natural logarithm ($e = 2.7189 \ldots$). The equation is the general formula for all possible normal curves because difference in the parameters of μ and σ account for an infinite variety of normal nonstandardized curves.

Because the interrelation between the random variable X and the corresponding parameters μ and σ constitutes the basic connection (Figure 19A.2, connection III) that determines the shape of the normal curve, namely, its central axis and the spread or deviation of its variables from its mean, it would thus be instructive to look at the bare bones of the curve stripped of its accouterment by locating its central axis at the origin of an x-y coordinate system (i.e., $\mu = 0$) and standardizing the degree of its spread to the single unit of 1 (i.e., $\sigma = 1$),

$$y = f(x) = \frac{1}{\sigma} \times \frac{1}{\sqrt{2\pi}} \times e^{-\frac{1}{2}\left(\frac{x-\mu}{\sigma}\right)^2}$$

$$y = f(x) = \frac{1}{1} \times \frac{1}{\sqrt{2\pi}} \times e^{-\frac{1}{2}\left(\frac{x-0}{1}\right)^2} = \frac{1}{\sqrt{2\pi}} \times e^{-\frac{x^2}{2}}$$

The equation now assumes a simplified format relating y, the height of the curve to a corresponding point x on the x axis or more precisely the value of the probability density, y, to a corresponding x value of the random variable X,

$$y = \frac{1}{\sqrt{2\pi}} \times e^{-\frac{x^2}{2}}$$

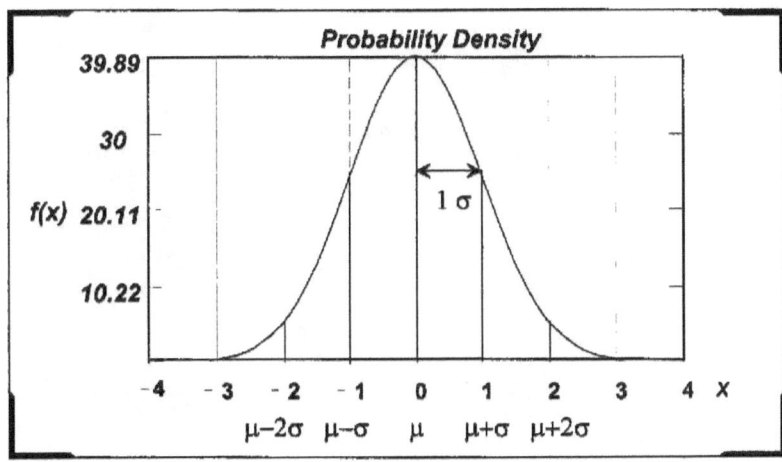

Figure 19A.1. Probability Density Vs. x value of the random variable

The maximal density, the height of the curve at its central axis, can be derived by equating x, the exponent of e, to 0. The expression is now further simplified as follows:

$$y = \frac{1}{\sqrt{2\pi}} \times e^{-\frac{x^2}{2}} = \frac{1}{\sqrt{2\pi}} \times e^{0} = \frac{1}{\sqrt{2\pi}} \times 1 = \frac{1}{\sqrt{2\pi}} = 0.3989$$

The height of the curve is then 0.3989 if the area is taken to be one, or equivalently 39.89 if the area is taken to be 100.

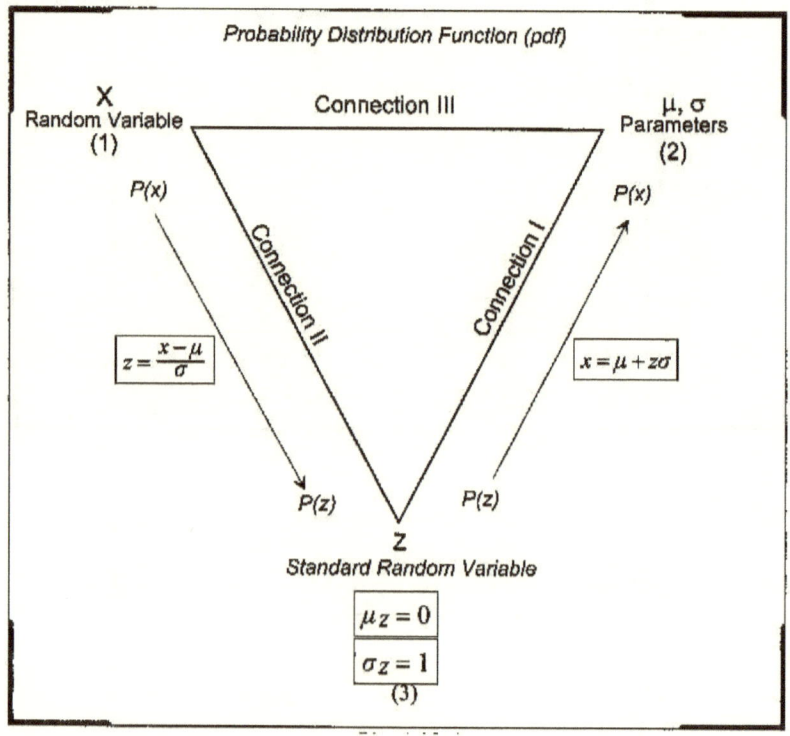

Figure 19A.2. The Connection involving The RV with
the Standard RV and the derived Parameters

The equation tends to lose its esoteric character when applied in practice to the distribution of measurements or scores derived from a given population. Figure 19A.3 is a case in point. It is an accurate PDF (relative frequency) depiction of the distribution of a continuous random variable, the heights in inches of all freshmen at a hypothetical New York University. In this case, x ranges from a minimum of fifty inches to a maximum of ninety inches. The two parameters that characterize the curve are its mean, μ, of seventy inches and its standard deviation, σ, of four inches.

As in the previous example, when $x = \mu = 70$ inches, the exponent of e collapses to 0, so that

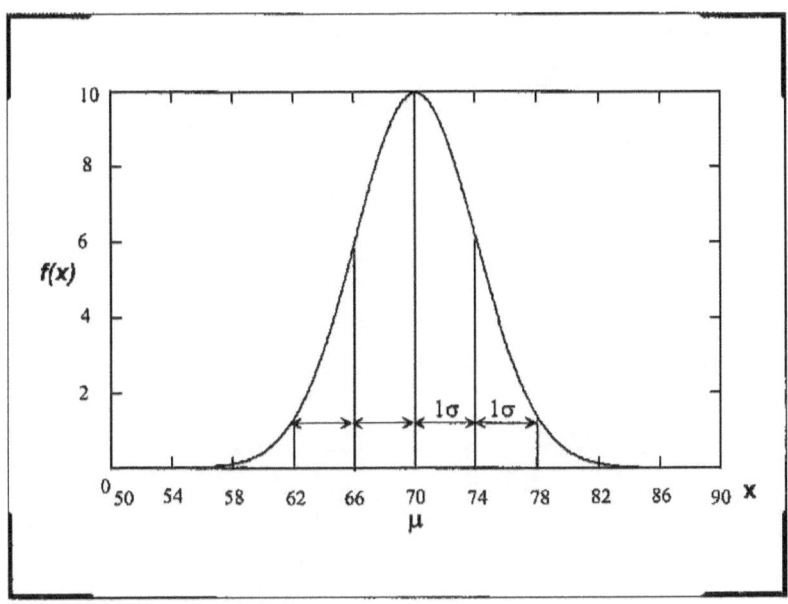

Figure 19A.3. Graph of the PDF of the heights distribution of the Freshmen Population

$$-\frac{1}{2}\left(\frac{x-\mu}{\sigma}\right)^2 = -\frac{1}{2}\left(\frac{70-70}{\sigma}\right)^2 = 0 \text{ and } e^0 = 1$$

The expression is reduced to the simple ratio noted as follows:

$$y = f(x) = \frac{1}{\sigma} \times \frac{1}{\sqrt{2\pi}} \times e^{-\frac{1}{2}\left(\frac{x-\mu}{\sigma}\right)^2} = \frac{1}{\sigma} \times \frac{1}{\sqrt{2\pi}} \times 1 = \frac{1}{\sigma\sqrt{2\pi}} = \frac{1}{4\sqrt{2\pi}} = 0.0997$$

y or $f(x)$ then assumes its maximal density (relative frequency). Note that the exponent of e in the equation is thus the key ratio that determines the center of the curve as well as the spread of the measurements around the central mean.

For any other value of the random variable X, that is, for any given height in x inches, the frequency density (relative frequency) of the particular measurement is determined by the corresponding y or $f(x)$.

The curve provides additional information common to all normal curves as follows (Figure 19A.4):

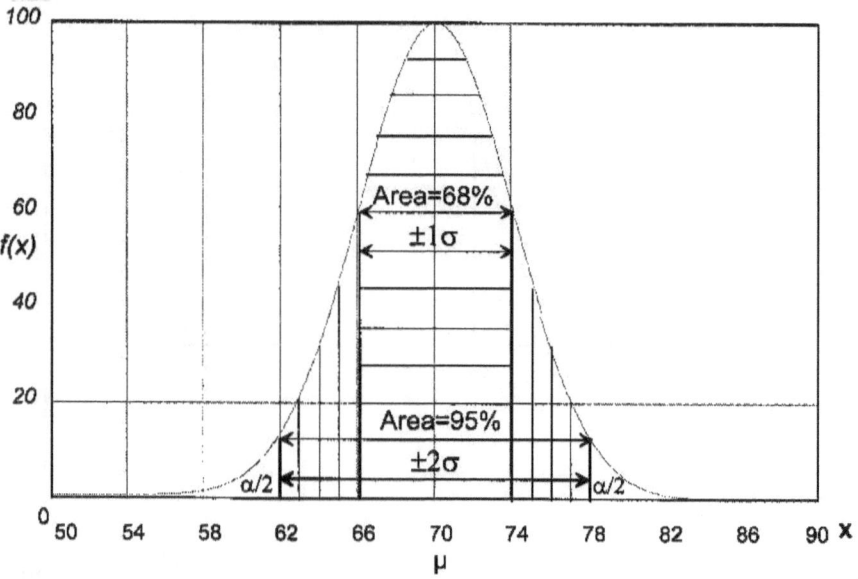

Figure 19A.4. Graph of the partition of the area under a normal curve bounded on either side of the central axis by a grid line corresponding to one or two standard deviates.

1. The total area under the normal distribution function or the PDF equals 1. A normal distribution is symmetrical about the mean and thus equally divided between the two halves.
2. The area enclosed between the mean (seventy inches) and one standard deviation on either side ($\mu \pm 1\sigma$), that is, the area enclosed between vertical grid lines at sixty-six inches and seventy-four inches, constitutes 68 percent of the total area under the curve ($0.3413 \times 2 = 0.6816$).

3. The area enclosed between the mean and the two standard deviations on either side ($\mu \pm 2\sigma$), that is, the area enclosed between vertical grid lines at sixty-two and seventy-eight inches, constitutes 95 percent of the total area under the curve ($0.4772 \times 2 = 0.9574$).

4. The area enclosed between the mean and the three standard deviations on either side ($\mu \pm 3\sigma$), that is, the area enclosed between vertical grid lines at fifty-eight and eighty-two inches, constitutes 99.7 percent of the total area under the curve ($0.4987 \times 2 = 0.9974$).

5. The balance of the area under the curve, $1 - 0.9974 = 0.0026 = 2 \times 0.0013$, is enclosed under the tails of the curves that extend to infinity on either side. Note that although the graphic curve touches the x axis and appears to close the area underneath it, in reality, however, a gradually diminishing but actual space extends under both tails up to $\pm\infty$.

The statements defining the specific areas under the normal curve noted previously may be restated in terms of the random variable X, being a measure of the heights of the male freshman class in inches. Thus,

2a. The area enclosed between the mean (seventy inches) and one standard deviation on either side ($\mu \pm 1\sigma$), that is, the area enclosed between vertical grid lines at sixty-six and seventy-four inches, constitutes the percentage of students exhibiting this range in height out of the total population of the freshman class. Thus, 68 percent (68.26 to be exact) of all freshmen, more accurately 68 percent of the measured heights, fall in the range between sixty-six and seventy-four inches.

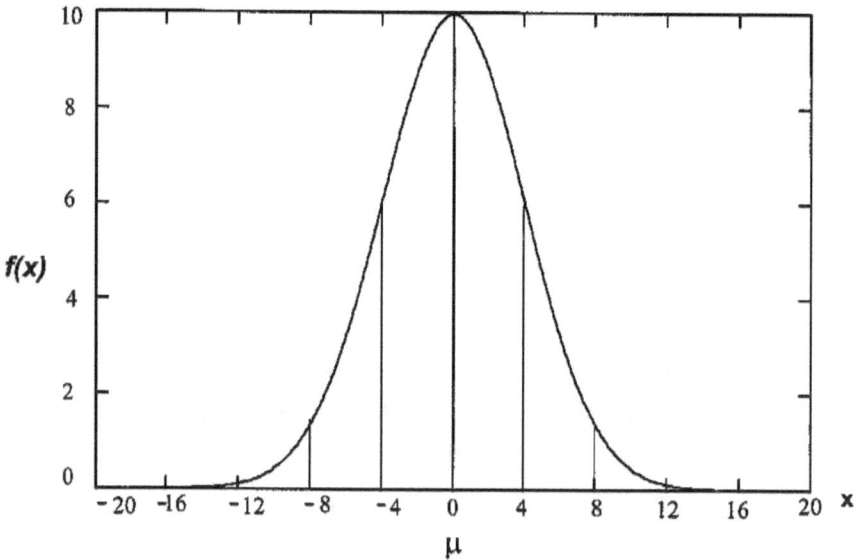

Figure 19A.5. Graph of the PDF of the heights distribution of the freshmen population plotted on the transformed x axis.

The curve so far described pertains to a specific set of measurements derived from a specific population. Comparison with other set of measurements, obtained from another specific population with different mean and standard deviation, for example, comparison with the heights of female students of the freshman class, is impossible because a common reference point of origin and a uniform measurement yardstick is lacking. Obviously, a generic format applicable to all measurements that may be described by the normal curve is necessary.

The transformation of normal distribution into a generic standard normal distribution requires addressing the two parameters that characterize the individual normal curves, namely, μ (the point of reference) and σ (the unit of spread or deviation from the mean) (Figure 19A.5).

The transformation of a specific μ, seventy inches in this case, into a generic μ of 0 is performed by subtracting the mean, μ, from each value of x, a manipulation that results in relocating the original curve to a new center at 0. As noted in Figure 19A.5, when μ is made equal to zero, the original equation is transformed into the following equation in which the exponent of e is a function of x and σ only:

$$y = f(x)\frac{1}{\sigma} \times e^{-\frac{1}{2}\cdot\frac{x^2}{\sigma^2}} \text{ where } \mu = 0, \sigma \neq 0.$$

The x axis now becomes a relative scale, still measured in inches, extending in the opposite directions with respect to a zero central point of origin.

The second requirement for standardization is the adoption of a common unit of measurement. In Figures 19A.3 and 19A.4, the unit of measurement displayed on the x axis is the same as the unit in which the measurements were carried out.

In Figure 19A.5, except for the transformation of the mean to 0, the scale of the x axis remained essentially unchanged because the unit inches remained in both cases, although differently displayed.

In order to standardize the unit of measurements, the dispersion parameter, σ, needs to be taken into consideration by adopting it as standard unit of measurement. Thus, if the distance of a measured value of x from the mean of all the x values, μ (i.e., $x - \mu$), is divided by σ (four inches in this case), the resulting unit is simply a ratio of two distances (measured in the same unit of inches), answering the question how many sigmas (σ's) or units of standard deviation, the given distance ($x - \mu$), contains or is equivalent to? This is analogous to 36 / 12 inches to derive a new unit arbitrarily named a foot. In this case, the nondimensional unit z is the standardized normal random variable, defined by the following relation, which as you might have noted is exactly the core ratio of the exponent of e in the normal curve expression detailed earlier (excluding the coefficient of $-\frac{1}{2}$ and the power of 2),

$$z = \frac{\overset{\text{Measured value of } X}{x} - \overset{\text{Mean of } x \text{ values}}{\mu}}{\underset{\text{Standard deviation}}{\sigma}},$$

The standard unit of measurement z in effect translates the distance on the x axis, irrespective of the units of measurements used previously into z standard units. With this transformation, the normal curve becomes the standard normal curve as shown in Figure 19A.6 and expressed by the following equation:

$$y = f(z) = \frac{1}{\sqrt{2\pi}} \times e^{-\frac{1}{2}z^2} \quad \text{where } \mu = 0, \sigma = 1; \text{ random variable } x \text{ is now } z,$$

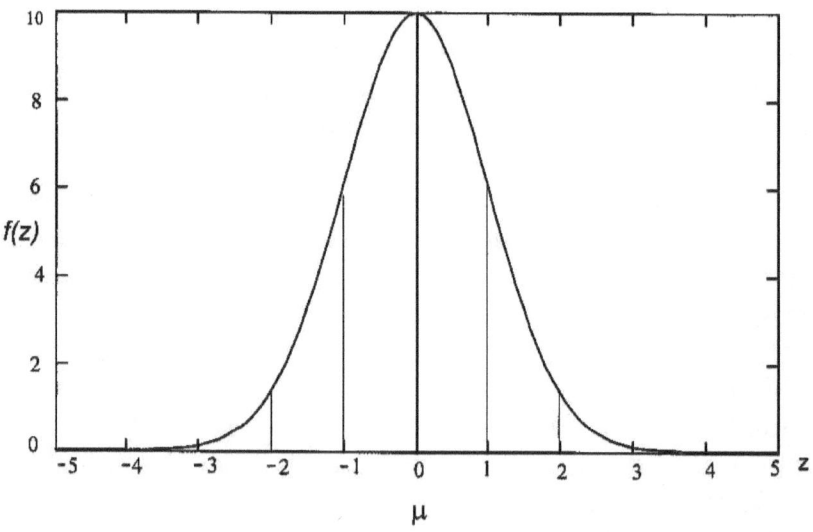

Figure 19A.6. Graph of the PDF of the heights distribution of the freshmen population transformed into a standard normal distribution.

where the standardized random variable is now z, the mean of the new random variable is $\mu_z = 0$, and its standard deviation is one unit, $\sigma_z = 1$. The exponent of the equation then becomes $-\frac{1}{2} z^2$. Note that the transformation left the normal curve essentially unchanged except for the adoption of zero as a point of reference for μ and z as a unit of measure for x.

This unique transformation corresponds to connection II of the triangular relationship binding the random variable to its standardized counterpart (Figure 19A.2, connection II).

The transformation is of course reversible, such that a given standard RV may be reconverted to its normal variant by reversing the standardization process as noted in connection I of Figure 19A.2. Thus, in order to retrieve the actual value of the random variable x, two standard deviations to the right of the mean, given $\sigma = 4$, and a $z = 2$, the first step, the reverse of connection II, arrive at the equivalent x point located eight units to the left of the 0 mean of Figure 19A.5.

$$x = u + z\sigma = 0 + 2 \times 4 = 8.$$

Finally, to retrieve the actual value of x, the reversal of substraction process is required to arrive at the original value; thus,

$$u + x = 70 + 8 = 78.$$

19A.3 The Standard Normal Distribution Curve

Once a normal curve is translated into a standardized format, all the x values on the original curve may be translated into z values so that the distance of an x value of seventy-four inches from the mean of seventy inches is equal to a corresponding distance of the z value from its mean of 0,

$$z = \frac{x - \mu}{\sigma} = \frac{74 - 70}{4} = 1 \text{ standard units.}$$

The areas under the curve delineated for the nonstandardized normal curve are identical to the areas defined by the corresponding standard z values.

From Figures 19A.3 and 19A.6, notice that a freshman seventy-four inches in height has a z score of 1, which means that his height is one standard deviation above the mean. A freshman whose height is sixty-four inches has a z score of $\dfrac{64-70}{4} = -\dfrac{6}{4} = -1.5$, which places his height at 1.5 standard deviation below the mean.

The main thrust of the standardized normal distribution curve is the ability to translate any range of randomly chosen x values into its standardized equivalent and thereby assign a probability value to the range of values under consideration. Thus, the probability that a student chosen at random from the freshman class population will be more that seventy-four inches tall may be formally expressed as follows:

$$P(X > 74") = P\left(\underbrace{\frac{74-70}{4}}_{} > \overset{z\,\text{score}}{1}\right) = \overset{\text{Probability}}{P}\ (z > 1).$$

Given the perusal of Figure 19A.4, $P(z > 1)$ is given by the area to the right of $z = 1$. Given that the area under the right half of the curve is coextensive with the tail that remains above the x axis, and given that the area under the either half of the curve is 0.5 or 50 percent of the area under the total curve, the area bounded by the z score of 1 is calculated as follows:

Without recourse to a table that shows the areas under the standard normal curve between zero (the mean of a standard normal variable) and a given z score, the perusal of the symmetrically divided curve into equal halves allows the visual estimation of the magnitude of the area involved. It can be readily appreciated that the area enclosed by $\pm 1z$ on either side of the mean is 68 percent of the area under the curve. Thus, half of the area between the central axis of the mean and the vertical grid line at $z = 1$ is 34 percent of the area under the curve. Accordingly, the area to the right of $z = 1$,

$P(x>4) = P(z > 1.0) = 0.5 - 0.3413 = 0.1587 \cong 0.16.$

Left half of the area under the curve	Area between $z =$ 1 and central axis	Area between $z =$ 1 and $+\infty$
0.5	$-$ 0.34	$=$ 0.16 or 16 percent.

Thus, the probability of a randomly selected freshman from the freshman population of the university taller than seventy-four inches is formally expressed as follows:

$P(x > 74 \text{ inches}) = P(z > 1) = 0.86.$

The probability of selecting a student shorter than or equal to seventy-four inches from the same population is expressed as follows:

$P(x \leq 74 \text{ inches}) = P(z \leq 1) = 0.86.$

Finally, the probability of selecting a student between seventy and seventy-five inches gets more complicated because we need to find the z value corresponding to seventy-five inches as follows:

$$z = \frac{x-\mu}{\sigma} = \frac{75-70}{4} = \frac{5}{4} = 1.25 \ z \text{ units.}$$

Reference to the table that shows the areas under the standard normal curve between zero (the mean of a standard normal variable) and the calculated z of 1.25 yields 0.3944, which is the exact probability of selecting a student whose height ranges from seventy to seventy-five inches.

Given a normal distribution, the use of standardized normal curve has made it possible to assign probabilities to areas under the curve cutoff by a vertical grid line passing through specifically designated z values, a fact that assumes a key role in statistical inference as will be seen later. As noted earlier, z is the standardized normal random variable unit that partitions the z axis into z units. Because a z of

±3.9 cuts off an area under the standard normal curve equivalent to 0.9999 of the total area, leaving 0.0001 of the area in the trailing tails on both sides, the values of z of practical concern normally fall within the range of ±3z, which accounts for 0.9974 of the total area, leaving just 0.0026 in both tails. Tables 19B.1-19B.3 and Figures 19A.7 and 19A.8 assign predefined percentages of the total area to the tail, areas, and their complements cutoff by specific z values that will find practical application later in the discussion.

In the discussion so far, the problem dealt with the conversion of the normal distribution to the standard normal distribution. The process can be equally reversed so that given an area of +0.16, it is possible to arrive at the original x value.

The process begins with the reverse subtraction: $0.5 - 0.16 = 0.3413$ = area to the left of the demarcated area of 0.16. Reverse consult of the z table assigns a score of 1 to the z parameter.

Finally, given $z = 1$ (and the prior knowledge of the normal distribution parameters of μ and σ), the original random variable x can now be determined as follows:

$$x = \mu - z\sigma = 70 + 1 \times 4 = 74.$$

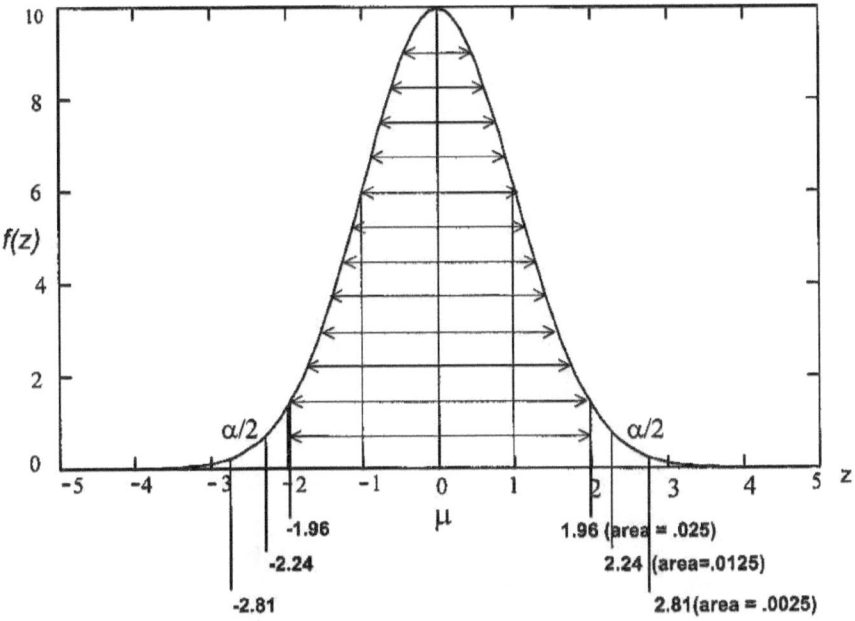

Figure 19A.7. Graph of the standard normal curve and three separate areas in both tails, marked off by their corresponding z values, each of which is the equivalent of $\alpha/2$.

Note that the tail areas marked off by specifically designated z values are referred to as α area of the curve to mark it off from the balance of the area designated as $1 - \alpha$. When considering both tails, the α area is obviously equally divided between the two tails, with each tail accounting for $\alpha/2$ so that the z value marking off the 5 percent for both tail ends is obviously not the same when the full 5 percent of the area is concentrated in one single tail. In the first case, a z value of ±1.96 accounts for 0.025 of the area in each tail; whereas for the single tail, a z value of 1.64 accounts for the full 5 percent in the single tail.

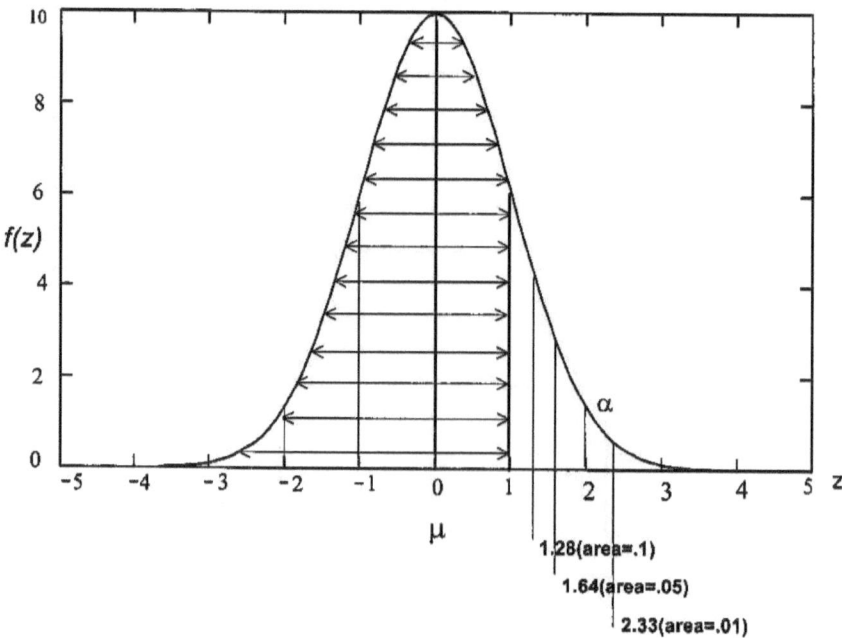

Figure 19A.8. Graph of the standard normal curve and three separate areas in one tail only, marked off by their corresponding z values, each of which is the equivalent of α.

Significance level. Total area in right tail of the standard normal curve between z and $+\infty$ from Table 19B.2	Corresponding complementary area between z and 0, the mean from Table 19B.1	Standard normal variable z_α marking off the right tail area
α	$0.5 - \alpha$	z_α
0.1 (0.1003)	0.4 (0.3997)	1.2817
0.05 (0.0505)	0.45 (0.4495)	1.645
0.025 (0.0250)	0.475 (0.4750)	1.96
0.01 (0.009)	0.49 (0.4901)	2.33
0.005 (0.0049)	0.495 (0.4951)	2.58

Table 19A.1. Critical normal deviate values: one-tailed tests

Significance level. Total area in the two tails of the standard normal curve	Area in one tail equivalent to one-half of the total area	Corresponding area between $\pm z$ and 0, the mean of the standard normal curve	Standard normal variable, $z_{\alpha/2}$, marking off one tail area only
α	$\alpha/2$	$0.5 - \alpha/2$	$z_{\alpha/2}$
0.1 (0.1010)	0.05 (0.0505)	0.45	1.64
0.05 (0.0500)	0.025 (0.0250)	0.4750	1.96
0.025 (0.0250)	0.0125 (0.0125)	0.4875	2.24
0.01 (0.0098)	0.005 (0.0049)	0.4950	2.58
0.005	0.0025	0.4975	2.81

Table 19A.2. Critical normal deviate values: two-tailed tests

Chapter 19B

Z Tables

Tables, normally relegated to the appendix, come under several formats, consistent with the demarcated area under the curve, which the author feels to be the most convenient to use. Irrespective of the format, the values in any one table may be derived from any other table because of the symmetry and standardization of the normal curve by simply adding or subtracting the given value to or from its complement.

The most common format is to table the area between a given z value and the mean of $f(z)$ or $\mu_z = 0$ as noted in Table 19B.1 and its corresponding normal curve. Tables 19B.2 and 19B.3 illustrate two complementary formats.

In Table 19B.2, the area between z and $+\infty$ is tabled. Table 19B.3 splits the area under the one tail of Table 19B.2 equally between the two tails.

As can be easily verified, the sum of any two corresponding values between Tables 19B.1, 19B.2, and 19B.3 adds up to 0.5 or one-half the total area under the curve. The values referred to in the text are printed in bold.

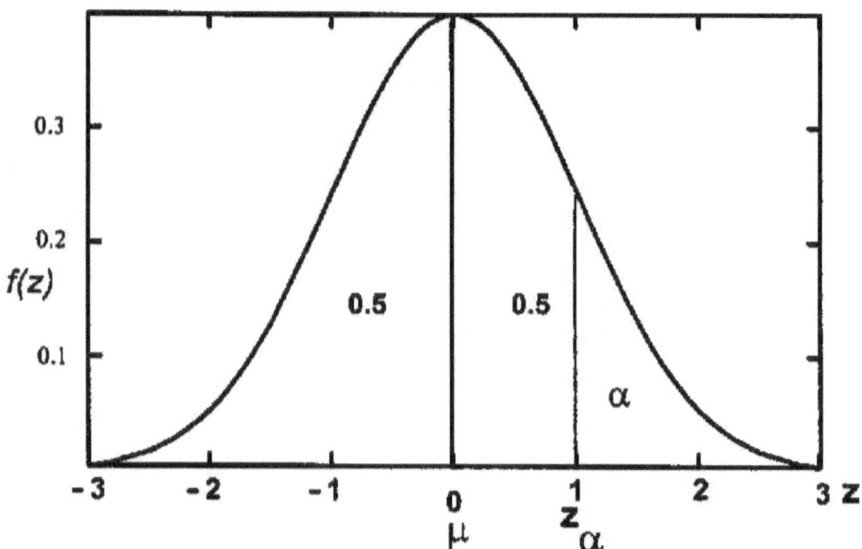

α or p refers to the single tail area partitioned off by the grid line through $|z|$ or the sum of the two tail areas partitioned by grid lines through $\pm z$.

To transform a one-tailed area into a two-tailed area, that is, to distribute the α area between the two tails such that each tail gets $\alpha/2$ area, divide the area by 2 and then locate the corresponding z for the $\alpha/2$. The z line will be pushed outward, resulting in greater numerical absolute value of $\uparrow|z|$. In other words, the smaller the tail area, the greater the absolute value of the z.

To transform a two-tailed area into a one-tailed area, double the size of the one-tailed area because the total area is now restricted to a one-tailed area. The z line is then pushed inward to accommodate the larger area, resulting in small numerical absolute value of $\downarrow|z|$. In other words, the larger the tail area, the smaller the $|z|$ value. For the same z value, that is, constant z line, to transform from one tail to two tails, simply double the α area in the one-tailed area.

Table 19B.1. An excerpted table of the area under the standard normal curve between the mean of 0 and the standard normal variable z

z	0.00	0.01	0.02	0.03	0.04	0.05	0.06	0.07	0.08	0.09
0.0	0.0000	0.0040	0.0080	0.0120	0.0160	0.0199	0.0239	0.0279	0.0319	0.359
1.0	**0.3413**	0.3438	0.3461	0.3485	0.3508	0.3531	0.3554	0.3577	0.399	0.3621
1.2	0.3849	0.3869	0.3888	0.3907	0.3925	**0.3944**	0.3962	0.3980	**0.3997**	0.4015
1.6	0.4452	0.4463	0.4474	0.4484	**0.4495**	0.4505	0.4515	0.4525	0.4535	0.4545
1.9	0.4713	0.4719	0.4726	0.4732	0.4738	0.4744	**0.4750**	0.4756	0.4761	0.4767
2.0	**0.4772**	0.4778	0.4783	0.4788	0.4793	0.4798	0.4803	0.4808	0.4812	0.4817
2.2	0.4861	0.4864	0.4868	0.4871	**0.4875**	0.4878	0.4881	0.4884	0.4887	0.4890
2.3	0.4893	0.4896	0.4898	**0.4901**	0.4904	0.4906	0.4909	0.4911	0.4913	0.4916
2.5	0.4938	0.4940	0.4941	0.4943	0.4945	0.4946	0.4948	0.4949	**0.4951**	0.4952
2.8	0.4974	**0.4975**	0.4976	0.4977	0.4977	0.4978	0.4979	0.4979	0.4980	0.4981
3.0	**0.4986**	0.4987	0.4987	0.4988	0.4988	0.4989	0.4989	0.4989	0.4990	0.4990

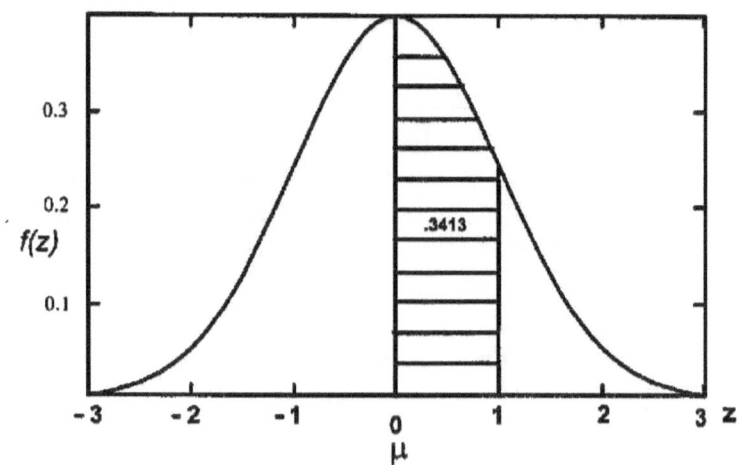

Table 19B.2. An excerpted table of the area under the standard normal curve (right tail) between the standard normal variable z and $+\infty$										
z	0.00	0.01	0.02	0.03	0.04	0.05	0.06	0.07	0.08	0.09
0.0	0.5000	0.4960	0.4920	0.4880	0.4840	0.4801	0.4761	0.4721	0.4681	0.4641
1.0	**0.1587**	0.1562	0.1539	0.1515	0.1492	0.1469	0.1446	0.1423	0.1401	0.1379
1.2	0.1151	0.1131	0.1112	0.1093	0.1075	0.1056	0.1038	0.1020	**0.1003**	0.0985
1.6	0.0548	0.0537	0.0526	0.0516	**0.0505**	0.0495	0.0485	0.0475	0.0465	0.0455
1.9	0.0287	0.0281	0.0274	0.0268	0.0262	0.0256	**0.0250**	0.0244	0.0239	0.0233
2.0	**0.0228**	0.0222	0.0217	0.0212	0.0207	0.0202	0.0197	0.0192	0.0188	0.0183
2.2	0.0139	0.0136	0.0132	0.0129	**0.0125**	0.0122	0.0091	0.0089	0.0087	0.0084
2.3	0.0107	0.0104	0.0102	**0.010**	0.0096	0.0094	0.0091	0.0089	0.0087	0.0084
2.5	0.0062	0.0060	0.0059	0.0057	0.0055	0.0054	0.0052	0.0051	**0.0049**	0.0048
2.8	0.0026	**0.0025**	0.0024	0.0023	0.0023	0.0022	0.0021	0.0021	0.0020	0.0019
3.0	**0.0014**	0.0013	0.0013	0.0012	0.0012	0.0011	0.0011	0.0011	0.0010	0.0010

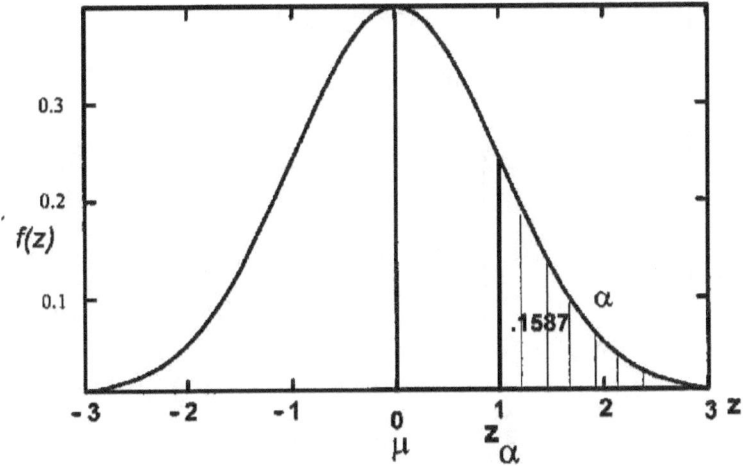

Table 19B.3. An excerpted table of the area under the standard normal curve (right and left tails) between the standard normal variable ±z and ±∞

z	0.00	0.01	0.02	0.03	0.04	0.05	0.06	0.07	0.08	0.09
0.0	1.000	0.9920	0.9840	0.9760	0.9680	0.9602	0.9522	0.9442	0.9462	0.9282
1.0	**0.3174**	0.3124	0.3078	0.3030	0.2984	0.2938	0.2892	0.2846	0.2802	0.2758
1.2	0.2302	0.2262	0.2224	0.2186	0.2150	0.2112	0.2076	0.2040	**0.2006**	0.1970
1.6	0.1096	0.1074	0.1052	0.1032	**0.1010**	0.0990	0.0970	0.0950	0.0930	0.0910
1.9	0.0574	0.0562	0.0548	0.0536	0.0524	0.0512	**0.0500**	0.0488	0.0478	0.0466
2.0	**0.0456**	0.0444	0.0434	0.0424	0.0414	0.0404	0.0394	0.0384	0.0376	0.0366
2.2	0.0278	0.0272	0.0264	0.0258	**0.0250**	0.0244	0.0238	0.0232	0.0226	0.0220
2.3	0.0214	0.0208	0.0204	**0.020**	0.0192	0.0188	0.0182	0.0178	0.0174	0.0168
2.5	0.0124	0.0120	0.0118	0.0114	0.0110	0.0108	0.0104	0.0102	**0.01**	0.0096
2.8	0.0052	**0.0050**	0.0048	0.0046	0.0046	0.0044	0.0042	0.0042	0.0040	0.0038
3.0	**0.0027**	0.0026	0.0026	0.0024	0.0024	0.0022	0.0022	0.0022	0.0020	0.0020

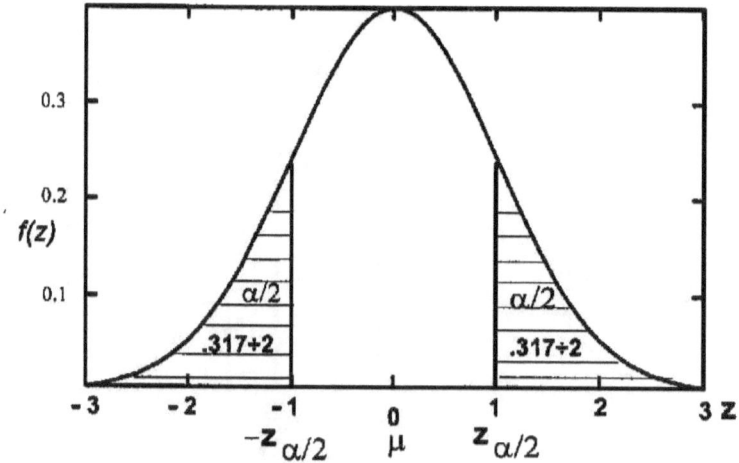

Table 19B.4. One-tailed tests		
Significance level. Total area in right tail of the standard normal curve between z and $+\infty$ from Table 19B.2	Corresponding complementary area between z and 0, the mean from Table 19B.1	Standard normal variable z_α marking off the right tail area
α	$0.5 - \alpha$	z_α
0.1 (0.1003)	0.4 (0.3997)	1.2817
0.05 (0.0505)	0.45 (0.4495)	1.645
0.025 (0.0250)	0.475 (0.4750)	1.96
0.01 (0.009)	0.49 (0.4901)	2.33
0.005 (0.0049)	0.495 (0.4951)	2.58

Table 19B.5. Two-tailed tests			
Significance level. Total area in the two tails of the standard normal curve	Area in one tail equivalent to one-half of the total area	Corresponding area between $\pm z$ and 0, the mean of the standard normal curve	Standard normal variable, $z_{\alpha/2}$, marking off one tail area only
α	$\alpha/2$	$0.5 - \alpha/2$	$z_{\alpha/2}$
0.1 (0.1010)	0.05 (0.0505)	0.45	1.64
0.05 (0.0500)	0.025 (0.0250)	0.4750	1.96
0.025 (0.0250)	0.0125 (0.0125)	0.4875	2.24
0.01 (0.0098)	0.005 (0.0049)	0.4950	2.58
0.005	0.0025	0.4975	2.81

Chapter 20

Statistical Inference
Estimation

20.1 Probability Revisited

The declared aim of this monograph is to help the reader from an intuitive grasp of the subtle and not-so-subtle meaning of probability. Note that the stress is on the intuitive, which the *Merriam-Webster's Dictionary of Synonyms* defines as "the highly personal capacity of passing directly from observation to comprehension without conscious intervention of reasoning . . ." The approach pursued in this monograph does not strictly comply with the given definition. However, the reasoning process involved has been sufficiently verbalized so as to bridge the logical gaps encountered in the assimilation process.

To this end, the initial approach in the formulation of probability was in terms the equally likely outcomes such that if an experiment had m equally likely outcomes, n of which are favorable to a given event, then the probability of that event is $\dfrac{n}{m}$. This approach, although intuitively obvious, is essentially a circular definition because the key words of "equally likely" is just another way of saying "equally probable" (Figure 20.1).

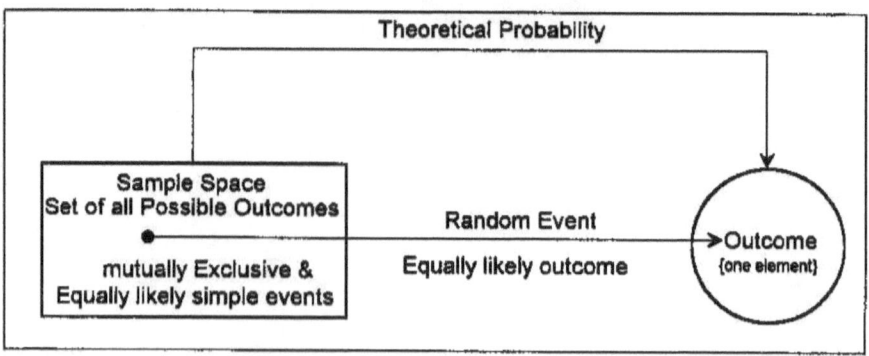

Figure 20.1. The equally likely outcome of a random event

The initial approach noted previously, largely based on the symmetry inherent in the games of chance, was further refined by introducing the concept of empirical probability where the phenomenon of frequency stabilization following repeated trials is bound to occur. In essence, the probability of an event is considered to be the relative frequency with which the event occurs over the long run, that is, following infinitely repeated trials (Figure 20.2).

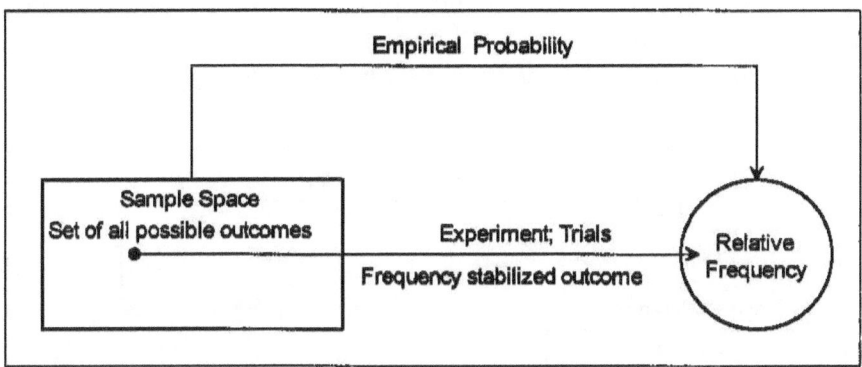

Figure 20.2. Empirical Relative frequency as function of infinitely repeated trials

In both the above "definitions," the probability of the event is a derivative of a well-defined sample space. In both cases, the probability of the event is conditional upon prior knowledge of the sample space.

In statistical terms, both attempts are geared to predict the probable occurrence or probable composition of a subset (sample) drawn from a defined sample space (population). It is manifestly obvious that the interest in the sample as derived from a given population is of limited practical use. The thrust of statistics, however, is exactly the reverse of what is collectively described as classical probability. The attempt in this case is to be able to infer the composition of the population (sample space) given the data provided by a sample, not just any sample (subset), but a "randomly" selected sample, that is, sample drawn in accordance with specific guidelines.

A partial attempt at such a reversal of priority is provided by Bayes' theorem. In here, as may have been made fairly clear, the population is estimated either subjectively or more often as obtained in clinical medicine, and the prevalence (estimated parameter) is known through experience or epidemiological survey. The sample data in this case offer a qualified entry (posterior probability) to modify and revise the initial tentative assumptions regarding the assumed parameter of the population. Bayes' theorem is thus a technique of inductive inference in which the opinion (prior probability) held before the experiment or test is integrated into the sample evidence, resulting in a modified or posterior probability (Figure 20.3).

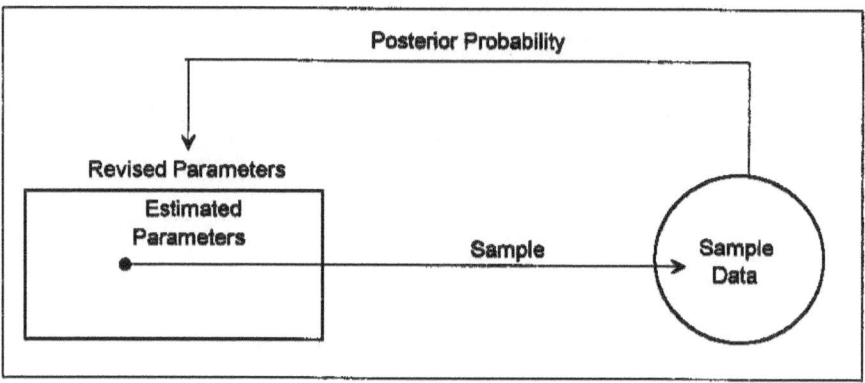

Figure 20.3

The final and the most comprehensive effort at complete reversal of priority, that is, to generalize from the known sample statistics to the unknown population at large, is provided by the powerful tools of statistical inference. Statistical inference as the name implies is a set of techniques of inductive inference based on the information obtained from a randomly selected sample that makes it possible to formulate predictive statements about the population from which the sample is derived (Figure 20.4).

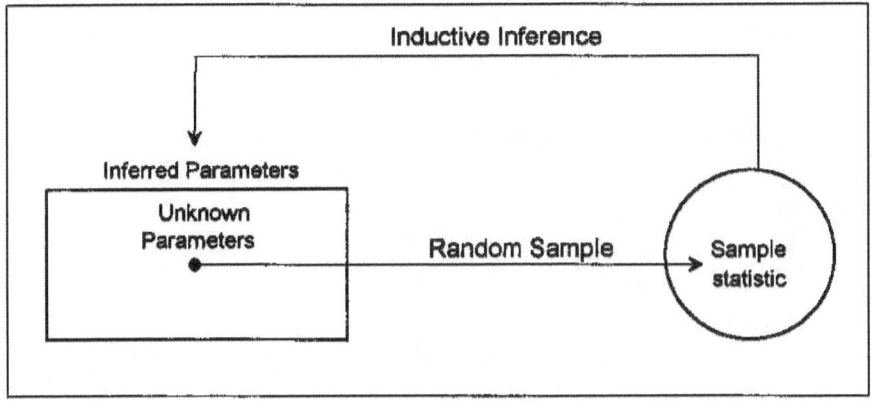

Figure 20.4

As an applied and practical technique, statistical inference develops into two related approaches that are normally separately covered. The first approach uses the technique of point and interval estimation as the inferential tool, whereas the second approach involves hypothesis testing within the framework of the null hypothesis as the tool of inductive inference.

20.2 The Interrelation Between Random Sample, Sampling Distribution, and Population

Statistical inference, the capacity to predict the hidden and sought after parameters of a given population from the simple statistic of a sample (a randomly selected sample to be specific), derives its potent power by the simple exploitation of the interrelation that obtains between the given sample, the sampling distribution, and the population from which the sample is purported to be derived. This trilogy of mutually related and interdependent themes uniting three interdependent entities comprised individual elements or members that form the infrastructure from which statistical inference inherits its claim for predictive authenticity (Figure 20.5).

The interdependent entities are defined by their statistic or their parameters as follows:

1. The random sample with $\overline{X}$ and s as the defining statistic
2. The population with μ and σ as the defining parameters
3. The sampling distribution of sample mean with $\mu_{\overline{x}}$ and $\sigma_{\overline{x}}$ as the defining parameters

The three connecting themes, on the other hand, define the linkage between the three entities:

1. The population-sampling distribution connection, relating the population to the sampling distribution of its sample means
2. The sample-sampling distribution connection, relating the random sample to its sampling origin
3. The sample-population connection, relating the random sample to the population, a process that defines the main thrust of statistical inference

20.3 Random Sample: The First Entity

The random sample is the first entity to be considered. In this context, the implication of random sampling needs to be fully appreciated. Its practical application mandates that every possible sample that could be derived from the population has an equal chance of being selected, which further begs the question as to how many samples are there in a given population. Because a sample can be defined as a single unique combination derived from the elements of the population being sampled, the possible number of samples, each consisting of r units, is the ubiquitous nCr, fully discussed in chapter 2. Stated in these terms, a random sample implies that each of the nCr samples has an equal opportunity of being selected.

To further put the problem of random selection and sampling in perspective note that given a population of twenty from which a sample of five elements is to be chosen, a total of 15,504 possible combinations of five units each are candidates for the choice of one random sample ($nCr = 20C5 = 15{,}504$).

From a population of fifty and a random sample of seven (a very modest enterprise), the number of possible samples is 99,884,400.00.

In dealing with real situations, the numbers are accordingly astronomical and irrelevant to the discussion, except as a prop to the understanding of the intricate relations of samples and population.

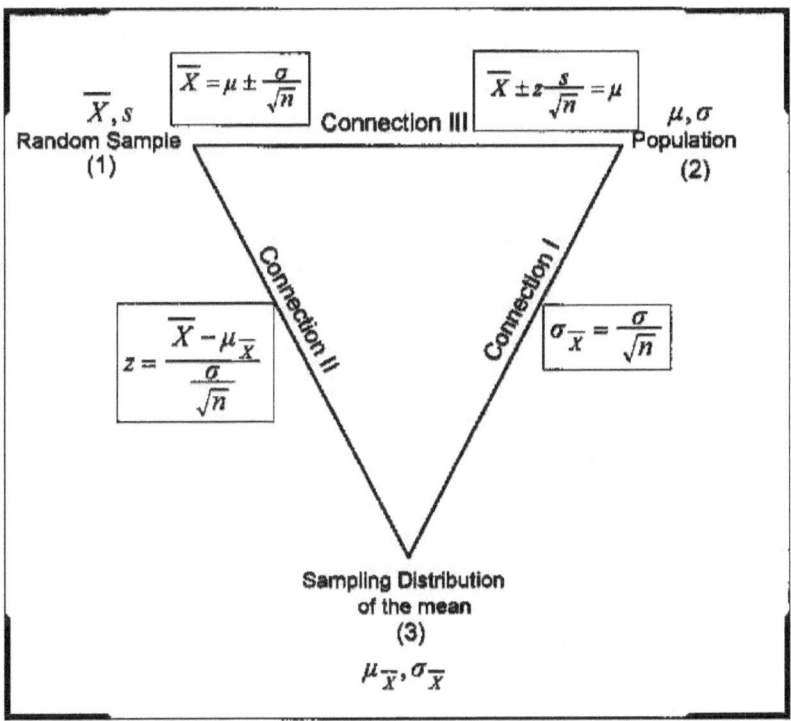

Figure 20.5. A schematic outline of the trilogy of connections, joining the interdependent statistical entities.

To highlight the relationship between sample, sampling distribution, and population, a crude physical analogy may serve as a bridge between the intuitive and the conceptual. A sample may be configured as a circular tent supported by a central pole with its tarpaulin roof sloping outward in the shape of a normal curve. In this sense, a vertical section through the tent with the central pole as its center is analogous to normal curve with the central axis at its center. The contents of the tent need to be made distinctly clear. A sample tent include individuals, units, and elements of a given population selected at random from the elements of the population such that every member of the population is as likely as any other member to be selected for this sample. In general, the number of units in the sample constitutes a small fraction of the population.

Now once the sample is thus selected, it becomes a random sample, which makes it perforce one particular sample out of the total number of possible samples of similar size dictated by nCr from the population. This is indeed a startling conclusion. An effort has been made to ensure that the sample obeys all the rules of random sampling so as to give equal opportunity of representation to every member of the population. Once done, the sample itself is pigeonholed as a specific member of the total number of possible samples that could be formed through the random selection process out of the total population.

This distribution guarantees that a random sample whose individual members were randomly selected may be considered in effect as a *preformed* sample randomly drawn from any one the available samples. To reiterate this point, the making of a random sample is equivalent to the drawing of the very same sample from the inventory of preformed possible samples.

20.4 Population: The Second Entity

To continue the analogy, the population tent from which the sample is derived may be similarly constructed, although as might be expected, it is now the big tent, which includes every member or element of the population under consideration. A census is the enumeration process that attempt to include every element of the targeted population. A finite population denotes the possibility of a count that includes all the elements of a targeted population. An infinite population, on the other hand, is a conceptual device used to account for repetitive data generated by an unending process. However, when the finite population is very large relative to the sample size, it is simpler to consider the finite population as infinite. In this case, sampling without replacement from an inexhaustible supply is theoretically identical to sampling with replacement from a finite population.

20.5 Sampling Distribution: The Third Entity

In order to categorize the linkage between the sample and the population, an intermediate distribution center is postulated that theoretically contains all the possible samples that can be chosen from the population. The distribution center does not contain samples as such because, as noted previously, 15,504 samples cannot be simultaneously selected from the population of twenty. The intermediate sampling center may be considered as a clearance station, under the roof of the population tent, for the storage and supply of the real random samples that can be drawn from the population on demand. In other words, the sampling center is unique in that it does not contain a specific number of the members of the population as in the sample tent nor the total number of the population as in the population tent. Its main content is the inventory of the samples that can be formed on demand from the population at large. In addition, the inventory of the samples is not just piled up haphazardly without any order inside the big tent. On the contrary, it is meticulously organized under a "normal"[20] roof around the central pole of the big tent (Figures 20.6 and 20.7).

The distribution center functions in this sense as an in-between station where all possible samples of a given size that can be formed from the population at large are stacked and arranged in such a way that those samples whose mean is closest to the population mean are stacked around the central pole, followed in descending order by the those whose means deviate from the population mean following the outline of the normal roof enclosing them. It is important to note that those samples whose mean is exactly the equivalent of the population mean are stacked within the central pole itself. The stacking order is continued until the distribution of the all the possible sample means of a given size that can be derived from the population are properly accounted for in the final inventory of the

---

[20] The assumption that the sampling distribution assumes a normal configuration is based on the central limit theorem, which predicts that the distribution of sample means approaches a normal distribution as the sample size increases, typically, $n = 30$ is considered large.

distribution of the sample means of a given size. A different stacking order and arrangement is automatically substituted for each sample size, such that the order and stacking spread is unique for every sample size that might be chosen.

The distribution of the stacks of sample means on and around the central pole of the big tent, which is in effect the mean of the population, is another way of saying that both the population and the sampling distribution share the same central pole as their central point of origin, so that the sample distribution and the population share the same identical mean. The only difference is that the stacking spread of the sample means is more concentrated around the center requiring greater height to accommodate all possible samples of a given size associated with a restricted lateral spread (Figures 20.6 and 20.7).

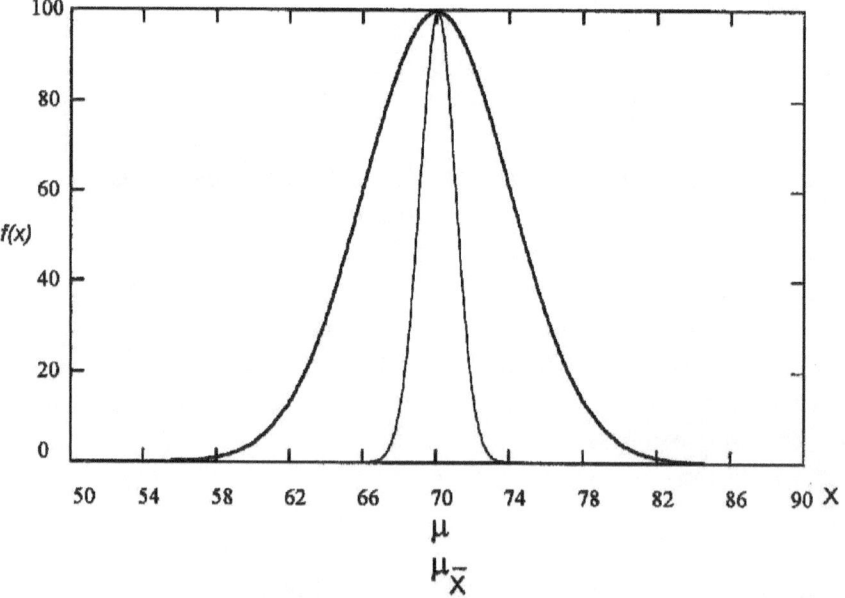

Figure 20.6. Distribution of sample means (light curve) derived from the student population, where $\mu = 70$ inches and n (sample size) $= 16$, resulting in a standard error of one inch compared with the population standard deviation of four inches. Note the narrow range of the standard error of the mean.

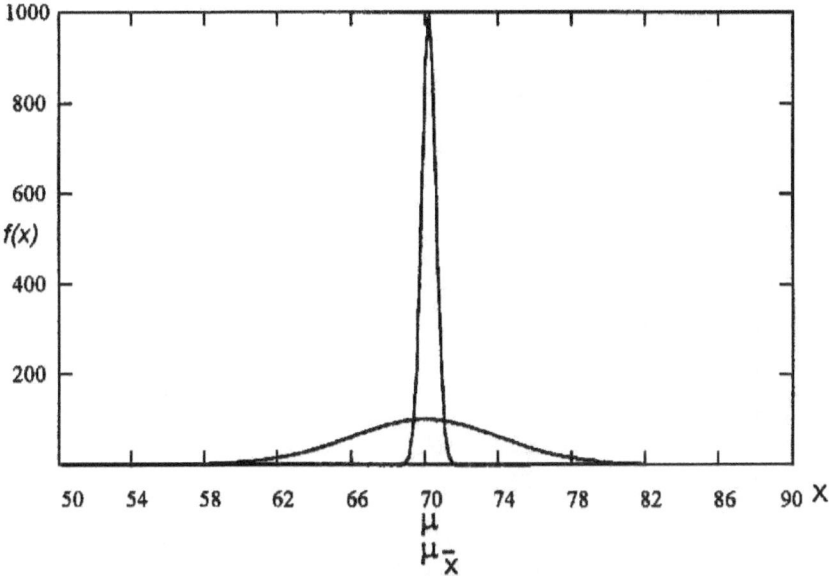

Figure 20.7. The sampling distribution of 1,000 sample means, derived from a sample of 1,000 students and plotted on the same scale. Note the narrow range of the standard error of the mean and the reduced area of the sample distribution relative to the sampling distribution.

20.6 The Population and Its Sampling Distribution: The First Connection

This stacking order can be better appreciated if the number of samples at a given distance from the central mean could be explicitly stated in terms of their distance from the central mean in standard units. Because the distribution of the sample means is similarly normal in configuration, it follows that all the sample means are stacked on both sides of the central axis with a frequency density in conformity with the height of the normal curve enclosing them. Within the constraints of the normal distribution, it follows that 68 percent of the total number of possible sample means that can be derived from the population are stacked within the range covered by one standard error of the mean (standard deviation) on both sides of the central mean of the population, μ, or its equivalent, the mean of the sampling distribution, $\mu_{\bar{x}}$ (Figure 20.8).

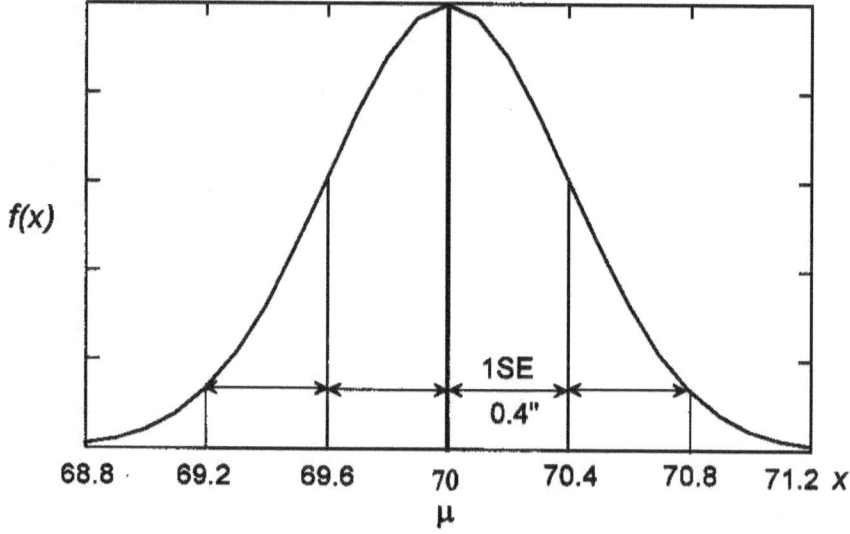

Figure 20.8. The sampling distribution of one hundred random sample means derived from the student population plotted on an amplified scale to show the narrow range of the standard error of the mean (standard deviation) ($\mu = 70$, $\sigma = 4$, $n = 100$).

Similarly, 95 percent of the total number of possible sample means would be contained within two standard errors and 99.7 within three standard errors. This last range of three standard errors on both sides of the population mean contains almost all, but not all, the possible sample means of the distribution. There remains 0.3 percent of the total number of possible samples whose mean extend beyond the ±3 standard error range.

The reader needs to be aware at all times that the distribution referred to concern sample means as distinct from the individual elements or units of measure that make up the population or the sample. In both cases, however, the percentage of the area under the normal curve marked off by corresponding standard deviation or z units remains the same (compare Graph 19-5 with Graph 19-6).

Note that the terms sampling distribution or distribution of the sample mean(s) refer only to the hypothetical distribution of the sample means referred to earlier. Similarly, the standard deviation of this hypothetical distribution is designated as standard error of the mean in order to mark its unique difference from the standard deviation of the real sample or population.

It is apparent that the population is less tightly distributed on and around the central pole than the sampling distribution. This in fact derived from the relationship of the standard deviation or dispersion of the population to the standard deviation or dispersion of its derived sample means as expressed in the following simple relation, which simply states that the larger the sample, the more likely that its sample mean will be sited nearer to the population mean and thus the shorter its displacement from the central pole (i.e., $\downarrow SE_{\overline{X}}$). On the other hand, for a given sample size, the spread of the population itself directly influences the proximity of the sample mean to the population mean (i.e., $\uparrow SE_{\overline{X}}$). As can be seen, the spread or dispersion of the sample means, that is, the standard error of sample means, is inversely proportional to the square root of the number of elements in the sample, that is, its assigned size, and directly proportional to the standard deviation of the population itself.

$$\underset{\substack{\text{Standard error} \\ \text{of sample mean}}}{SE_{\overline{X}}} = \underset{\substack{\text{Standard deviation} \\ \text{of sample mean}}}{\sigma_{\overline{X}}} = \frac{\overset{\substack{\text{Standard deviation} \\ \text{of the population}}}{\sigma}}{\sqrt{\underset{\substack{\text{Number of elements} \\ \text{in a sample}}}{n}}}$$

This relationship results in a tighter sampling spread with increase in sample size. Thus, quadrupling the sample size ($n \times 4$) reduces the standard error to one-half of its previous value. Despite this difference, the mean of the population and the mean of the sampling distribution remain one and the same.

$$\underset{\substack{\text{Population} \\ \text{mean}}}{\mu} = \underset{\substack{\text{Sampling distribution} \\ \text{mean}}}{\mu_{\overline{X}}}$$

20.7 Relation of the Sample Mean to the Sampling Distribution: The Second Connection (Known Population Parameters)

Recapitulating, given the population mean, μ, and given the standard deviation of the population, σ, a random sample of a given size, n, picked from the same population may be considered as derived from any one of the stacks surrounding the central mean, which literally extends to infinity on both sides at a gradually diminishing height.

Faced with a sample of a given size, known to be derived from a population whose mean and spread around the central axis (standard deviation) are known either through census or historical data, we are in the unique position of being able to precisely locate the point of origin of the mean of any randomly selected sample (once its mean has been calculated), that is, the location on the x axis of the stacking rank of the distribution of all the sample means from which this particular sample mean originated.

The mean of this sample is thus a point on the common x axis of both the total population and the distribution of the sample means where the central pole or y axis is also identically shared by both.

Our ability to pinpoint the exact location of the sample mean on the x axis of the sampling distribution was derived from the key relationship noted previously, relating the sample size to the sampling distribution, given that the standard deviation of the population, σ, is known, such that

$$SE_{\overline{X}} = \sigma_{\overline{X}} = \frac{\overset{\text{Known}}{\sigma}}{\underset{\text{Known}}{\sqrt{n}}}$$

This relationship is the formal recognition that the stacking order of the samples of a given size, that is, their dispersion or spread, $\sigma_{\overline{X}}$, from the common central axis of the sampling distribution and the population is directly related to the spread or standard deviation of the population itself, σ, so that the wider the population spread or dispersion, the more disperse the sampling distribution.

Conversely, the bigger the sample size, the more likely its contents are in effect a semireplica of the actual population spread itself and thus the more concentrated is its stacking order around the mean or the less disperse is its spread from the mean as symbolized by a smaller standard error of the mean or $\downarrow \text{SE}_{\bar{X}}$.

The logic of this analysis requires a revision that may have been apparent to the reader. The fact is that we have been able to pinpoint the location of our sample mean $\bar{X}$, only because we were able to derive the standard error of the mean, $\text{SE}_{\bar{X}}$, from the above relation, based on our prior knowledge of the population standard deviation and the sample size, which in turn allowed us to plot the sampling distribution that allowed us to pinpoint the location of the sample mean, $\bar{X}$ (Figure 20.9).

Once the sample mean is placed at its proper address, its relation to the population mean, μ, or the equivalent mean of the means, $\mu_{\bar{X}}$, becomes explicit. The sample mean may be smaller or larger than the sampling distribution mean, which places it to the left or to the right of the common mean, μ. More important, its actual distance from the common mean may be derived or measured either in terms of the units of the x axis or in terms of the standard error of the mean, $\sigma_{\bar{X}}$, or fraction thereof. It is the measurement of the actual distance that allows us to locate the particular stack from which this particular sample mean is derived. And what is more important to consider is the probability of its occurrence, which is the probability of deriving this particular random sample from the stacks that are normally distributed around the common mean.

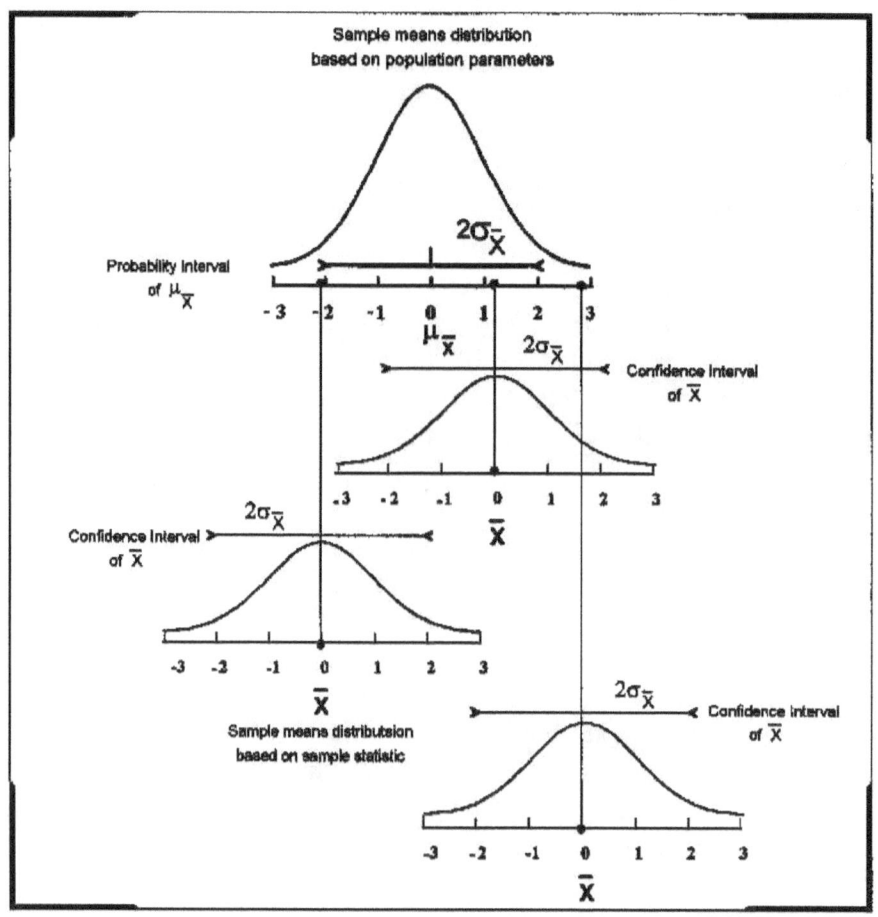

Figure 20.9. Chart of the relationship of probability interval to confidence interval.

The critical link is derived from the relationship of the sample mean, $\overline{X}$, to the mean of the sampling distribution, $\mu_{\overline{x}}$. In other words, the sample mean is in fact just one of the many means that cluster (stacked in an ordered sequence in conformity with the height of the normal curve defining the sampling distribution) on and around the sampling mean or identically the population mean $\mu_{\overline{x}} = \mu$.

In practical terms, the actual distance of the sample mean from the sampling mean (i.e., $\overline{X} - \mu_{\overline{x}}$) when divided by the standard error of the mean ($\sigma_{\overline{x}}$) translates the distance multiple of the standard error, expressed as standard z units. Simply stated, the ratio divides the distance $\left(\overline{X} - \mu_{\overline{X}}\right)$ by ($\sigma_{\overline{X}}$) to convert its original units into units of standard error.

$$\underset{\substack{\text{Sample} \\ \text{mean}}}{\overline{X}} - \underset{\substack{\text{Population} \\ \text{mean}}}{\mu} \over \dfrac{\sigma}{\sqrt{n}} = \frac{\overline{X} - \underset{\substack{\text{Sampling} \\ \text{mean}}}{\mu_{\overline{X}}}}{\underset{\substack{\text{Standard error} \\ \text{of the mean}}}{\sigma_{\overline{X}}}} = \pm z \ \text{standard error unit.}$$

This of course is the same analogous technique employed in the conversion of the normal curve into its standard format, where the x distance from μ was translated into standard z units.

$$\frac{\underset{\substack{\text{Measured} \\ \text{value of } X}}{x} - \underset{\substack{\text{Mean} \\ \text{of } x \text{ values}}}{\mu}}{\underset{\text{Standard deviation}}{\sigma}} = \pm z \ \text{standard unit.}$$

20.7.1 Probability versus Confidence

This last point requires further clarification. We are dealing here with a random sample derived from a known population. With the available data at our disposal in this given situation, we have been able to place the sample mean, $\overline{X}$, at its exact addressable stack, in exact mathematical relation to the common mean (population mean and sampling distribution mean). Moreover, because the sampling distribution is bell shaped or normal, the probability of drawing such a random sample is obviously related to its proximity to the central axis because the stacking height is proportionally less further from the central axis the sample mean is located. In other words, the probability of drawing a sample from within the area bounded by ±2 standard errors of the mean accounts for 95 percent of all the samples that may be randomly drawn. A sample mean located beyond two standard errors of the mean on either side of the central axis is really a rare occurrence because it accounts for only 5 percent of all the possible samples of a given size that can be randomly drawn from the population.

Nevertheless, in this scenario so far detailed, should the mean of our sample turns out to be placed beyond two standard errors of the mean, we are still obliged to conclude that the sample is in fact derived from the same population, although it happens to be a sample that is much less often, if not rarely, drawn from the population at large, that is, twenty-seven times out of 10,000 draws if the mean happens to be in either tail beyond three standard deviations.

20.8 Relation of the Sample Mean to the Sampling Distribution: The Second Connection (Unknown Population Parameters)

This verbose exposition may appear to be aiming at the wrong target because, as noted previously, we are neither in possession of the population mean, μ (a parameter that in real life is rarely known for sure unless a meticulous census is undertaken to include every possible member of the population), nor its standard deviation, σ (again essentially unknown in real life).

What we do have is a random sample, of a given size, n, knowingly derived from a certain designated population of our choice. In addition to the number of its elements or size, n, the sample yields on examination three additional pieces of information, two of which are solid exact data and the third is an estimated datum. Obviously, the sample mean, $\overline{X}$, and its standard deviation, s, are the two solid derived data calculated from the sample. The third estimated datum is the analog of the standard error of the mean derived normally from the population standard deviation, σ, and the sample size, n. Under the circumstances, in the absence of the critical population parameters of σ, we have no option but to substitute its cousin, s, the standard deviation of the sample itself, in order to obtain an estimated standard error of the mean.

The substitution of s for σ is not an irrational act as may seem on first sight. The fact that is readily appreciated is that a large sample tends to reflect the spread of its parent population, thus serving as a mini or semireplica of the population at large from which it is derived.

In this sense, the sample, if large enough, is considered as miniaturized version of the parent population, which allows us to forge the crucial link between population and sample.

From the sample data at hand, we were able to calculate the sample mean, $\overline{X}$, although we are unable so far to pinpoint its location on the sampling distribution of the means. The calculated standard deviation, s, is similarly a measure of how packed around the central axis the elements (not the means) of the sample are arrayed. The missing link that enables us to place the sample mean in exact relation to the sampling distribution of all the possible means is of course the population parameter σ that ties in $\overline{X}$ to the standard error of the sampling distribution. Now if the standard error of the sampling distribution could be based on the sample statistic of the calculated standard deviation, s, instead of σ of the population, the sought out linkage between sample and population may be bridged; thus,

$$\underbrace{\frac{s}{\sqrt{n}}}_{\substack{\text{Standard deviation}\\\text{of sample}}} = \underbrace{s_{\overline{X}}}_{\substack{\text{Standard deviation}\\\text{of sample mean}\\\text{sample}}} \cong \underbrace{\sigma_{\overline{X}}}_{\substack{\text{Standard deviation}\\\text{of sample mean}\\\text{population}}} = \underbrace{\frac{\sigma}{\sqrt{n}}}_{\substack{\text{Standard deviation}\\\text{of population}}}.$$

20.8.1 Probability versus Confidence

It is essential to grasp the implication of this substitution as to the actual placement of the sample mean in relation to the common central axis of the population mean or its equivalent, the mean of the sampling distribution of the means. Note that in this derivation, the sample mean $\overline{X}$ was in effect presumed to be the analog of the population mean, μ, so that $\overline{X}$ becomes the standard error of the mean derived from the sample n and s, in which s represents the analog of the population σ. In this context, $s_{\overline{X}}$ is the expression of the stacking order of the means centered at $\overline{X}$. However, because $s_{\overline{X}} \cong \sigma_{\overline{X}}$, we are now in a position to project $\overline{X}$ on the population axis and to infer that because the probability of drawing a given sample from the distribution of the sample means accounts for 95 percent of the total possible samples drawn, the inverse of this argument is that given a sample mean, $\overline{X}$, centered within a range of two standard errors, we may assume that the population mean, μ, or its equivalent the sampling distribution mean, $\mu_{\overline{X}}$, is to be found within this range with a confidence of 95 percent (Figure 20.10).

The logic of this proposition is important enough to repeat in different words; thus, if the sample mean drawn from within the range of ± 2 standard errors was removed from the central axis, that is, within $\pm 1.96\sigma_{\overline{x}}$ from the mean of the sampling distribution, $\mu_{\overline{X}}$, or its equivalent the population mean μ, then it can be correctly inferred that 95 percent of the sample means are within the $\pm 1.96\sigma_{\overline{x}}$ interval, which should include or just border on the population mean or its equivalent, the sampling distribution mean.

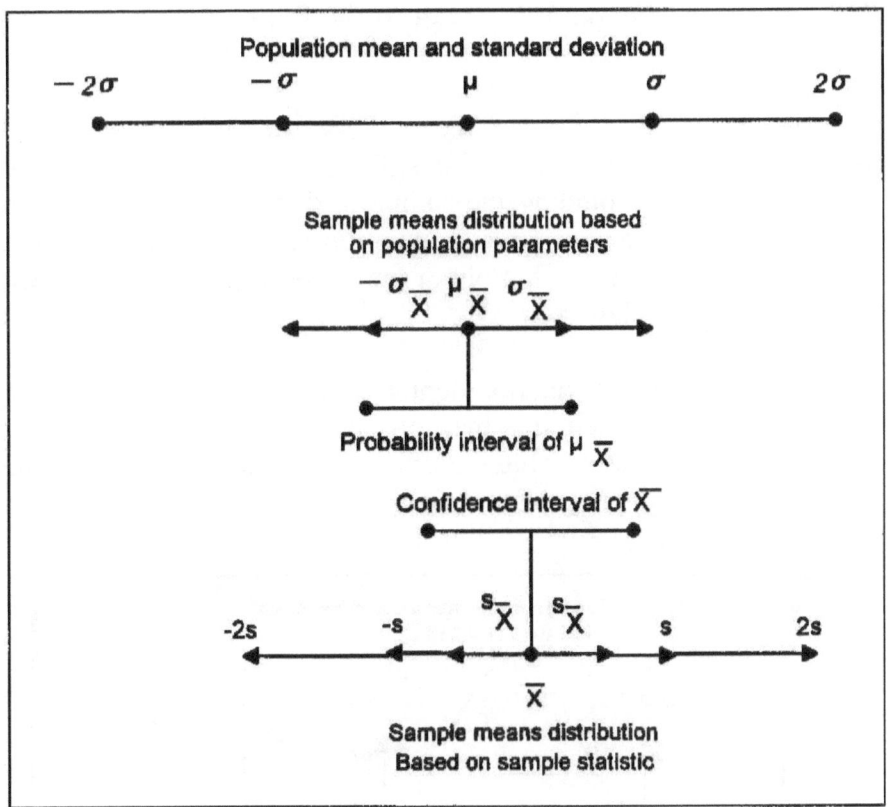

Figure 20.10

20.9 Relation of the Sample Mean to the Population Mean: The Third Connection (Known Population Parameters)

The critical linkage between the solitary sample mean and the population mean comes into focus from an appreciation of the intimate connection binding the sampling distribution of the mean for a given sample size in a population and the corresponding sampling distribution in a sample of the same size, randomly drawn from the same population.

As noted in the tripolar relation depicted in Figure 20.5, the linkage tying the two means requires the unifying concept of the sampling distribution of the mean, which in effect ties the sample mean to the population mean via the standard error of the mean, $\dfrac{\sigma}{\sqrt{n}}; \dfrac{s}{\sqrt{n}}$.

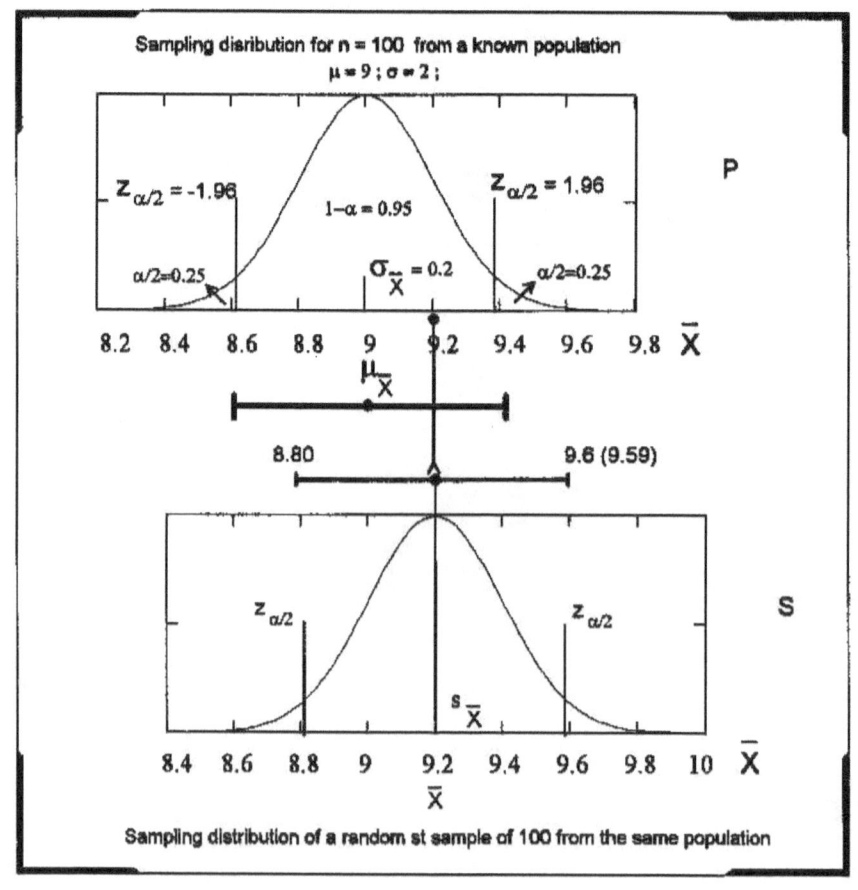

Figure 20.11A

To put the relation in a practical perspective, consider the average response time of nine minutes with a standard deviation of two minutes computed from the log entries of an emergency medical unit over a period of several years (population).

Given the standard deviation of the population, the standard error of the mean of the sampling distribution of a sample for $n = 100$ is readily derived as follows:

$$\sigma_{\overline{X}} = \frac{\sigma}{\sqrt{n}} = \frac{2}{\sqrt{100}} = 0.2 \text{ standard error of the mean.}$$

The normal density curve of the sampling distribution of samples of size $n = 100$ may now be plotted given $\sigma_{\overline{X}} = 0.$ and $\mu_{\overline{X}} =$, as shown in the distribution curve P of Figure 20.11A. From P, it can be readily noted that 95 percent of the samples are stacked under the density curve between $\pm z_{\alpha/2} = \pm 1.96$ The balance of 5 percent is split between the wings of the curve.

The boundaries of the interval accounting for 95 percent of all the sample means of $n = 100$, $\overline{X}$, may be computed as follows:

Upper limit of $\overline{X} : \mu_{\overline{X}} + \left[1.96 \cdot \sigma_{\overline{X}}\right] = 9 + [1.96 \times 0.2] = 9 + 0.392 = 9.392 \cong 9.4$ minutes

Lower limit of $\overline{X} : \mu_{\overline{X}} - \left[1.96 \cdot \sigma_{\overline{X}}\right] = 9 - [1.96 \times 0.2] = 9 - 0.392 = 8.608 \cong 8.6$ minutes

This effectively states that 95 percent of all the sample means of size $n = 100$ fall within a range of 8.6 to 9.4 minutes.

Consider now a random sample of one hundred calls, collected during the same time from the same population as a quality control measure. A sample mean $\overline{X}$ of 9.2 minutes was obtained. Because the standard deviation was considered the same as that of the population from which it was drawn, the sampling distribution was plotted based on the same scale as shown in the normal density curve S of Figure 20.11A.

From S, it can be similarly shown, that the area bounded by 9.2 + 0.392 = 9.592 ≅ 9.6 minutes on the right and by 9.2 − 0.392 = 8.808 ≅ 8.8 minutes on the left accounts for 95 percent of the samples in a sampling distribution based on the statistic of one random sample of $n = 100$.

The relationship between the sampling distribution of the mean based on the population parameters for samples of $n = 100$ size and the sampling distribution of the mean for the same size samples based on the statistic of a random sample ($\overline{X}$ of 9.2 minutes and $\sigma_{\overline{X}}$ of 0.2) known to be derived from the same population bears a closer scrutiny.

- Note that the sample mean of 9.2 in S is derived from the $1 - \alpha$ area of the population-sampling distribution P. Furthermore, its exact site of origin can be pinpointed with accuracy on the $\overline{X}$ axis of P.
- All sample means in the range of 8.6 to 9.4 minutes from the $1 - \alpha$ area of P are the potential candidates of random sampling, and as such, it is possible to pinpoint their origin on the $\overline{X}$ axis of P, and what is more significant is that the probability interval of which they are the central point always includes the population mean in its range.
- The interval centered at 9.2 and bounded by 9.6 minutes on the right and 8.8 minutes on the left is accordingly wide enough to include the population mean in its range.
- Recall that the stacking order (distance from the central axis or density) of the sampling distribution determine the probability of a given sample, which is another way of saying that random sampling is selectively biased in favor of samples in the $1 - \alpha$ area and even more so from the central area surrounding the central axis.

Thus, given a sample whose origin from a known population is confirmed, the following conclusions may be derived from the relationship:

1. The sample mean, $\overline{X}$, is a close approximation of the population mean, μ, because it can be placed in close proximity to μ, on the sampling distribution $\overline{X}$ axis of P.
2. The range of values within which the sample mean is centered is guaranteed to include the population mean in its range with a high degree of confidence.

This linkage between the sample mean and the mean of the sampling distribution given the sample size is formalized in the following equation reprinted from previous discussion.

$$\underset{\substack{\text{Standard Error}\\\text{of the mean}}}{\underset{\sigma_{\overline{X}}}{\underbrace{\frac{\overset{\substack{\text{Sample}\\\text{Mean}}}{\overline{X}} - \overset{\substack{\text{Sampling}\\\text{Mean}}}{\mu_{\overline{X}}}}{}}} = \overset{\substack{\text{Distance of }\overline{X}\\\text{from }\mu_{\overline{X}}}}{\frac{\overline{X} - \mu_{\overline{X}}}{\frac{\sigma}{\sqrt{n}}}} = \overset{\substack{\text{Distance of }\overline{X}\\\text{from }\mu}}{\frac{\overline{X} - \mu}{\frac{\sigma}{\sqrt{n}}}} = \pm z \text{ standard error units.} \quad (20.1)$$

As noted earlier, the above-mentioned relation converts the distance of the sample mean $\overline{X}$ from the sampling distribution mean $\mu_{\overline{X}}$ or its equivalent the population mean μ into standard error units or its equivalent standard z units. The conversion in effect pinpoints the site of origin of the sample mean, $\overline{X}$, on the $\overline{X}$ axis of P in z standard units, on either sides of $\mu_{\overline{X}}$. Thus, $\dfrac{9.2 - 9}{0.2} =$ which places the sample mean of 9.2 at its exact point of origin from the bounded interval of $1 - \alpha$. It would be desirable and more informative if the distance of $\overline{X}$ from $\mu_{\overline{X}}$ can be explicitly stated. A simple transformation of equation (20.1) yields

$$\boxed{\overline{X} - \mu_{\overline{X}} = \pm z \cdot \sigma_{\overline{X}} = \pm z \cdot \frac{\sigma}{\sqrt{n}}}$$

$$\overline{X} = \mu_{\overline{X}} \pm \left[z \bullet \sigma_{\overline{X}} \right] = \mu_{\overline{X}} \pm \left[z \bullet \frac{\sigma}{\sqrt{n}} \right] \qquad (20.2)$$

Transposing and rearranging yields

$$\mu_{\overline{X}} - \left[z \bullet \frac{\sigma}{\sqrt{n}} \right] \leq \overset{\text{Sample mean}}{\overline{X}} \leq \mu_{\overline{X}} \pm \left[z \bullet \frac{\sigma}{\sqrt{n}} \right]$$

This now states that the sample mean $\overline{X}$ is located between the two values of $\pm z_{\alpha/2}$ on either side of $\mu_{\overline{X}}$.

From the above-mentioned relation, the exact location of $\overline{X}$, relative to the mean of the sampling distribution $\mu_{\overline{X}}$, may now be computed as $(9 + (1 \times 0.2) = 9.2$. Note that the solution of the equation, that is, the exact localization of the sample mean, $\overline{X}$, requires prior knowledge of the population parameters μ and σ as well as the sample statistic, n (Figure 20.11B).

For an assigned z value (Tables 19B.3 and 19B.5, chapter 19B) of ± 1.96, $\overline{X}$ can be addressed to its location on the $\overline{X}$ axis between $\mu_{\overline{X}} \pm \left[1.96 \bullet \sigma / \sqrt{n} \right]$.

$$\mu_{\overline{X}} - \left[1.96 \bullet \frac{\sigma}{\sqrt{n}} \right] \leq \overline{X} \leq \mu_{\overline{X}} \pm \left[1.96 \bullet \frac{\sigma}{\sqrt{n}} \right]$$

The probability that a sample mean, $\overline{X}$, will be found lying within the bounded interval on the $\overline{X}$ axis of the sampling distribution may then be derived from the following relation:

$$P \left(\mu_{\overline{X}} - \left[1.96 \times \sigma_{\overline{X}} \right] \leq \overline{X} \leq \mu_{\overline{X}} \pm \left[1.96 \times \sigma_{\overline{X}} \right] \right) = 1 - a = 1 - 0.05 = 0.95$$

Thus, the boundaries of the probability interval within which there is a 95 percent probability that the sample mean $\overline{X}$ would lie corresponding to the 95 percent of the area under the standard normal curve may be computed as follows:

$$\text{Upper limit of } \overline{X}: \mu_{\overline{X}} + \left[1.96 \cdot \sigma_{\overline{X}}\right] = \mu_{\overline{X}} + \left[1.96 \cdot \frac{\sigma}{\sqrt{n}}\right]$$

$$\text{Lower limit of } \overline{X}: \mu_{\overline{X}} - \left[1.96 \cdot \sigma_{\overline{X}}\right] = \mu_{\overline{X}} - \left[1.96 \cdot \frac{\sigma}{\sqrt{n}}\right]$$

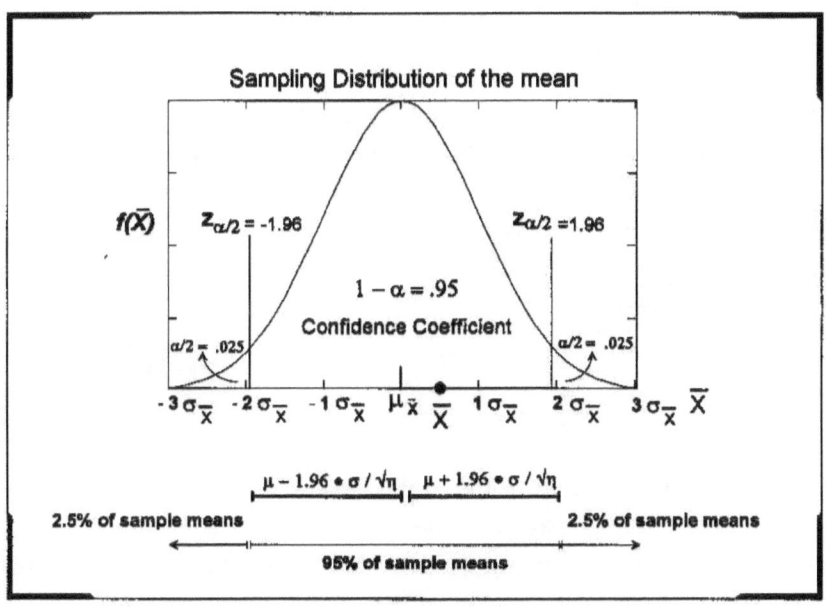

Figure 20.11B

By defining the probability interval in terms of the known population parameters, μ and σ, we were able to assert that a randomly chosen $\overline{X}$ lies within the bounded interval with 95 percent probability.

A more pertinent question would be to define the interval within which μ would lie given a sample mean $\overline{X}$ at its center. In other words, define the boundaries of the interval in terms of the known $\overline{X}$ and σ, which would include μ with a certain measure of confidence.

In this ideal setup, where the parameters of the population are given, the same equation defining $\overline{X}$ is applicable by simply switching the variables in equation (20.2) to reformat the equation in terms of μ as $\overline{X}$ and σ as follows:

$$\mu = \overline{X} \pm z \bullet \sigma_{\overline{X}} = \overline{X} \pm z \bullet \frac{\sigma}{\sqrt{n}}$$

(20.3)

Equation (20.3) establishes an interval within which μ would lie, which in turn may be rewritten to stress that μ is now located within an interval on either side of the sample mean $\overline{X}$ between values $\overline{X} \pm [z \bullet \frac{\sigma}{\sqrt{n}}]$, as follows:

$$\overline{X} - \left[z \bullet \frac{\sigma}{\sqrt{n}} \right] \leq \overset{\text{Population}}{\underset{\text{mean}}{\mu}} \leq \overline{X} + \left[z \bullet \frac{\sigma}{\sqrt{n}} \right]$$

From the previously mentioned relation, the location of μ, relative to the sample mean, may now be computed ($9.2 + [1.96 \times 0.2] = 9.592 \cong 9.6$). Note once again that the solution of the equation, that is, the localization of μ relative to the sample mean, requires prior knowledge of the sample mean $\overline{X}$, the population standard deviation σ, as well as the sample number n.

For an assigned z value (Tables 19B.3 and 19B.5, chapter 19B) of ± 1.96, the probability that the population mean or its equivalent the sampling distribution mean $\mu = \mu_{\overline{X}}$ will lie within the bounded interval centered at $\overline{X}$ is stated with 0.95 confidence, as follows:

$$P\left(\overline{X}-\left[1.96 \cdot \frac{\sigma}{\sqrt{n}}\right] \le \mu \le \overline{X}+\left[1.96 \cdot \frac{\sigma}{\sqrt{n}}\right]\right)=1-a=1-0.5=.95$$

Thus, the confidence interval centered at $\overline{X}$ within which the population mean would lie with 95 percent confidence may be computed as follows:

Lower confidence limit of $\mu : \overline{X}-\left[1.96 \cdot \dfrac{\sigma}{\sqrt{n}}\right]$
Upper confidence limit of $\mu : \overline{X}+\left[1.96 \cdot \dfrac{\sigma}{\sqrt{n}}\right]$

We are dealing here with two separate intervals of equal width. The one centered at the population mean, μ, corresponds to the probability of a randomly drawn sample from the population-sampling distribution of sample means. The second interval centered at the sample mean $\overline{X}$ corresponds to the probability of containing μ within its span of equivalent range. And because the sample mean may be retraced to its site of origin on the probability interval of the population-sampling distribution with a probability of 95 percent, then its span would include μ with 95 percent probability.

In this instance, the question might be raised as to how confident are we that the interval would indeed contain μ? If $\pm z$ is made to equal 1.96, we are in effect 95 percent confident that μ would be contained within the interval. Because 95 percent of all samples of size n are contained within the $1 - \alpha$ area, and because the probability of randomly drawing a sample from the sampling distribution is similarly 95 percent, then the probability of that the interval spanning the sample mean includes μ in its range is equally 95 percent.

However, in the unrealistic situation under discussion, given $\overline{X}$ and the population parameters μ and σ, we are in a position to place $\overline{X}$ at the very same site from which it was derived. Once placed, its actual distance from the population mean, μ, may be determined in standard units from equation (20.1). In this case, because σ, z, and $\overline{X}$ are defined, we are 100 percent confident that μ is within the interval.

The interplay of these two intervals depend of course on the site of origin of $\overline{X}$. Should $\overline{X}$ by chance be identical to the population mean, μ, the two intervals are coextensive and on overlapping.

At the other extreme, $\overline{X}$ may be derived from the very margin of the interval. In this case, the confidence interval would just include the population mean, μ. For any $\overline{X}$ originating from within, the probability interval would most certainly include the μ in its range.

20.10 Relation of the Sample Mean to the Population Mean: The Third Connection (Unknown Population Parameters)

To return to the real world in which the only available information is to be derived from the sample at hand, we are forced to resort to the linkage established earlier between s and σ, allowing us to substitute the following practical relation for the unavailable ideal one:

$$
\underset{\substack{\text{Standard deviation} \\ \text{of sample}}}{\frac{s}{\sqrt{n}}} = \underset{\substack{\text{Standard deviation} \\ \text{of sample means} \\ \text{Sample}}}{s_{\overline{X}}} \cong \underset{\substack{\text{Standard deviation} \\ \text{of sample means} \\ \text{Population}}}{\sigma_{\overline{X}}} = \underset{\substack{\text{Standard deviation} \\ \text{of population}}}{\frac{\sigma}{\sqrt{n}}}
$$

In this case, the probability interval for $\overline{X}$ is restated in terms of s rather than σ as noted below, in which case we are assuming that $s \cong \sigma = (\sigma_{\overline{X}} \times \sqrt{n})$,

$$\boxed{\text{Sample mean}\;\; \overline{X} \;\; = \mu \pm \left[z{\scriptstyle\bullet} s_{\overline{X}} \right] = \mu \pm \left[z{\scriptstyle\bullet}\dfrac{\overset{\text{Standard deviation of sample}}{s}}{\underset{\text{Number of elements}}{\sqrt{n}}} \right]}$$

Similarly, in order to address the more pertinent question of defining the interval within which μ would lie given s and $\overline{X}$, we are forced once more to make the necessary substitution in equation (20.3), noted as follows:

$$\mu = \overline{X} \pm z{\scriptstyle\bullet} s_{\overline{X}} = \overline{X} \pm z{\scriptstyle\bullet}\frac{s}{\sqrt{n}} \qquad\qquad (20.3a)$$

Equation (20.3a) establishes an interval within which μ would lie, which in turn may be rewritten to stress that μ is now located within an interval on either side of the sample mean $\overline{X}$ between values $\overline{X} \pm [z{\scriptstyle\bullet}\frac{s}{\sqrt{n}}]$,

$$\overline{X} - \left[z{\scriptstyle\bullet}\frac{s}{\sqrt{n}} \right] \leq \mu \leq \overline{X} + \left[z{\scriptstyle\bullet}\frac{s}{\sqrt{n}} \right]$$

Unlike the previous hypothetical case, we are dealing here with the implicit relationship between two distinct separate intervals derived from two distribution curves. The first is derived from the distribution of the sample means given the population standard deviation σ and the size n of the samples centered at the population mean μ, whereas the second interval centered at the sample mean $\overline{X}$ is derived from the sampling distribution based on the sample standard deviation s and the size n of the sample.

As in the previous case, the probability interval encloses 95 percent of all the possible samples of size n that can be derived from the population. Its boundaries remain the same as in the previous case. The confidence interval, on the other hand, is derived from the distribution of the sample means based on the standard deviation of the sample, s, and its size, n.

In this case, $\overline{X}$ is the point estimate of μ and the confidence interval centered at $\overline{X}$ within which the population mean would lie 95 percent confidence may be computed as follows:

Lower confidence limit of $\mu : \overline{X} - \left[1.96 \bullet \dfrac{s}{\sqrt{n}} \right]$
Upper confidence limit of $\mu : \overline{X} + \left[1.96 \bullet \dfrac{s}{\sqrt{n}} \right]$

In the first case, given knowledge of the population, 95 percent of all sample means are stacked in the interval extending $1.96\sigma_{\overline{x}}$ on either side of the population mean, μ, or its equivalent the sampling distribution mean, $\mu_{\overline{x}}$.

In the second case, $\overline{X}$ is at the center of an interval extending on both sides of the sample mean assumed to be approximately of equal width with the first interval. Because 95 percent of all possible samples are derived from the stacks bounded by the sampling distribution interval $\mu \pm 2\sigma_{\overline{x}}$, the reverse inference is that a given sample mean is assumed to be derived from the stacks bounded by the first interval with 95 percent probability. Stated differently, because 95 percent of all sample means are within 1.96 standard error of the mean from the population mean, it follows that a given random sample is most likely to be one of the 95 percent of the samples surrounding the population mean.

Therefore, we can state with 95 percent confidence that the population mean (not the sample mean) is within $\pm$ 1.96 standard error of the mean from the sample mean.

Subsequently, when $\overline{X}$ is located on the common population-sample distribution axis anywhere within the $\mu \pm 2\sigma_{\overline{x}}$ interval, one can be confident that the interval centered at $\overline{X}$ will include μ in its span as well, with a 95 percent confidence. In 5 percent of the cases, the $\overline{X}$ will fall beyond the limits of $\mu \pm 1.96\sigma_{\overline{x}}$, and its interval will not include the population mean, μ.

The exact location of $\overline{X}$ on the common population-sampling axis cannot be determined with certainty if σ is unknown. However, because $s_{\overline{x}}$ is an estimate of $\sigma_{\overline{x}}$, $\overline{X}$ may be derived from any one stack within $1.96\sigma_{\overline{x}}$ range of the actual sampling distribution. Nevertheless, irrespective of its position with respect to the population-sampling mean, one can ascertain with 95 percent confidence that the population-distribution mean is to be found within the range of designated interval.

When μ and σ are known, the standard deviation of the sample means, that is, $\left(\sigma_{\overline{x}} = \dfrac{\sigma}{\sqrt{n}}\right)$, can be easily computed. With this new information, any $\overline{X}$ can now be assured to be the center of an interval roughly equivalent to the interval enclosing $\mu_{\overline{x}}$. It now can be said with 95 percent confidence that the interval $\overline{X} \pm z \times \sigma_{\overline{x}} = 1.96 \times \sigma_{\overline{x}}$ will contain within its boundary, the mean of the population, μ.

20.11 Statistical Estimation

The previously mentioned exposition was intended to provide the necessary theoretical background to the first of two statistical inference procedures that go under the name of estimation, which may take the form of either a point estimation or an interval estimation. An estimate is thus a specific numerical value designed to answer a query concerning a population parameter, as represented by the following examples.

1. The average amount of time hospital patients (population) spend in the ICU prior to transfer
2. The SAT score of all applicants for admission to medical school A
3. The proportion of patients in a hospital who are HMO subscribers

The scenario in this case differs from the one postulated earlier where the parameters of the population were a given. In this setup, a random sample is drawn from a defined population whose parameters are unknown. Once the sample statistics are calculated, an estimate of the unknown population parameters is considered.

At the simplest level, the question requires an estimate, that is, a single numerical value categorizing the mean or proportion of the population, given the statistic of a single random sample.

At a more appropriate level, the estimate requires defining an interval specified by an upper and lower boundary within which the population parameter, the mean or proportion in the above cases, is supposed to lie. Furthermore, it is important to assign a confidence level to the assumptions involved in the proposed interval.

20.11.1 The Point Estimate

Point estimate is a straightforward attempt at statistical inference designed to estimate the parameters of the population from the available statistics of a sample. As such, it represents the simplest and most obvious corollary of the connection between sample and population. Because the estimate involves a single value calculated from the sample, the designation of a point estimate is apt.

Point estimate is thus a literal estimate of the population parameters σ and μ calculated from the sample such that $\overline{X}$, the sample mean, is an estimate of the population mean, μ, and the sample standard deviation, s, is an estimate of the population standard deviation, σ.
This is a rough estimation of population parameters based on data derived from one sample. It is unrealistic to expect that any one of the thousands of possible samples to have the exact mean and standard deviation of the population from which it is derived. What can be expected, based on the sampling distribution of all possible sample means of size n on and around the population mean, is that the sample mean of a random sample $\overline{X}$ is more often than not to be a close neighbor of the population mean and thus a good estimate of the population μ.

A study was ordered to investigate the average response time of the Emergency Ambulance Service because of recent allegations claiming unusual delays. Accordingly, from the dispatcher's log book, a random sample of one hundred calls was selected for evaluation and analysis from the roster of calls covering the recent period of 1 month.

Following standard procedure, the response time of each call was calculated as the elapsed period starting with the receipt of the 911 call at the dispatcher's console and ending with the return call from the EMS on arrival at the scene.

From the individual response time of each call, an average response time of ten minutes was obtained. The sample standard deviation was calculated at three minutes (Figure 20.12).

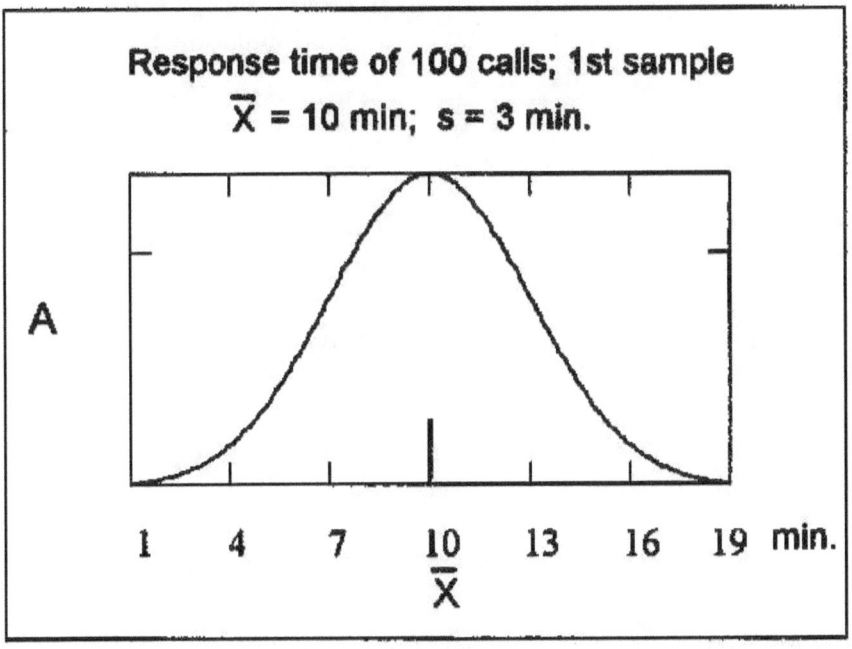

Figure 20.12

From these initial sample statistics, the corresponding point estimates of the population parameters μ (population mean) and σ (population standard deviation) were suggested to be identically ten and three minutes, respectively.

The formula used to compute the estimate from the given sample is the same employed in deriving the sample mean and its standard deviation, so that

$$\mu(\text{estimated}) = \overline{X},$$
$$\sigma(\text{estimated}) = s.$$

It is important to realize that the estimates of the population parameters will vary from one sample to another. However, the formula used to compute the estimate will be the same for each sample. The inherent variability in the sampling process will thus result in different point estimates of the population parameters as derived from the sample statistic.

20.11.2 The Interval Estimate

Interval estimate is the second major procedure that attempts to systematize the sample-population connection. The logical underpinning in this method is the probability associated with the normal distribution because as has been repeatedly emphasized, 95 percent of all sample means are clustered in between $\pm z_{\alpha/2} =$ 1.9. Such being the case, the interval surrounding the population μ accounts for 95 percent of all sample means of a given size, n, that may be derived from the given population.

To repeat, a randomly drawn sample thus has a 95 percent chance of being one of the sample means stacked in between the interval boundaries. The implication of this assumed derivation is twofold:

1. A given sample may be assumed to be one of those derived from within the interval surrounding, $\mu_{\overline{X}}$.
2. Under the circumstances, that is, because a given sample $\overline{X}$ may be presumed to be derived from the interval surrounding

$\mu_{\overline{x}}$ with 95 percent probability, it would be logical to assume that the probability of the interval spanning $\overline{X}$ includes μ in its span with a probability of 95 percent.

In contrast to the single valued point estimate, the interval estimate is made of two complementary values: the first is the interval estimate bounded by and upper and lower limits, within which the targeted population parameter (e.g., the population mean, μ) is supposed to lie. The second value is the confidence with which the estimated interval is weighted.

In order to supplement the point estimate with a confidence interval, the sampling distribution of the mean was derived based on the data provided by the first sample (one hundred calls). Based on the sample statistic, the point estimate of the population mean μ was rated as 10 minutes, associated with a 95 percent confidence interval bounded by 9.4 minutes as its lower limit and 10.6 minutes as its upper limit (Figure 20.13C).

Lower confidence limit of $\overline{X} - \left[1.96 \cdot \dfrac{s}{\sqrt{n}} \right] = 10 - 1.96 \cdot \dfrac{3}{\sqrt{100}} = 9.41 \cong 9.4$
Upper confidence limit of $\overline{X} + \left[1.96 \cdot \dfrac{s}{\sqrt{n}} \right] = 10 + 1.96 \cdot \dfrac{3}{\sqrt{100}} = 10.58 \cong 10.$

In the absence of actual population parameters, the interval estimate is presumed to enclose the population mean with 95 percent confidence level.

In this case, however, both the mean and the standard deviation of the response time for the whole past year, representing the actual population parameters, have been computed and are known.

We are now in the ideal situation where the actual sampling distribution of the population may be derived and compared with the sampling distribution derived from the one hundred calls sample of the past one month.

Given the population average response time of nine minutes and a standard deviation of two minutes, the standard error of the mean for a sample of one hundred was calculated at 0.2 and plotted in Figure 20.13B. Thus,

Upper limit of $\overline{X}:\mu_{\overline{x}}+\left[1.96{\bullet}\sigma_{\overline{x}}\right]=9+[1.96\times0.2]=9+0.392=9.392\cong9.4$ minutes

Lower limit of $\overline{X}:\mu_{\overline{x}}-\left[1.96{\bullet}\sigma_{\overline{x}}\right]=9-[1.96\times0.2]=9-0.392=8.608\cong8.6$ minutes

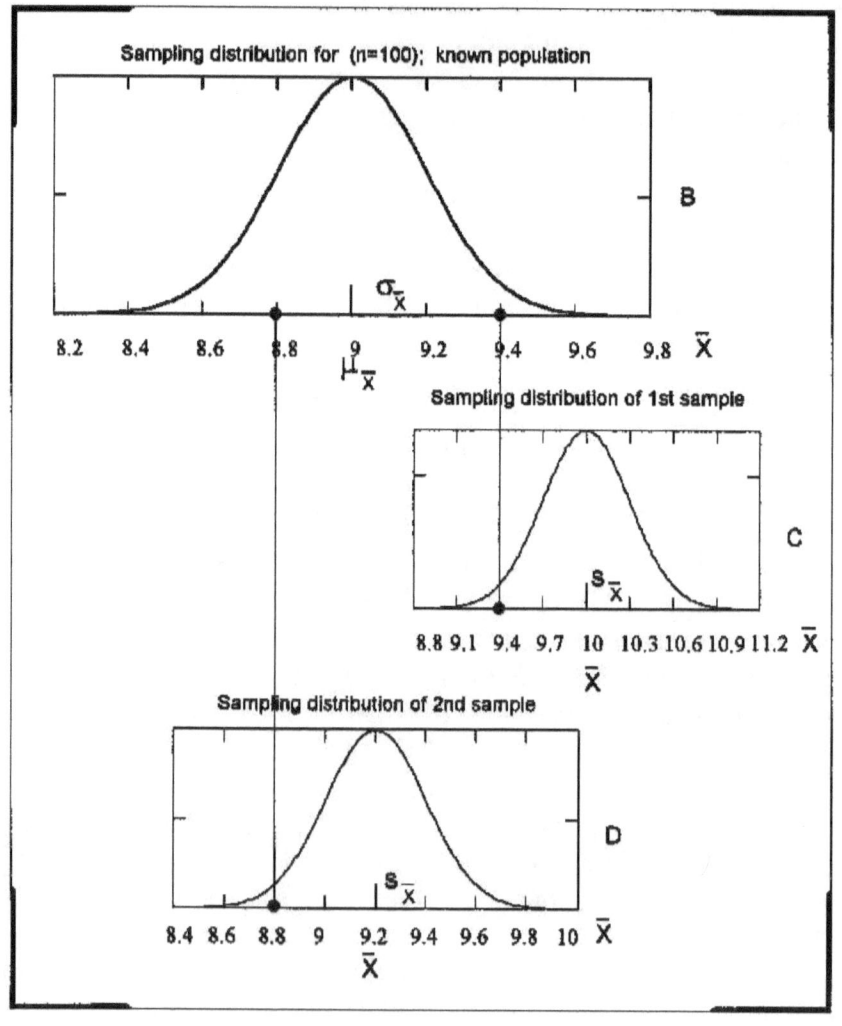

Figure 20.13

As can be readily appreciated, the estimated 95 percent confidence interval based on the first sample missed enclosing the mean of the population, μ, by a wide margin (compare Figure 20.13C with 20.13B). Note that the lower limit of the interval (9.4) in Figure 20.13C is two standard errors of the mean removed from the population mean.

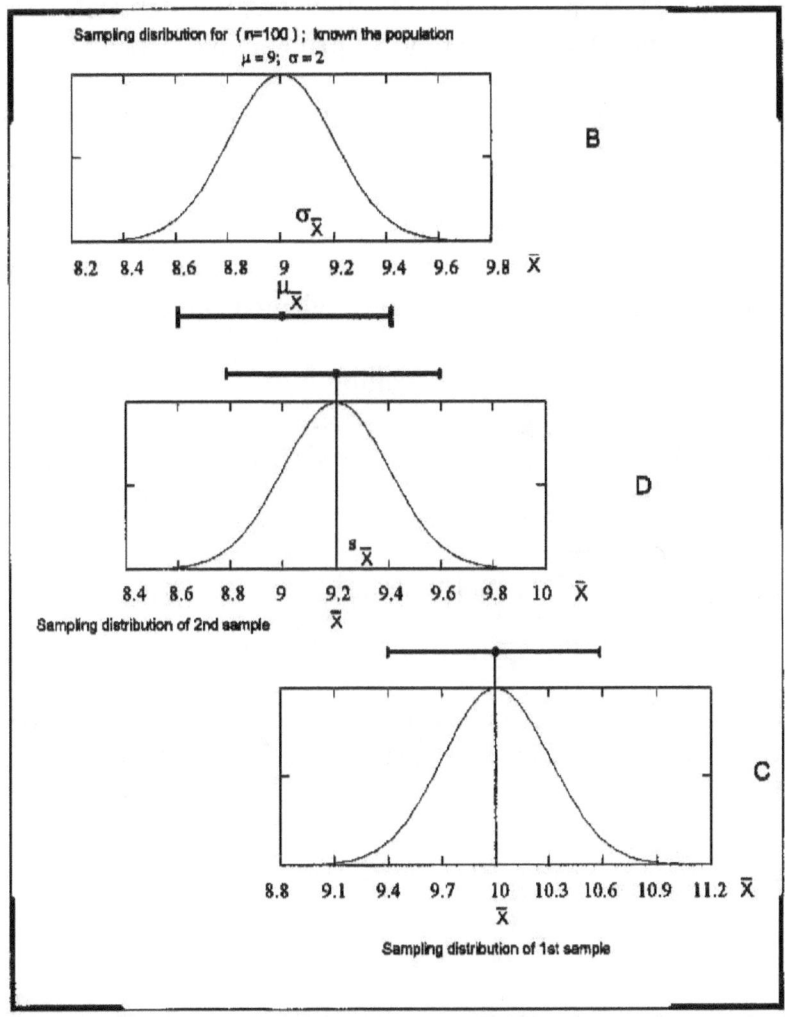

Figure 20.14

Faced with this divergent outcome, we are forced to conclude that the estimated interval derived from the one hundred calls sample enclosed a population mean that differed from the established population mean. In other words, the population mean presumed to lie within the interval of 9.4 to 10.6 minutes with 95 percent confidence may not be related to the established mean. It is, however, remotely conceivable that the sample represents a way out sample derived from the upper tail and thus missed enclosing the established population mean at the 95 percent confidence level.

It was thus concluded that the estimate from the one hundred calls sample confirmed the suspicion that the population mean has recently increased above the established norm.

Following an administrative overhaul, a second sample of one hundred response times was randomly selected and analyzed.

An average response time of 9.2 minutes and a standard deviation of two minutes were obtained. The sampling distribution depicted in Figure 20.13D yields a 95 percent confidence interval bounded by 8.8 $\leftrightarrow$ 9.6 minutes. Thus,

$$\text{Confidence limits: } \overline{X} + \left[z \bullet \frac{s}{\sqrt{n}} \right] = 9.2 \pm \left[1.96 \times \frac{2}{\sqrt{100}} \right] = 9.2 \pm 0.392 \cong (8.8 - 9.6) \text{ minutes.}$$

As noted in Figure 20.13D, the estimated confidence interval encloses the population mean, μ, at the 95 percent confidence interval.

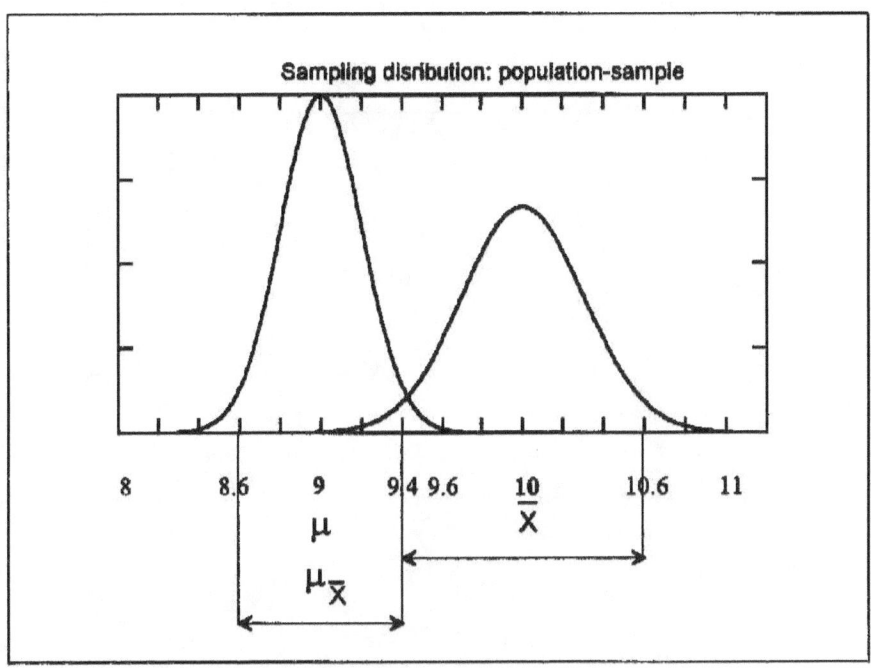

Figure 20.15

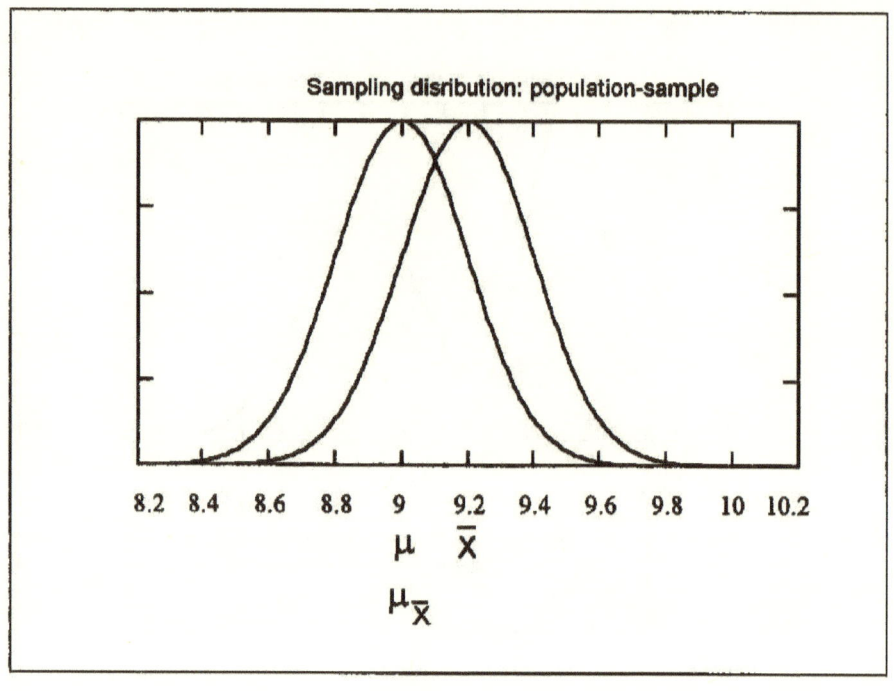

Figure 20.16

Chapter 21A

Statistical Inference: Hypothesis Testing

The introduction to hypothesis testing confronts the author with the agonizing choice of defining the test in allegorical, philosophical, or practical terminology. A common approach is to define hypothesis testing as a structured method for the evaluation of tentatively assumed beliefs about reality, often referred to as the state of nature, actual situation, and so on.

It thus divides the state of reality or truth into two mutually exclusive and exhaustive subsets. In other words, hypothesis testing is a procedure designed to resolve the conflict between two opposing views of reality or alternative courses of action.

The proposition tentatively assumed to be true is called the null hypothesis and is symbolized by H_0, whereas the proposition initially assumed to be false is called the alternative hypothesis and is symbolized by H_1.

In effect, the decision implies a choice, in the light of available evidence, between two, and only two, complementary states of reality that are mutually exclusive and exhaustive, such that the truth in one implies the falsity of the other.

The graphic equivalent of the idealized actual situation or states of nature may be represented by Figure 21A.1, where H_0 is the acceptance region and H_1 is the rejection region.

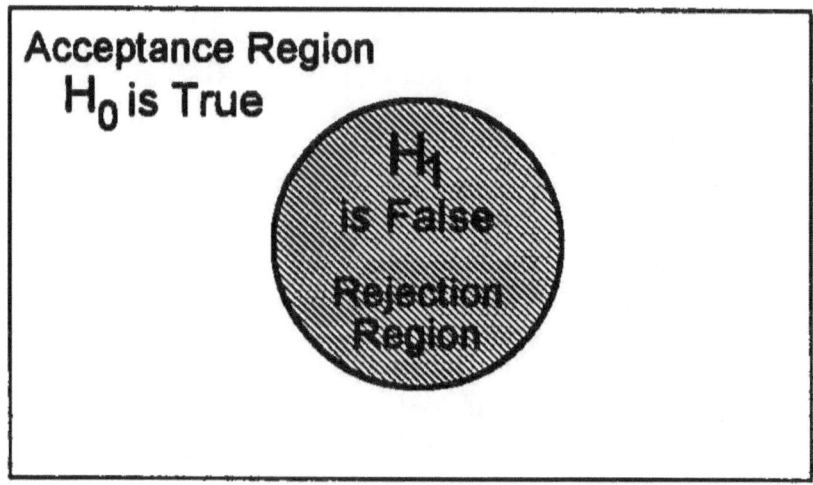

Figure 21A.1 Venn diagram of the partition of
the sample space into two mutually exclusive and
exhaustive acceptance and rejection regions.

Given the stated objective, the decision-making technique is
designed to establish within the limits of certainty the truth or fallacy
of a given proposition or hypothesis.

The judicial process in which the defendant is assumed to be
innocent (H_0 is true) until proven otherwise (H_0 is false, H_1 is true)
offers the perfect and realistic setup in which the decision-making
process is carried out when confronted by the evidence (Table
21A.1).

From the table and the associated graph, the two possible decisions
(accept the null or reject the null) are clearly demarcated. The simple
dichotomous yes and no decision leads to four distinct outcomes,
two of which, unknown to the jurors, are in conflict with the true
state of reality and thus represent a miscarriage of justice or an error
in the decision-making process.

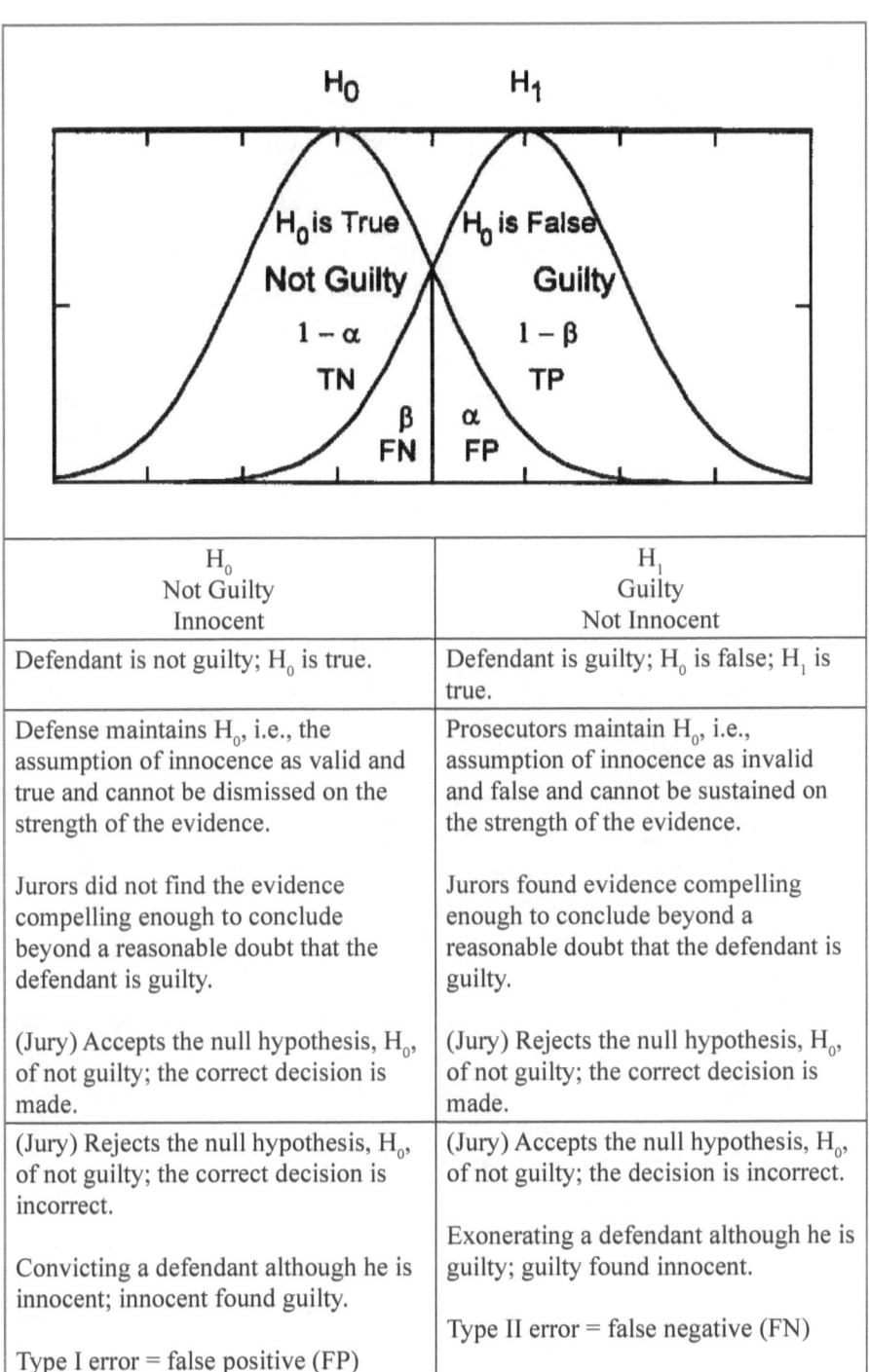

H_0 Not Guilty Innocent	H_1 Guilty Not Innocent
Defendant is not guilty; H_0 is true.	Defendant is guilty; H_0 is false; H_1 is true.
Defense maintains H_0, i.e., the assumption of innocence as valid and true and cannot be dismissed on the strength of the evidence. Jurors did not find the evidence compelling enough to conclude beyond a reasonable doubt that the defendant is guilty. (Jury) Accepts the null hypothesis, H_0, of not guilty; the correct decision is made.	Prosecutors maintain H_0, i.e., assumption of innocence as invalid and false and cannot be sustained on the strength of the evidence. Jurors found evidence compelling enough to conclude beyond a reasonable doubt that the defendant is guilty. (Jury) Rejects the null hypothesis, H_0, of not guilty; the correct decision is made.
(Jury) Rejects the null hypothesis, H_0, of not guilty; the correct decision is incorrect. Convicting a defendant although he is innocent; innocent found guilty. Type I error = false positive (FP)	(Jury) Accepts the null hypothesis, H_0, of not guilty; the decision is incorrect. Exonerating a defendant although he is guilty; guilty found innocent. Type II error = false negative (FN)

Table 21A.1.

Crossing over from the judicial world to the real world, the defendant in this case is none other than our lone sample that was initially assumed to be drawn from the known population (not guilty in accordance with the null hypothesis), pending the collection and evaluation of the evidence (Table 21A.2).

This overview of the decision-making process may give the impression of a straightforward procedure that needs no further elaboration. On closer examination, the practical application of the process proves to be more involved, allowing the decision maker the leeway to devise a strategy that will mitigate the impact of the unforeseen and unavoidable errors to which the process is liable.

Before detailing the technical aspect of the process, a sampling of its possible application should underline the relevance of the hypothesis testing process in clinical medicine.

The survival time of forty-nine patients treated with a new drug (sample) is reported to be longer than the known (based on cumulative data and experience) survival time in patients (population) hither to be treated in the standard mode. The null hypothesis addressed the question whether the observed difference between the mean (average) survival time of the sample of forty-nine patients, $\overline{X}$, and the average survival time of the population, μ, is real or just outwardly apparent. The answer will influence our decision to either maintain that the observed difference is only apparent and can be accounted for by the laws of probability, thus accepting the null hypothesis of no difference (i.e., declaring that the sample is just another random sample drawn from the hypothesized population), or alternatively to decide that chance factors, although possible, are so small that we are forced to reject the null (no difference) hypothesis as false and accept the alternate hypothesis (real difference) as the possible source population from which the sample is actually drawn.

21A.1 The Sample-Population Relation

At the simplest level, the relationship of the sample to its parent population may be graphically depicted by the following flow chart (Figure 21A.2).

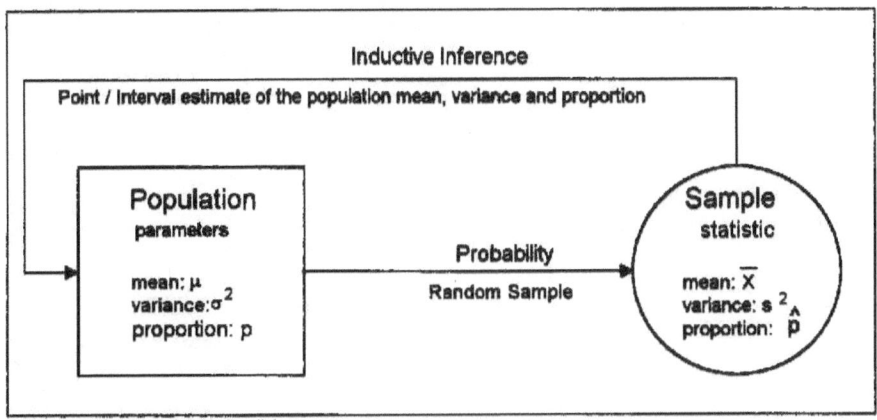

Figure 21A.2. Flow chart of the direct (random sample) and indirect (inference) relation of population and sample.

In reality, the closed loop configuration is meant only to dramatize the relationship and to categorize the possible combinations that may actually be encountered. In this sense, the chart is an attempt to portray the interconnection obtained in the estimation process.

This common situation is that of a sole random sample known to be derived (i.e., randomly drawn) from a given population. As such, the sample may be used as the basis from which to infer the population parameters. The sample in this case provides the necessary data from which to compute the sample statistic of mean and standard deviation.

The relationship of sample to population is, however, not always as straightforward as depicted in Figure 21A.2. A more relevant situation and one that closely parallels commonly encountered situations is depicted in Figure 21A.3.

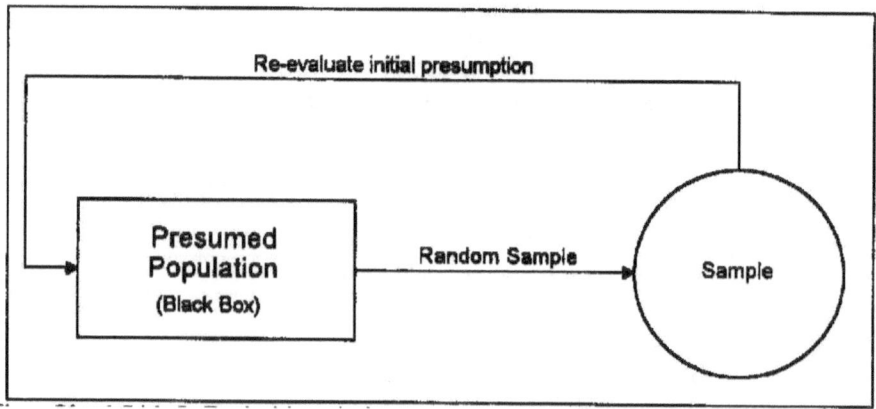

Figure 21A.3. Flow chart of the probable relation of random sample to presumed population subject to hypothesis testing.

In this situation, we are in possession of a sample with a presumed lineage (i.e., assumed to be a random sample derived from the given population). To continue the metaphor, the question to be resolved is to establish beyond a reasonable doubt the parenthood of the presumed population. Failing that, the validity of the claim is cast in doubt (H_1).

This simple proposition takes on the name of the null hypothesis, which decrees that until otherwise proven, the paternity claim between the sample and the presumed population is assumed to be valid (H_0).

A less common situation is encountered when the population parameters are known. This fact makes it possible to predict the probability of selecting a random sample of a given mean, standard deviation, and size. This of course is derived from the fact that, given the parameters of the population, the sampling distribution is determined. Given the distribution (from the stacks surrounding the central mean), random sampling becomes a function of the probability of the spread of the sample means. The population parameters by themselves are of course the source of infinite relevant statistical data.

Finally, an unlikely situation (of theoretical interest only) may be encountered when both the population parameter and the derived random sample statistic are known. This is the only situation where the relationship can be determined with precision so as to place the sample mean precisely on the sample distribution $\overline{X}$ axis from which it was drawn.

21A.2 Formal Approach to Hypothesis Testing

Hypothesis testing is the second of two statistical inferential techniques designed to explore the connection between a given sample and a hypothesized population, the first being the statistical estimate, fully explored in the last chapter.

Textbooks approach hypothesis testing by following a set of steps beginning with the formulation of the null hypothesis that is being tested and assumed to be true, leading to the final step of arriving at a conclusion concerning the disposition of the original null hypothesis.

In practice, this is certainly the desired path of testing a given null hypothesis. This approach, however, may conceal the intricate roundabout way by which the practical evaluation is carried out.

The interrelationship between the components of the "triad," (sample, sampling, and population) detailed in the last chapter as the necessary background for a clear understanding of inference estimation procedure, is applied with equal relevance to the inference procedure of hypothesis testing.

What is more to the point is that both procedures target the same objective, using the same theoretical background and differing only in the procedural approach. This subtle difference will become clearer as the technical aspect of the hypothesis testing method unfolds.

Recall that the interval estimate sought to place the population mean in the neighborhood of the sample mean (i.e., within a defined interval centered on $\overline{X}$, the sample mean), implying the common origin of the sample from the immediate vicinity of the population-sampling mean, $\mu = \mu_{\overline{x}}$, and further implying that the sample mean may be considered as a fair representative of the population mean.

In certain percentages of the cases, depending on the width assigned to the interval, the assumption proved faulty, such that the sample mean did not originate from the $1 - \alpha$ area surrounding the population-sampling mean, but from the remote $\alpha/2$ tail area, so that the specified interval fell short of enclosing and in essence failing to predict the magnitude of the population-distribution mean with the degree of confidence attached to the interval limits (Figure 21A.4).

In hypothesis testing, the procedure is more direct, although it appears to be more circuitous. The objective is the exact placement of the sample mean, $\overline{X}$, on the population-sampling axis, $\mu = \mu_{\overline{x}}$. In this case, depending on the extent of the partition of the sampling distribution into a proposed or predefined α tail area and a central core area of $1 - \alpha$, the sample mean falling into the central core area would be considered not particularly different from the central population-sampling mean. On the other hand, a sample mean value that would place it way out into the tail end area would put into question its relationship to the population-sampling mean.

Thus, in interval estimation, the question addressed stated in colorful language may be phrased as follows:

"Is $\overline{X}$, the sample mean, a close neighbor of the population mean, μ?"

In hypothesis testing, the same question in a different guise takes the following format:

"How far is $\overline{X}$, the sample mean, from the population mean, μ?"

To repeat, in both procedures, the aim is to investigate the site of origin of the sample mean from the sampling distribution. The route followed differed marginally, although the aim remains essentially the same in the two procedures. In both cases, the judgment that follows is simply the outcome of the placement strategy.

In terms of the "trilogy" construct, it may be considered as an extension or variation on the process of interval estimation connecting sample and population.

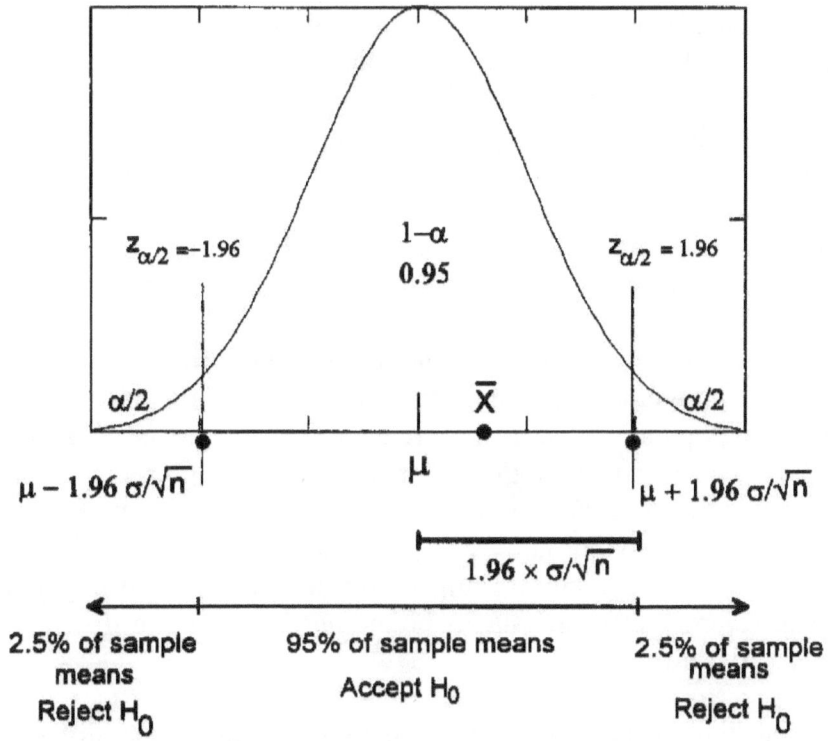

Figure 21A.4. Sampling Distribution of the Mean

As such, it represents the logical corollary of the sampling distribution. Although on the surface it does appear that we are relating the sample to a presumed known population, in actual fact, we are checking the probable origin of the sample from the sampling distribution of the known population.

1. Statement of the hypothesis: formulation of two opposing hypotheses

In practical terms, the statement that the Null Hypothesis proclaims assumes one of three possible formats (Table 21A.2). In the first format, the null hypothesis asserts that the mean of the sample's population, μ, is exactly equal to a given value, μ_0, which is the mean of a hypothesized population whose value come from some external reference system, such as a previous value, a laboratory average based on extensive cumulative data, or a mean value derived from a comprehensive survey (i.e., $\mu = \mu_0$). The implication of the statement asserts that the mean of the parent population of the given sample at hand, μ, is thus no different from the population whose mean is proclaimed by the null hypothesis, μ_0. Stated in terms of the sampling distribution, the null hypothesis maintains that mean of the sample at hand is not far off from the sampling distribution mean, $\mu_{\bar{x}}$, and thus may be considered as a random sample derived from the very same population whose mean is proclaimed by the null hypothesis.

The alternate hypothesis, on the other hand, denies the above assertion altogether and maintains instead that the mean of the sample's population, μ, is not related to the alleged population whose mean is given by the null hypothesis (i.e., $\mu \neq \mu_0$). In other words, the mean of the sample at hand is far removed from the mean of the alleged population mean, μ_0, as to render the possibility of its being just another random sample from the alleged null population or equivalently from the stacks bounding the sampling distribution mean very unlikely.

The null hypothesis is thus the verbal equivalent of this probability exercise. The hypothesis as set forth assumes that the sample is in fact a derivative of the hypothesized population, by virtue of the fact that its score of say $z = 1$ does not justify the claim of separate identity because such a score is likely to occur by the nature of the distribution of the sample statistic (densely packed around the distribution mean) in compliance with the laws of probability.

The logical frame of this relation is to proclaim via the null hypothesis that the observed difference in the sample mean represents only a chance variation of a random draw from the sampling distribution of sample means, and by implication, its parent population is no different from the presumed population, so that

$$H_0: \quad \underset{\substack{\text{Mean of the}\\ \text{sample's population}}}{\mu} \quad = \quad \underset{\substack{\text{Mean of the}\\ \text{hypothesized population}}}{\mu_0} \quad .$$

The alternative hypothesis, the fallback hypothesis, is invoked when it is realized that the derived score represents a value as extreme or more extreme, that is, it partitions a tail area so small (e.g., smaller than 5 percent of the total area under the sampling curve), which in effect makes it very unlikely (less than 5 percent probability) that the sample population and the presumed population are one and the same, and by implication, the population represented by the sample is different from the population we have initially assumed to be its parent population, so that

$$H_1: \quad \underset{\substack{\text{Mean of the}\\ \text{sample's population}}}{\mu} \quad \neq \quad \underset{\substack{\text{Mean of the}\\ \text{hypothesized population}}}{\mu_0} \quad .$$

True State: Actual Situation Unknown to Decision Maker	
H_1 is true H_0 is false	H_0 is true H_1 is false
$\mu_1 = \mu_{\text{True}} \neq \mu_{\text{Hypo}}$ $\mu_{\text{True}} < \mu_{\text{Hypo}}$ $\mu_{\text{True}} > \mu_{\text{Hypo}}$ Significant difference Significant effect	$\mu_0 = \mu_{\text{True}} = \mu_{\text{Hypo}}$ two-tailed $\mu_{\text{True}} \geq \mu_{\text{Hypo}}$ lower-tailed $\mu_{\text{True}} \leq \mu_{\text{Hypo}}$ upper tailed No significant difference No significant effect

	Correct decision Inference of difference P(rejecting H_0 | H_1 is true) P(No error | H_1 is true) $1 - \beta$ = Power	Erroneous prediction Inference of difference P(rejecting H_0 | H_0 is true) P(Type I error | H_0 is true) α	Reject H_0	
$\mu_{True} \neq \mu_{Hypo}$ $\mu_{True} < \mu_{Hypo}$ $\mu_{True} > \mu_{Hypo}$				Decision
$\mu_{True} = \mu_{Hypo}$ $\mu_{True} \geq \mu_{Hypo}$ $\mu_{True} \leq \mu_{Hypo}$	Erroneous prediction Inference of No difference P(accepting H_0 | H_1 is true) $= P$(Type I error | H_1 is true) $= \beta$	Correct decision Inference of No difference P(accepting H_0 | H_0 is true) $=P$(No error | H_0 is true) $= 1 - \alpha$	Accept H_0	

Table 21A.2. The four possible outcomes resulting from a binary decision coupled to a binary true state of nature

2. Placement and siting of the sample mean on the axis of the sampling distribution of the hypothesized population (known population parameters)

Recall that the standard unit of measurement, z, is in effect a translation of the original x axis units of measurements into standard z units. The result is the conversion of the distance from μ into multiple or fraction of σ, that is, z units, representing a generic unit of measurement for all x values (Figure 19A.6),

$$\frac{\overset{\text{Measured value of } X}{x} - \overset{\text{Mean of } x \text{ values}}{\mu}}{\underset{\text{Standard deviation}}{\sigma}} = z \text{ standard units.}$$

The standard error of sample means can be derived from the standard deviation of the population given the number of elements in the sample, as per the following relation,

$$
\begin{array}{c}
\text{Standard error of} \\
\text{sample means}
\end{array}
\quad
\begin{array}{c}
\text{Standard eeviation} \\
\text{of population}
\end{array}
$$

$$
\text{SE}_{\overline{X}} = \sigma_{\overline{X}} = \dfrac{\sigma}{\sqrt{\underset{\text{No. of elements}}{n}}}.
$$

The distance of the sample mean, $\overline{X}$, from the hypothesized population mean, μ_0, or its equivalent the mean of the sampling distribution, $\mu_{\overline{X}}$, may now be converted into multiple or fraction of the standard error of the mean, $\text{SE}_{\overline{X}}$, using the conversion formula noted previously. The results are then similarly expressed in z standard units; in other words, the sampling distribution curve is now calibrated in standard z units as follows:

$$
\underset{\substack{\text{How far } \overline{X} \text{ from } \mu_0 \\ \text{in terms of SE}}}{\dfrac{\overline{X} - \mu_0}{\sigma_{\overline{X}}(= \text{SE})}} = \underset{\substack{\text{Population} \\ \text{mean}}}{\dfrac{\overline{X} - \mu_0}{\dfrac{\sigma}{\sqrt{n}}}} = \underset{\substack{\text{Sample} \\ \text{mean}}}{\dfrac{\overline{X} - \underset{\substack{\text{Sampling} \\ \text{mean}}}{\mu_{\overline{X}}}}{\dfrac{\sigma}{\sqrt{n}}}} = z \text{ standard units} \quad \text{(Test statistic)}
$$

The test statistic in this case places the sample mean, $\overline{X}$, at its corresponding distance in z units from $\mu_{\overline{X}}$. This transformation allows us to focus on the site of origin of the sample mean and to determine the probability with which it could realistically be considered a sample derived from the alleged population whose hypothesized mean was postulated to be equal to μ_0 (Figure 21A.5). This transformation takes for granted the fact than the population mean is what the null hypothesis states.

All hypothesis testing implies the targeting and positioning the sample mean on the corresponding sampling distribution $\overline{X}$ axis in order to measure the resultant distance from the sampling mean of the hypothesized population $\mu_{\overline{X}}$, in z standard units or score. The derived z score in turn determines the probability of origin of a similar sample or one even more extreme from stacks beyond its actual siting or location on the z axis, in either tail.

In more practical terms, the derived score in z units divides the area under the normal curve of the sampling distribution into two regions, a main body region proximal to the mean of the sampling distribution and a distal tail region. In the more formal language of statistical hypothesis testing, the probability of a z score is considered to be equal to the demarcated tail area, which accounts for the actual as well as the more extreme z scores, that is, all possible scores extending further into the tail of the sampling distribution curve. The tail area then is the probability of scoring a value the equal of the actual sample statistic or any other value more extreme sample statistic, given that the null hypothesis is true.

3. Placement and siting of the sample mean on the axis of the sampling distribution of the hypothesized population (unknown population parameters)

In this fairly common situation, we are given a hypothesized mean only but not the standard deviation of the population. Accordingly, if the sample is large enough, we are forced to substitute the standard deviation of the sample itself for standard deviation of the hypothesized population, so that

$$\underset{\substack{\text{Standard error} \\ \text{of sample means}}}{\text{SE}_{\overline{X}}} = \sigma_{\overline{X}} = \frac{\overset{\substack{\text{Standard deviation} \\ \text{of the sample}}}{s}}{\sqrt{\underset{\text{No. of elements}}{n}}}$$

With this substitution, the sampling distribution curve is now determined, and the placement of the sample mean follows the same prescribed pattern noted earlier.

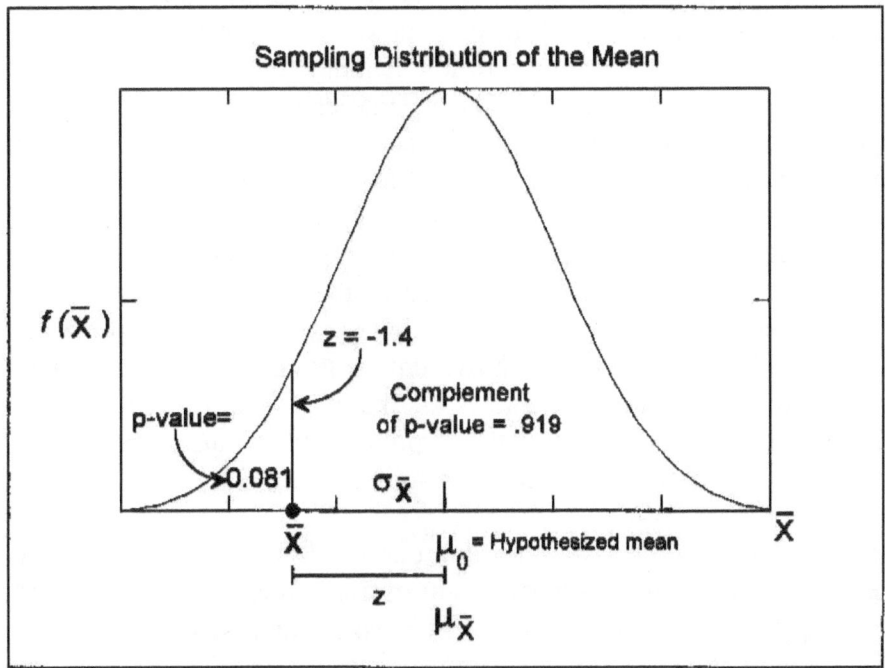

Figure 21A.6. Placement of the Sample Mean

21A.3 The *p* Value and the Observed Significance Level

It is important to realize that the computed *z* axis of the sampling distribution is a directed line in which the directed numbers are ordered, so that any *z* number on the number line, whether positive, negative, or zero, is greater than any number to its left and less than any number to its right (Figure 21A.7).

Once the calculated value of the test statistic, *z*, is derived, the sample mean, $\overline{X}$, is then sited at its corresponding *z* transform on the $\overline{X}$ axis,

$$z = \frac{\overline{X} - \mu_{\overline{X}}}{\sigma_{\overline{X}}}$$

As noted form Figure 21A.6, the vertical line through the placed sample mean $\overline{X}$ divides the area under the normal curve at the designated z value into two complementary areas. A left area that includes all sample means equal or smaller in value that the mean value of $\overline{X}$, placed at $z = -1.4$. The complementary area to the right of the z line running through $z = -1.4$ includes all sample means that are greater than the mean value of $\overline{X}$ placed at z of -1.4. More to the point, this division into the two complementary areas carries with it a far-reaching implication as to the probability of such an occurrence. In essence, the lower-tailed area to the left of the z line designated as the p value is equivalent to the probability of drawing a random sample whose mean is as extreme or more extreme than the one actually noted given the hypothesized population mean, μ_0, or its equivalent the sampling distribution mean, $\mu_{\overline{X}}$.

Because areas under the normal curve of sampling distribution represent the probable site of origin of a given random sample and, consequently, the probability of drawing such sample from the stacks contained within the same partitioned area, it follows that the partitioned tail areas represent a small segment of the total area and thus a corresponding minimal probability of drawing a random sample of extreme $\pm z$ values

The p value may thus be defined as the probability of obtaining a value of the sample mean equal to or more extreme than actually obtained given the null hypothesis is true.

In formal notation, the p value and its associated probability is simplified as follows:

$P(\text{This sample result or one more extreme}| \text{ Null hypothesis is true}) = p \text{ value.}$

$P(z \leq -1.4) = 0.081 \text{ (lower-tailed area)} = p \text{ value.}$

The derived probability, that is, the p value, is the measure with which the sample can be said to be part of the presumed population (i.e., on target) or, otherwise, unlikely to be derived from the said population (i.e., off target).

In this context, the p value is the direct answer to the chance occurrence of such a sample mean given the hypothesized value of the population mean. In terms of the stacking order of the sample means surrounding the sampling distribution, the p value of 0.08 or 8 percent account for all the sample means confined to the tail area marked off by the z value. The significance of the p value, however, is not definitive in that it is associated with an objective decision and subjective conclusion. Would you consider a sample derived from the lower 8 percent of all the possible samples of size n, surrounding the sampling distribution mean as an unlikely event? Or would you consider such a derivation from the sampling distribution as a somewhat common occurrence? If the first option is the choice, then one is likely to conclude that the sample in question may not be related to the hypothesized mean and as such needs to be viewed as an alien sample which in reality belongs to a different sampling distribution. This is another way of saying that the initial proposition of null difference is null and void and must be rejected in favor the alternate hypothesis (i.e., real difference). If the second option is the choice, then one is likely to conclude that the sample in question is not really different from other samples clustering around the distribution mean, which is another way of saying that the null hypothesis is valid and must be maintained until proven otherwise.

For a p value of ≤ 0.01 on the other hand, it would be logical to assume that the sample is not a derivative of the population under consideration because to claim otherwise is to assert that a chance of one in one hundred is good enough for such a claim, which obviously is not.

The p value is thus the actual level of significance calculated from the test statistic. Whether it is significant or otherwise depends on the level that we choose to use. The lower the p value, the smaller the cutoff tail area, the more certain is one of having made a correct decision in rejecting the null hypothesis.

4. The α value and the predetermined significance level

The sequence of steps leading to the p value beginning with the statement of the null hypothesis detailed earlier appears to be the logical pattern of assessing the significance level of the observed sample mean.

The classic alternative to the previously mentioned sequence is to simply reverse steps 2 and 3. In this sequence, once the hypothesis has been formulated, the distribution curve is then artificially partitioned into a predetermined and fixed tail area corresponding to a specified probability, set in advance, considered to be appropriate and necessary in order to circumvent the inherent errors involved as will be discussed later.

Usually, a value ranging from 5 to 0.5 percent of the total area under the distribution curve is assigned to the relevant tail area, now designated as α, the significance level or critical level.

In order to mark off the assigned area from its complement under the normal distribution curve, the corresponding critical z value, z_α, is derived from the tables. The vertical ordinate, the line of demarcation, through the critical z_α value now partitions the area under the curve into the predetermined significant α and its complement, $1 - \alpha$, the insignificant level (Figure 21A.7).

But what exactly is α? By definition, α is the area in one or two tails of the normal curve (depending on the way the null hypothesis is defined) comprising a small percentage of the total area under the curve, usually set at less than 0.05 or 5 percent of the total. For a two-tailed test, this accounts for 0.025 or 2.5 percent of the area in each tail.

What is not explicitly stated is that the normal curve of which α is a predefined tail area is the sampling distribution curve derived from the population whose mean and standard deviations are known or calculated.

From Table 19B.2 (chapter 19B), the critical z value, z_α, corresponding to the α demarcation line in an upper-tailed hypothesis, equals 1.645. The specification of α sets the stage for the decision that follows the acquisition and calculation of the sample statistic, as will be detailed later.

For the moment, suffice to note that the central area bounded by the demarcation line, z_α, and the central line through z_0 account for the bulk of all possible sample means (of size n) that are most likely to be drawn as a random sample whose mean is equal or greater than the hypothesized mean μ_0, and as such defines the acceptance region whereby a sample mean so placed is assumed to be derived from the hypothesized population and accepted as confirmation of the null hypothesis, whereas the tail areas include the sample means that are thought most unlikely to be drawn as a random sample and as such are to be considered as samples from an alternative population. Note the implicit uncertainty in the statement that suggests that after all, the tail sample, although rare, is still a viable possibility as a genuine sample drawn from the hypothesized population (Figure 21A.7).

With the partition in place, and the critical z value separating the significant from the insignificant levels, the placement of a sample mean now becomes a simple binary choice. The test statistic of the sample mean, z, may turn out either larger than the critical z value, z_a, or smaller. For the upper tail partition, the sample mean would be placed in the tail area, to the right of the cutoff line, or to the left of the cutoff line, proximal to the mean of the sampling distribution. The reverse situation obtains for the lower tail partition, so that for the lower tail partition the sample mean would be placed in the tail area, to the left of the cutoff line, or to the right of the cutoff line, proximal to the mean of the sampling distribution.

Note that the upper tail is associated with z values greater than the critical z_a, whereas the lower tail is associated with values smaller than z_a.

This allocation of probabilities gives the α area double status. On the one hand, a random sample whose mean happens to fall within the α area, that is, within the rejection region, is automatically considered unlikely to be a genuine random sample from the assumed population and thus consigned to an alternative population. On the other hand, should the random sample mean be in fact, although rarely, drawn from the sample means of the α area, an error has been committed by denying reality when it is a true fact.

Accordingly, the α area accounts for the following definitions:

z_α	α	Computed z	p value	H_0
1.645	0.05	1.96	0.025	$p \le \alpha \Rightarrow$ Reject H_0
2.33	0.01	1.96	0.025	$p > \alpha \Rightarrow$ Accept H_0

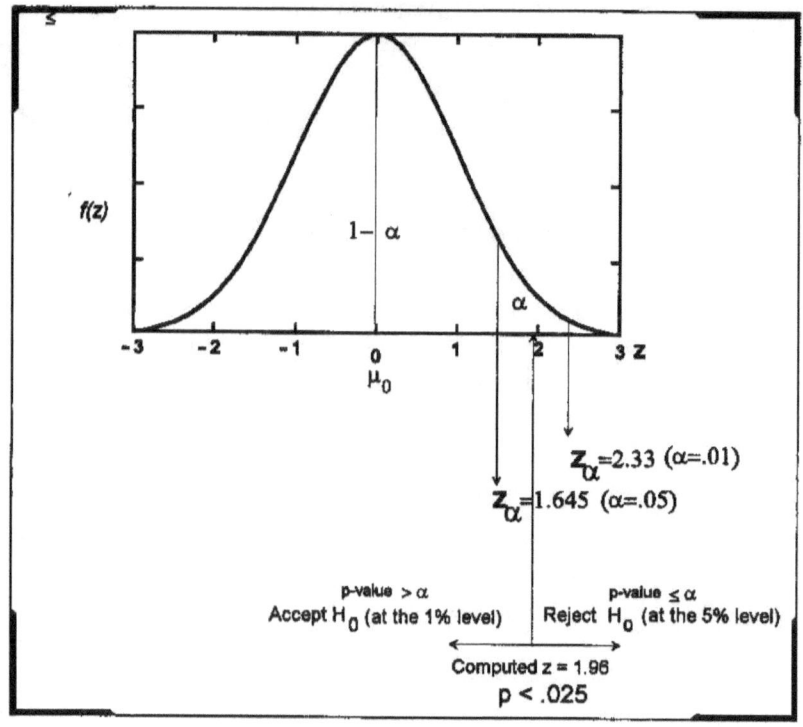

Figure 21A.7

21A.4 Definitions of α

The following are definitions of α:

- Percentage of area under the sampling distribution curve arbitrarily set in advance
- Level of significance
- Maximum probability of committing Type I or α error
- Amount of risk tolerated by incorrectly rejecting H_0 (setting the α level)

21A.5 The Interrelationship of p and α

The relation of α to p is a subject that may appear to be unnecessarily complex. We are dealing here with two simultaneous probabilities, one set a priori, and one determined a posteriori. In other words, we are faced with two simultaneous probabilities, a preset and predetermined probability or significance level and a computed probability level derived from the actual and observed test statistic where the relation between one and the other may be in accordance or in conflict.

The relative placement of the computed z in relation to the critical z_α or, alternatively, the relative magnitude of the α significance level to the tail area cutoff by the computed z, namely, the p value, may assume one of three possible outcomes.

Thus, three possibilities may be entertained by considering the relative magnitude of the computed z versus the critical z_α or, alternatively, by considering the p value versus the α significance level.

Comparing the computed z to the critical z_α, the following inequalities are possible (Figure 21A.8):

1. Computed $z <$ Critical $z_\alpha \Rightarrow$ reject H_0
2. Computed $z >$ Critical $z_\alpha \Rightarrow$ accept H_0
3. Computed $z =$ Critical $z_\alpha \Rightarrow$ accept H_0

In terms of the cutoff tail areas, the comparison assumes the following corresponding inequalities:

1. p value $<$ significance level; p to the right of α, i.e., $p \leq \alpha \Rightarrow$ reject H_0.
2. p value $>$ significance level; p to the left of α, i.e., $p > \alpha \Rightarrow$ accept H_0.
3. p value $=$ significance level; p same area as α, i.e., $p = \alpha \Rightarrow$ reject H_0.

In Figure 21A.7, two critical z_α values are postulated: the first set at $z_\alpha = 1.645$ corresponding to an α significance level of 5 percent, and the second set at $z_\alpha = 2.33$ corresponding to an α significance level of 1 percent. The test statistic in this instance was computed at

$z = 1.96$, corresponding to a p value of 0.025. As can be appreciated from the chart and the appended table, the decision under the first postulate of $z_\alpha = 1.645$ is to reject the null hypothesis because the computed z is greater than the critical z_α value or, alternatively, the p value is smaller than the α significance level.

Under the second postulate of $z_\alpha = 2.33$, a reverse situation obtains. In this instance, the computed z value is smaller than the critical z_α value; or alternatively, the p value is greater than the α significance level. In this case, the decision is to accept the null hypothesis.

21A.6 Difference between p and α

Both p and α partitions the area under the distribution normal curve into a left and right regional areas. The difference is that while α is preset and constant for the hypothesis being tested, p is computed and thus is a variable that may assume any magnitude larger or smaller than α, the significance level.

More to the point, by dividing the area under the sampling distribution into an acceptance and rejection regions, the distinct boundary as to what range of values of a sample mean may be accepted and what range of values is to be rejected is set.

The p allows the observer the freedom to treat the p value, that is, the probability associated with the computed z as a derived variable whose significance needs to be assessed in the context at hand, keeping in mind the degree of error tolerated.

Note that although the level of significance is predetermined, the computed z of the sample mean will just the same define its own p value, which needs to be related to the level of significance.

To Backtrack for a Moment

The sampling distribution was assumed to center on hypothesized parameters μ_0 and $\mu_{\bar{x}}$. In this case, its sample distribution was partitioned into two regions, and an acceptance region of $1 - \alpha$ and a rejection region of α demarcated by a given z_α value.

If the sample statistic, $\overline{X}$, fell beyond z_α (in either direction), that is, under the α area, the assumed H_0 was rejected, and the sample mean was considered as being derived from another distribution different from our original assumption.

If per chance $\overline{X}$ did in fact (unknown to us) come from the tail end of the distribution and in accordance with decision rule placed it in a different distribution, then unknowingly we have committed an α error.

The problem takes an entirely different aspect when our hypothesized population mean is not what it was presumed to be, the real population mean, thus making our null hypothesis false. In this case, the relation of the real sample mean, $\overline{X}$, to the hypothesized μ is not what we initially were led to believe based on the original μ_0. However, unknowingly, we continue to place our sample mean in accordance with the constraints of the hypothesized false mean, as will be detailed later. Under the circumstances, we are committing a β error.

21A.7 Reporting p and/or α

5. Weighing and reporting the observed versus the predetermined significance level

The above consideration regarding the intricate relation of α and p allows the investigator a certain latitude of reporting the actual computed z values, leading to the statistical decision of either rejecting or accepting the null hypothesis.

To be more specific, an investigator may chose any one of three modes of reporting the results of hypothesis testing analysis. The optimal format for reporting is as much a subjective as well as a deliberate decision reflecting the investigator's choice.

I. In this commonly reported format, the significance level α is exclusively specified. The computed z is not explicitly mentioned, and the decision is implicitly based on the computed z relation to the predetermined significance level.

In this case, the report of the hypothesis testing analysis simply states whether the null hypothesis was rejected at a specified level of significance or otherwise accepted. The decision is based on the position of the z value derived from the test statistic in relation to the α area and subsequent derivation of the conclusion from this relationship.

The statement as reported "H_0 rejected at the significance level of 0.05" fails to indicate whether by intent or neglect the degree or extent of deviation of the computed z value of the test statistic from the critical z value.

What is perhaps more objectionable is that in the absence of a an explicit computed z value, we are obliged to accept the author's imposed significance level. The reader is thus restricted from a critical evaluation of the results by substituting a significance level different from the author's own and thus arriving at a different statistical conclusion.

Type of z Test	Null Hypothesis H_0	Accept the Null Hypothesis H_0 if	Alternative Hypothesis H_1	Reject the Null Hypothesis H_0 if
Lower-tailed test	$\mu \geq \mu_0$	$z \geq -z_\alpha$	$\mu < \mu_0$	$z < -z_\alpha$
Upper-tailed test	$\mu \leq \mu_0$	$z \leq -z_\alpha$	$\mu > \mu_0$	$z > -z_\alpha$
Two-tailed test	$\mu = \mu_0$	$-z_{\alpha/2} \leq z \leq z_{\alpha/2}$	$\mu \neq \mu_0$	$z < -z_{\alpha/2}$ or $z > z_{\alpha/2}$

Table 21A.4. Decision rules for large-sample hypothesis tests about a mean based on the relation of computed z to the critical value, z_α

II. In this format, the p value is exclusively specified. No predetermined significance level is assigned or assumed. Decision is solely based on the p value derived from the computed z.

The p value in this reporting format refer similarly to a tail area. In this case, however, the tail area is not cutoff at a designated point on the z axis; it is instead the specific area marked off by the calculated z value of the test statistic. This value is a derived value and is not related directly to the α areas, which are arbitrarily set prior to the experimental setup.

Although the decision in the level of significance reporting format is to position the z value derived from the test statistic in relation to the α area and derive the final conclusion from this relationship, in the p-reporting format, the area demarcated by the z value is calculated and its absolute value evaluated in relation to arbitrary limits.

In the research fields including the medical field, the reporting of the p value takes on a compact format such as $p < 0.01$, $p < 0.025$, and so on. At the risk of being overly repetitious, it is of the utmost importance that the reader of current journals should be able to put the p value in context, in particular, with regard to the conclusion advanced by the author. As a first impression, one needs to keep in mind that the p value represents in effect the smallest significance level at which the null hypothesis, H_0, can be rejected.

More to the point, the statement $p < 0.01$ is a shorthand notation for the fact that given a true null hypothesis, the probability of obtaining the same or more extreme (i.e., at least as extreme) value of the test statistic, for example, $\overline{X}$, than the one actually obtained is less than 0.01, a mere 1 percent chance. Thus, for an upper-tailed test of the mean, a $p < 0.025$ is the probability that the sample mean $\overline{X}$ computed from any other random sample will be greater than or equal to the actual observed sample mean $\overline{X}$ or its z transform 1.96 (Figure 21A.7).

The p value is thus reported as follows:

$$\boxed{P(z \geq 2.33 \mid H_0 \text{ is true}) = 0.010.}$$

$p \leq 0.010.$

The probability notation means that the computed z statistic of the sample mean is 2.33 z standard units or 2.33 standard errors above the mean, assuming the null hypothesis is true. The probability of obtaining such a computed sample mean or larger is less than 0.010. The statement $p \leq 0.010$ implies that if the null hypothesis is true, the probability of obtaining a computed z value as extreme or more extreme than that actually observed is less than 0.010, that is, the area to the right of the computed z value of 2.33.

In this mode of reporting, α is not mentioned directly. the whole evidence presented is the value of the cutoff area as the relevant finding to accept or reject H_0 in view of a given p value particularly if the value is border line i.e., between 0.05 and 0.01, making it essentially a value judgment

It is becoming increasingly common to report the result of a test by giving calculated value of the test statistic with the corresponding tail probability, or p value, namely, with the probability of getting a difference between $\overline{X}$ and μ_0, which is numerically greater than or equal to that actually observed.

The information contained in the p value is central to the resolution of the null hypothesis. Its actual value is a measure of the strength of evidence against H_0. Rather than being bound by a predetermined α value, the investigator is able to gauge the result against any specified α level.

The stress on the probabilistic aspect of the p value in rejecting the null given a p value less than 0.010 need not obscure the fact that it is also the actual probability of making a Type I error. If the p value is less than 0.010, the probability of rejecting the null when in fact it is true corresponds to the same probability of making a Type I error, that is, less than 10 times in 1,000.

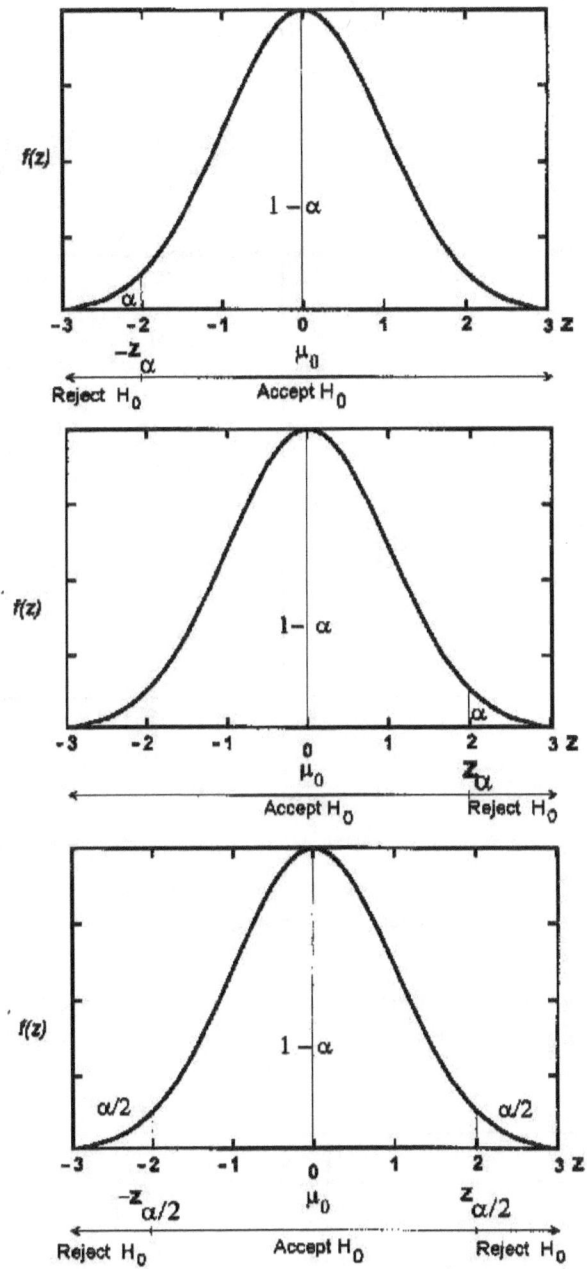

Figure 21A.9. The Partition of the distribution curve into a predetermined tail area corresponding to the probability set in advance, for the three types of the z test in Table 21A.4.

III. In this third mode of reporting, both p and α are explicitly stated. The decision is based on the relation of the p value to the assigned significance level.

Suppose that $z = 2.33$, the accompanying table displays the rejection region for each of four different values of α along with the resulting conclusion (Table 21A.5).

z_α Critical value	α Level of Significance = Percentage of Area to the Right of Critical z_α	Computed z	p value Lowest Level of Significance = Percentage of Area to the Right of Computed	Conclusion p value vs. α or Computed z vs. Critical z_α
1.64	0.05	2.33	$p \leq 0.010$	$p \leq \alpha \Rightarrow$ Reject H_0
1.96	0.025	2.33	$p \leq 0.010$	$p \leq \alpha \Rightarrow$ Reject H_0
2.58	0.005	2.33	$p \leq 0.010$	$p > \alpha \Rightarrow$ Accept H_0
2.81	0.0025	2.33	$p \leq 0.010$	$p > \alpha \Rightarrow$ Accept H_0

Table 21A.5 The interrelationship of an observed p value and four levels of α significance

Once the p value has been determined, the conclusion at any particular level α results from comparing the p value to α, as follows:

Accept H_θ $0.05 > p$ value ≤ 0.01 Reject H_0.

In other words, if the z value marks off an area in either tail that is smaller than 0.01, the evidence is against chance occurrence and H_0 should be rejected. On the other hand, if the marked off area is bigger than 0.05 of the enclosed normal area, the chance occurrence is possible and H_0 should not be rejected (Table 21A.6).

If the test is upper tailed, the p value is the area captured under the z curve to the right of the computed value of z. If the test had been lower tailed, the p value would have been the area under the z curve to the left of the computed z (lower-tail area). For two-tailed test, finding the area captured in the tail in which z falls, for example, the upper tail or the lower tail, determines $\alpha/2$ (because α is the sum of the upper and lower tail areas). In this case, the p value is twice the captured area. This is summarized in the accompanying box.

Note that p value and significance level are different. The decision maker sets the significance level, α, before running the study. It is the maximum probability of making a Type I error that a decision maker can tolerate, given its costs. The p value can be determined only *after* computing the sample mean once the study data have been collected.

With α, you set the area α and then check the z. With p, you determine the z and then check the area, α.

α = level of significance	p value = lowest (smallest) level of significance at which H_0 can be rejected
α = risk of incorrectly rejecting H_0 = maximum probability of Type I error	= Maximum probability of Type I error = Maximum credibility of H_0
$\alpha = P(\text{rejecting } H_0 \mid H_0 \text{ is true})$ $\alpha = P(\text{Type I error} \mid H_0 \text{ is true}$	p value = probability (this sample result or one more extreme | null hypothesis is true) = Probability of obtaining a value of the test statistic as extreme as or more extreme than that actually obtained given that H_0 is true = Probability of getting a value of the sample mean $\overline{X}$ that is at least as extreme as the $\overline{X}$ obtained from the sample data given that H_0 is correct

The conclusion at any particular level α results from comparing the p value to α:
Reject the null hypothesis if the p value is less than
or equal to the significance level α:
p value $\leq \alpha \Rightarrow$ reject H_0 at α level.
Do not reject the null hypothesis if the p value is
greater than the significance level α:
p value $> \alpha \Rightarrow$ accept H_0 at α level
Alternatively.
If α is greater than or equal to the p value,
$\alpha \geq p$ value $\Rightarrow$ reject H_0.
If α is less than the p value
$\alpha < p$ value $\Rightarrow$ accept H_0.

Table 21A.3 Definition of the p value juxtaposed to that of the α significance and the resultant conclusion that may be derived from their interrelationship.

Chapter 21B

Hypothesis Testing in Action

The null hypothesis is commonly defined as the process of making statements about a population on the basis of information derived from a sample. The data listed earlier for the resting heart rate of marathon runners will be used as the background in order to highlight the essential elements of the hypothesis.

Recall (chapter 11) that the mean resting heart rate of the ninety marathon runners was calculated to be $60.289 \cong 60.29$ beats per minute (bpm). The measure of dispersion around this central tendency is best defined by calculating the sample standard deviation, s. This was done using a standard formula as follows:

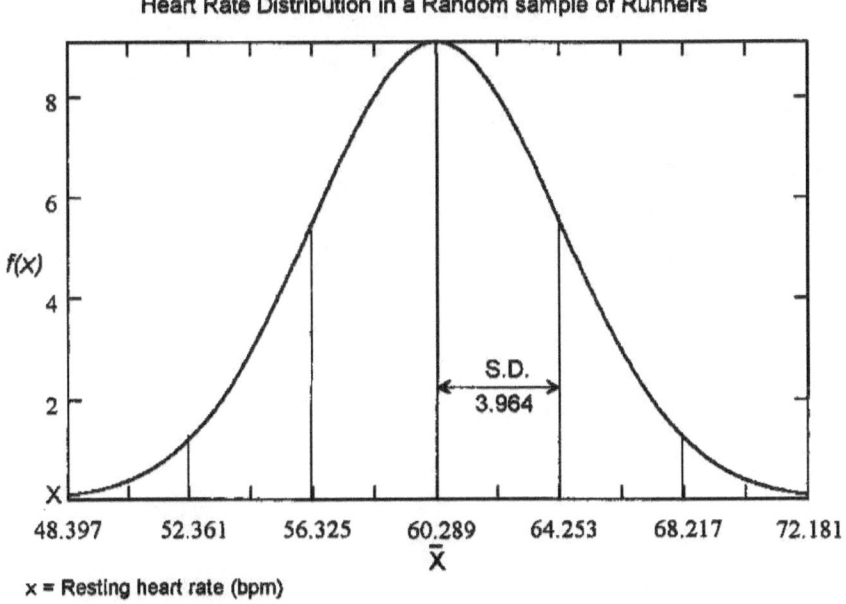

Figure 21B.1. Graph of the distribution of the resting heart rate of the ninety marathon runners, given the sample mean of 60.289 bpm and the standard deviation of 3.964.

$$s = \sqrt{\frac{\sum_{i=1}^{n}\left(x_i - \overline{X}\right)^2}{n-1}} = \pm 3.964 \text{ bpm} = \text{sample (runners) standard deviation.}$$

$\overline{X}_{\text{Runners}} = 60.289 \text{ bpm}; \ s = 3.964 \text{ bpm}.$

Given the mean of 60.289 bpm, the range defined by one standard deviation extends from $60.289 - 3.964 = 56.325$ below the mean to $60.289 + 3.964 = 64.253$ above the mean (Figure 21B.1).

Sample mean $\overline{X}$	Standard deviation s	
60.289 +	3.964	= 64.253 bpm

Sample mean $\overline{X}$	Standard deviation s	
60.289 −	3.964	= 56.325 bpm

Which is a precise way of saying that 68 percent (68.26 percent to be exact) of the ninety runners exhibit this range of resting heart rates.

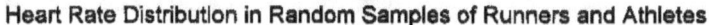

Heart Rate Distribution in Random Samples of Runners and Athletes

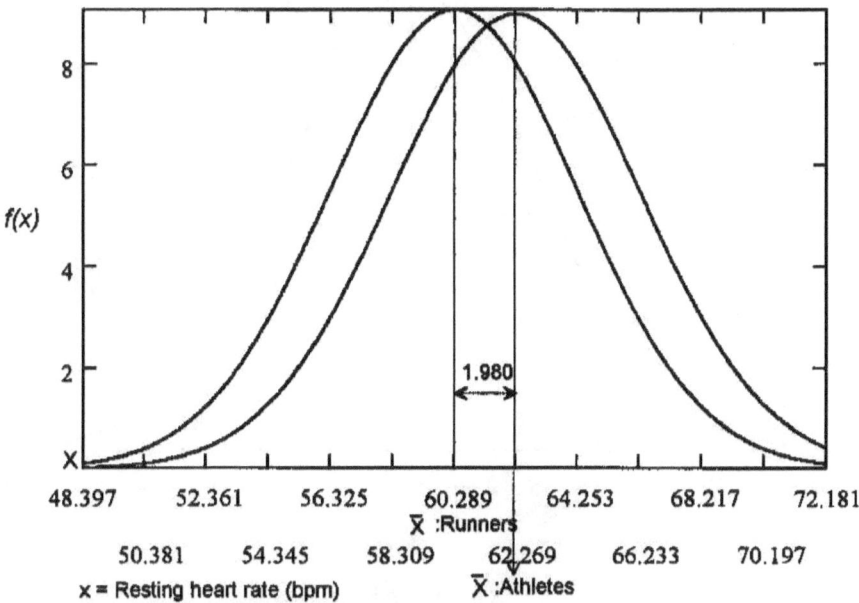

Figure 21B.2. Graph of the distribution of the resting heart rate of a random sample of ninety athletes drawn from the athletic population with a mean of 62.269 bpm and a standard deviation of 4, plotted on the same axis with the distribution of the random sample of the ninety runners whose mean is 60.289 bpm and the standard deviation of 3.964.

By the same token, 95 percent (95.44 percent to be exact) of the ninety runners exhibit a range of resting heart rates defined by two standard deviations, extending from 52.361 below the mean to 68.217 above the mean of the resting heart rates.

Sample mean $\overline{X}$	Standard deviation $2s$	
60.289 $+$	7.928	$= 68.217$ bpm
Sample mean $\overline{X}$	Standard deviation $2s$	
60.289 $-$	7.928	$= 52.361$ bpm

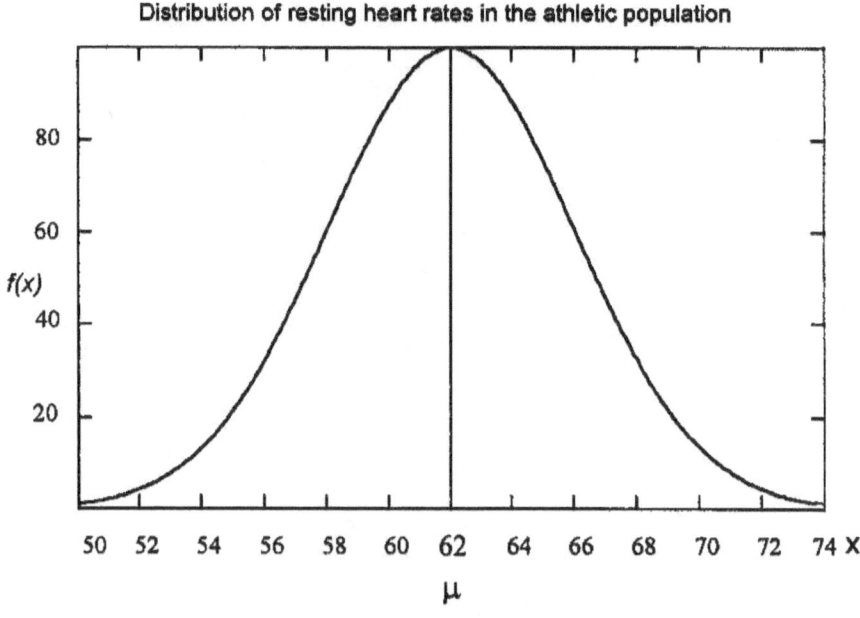

Distribution of resting heart rates in the athletic population

x = Resting Heart rate

μ = Mean Resting heart of the athletic population

Figure 21B.3. Graph of the distribution of the resting heart rates in the athletic population, based on a census involving a very large segment of the athletic population. A mean of 62 bpm and a standard deviation of 4 was determined from the census data.

Of the many questions that may be raised regarding this rather low mean resting heart rate, one in particular is relevant as to whether it equally applies to the athletic population in general and not exclusively to the marathon runners. Accordingly, a random sample similar in characteristics to the runners (as to age, sex ethnic background, etc.) revealed a mean heart rate of 62.269 bpm,[21] with a standard deviation, σ, of 4 bpm (Figure 21B.2). The difference between the means of the two samples equaled 1.980 bpm.

---

[21] Please note that the figures are not based on data from the literature.

Athletes sample mean	Runners sample mean	Difference between the means
62.269 −	60.289 =	1.980

Given these results, one might be tempted to conclude that the difference of less than 2 bpm between the runners and the athletic sample means is really a chance occurrence and that in fact the runners represent an errant sample of the athletic population. In the case of the athletic sample, however, a comprehensive census conducted earlier involving a large segment of the athletic population revealed a mean resting heart rate of 62 bpm with a standard deviation, σ, of 4 bpm (Figure 21B.3).

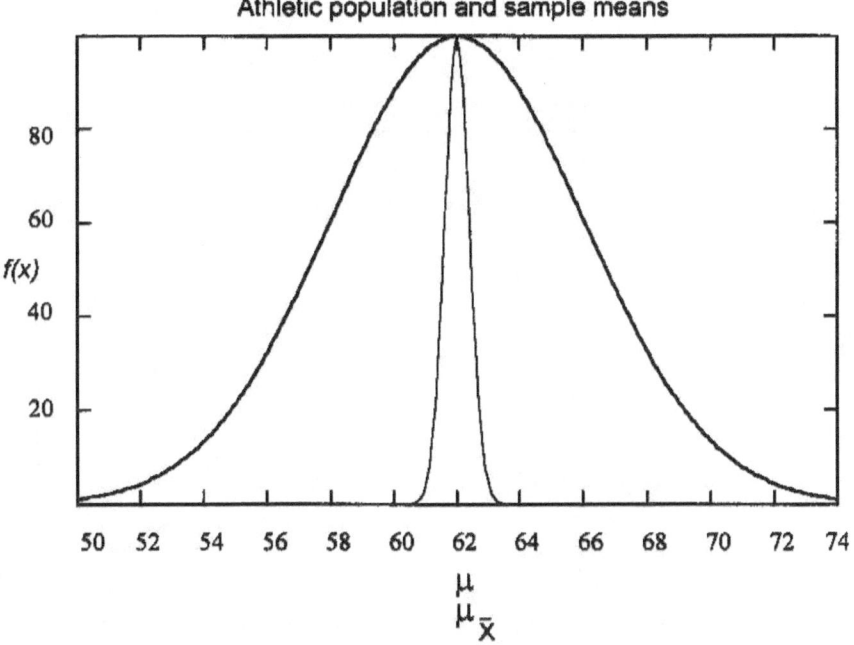

Figure 21B.4. Graph of the distribution of resting heart rate in the athletic population superimposed on the sampling distribution of the mean for samples of size $n = 100$, drawn from the same population. Population and sampling distribution are drawn to a different Y scale (10:1) for emphasis. Population: $\mu = 62$, $\sigma = 4$. Distribution: $\mu = 62$, $\sigma = 0.4$.

Before a structured approach to hypothesis testing is formalized, the triangular relationship of sample, sampling distribution, and population that forms the backdrop to the operational foreground will be examined in detail.

21B.1 Population versus Sampling Distribution

The stacking order of the sample means around the population mean, or its equivalent the mean of the sampling distribution, for a samples of size $n = 100$ and $n = 16$ randomly drawn from an athletic population, is depicted in Figures 21B.4 and 21B.5. Note that while the population heart rates extend over a wide band, 50-74 bpm, covering a span of 24 bpm, the sampling distribution encompass a much narrower band, which even for a small sample of 16 extends over a span of less than 8 bpm.

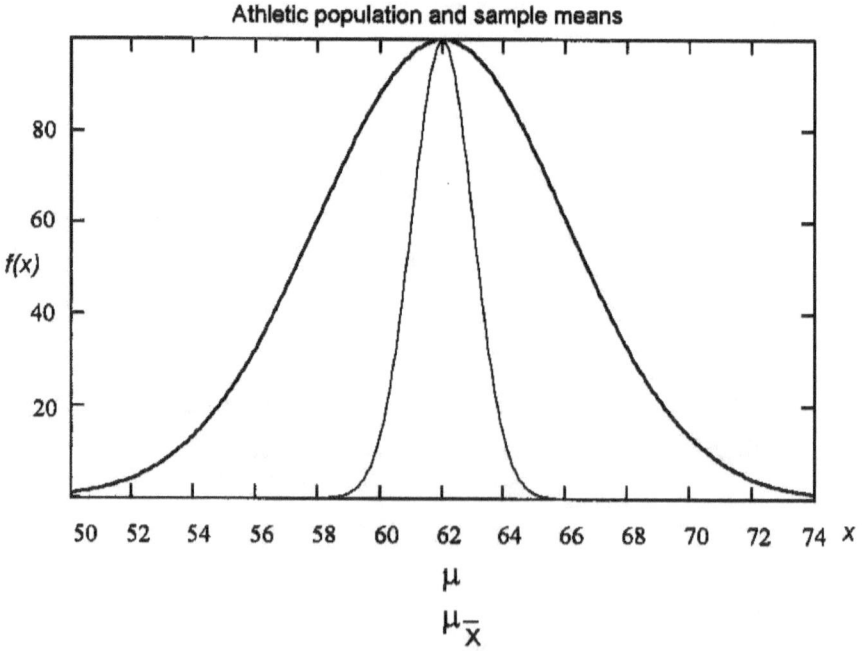

Figure 21B.5. Graph of the distribution of the resting heart rate in the athletic population superimposed on the sampling distribution of the mean for samples of size $n = 16$ drawn from the same population. Population and sampling distribution are drawn to a different Y scale for emphasis (4:1). Population: $\mu = 62$, $\sigma = 4$. Distribution: $\mu = 62$, $\sigma = 1$.

21B.2 Population Mean versus Sample Mean

This is depicted in Figure 21B.6, where the distribution of a random sample drawn from the athletic population is superimposed on the distribution pattern of its parent population at the same scale of measurements. Note that the sample parameters differ from the population parameters, given that the sample is randomly drawn from the defined population.

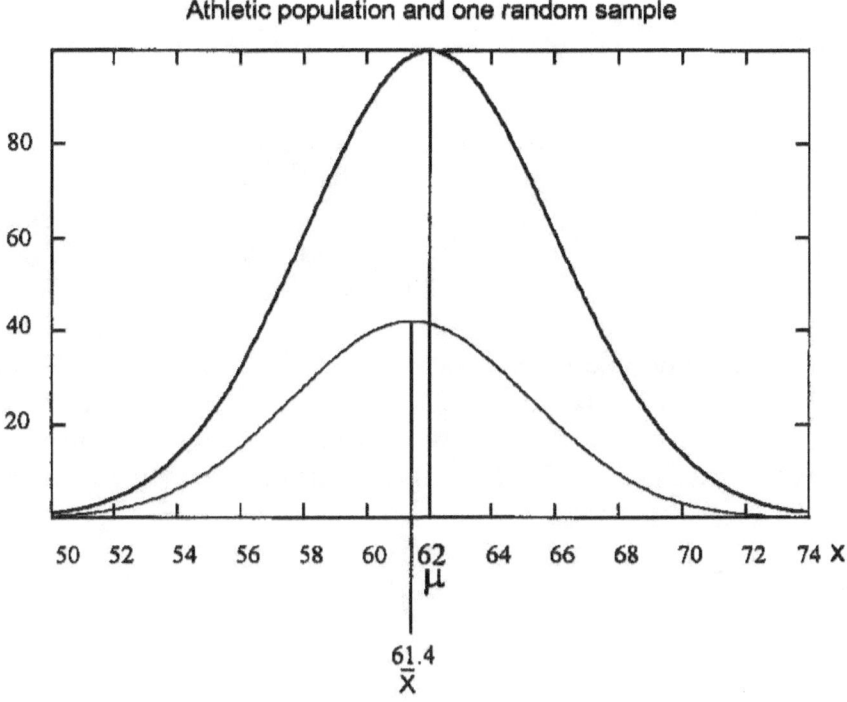

Figure 21B.6. Graph of the superimposed distribution of the resting heart rate in the athletic population and a random sample drawn from the same population. Note that the sample mean of 61.4 is below the population mean of 62 bpm, and its standard deviation is similarly different from that of the population (3.8 versus 4).

21B.3 Sample Mean vs. Sampling Distribution of the Mean

The sampling distribution of the mean for samples of ninety athletes drawn from the athletic population is graphed on an amplified scale in order to bring into focus the salient features of the distribution. For a sample size of 90 (n = 90) and standard deviation of 4, the standard error of the mean for this distribution is calculated as follows:

$$\frac{4}{\sqrt{90}} = 0.4216 = SE$$

Given the standard deviation of 0.4216, the graph makes it clear that 95 percent (95.44 percent to be exact) of all possible samples of size 90 drawn from this population would have their means spanning a range of two standard deviations on either side of $\mu_{\bar{x}}$, covering a band between 61.16 → 62.84. Thus, the sample depicted in Figure 21B.6, whose mean was calculated at 61.4, may be placed with confidence within the 95 percent span, certifying its origin from the 95 percent of the surrounding stacks. By contrast, the distribution for samples of ninety runners drawn from the marathon population centered on a mean of 60.289 yielded a standard error of the mean of 0.4179.

$$\frac{3.964}{\sqrt{90}} = 0.4178 = SE$$

	Runners	Athletes
Mean resting heart rate; sample $n = 90$	$\overline{X} = 60.289 \cong 60.29$	$\overline{X} = 62.269 \cong 62.27$
Standard deviation	$\sigma = 3.964$	$\sigma = 4$
Range for two standard deviations	$52.361 - 68.217$	$54.269 - 66.269$
Population		$\mu = 62; \sigma = 4$
Standard error for $n = 90$	$\sigma_{\overline{X}} = .4178$	$\sigma_{\overline{X}} = .4216$
Range for two standard errors	$59.4534 - 61.1246$	$61.1568 - 62.8432$

Table 21B.1. Statistic of equal samples from runners and athletes; population parameters of athletes. Sampling distribution of the mean ($n = 90$) in the athletic population.

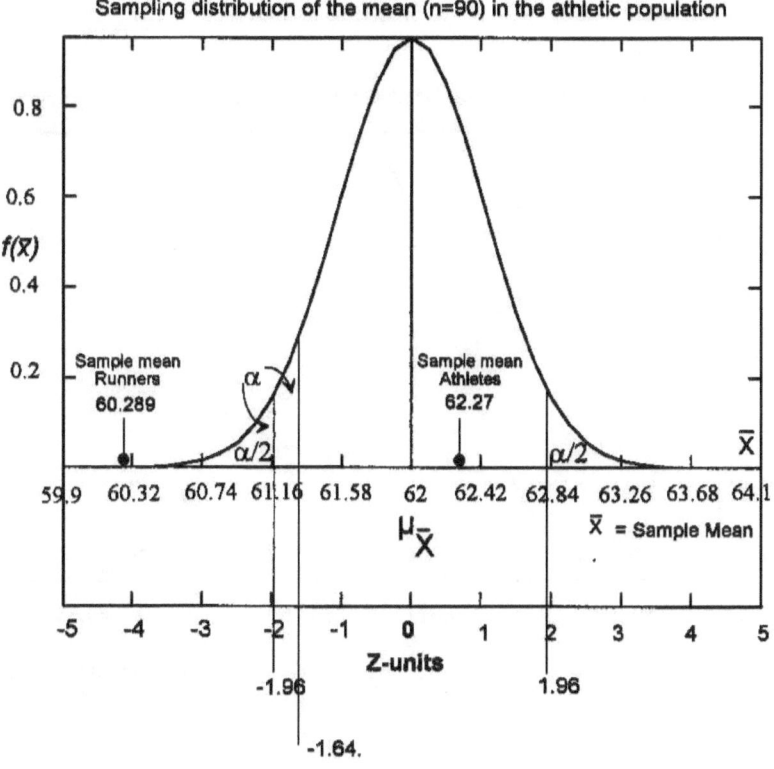

Figure 21B.7. Graph of the Distribution of sample means of $n = 90$, drawn from a population of athletes. The distribution of the sample means indicates that almost all the mean resting heart rates (95.44 percent in fact) exhibited by the samples lie within the interval of 61.16 to 62.84. A mere 2.5 percent of athletes mean resting heart rate will exceed 62.84 bpm, whereas another 2.5 percent of the mean resting rates will fall below 61.16 bpm.

In other words, 95 percent of all possible samples of ninety athletes drawn from the population of all the athletes will exhibit a mean resting hear rate within 62 ± 2SE of the mean that is between 61.16 and 62.84. On the other hand, 2.5 percent of the possible sample means will have a resting heart rate above the 62.84, whereas another 2.5 percent of the sample means will have a mean heart rate below 61.16.

Sampling distribution: $\mu = 62$; $\sigma = 0.42$; sampling distribution of the mean ($n = 90$) in the population of the runners

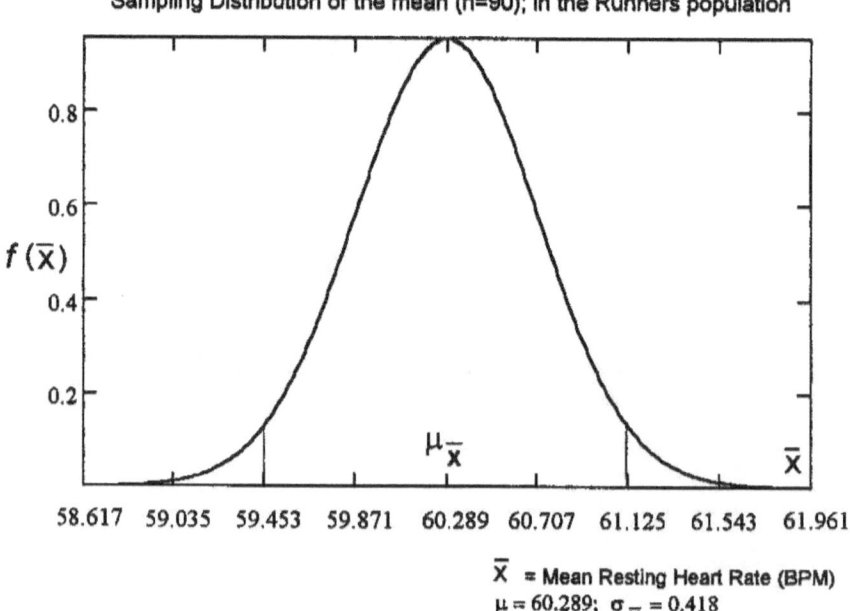

Figure 21B.8. Graph of the distribution of sample means for $n = 90$, drawn from a population of marathon runners.

The distribution of the sample means indicates that almost all the mean resting heart rates (95.44 percent in fact) exhibited by the marathon runners lie within the interval of 59.453 to 61.125 bpm. A mere 2.5 percent of runner's mean resting heart rates will exceed 61.125 bpm, while another 2.5 percent of the mean resting rates will fall below 59.453.

In other words, 95 percent of all possible samples of ninety runners drawn from the population of all the marathon runners will exhibit a mean resting heart rate within 60.289 ± 2SE of the mean, which is between 59.453 and 61.125.

On the other hand, 2.5 percent of the possible sample means will have a resting heart rate above 61.125, whereas another 2.5 percent of the sample means will have a mean heart rate below 59.453.

The difference between the two distribution may not appear to be significant. What is made clear by this triad of interconnections is the central role of the sampling distribution in determining whether a given sample mean falls within its assigned band width and thus qualifies as a genuine sample of the said population. Witness the siting of the sample mean of the ninety athletes on the sampling distribution of the mean in the athletic population compared with the siting of the sample mean of the ninety runners on the same distribution (Figure 21B.2 vs. Graph 21-7). The disparity in the siting location with respect to the population mean of the athletes or its equivalent the mean of the sampling distribution is striking. For the athletic sample, the siting is well within the central 95 percent of the stacking order, whereas runners in the sample are more than four standard errors to the left of the central population mean. In contrast to Figure 21B.2, where the difference of 1.980 in the sample means did not appear to be significant, the siting relationship with respect to the to the alleged population defines the criterion that establishes the nature of the sample-population relationship.

21B.4 Statement and Formulation of Two Opposing Hypotheses

What is being asserted then is that in reality the average resting heart rates of all the Marathon runners, not just the sample of ninety runners under consideration is not different from the average heart rate of the general athletic population, that is,

Mean resting heart rate μ Runners	=	Mean resting heart rate μ_0 Athletes

This simple initial assertion of no difference or null difference (between the means in this case) is titled the null hypothesis, H_0, which maintains that,

$$\mu_{Runners} = \mu_{Athletes} = 62 \text{ bpm}$$

The challenge to this initial assertion of the null hypothesis comes from those who maintain that although the difference in heart rate is small, there is no justification in dismissing it as a chance occurrence of a sample picked at random from the main body or universe of the athletic population without a weighted measure of such a probability. The proposed relation thus takes the following alternate format:

Mean resting heart rate μ Runners	$\neq$	Mean resting heart rate μ_0 Athletes

The challenging theory goes under the title of alternate hypothesis, H_1, which maintains that

$$\mu_{Runners} \neq \mu_{Athletes} \neq 62 \text{ bpm.}$$

The resolution of this argument is the basis of the type of statistical inference referred to as hypothesis testing to be differentiated from the point and interval estimates.

The previously mentioned two-tailed format (Table 21A, Chart 21A-4) used in stating the null hypothesis postulates an exact equality between the mean heart rate of runners and athletes at large. This format carries with it the implication that failure to support the proclaimed null hypothesis may end up in two possible sequences that make up the alternate hypothesis—either the runners exhibiting a much higher heart rate than the athletic population or, alternatively, a much lower heart rate, because the inequality sign is nondirectional.

From a physiologic point of view, however, the likelihood of the first alternative, that is, higher heart rate rates in the runners population, is unlikely. Accordingly, a more appropriate way of phrasing the null hypothesis would be to state the hypothesis in a contradictory or provocative manner, which is contrary to expectation, hoping that the results would knock it down, lower-tailed format (Table 21B.2, Chart 21-5). In other words, to proclaim that the mean heart rate of the runners is at least equal if not greater to the mean heart rate of the athletes. Thus,

$$\underset{\text{Runners}}{\mu} \geq \underset{\text{Athletes}}{\mu_0}$$

In which case, failure to support the claim results in the adoption of the alternative hypothesis which maintains that the runners heart rate is lower than that of the athletes heart rate.

$$\underset{\text{Runners}}{\mu} < \underset{\text{Athletes}}{\mu_0}$$

The questions posed by the challengers may take any one of the following forms:

☑ What is the probability that the ninety runners are in reality a sample, albeit one with an extremely deviated sample mean, drawn by chance from the athletic population?

☑ Or, alternatively, is the sample of ninety runners representative of a totally different parent population distinct from the universal set of athletic population whose mean resting hear rate was determined by a large scale census to be 62?

21B.5 Placement and Siting of the Sample Mean (Runners) on the Axis of the Sampling Distribution of the Mean (Athletes) | Given H0 is true: Conditional Probability—p Value

In order to place the sample mean of the ninety runners, $\overline{X}$, in juxtaposition to the sampling distribution of the mean of the athletic population, one needs to be able to measure the exact siting point in standard units (Figures 21B.1 and 21B.7, Chart 21-5).

In other words, one needs to determine how far is $\overline{X}$ (runners) placed from $\mu_0 = \mu_{\overline{x}}$ (sampling mean of athletes) in z units. The measure of this distance from the central axis translates into the probability of drawing or selecting the given mean $\overline{X}$ from the assumed sampling distribution given that H_0 is true. Thus, the smaller the derived z, the test statistic transform, that is, the nearer to the sampling distribution mean the sample mean is sited, the greater the probability that the sample was derived from the central stacks surrounding the central mean. A $|z|$ of three units or more translates into a significant distance from the central sampling distribution mean, denoting a very small probability that the sample is a random sample from the parent population.

Sampling distribution of the mean values ($n = 90$): athletic population

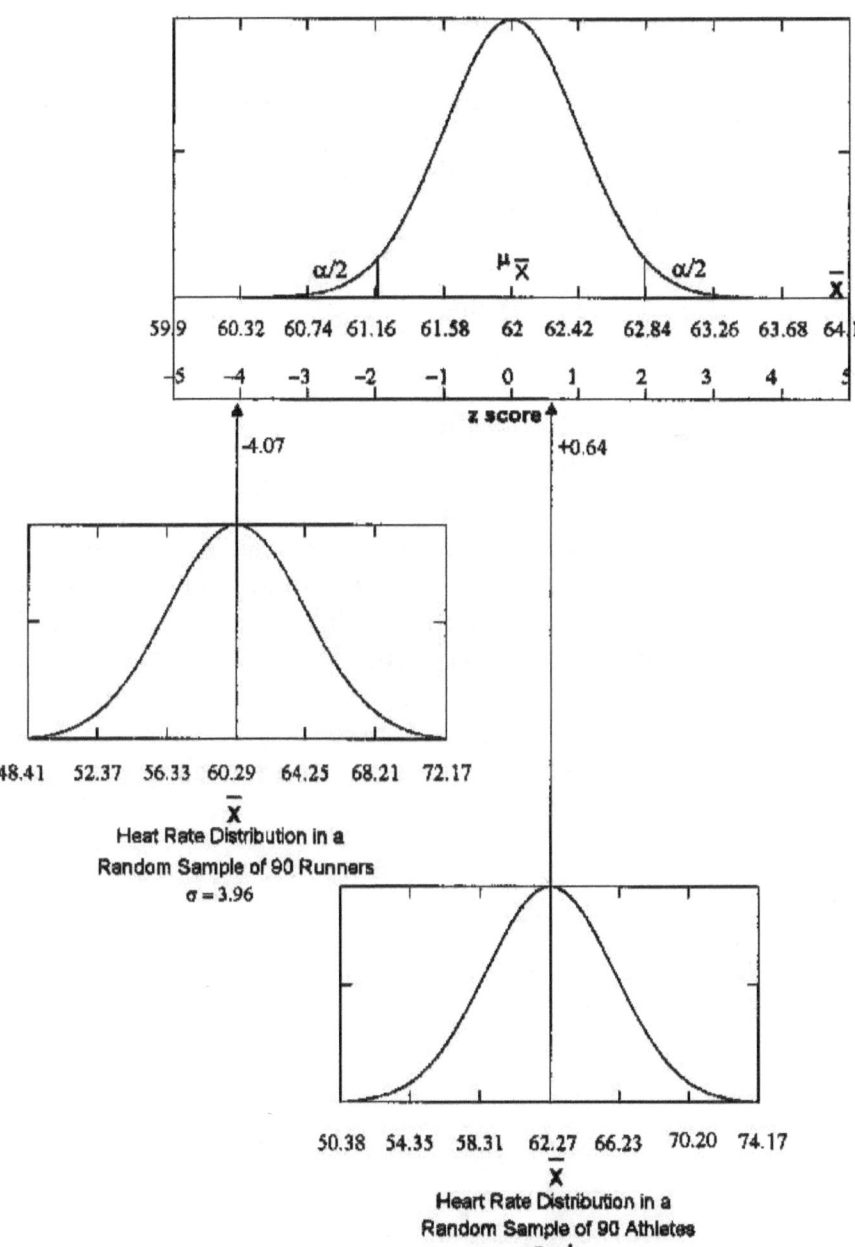

Chart 21-5. Sampling distribution of the mean for all samples of $n = 90$ based on the known population parameters "targeted" by the sample mean of ninety runners and ninety athletes.

In precise language, the conditional probability of obtaining this sample result, $\overline{X} = 60.289$, or one more extreme, given that the null hypothesis is true, may be expressed as follows:

P(This sample result or one more extreme | Null hypothesis is true) $= p$ value.

In symbolic notation, the verbal statement of the conditional probability is abbreviated to

$$P\left(\overline{X} \leq 60.289 \,|\, \mu = 62\right) = p \text{ value}$$

This elegantly states the probability of placing $\overline{X}$ at its allocated site on the sampling distribution scale. It is this calculated probability that determines the p value of the siting.

The distance of the sample mean from the mean of the sampling distribution, $\mu_{\overline{x}}$, may now be converted into multiple or fraction of the standard error of the mean, $SE_{\overline{x}}$, using the classical conversion formula. This transformation allows us to focus on the site of origin of the sample mean and to determine the probability with which it could realistically be considered a sample derived from the alleged population whose hypothesized mean was postulated to be equal to μ_0 (Figure 21A.5).

$$P\left(z \leq 60.289 \,|\, \mu_0 = 62\right) = P\left(z \leq \dfrac{\overset{\text{Sample mean}}{\overline{X}} - \overset{\substack{\text{Population mean} \\ \text{Sampling mean}}}{\mu_{\overline{X}}}}{\dfrac{\overset{\text{Population SD}}{\sigma}}{\sqrt{\underset{\text{sample size}}{n}}}}\right) = P\left(z \leq \dfrac{60.289 - 62}{\dfrac{4}{\sqrt{90}}}\right) = P\left(z \leq \dfrac{-1.71}{0.42}\right)$$

$$= P(z \leq -4.07) = <<0.0001$$

p value < 0.00001

Therefore, given the sample mean, $\overline{X}$, of the runners and the parameters of the athletic population, μ_0 and σ, it can be stated that the probability of such a sample as the ninety runners being drawn from the general athletic population occurs less than once in a hundred thousand draws.

Because such an outcome is very rare, we are justified in rejecting the null and concluding that the population of marathon runners is indeed a distinct population different from the general athletic population.

Given that the mean of samples drawn from the athletic population normally congregate about the expected mean of 62 bpm (Figures 21B.5-21B.7), it is still conceivably possible to draw a sample of ninety members whose mean is as extreme as 60.289 found in the current sample. However, this probability located way out into the left tail of the sampling distribution curve (Figure 21B.7) is very small; in fact, it is less than 0.00001, so that $p \ll 0.00001$ of the area under the sampling distribution curve. Such being the case, it is very unlikely that the sample of ninety runners is a derivative of the general athletic population whose mean resting heart rate equals 62 bpm. Accordingly, because the chance of selecting such a sample from the athletic population is so remote, the null hypothesis of equal or greater difference is rejected in favor of the alternate hypothesis of smaller difference.

Nevertheless, if we know for sure that the sample meets all the criteria of a genuine random sample, we are obliged to conclude that the sample belongs to the same population and the minuscule probability of drawing it is just that, a statistical fluke.

In order to demonstrate the effect of a minor change in the population parameter as stipulated in the null hypothesis, consider a population mean of 61 bpm instead of the 62 bpm postulated earlier.

In this case, the conditional probability is expressed and calculated as follows:

$$P\left(\overline{X} \le 60.289 \,|\, \mu = 61\right) = p \text{ value}$$

$$P\left(z \le \dfrac{\overset{\substack{\text{Sample}\\\text{mean}}}{\overline{X}} - \overset{\substack{\text{Population mean}\\\text{Sampling mean}}}{\mu_{\overline{X}}}}{\dfrac{\underset{\text{Population SD}}{\sigma}}{\underset{\text{sample size}}{\sqrt{n}}}} \right) = P\left(z \le \dfrac{60.289 - 61}{\dfrac{4}{\sqrt{90}}} \right) = P\left(z \le \dfrac{-0.71}{0.42} \right) = P(z \le -1.69) = 0.455$$

p value $= 0.0455$

The probability of such an occurrence, that is, probability of drawing a sample of ninety runners from the general athletic population whose mean heart rate turns out to be 60.289 bpm, is now given at 4.5 percent. This new figure is less extreme than the original probability. It does not actually reverse the initial contention of difference, but it now seems plausible to suggest that the sample of runners may actually be a subset of the general athletic population, bearing in mind that this is again a remote probability that does not justify such a conclusion. If this, however, turns out to be the true but unforeseen situation, we would have committed an α error in our assumption of difference where none existed in reality (Figure 21B.10).

In both the above cases, the derived probability in terms of the p value was sufficient to resolve the conflict in the formulation of the two opposing hypotheses in favor of one at the expense of the other.

21B.6 Prior Specification and Setting of the Significance Level

The hypothesis testing procedure noted above can be described as a straightforward process of statistical inference that leaves the ultimate disposition of the null hypothesis (accept or reject), particularly in marginal situation, in the hands of the observer.

In order to circumvent the subjective element from the final statistical decision, the classical approach is designed to mitigate the subjective element from the decision-making process.

It is now possible to put the believers and doubters of the null to the test. Before settling the problem for or against, we need to agree on a criterion or level that would settle the argument in favor of the null, that is, no difference, or against it. We could for example ascertain a priori that if the mean of a random sample derived from the runners population at large should fall below or beyond three standard errors of the mean to the left of the mean of the sampling distribution (≤ -3 z units), that is, less than 60.74 bpm (Figure 21B.7), we are likely to conclude that the sample may not have been derived from the alleged parent athletic population. In other words, we might be tempted to rule against the null and conclude that this small probability does not justify us in maintaining that no difference exists and that the runners are a subset of the athletic population.

by rejecting the null, we now adopt the alternative hypothesis and assert that the ninety runners belong indeed to a different category of athletes.

With this in mind, the process begins by assigning, a priori, a level of significance α, the equivalent of the probability level obtained in the previous direct placement procedure. The specific value assigned to α divides the area under the sampling distribution curve into contiguous complementary regions of α and $1 - \alpha$. With the division thus arbitrarily set, the placement of all possible sample means turns out into a binary alternative as to whether the siting is within the α or the $1 - \alpha$ area.

This initial setting of probability reverses the sequence of the final step prescribed for the p value procedure from last to first. Thus, the setting of a significant α level implies the demarcation of a tail area as a percent of the area under the distribution curve equivalent to the predetermined significance level. From the appropriate z tables, the critical z value bounding the cutoff tail area is derived. For a lower tail area, a significance level of 5 percent places the critical z value at ± 1.645 on the $\overline{X}$ axis. For a two-tailed 5 percent area, the critical z value is placed at ± 1.96.

With the α significance level clearly marked off by the critical z value, and the probability of this sample result or one more extreme marked off by the p value, given that the null hypothesis is correct, we are faced with two concurrent data values: a level of significance, α, and a calculated probability level of the observed sample result, p value.

For the athletic population whose sampling distribution curve is shown in Figure 21B.7, α is composed of the tail area bounded by 62.84 bpm on the upper side and 61.16 bpm on the lower side. The distribution makes it clear that the probability of drawing a sample with a mean heart rate greater than 62.84 bpm or smaller than 61.16 bpm from the athletic population is less than 5 percent, whereas the probability of drawing a sample equal or greater than 61.16 bpm or equal and smaller than 62.84 accounts for 95 percent of the total.

21B.7 Weighing the Observed versus the Assigned Significance Lever

- This introduction was begun by assigning a critical value of $\leq-3z$ standard units corresponding to a significance level of $\alpha = 0.0013$, in order to guide the decision regarding the acceptance or rejection of the null hypothesis, H_0.
- The probability, p, of the occurrence of such a sample or more extreme as the one under consideration is calculated.
- Comparison of the calculated p value with the initially set level of significance, α, determines the final decision and settles the argument for or against.

The decision in all the above cases is determined by the level at which α is set. Thus, setting the α level defines the maximum probability of rejecting a true null because $p < \alpha$ is considered significant enough to reject H_0. On the other side, α defines the maximum probability of Type I error that may be tolerated because $p > \alpha$ results in the opposite decision by accepting the null, H_0. α then is a measure of the acceptable level of error tolerated in making a decision.

To recapitulate,

A. Specify the level of significance, that is, the probability level, α, as a criterion for rejection.

B. Compare the conditional probability of the sample results by calculating the observed difference.

1. If the calculated probability is smaller than the rejection criterion $p < \alpha$ (significant), reject H_0.
2. If the calculated probability exceeds or equals the rejection criterion $p \geq \alpha$ (insignificant), accept H_0.
3. If a significant result is obtained when the null hypothesis is correct, Type I error is made.
4. If an insignificant result is obtained when the null is false, Type II error is made.

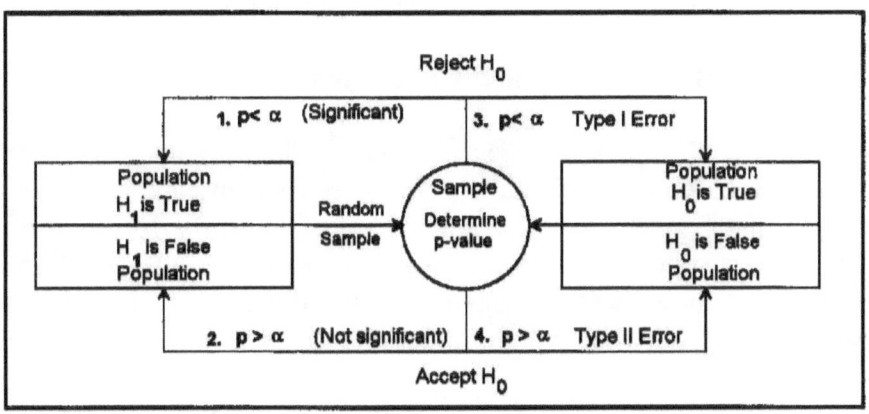

Flow Chart 21-3. Graphic equivalent to one variant of the null hypothesis

True State: Actual Situation	
H_1 is true H_0 is false	H_0 is true H_1 is false
$\mu_1 = \mu_{True}$	$\mu_{Hypo} = \mu_0$
$\mu_{True} < \mu_{Hypo}$	$\mu_{True} < \mu_{Hypo}$
Significant difference	No significant difference

$\mu_{True} < \mu_{Hypo}$	Correct decision Inference of difference	Erroneous prediction Inference of difference		
	$P(\text{rejecting } H_0 \mid H_1 \text{ is true})$ $= 1 - \beta = \text{Power}$	$P(\text{rejecting } H_0 \mid H_0 \text{ is true})$ $= \alpha$	Reject H_0	
	No error	Type I error		Decision
$\mu_{True} \geq \mu_{Hypo}$	Erroneous prediction Inference of no difference	Correct decision Inference of no difference		
	$P(\text{accepting } H_0 \mid H_1 \text{ is true}) = \beta$ Type II error	$P(\text{accepting } H_0 \mid H_0 \text{ is true})$ $= 1 - \alpha$ No error	Accept H_0	

Table 21B.3. The four possible outcomes in a lower-tailed hypothesis

21B.8 Statistical Decision and Conclusion

We are never 100 percent sure as to whether the sample of the ninety runners is essentially different from an equivalent random athletic sample that happens to exhibit an identical or similarly low mean resting heart rate. The question that needs to be addressed in the language of the null hypothesis is whether the sample of runners is no different from other random samples derived from the athletic population.

Stated differently, the mean heart rate of the sample of runners could be equally accounted for as a random sample from the left tail end of the sampling distribution of the athletic population. On the other hand, the same mean heart rate of the sample of runners may as well be a random sample derived from a unique and different sampling distribution that characterize the population of the marathon runners.

On the strength of the evidence, we are more than 99 percent sure that the latter interpretation is the correct answer. Nonetheless, the rare possibility cannot be escaped that our sample of runners is really a sample drawn from the athletic population, and although somewhat rare and highly improbable, its occurrence remain possible.

This trivial example turns into what is essentially the main thesis of statistical inference when the parenthood of the sample in question is investigated as to whether (despite what appears to be otherwise) the sample is just another random sample drawn from the its parent population or whether it is unlikely or very unlikely to belong to the alleged or suspected population.

In the case of the marathon runners, we may conclude that the athletic population is very unlikely to be the parent population and that indeed it is very likely that the ninety runners are a random sample drawn from a population we will designate as exclusively made of runners.

In quantitative terms, the sample mean of the ninety runners is to be found at one precise location on the $\overline{X}$ axis of the distribution of the sample means of size 90 as noted in the magnified normal distribution of the means (Chart 21-7).

Sampling distribution of the mean values ($n = 90$);
athletic population presumed mean = 62 bpm.

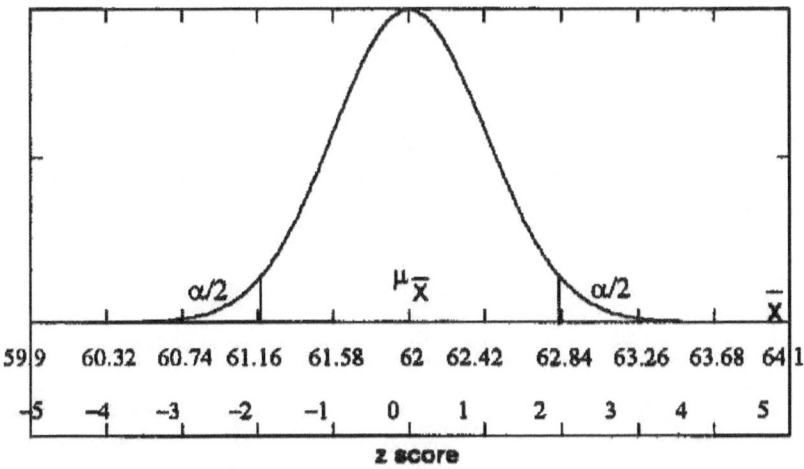

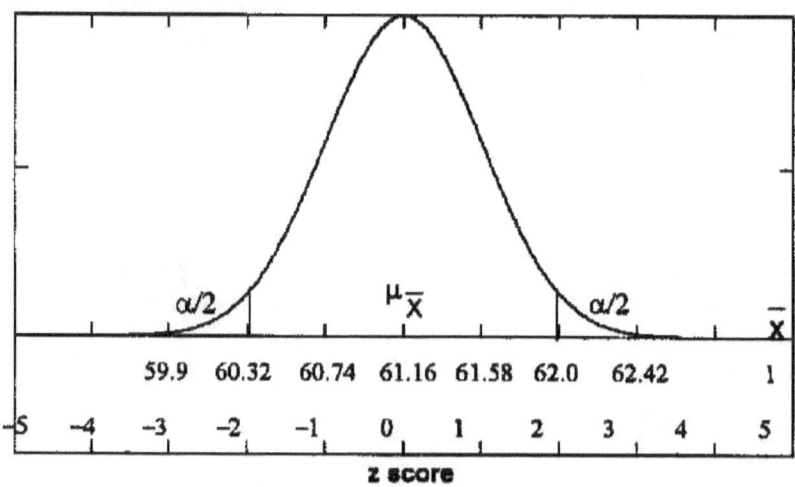

Sampling distribution of the mean values (*n*=90);
athletic population true mean = 61.16 bpm.

Chart 21.6. Relationship of the sampling distribution of the mean for
the same population and sample size based on presumed (hypothesized)
population mean and true but unknown population mean

**21B.8.1 P(Rejecting H_0 | H_0 Is True) = P(Type I Error | H_0 Is True)
= α: α Error**

If we took 10,000 random samples from the athletic population, it
is likely that at least one of them would have a mean heart rate of ≤
60.29 bpm (Figure 21B.7).

Small as the calculated probability turns out to be, the far-off
possibility cannot be ruled out completely (ruling completely
out the possibility is equivalent to saying that winning the lotto is
impossible despite the odds of) that the sample is in fact a subset of
the athletic population, belonging to the left tail end of the sampling
distribution of the same population. In other words, the sample is in
fact an odd but nevertheless a genuine random sample drawn from
the athletic population.

If this is the case, we did commit an error by ascertaining that the sample belongs to a distinct population of runners rather than the main athletic population.

The size of this error is equivalent to the cutoff area under the normal curve of the sampling distribution of the athletic population.

In the terminology of the null hypothesis, we have committed an alpha error equivalent to the set value we initially postulated as the cutoff level or significance level.

Unknown to us, we have inadvertently committed a classical α error. We have labeled a normal sample, in our parlance a true-negative sample, a positive sample, that is, false-positive sample.

Sampling distribution of the mean: runners and athletes

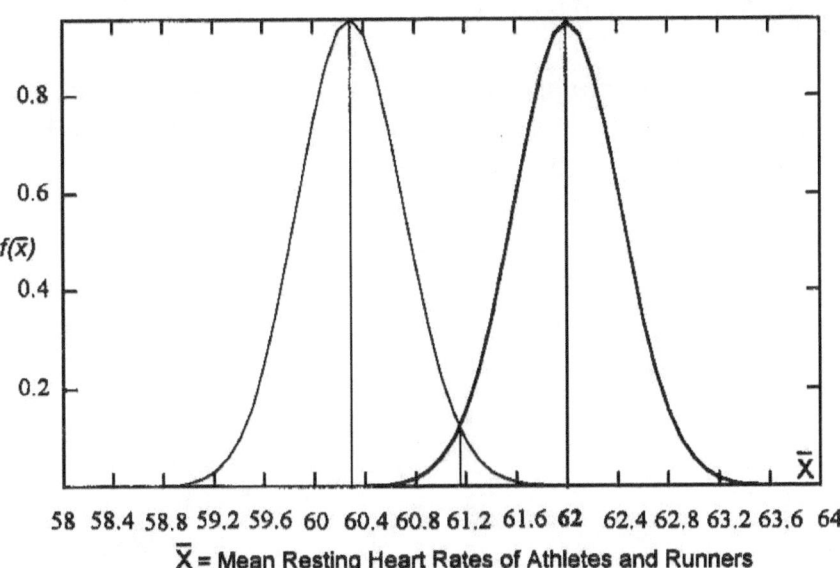

58 58.4 58.8 59.2 59.6 60 60.4 60.8 61.2 61.6 62 62.4 62.8 63.2 63.6 64

$\overline{X}$ = Mean Resting Heart Rates of Athletes and Runners

Figure 21B.9. Graph of the juxtaposed distribution of the sample means of runners and athletes based on equal samples of ninety drawn from their respective population. The athletic population mean resting heart rate of 62 bpm and the standard deviation of 4 were known from a previous census. The solid curve is based on standard error of the mean 0.42. The ninety runners were randomly drawn from the population of participating marathon runners. Their resting mean heart rate was calculated at 60.289 bpm with a standard deviation of 3.964 and standard error of the mean of 0.418.

21B.8.2 P(Accepting H_0 | H_1 Is True) = P(Type II Error | H_1 Is True) = β: β Error

A final twist in the scenario may be construed as follows: What if our belief in the result of the census survey not supported by the true facts, such that our null hypothesis of $\mu = 62$ bpm is false. It is conceivable that through some unforeseen bias in the selection process, the results initially presented are flawed and that the real athletic population mean is 61.16 bpm and not the previous figure of 62 bpm. Yet being unaware of the facts, we continue to relate the sample means of the runners population to the assumed but faulty formulation of the null hypothesis.

In other words, we are in effect drawing samples from the sampling distribution of the real population and assigning them to the faulty but assumed distribution based on the null hypothesis.

Sampling distribution of the mean: runners and athletes

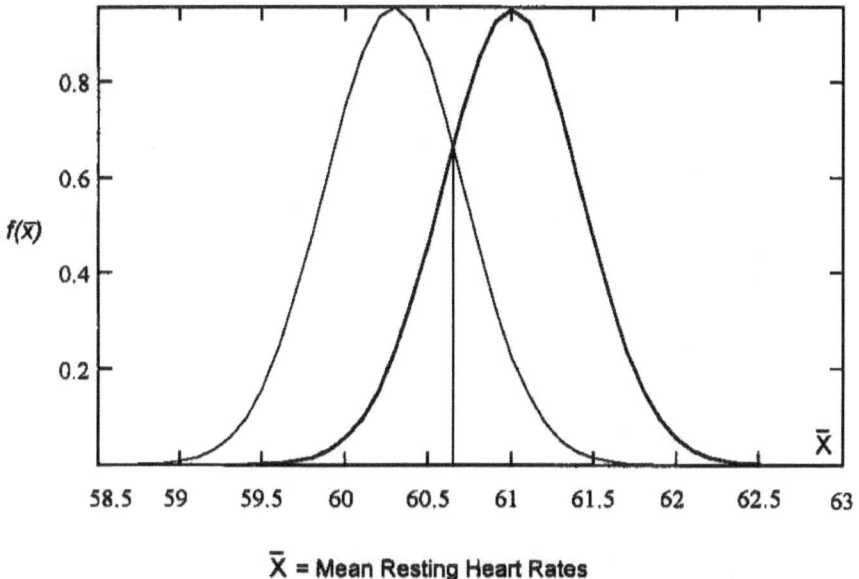

X = Mean Resting Heart Rates

Figure 21B.10. Graph of the juxtaposed distribution of the sample means of runners and athletes based on equal samples of ninety drawn from their respective population. The athletic population mean resting heart rate of 61 bpm and standard deviation of 4 are based on the assumption that the results of the previous census were flawed and the actual parameters are those noted above. The solid curve is based on standard error of the mean (0.42). The ninety runners were randomly drawn from the population of participating marathon runners. Their resting mean heart rate was calculated at 60.289 bpm with a standard deviation of 3.964 and standard error of the mean of 0.418. Note the degree of overlap between the means in this case compared with that of the previous case graphed in 19-8.

As noted in Figure 21B.6, all samples derived from the true sampling distribution to the right of the sampling mean of 61.16, which account for approximately 50 percent of all samples derived from the true sampling distribution, would fall in the acceptance region of the assumed but false sampling distribution of the null hypothesis and would thus be considered as representative of the athletic population. However, all samples derived from the true sampling distribution to the left of the sampling mean of 61.16 which account for approximately 50 percent of all samples derived from the true sampling distribution, would fall in the rejection region of the assumed but false null hypothesis and would thus be considered as unlikely to be derived from the athletic population.

In the first instance, we have concluded that the population from which the sample is drawn is no different from the assumed null; thus, we have committed a β error.

In the second instance, we have correctly rejected the null hypothesis and concluded the parent population of the sample is different from the assumed null hypothesis.

Chapter 21C

Controlling Errors in Hypothesis Testing

In the formulation of the null hypothesis detailed in the previous chapter, only two possibilities or outcomes were initially taken into consideration: either to accept the null hypothesis of no difference when it is true or to reject the null when it is false in favor of an alternate hypothesis of difference. Had this been always the case, the possibility of error would have been literally nonexistent. This, however, is not the case. This simple dichotomy of assigning a specific value to the null and accepting it or rejecting it on the evidence of sample statistic conceals the two errors, inherent in the probabilistic nature of hypothesis testing, which may have been committed without one being aware of either.

Thus, when the null hypothesis is rejected and it is indeed true, a Type I error has been committed. On the other side of the coin, when failure to reject the null hypothesis when it is indeed false, a Type II error has been committed. With this in mind, the capacity to control the magnitude of Type I and Type II errors must be taken into consideration, in the design and execution of hypothesis testing. The concepts noted previously are best expressed through the data of a realistic example.

21C.1 Two-Tailed Test

Consider a pharmaceutical manufacturing process designed to produce 30.0 mg capsules of a potent CV drug. Based on previous experience, the mean weight of the capsule in a production run averaged 30 mg with a standard deviation of 1 mg (Figure 21C.1). The capsule is thus considered safe and in compliance with FDA dosage specification if its sample mean remains within an acceptable range of the target weight of 30.0 mg deemed to be tolerable.

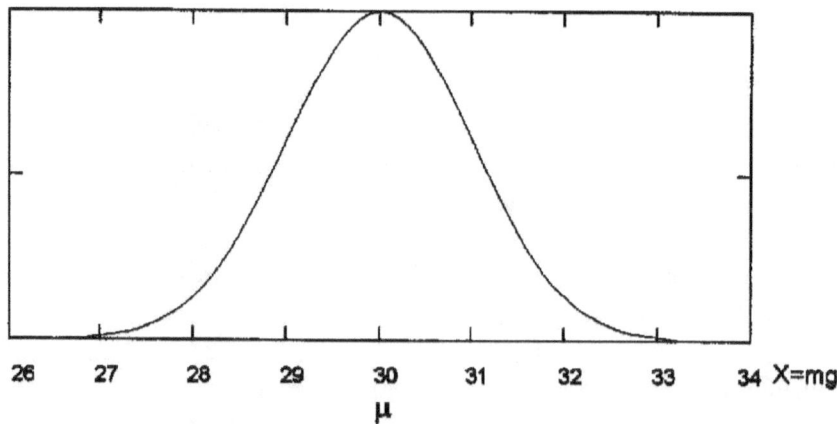

26 27 28 29 30 31 32 33 34 X=mg
μ

Figure 21C.1. Graph of the population parameters of the
capsules in production: A mean of 30 mg and a standard
deviation of 1 mg were observed over the long run

In order to ascertain that the capsules that finally reach the pharmacy
meet the above specification, a random sample of one hundred
capsules out of the thousands in stock is tested in order to verify that
the stock is in compliance with the allowed dosage. The proposed
null hypotheses is the basic hypothesis that is being challenged
for possible rejection by assuming that the mean capsular weight
remains unchanged in either direction. The null hypothesis, H_0, is
thus an affirmative statement of this fact, whereas the alternative
hypothesis, H_1, is the denial of the same fact. The two statements are
expressed as follows:

$$H_0: \mu = \mu_0 = 30$$

$$H_1: \mu \neq \mu_0 = 30$$

A hypothesis is an assumption about a population parameter, a mean
value in this case. A hypothesis test consists of taking a sample from
the population, calculating the sample mean, $\overline{X}$, and then deciding

if the sample mean could have come from a population whose mean $\mu = \mu_0 = \mu_{hypo}$, the hypothesized mean.

Because the average weight of a sample hovers around 30.0 mg but is rarely if ever 30 mg on the dot, the question that needs to be addressed is how far from 30.0 mg a sample mean may deviate and still be considered a sample from parent population whose mean is 30.0 mg. In other words, how many standard error of the mean, $SE_{\bar{X}} = \sigma_{\bar{X}}$, can a sample mean be removed from the sampling distribution mean, $\mu_{\bar{X}}$, to ensure that it is indeed a sample from the population whose mean is 30.0 mg and thus in compliance with the prescribed dosage? From the following relation,

$$\begin{matrix} \text{Standard error} \\ \text{of the mean} \\ \sigma_{\bar{X}} \end{matrix} = \begin{matrix} \text{Standard} \\ \text{deviation} \\ \dfrac{\sigma}{\sqrt{n}} \end{matrix} = \begin{matrix} \text{mg} \\ \dfrac{\sigma}{\sqrt{100}} \end{matrix} = 0.1 \text{ mg; therefore, } 2s_{\bar{X}} = 0.2 \text{ mg.}$$

It is now possible to ascertain that a sample of one hundred caps whose mean, $\bar{X}$, ranges between 29.8 and 30.2 mg may be considered as a random sample derived from a population whose mean is equal to 30.0 mg and thus certifying that the stock being tested is acceptable for patient's usage (Figure 21C.2). The decision rule in this case is simple. A random sample from the current stock is inspected. If the sample mean turns out between 29.8 and 30.2 mg, the stock (i.e., the population from which the random sample is derived) is considered safe for prescribing.

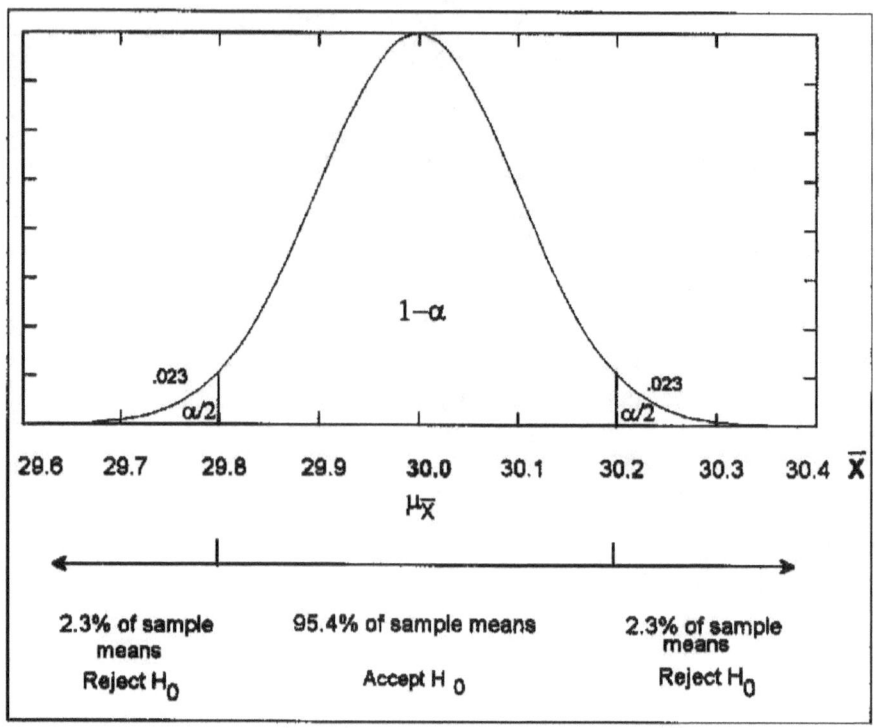

Figure 21C.2. Graph of the sampling distribution of the mean of the capsular population; A mean of 30 mg with a standard error of the mean of 0.1 mg was obtained.

21C.2 Type I Error: α Error (Rejecting a True Null Hypothesis)

Because the sample size is large, the sample mean will be normally distributed. It can thus be asserted that with a population whose actual mean is $\mu = \mu_0 = 30.0$ mg, that is, $\mu_{true} = \mu_{hypo}$, it is likely that 95.4 percent of all sample means whose $n = 100$ will lie in the interval between 29.8 and 30.2 mg (Figure 21C.4).

This implies that out of a one hundred random samples of one hundred capsules each, five sample means will lie outside the stated interval of 29.8 to 30.2 mg. Thus, 4.6 percent of the time (once in twenty-two times), a perfectly safe stock of capsules will be rejected for having its sample mean fall outside the prescribed boundaries stated previously. Such being the case, an α or Type I error would be committed at the 4.6 percent level of significance, equivalent to the areas under both tails of the sampling distribution.

The 1 percent significance level, that is, reducing the tail areas to 0.01 (0.005 in each tail) of the total under the normal curve, implies extending the control limits from the present 29.8-30.2 to 29.75-30.25 (critical $z_{a/2}$ = ±2.58; Table19B.3, Chapter 19B) in order to incur fewer costly false rejections. This less restrictive significance level was requested in order to meet the demand for fewer costly false rejections. As will be shown later, this may not have been a wise course to follow considering the dosage requirements and the unforeseen Type II error that needs to be taken into consideration.

21C.3 Type II Error: β Error (Failing to Reject a False Null Hypothesis)

Consider for a moment that due to a combination of factors affecting the manufacturing process, the true mean of the capsular stock has shifted from its established norm of 30.0 mg. This fact, of which the pharmacist is unaware, renders the assumption underlying the null hypothesis actually false (i.e., a true difference does exist, μ_{true} ≠ μ_{hypo}). However, in this case the real distribution of the mean is still judged in accordance with the constraints of the hypothesized distribution, so that the real sample mean is "placed" by the terms of the assumed and false hypothesis.

Such being the case, all outcomes of the samples are tested against the "assumed" null hypothesis sampling distribution curve. That is, the sample outcome is "placed" at the site of origin dictated by the assumed null distribution, so that a sample outcome may fall on either side of the assigned $a/2$ demarcation line which in reality places the sample mean either in the nonrejection region of the null distribution or in the rejection regions. When placed within the acceptance region, it is falsely accepted as a sample from within the main assumed distribution, thus committing a Type II or β error by asserting that the mean of the stock (population) being tested is no different from the standard historical mean.

If, on the other hand, the sample mean should fall within the $\alpha/2$ region outside the demarcation (cutoff) line, it will be classified as a reject with respect to the original null assumption and correctly assessed as a sample from a distribution whose mean differ from the hitherto assumed norm, thus correctly categorizing the mean of the stock as being outside the accepted mean dosage restriction. In this case, the probability of rejecting the null is the exact complement of β, or $1 - \beta$.

Suppose that, unknown to the pharmacist, the actual mean of the population of the stock being tested is $\mu = \mu_1 = 29.6$ mg, $\mu_{true} \neq \mu_{hypo}$. In this case, at the 4.6 percent significance level, the upper control limit is actually 29.8 mg; therefore, the stock being tested should be rejected. However, the hypothesized value of the population mean is still presumed to be 30.0 mg as per the null hypothesis, such that $\mu = \mu_0 = 30$ mg (Figure 21C.3).

A random sample drawn from the sampling distribution under H_1 yields as might be expected, a mean less than 29.8 mg with a probability of 97.7 percent. In only 2.3 percent of one hundred draws would the sample mean be expected to exceed 29.8 mg. Judged by the assumed null hypothesis, the samples drawn from the upper tail of H_1 (≥ 29.8 mg) would qualify as bona fide random samples assumed to be drawn from the main body or the acceptance region of H_0, that is, the central area bounded by the cutoff values of 29.8 and 30.2. A β error has been committed. The mitigating factor to consider is that the probability of such mishap or β error is rarely encountered, because 97.7 percent of the samples drawn from H_1 would exhibit a mean < 29.8 and thus would be correctly rejected as samples from a different population mean by the criteria of the null hypothesis with a probability of 0.977. Nevertheless, the probability of such an error although less than 0.023 is real and must be taken into consideration and balanced against the probability of the α error.

Consider a random sample drawn from yet another sampling distribution labeled H_2, whose actual sampling mean $= 29.7$ mg. Here again as might be expected, the area under the normal curve to the left of the demarcation or cutoff line comprising 84 percent of the total area and accounting similarly for 84 percent of all possible random samples drawn, whose mean <29.8 mg, would be rejected[22] because they fall beyond the cutoff line of the presumed null hypothesis. The complementary area of 16 percent to the right of the cutoff line accounting for 16 percent of all sample means drawn from H_2 whose mean ≥29.8 mg would fall in the acceptance region of the presumed but false null hypothesis, implying that the H_2 population is no different from the H_0 hypothesized population. In this case, the probability of β error is larger while the probability of rejecting the false hypothesis is smaller.

The decision not to reject a false null is not as innocent as it may appear. What in fact transpired is that the entire stock of capsules whose mean is 29.7 is accepted as a certified stock ready for prescription orders with a probability of 0.16, while in actual fact the whole stock is beyond the specified mean dosage range. A serious β or Type II error has been committed of which the pharmacist is not aware. In effect, we have mistakenly labeled a sample derived from the true distribution as being one derived from the alleged true (i.e., false) distribution, thus concluding that the mean of the stock being considered is not different form the assumed currently accepted mean. Crossing over to sampling distributions of H_3 whose mean of 30.1 mg exceed the hypothesized mean by 0.1 mg, we note that the β error involved now occurs with a frequency of 84 percent. In other words, a stock whose mean is 30.1 has been erroneously labeled as the same as the currently accepted mean with a solid probability of 0.84, leaving the probability of correctly rejecting the assertion to a mere 0.16 of the total.

Finally, at the other end in H_4, whose actual sampling distribution mean equals 30.4 mg., the acceptance and rejection regions are the reverse of those obtained in the H_1 distribution accounting for identical β error of 2.3 percent, while correctly rejecting the balance as representative of a different population.

---

[22]   Note that sample mean ≥30.2, that is, 5 SE of the mean beyond the sampling mean of H_2 would similarly fall in the rejection region of H_0. This fact is not included in the discussion for brevity and clarity.

Sampling distribution of assumed null hypothesis

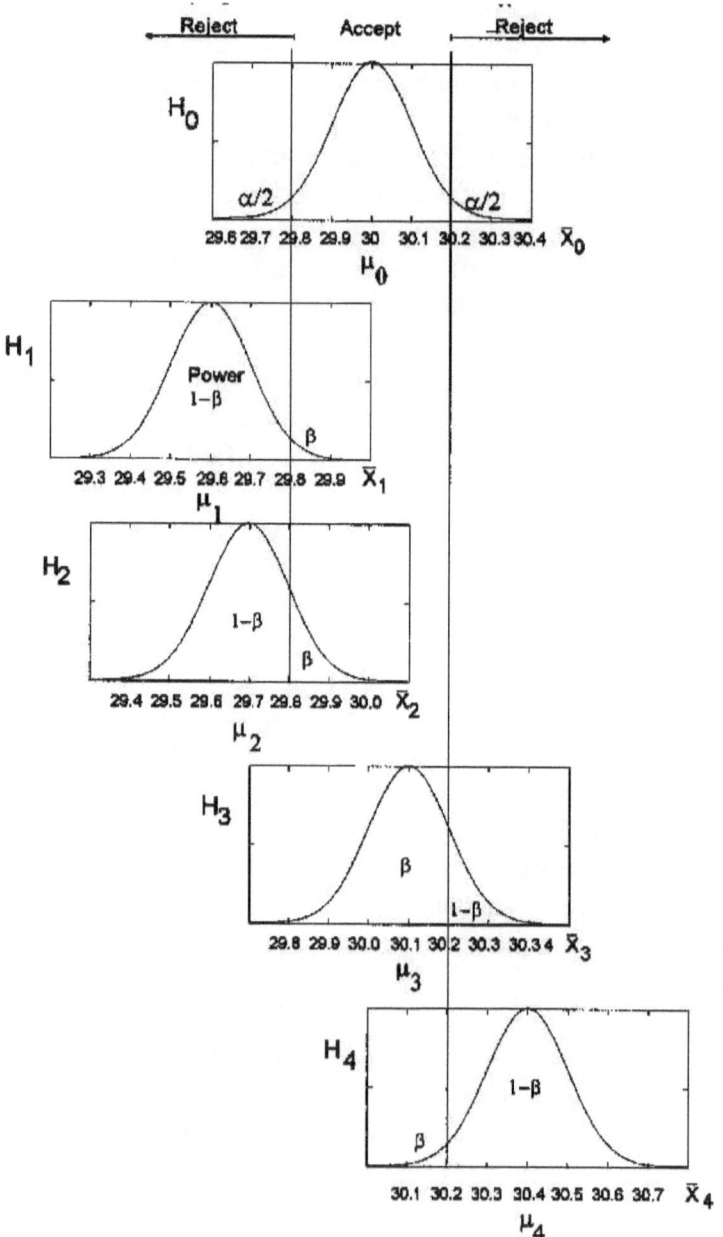

Figure 21C.3. Chart of the juxtaposed sampling distribution of assumed and false hypothesis to the true sampling distribution of four possible and true population means.

The four alternate or actual sampling distributions illustrated are in reality part of a continuum of sampling distributions that stretch in between the extremes of the assumed and faulty null distribution, none of which is known a priori to the person formulating the initial statement of the null hypothesis.

The classification or siting of the sample outcome may thus be divided into two subsets: the one falling inside the demarcation lines, within the nonrejection region, falsely assumed to originate from the sampling distribution whose mean $\mu_{\bar{x}} = \mu_0$, that is, from the hypothesized population. The other falling outside the demarcation line, outside the demarcation region, correctly classified as originating from a different population whose mean μ_1, μ_2, and so on, is the true population mean.

In other words, accepting the null given the assigned critical value and the original hypothesized mean μ_0, without knowing that the real mean is displaced resulted in our rejecting $1 - \beta$ of the area under the true sampling distribution and accepting the β area of the true distribution.

Initially, as the mean of the real distribution diverges from the mean of the hypothesized mean, μ_0, the rejection area, $1 - \beta$, is small. In other words, if the difference between the hypothesized mean and the actual mean is small, β is large, that is, a big chunk of the alternative curve falls within the nonrejection region of μ_0, and thus the rejection region of $1 - \beta$ will be accordingly small.

As the true mean moves further away from the assumed mean, we end up correctly rejecting a greater and greater percentage of the sample means, except for the small fraction in the tails that falls within the acceptance region of μ_0.

Recall that we are dealing with one distribution as mandated by H_0. All the outcomes will be classified either in β or $1 - \beta$. What this amounts to is that the data are split into β and $1 - \beta$, that is, false negative and true positive. No other possibility exists. In other words, none of the data in the $1 - \beta$ region are considered α or false positive. In this sense, because H_0 is false, there is no Type I or α error.

By the same token, the $1 - \alpha$ acceptance area of the assumed null now cover β only, the false negative.

In other words, accepting the Null given the assumed critical value and the original hypothesized mean μ_0, without knowing that the real mean is displaced resulted in our rejecting all sample means derived from $1 - \beta$ of the area under the true distribution while accepting sample means derived from the β area as legitimate samples from the assumed null distribution. We have in effect falsely certified that the tested stock will not be rejected with a probability equivalent to the β area, which translates into a Type II error of equivalent probability.

In order to appreciate the genesis and magnitude of the β error, one must keep in mind the fact, of which we are unaware, that the true and actual population mean from which a sample is derived depart from the assumed mean of the null hypothesis both as to its magnitude and direction. Thus, with the assumed but false null hypothesis as the rule, all samples outcomes are tested against the assumed null hypothesis, with the result, that the sample outcome placement in relation to the assumed null is not in accord with the facts of the prevailing but unknown situation.

21C.4 Control of the Type I Error, α

P(rejecting H_0 | H_0 is true) = P(rejecting true H_0) = P(Type I error | H_0 is true) = α
P(accepting H_0 | H_0 is true) = P(accepting true H_0) = P(No error | H_0 is true) = $(1 - \alpha)$

The statistical standard used as the basis for the control of α is the assigned or predetermined level of significance, which in effect predetermines the probability of rejecting the null hypothesis, given that the null hypothesis is true. Thus, at the 4.6 percent significance level, the sample result needs to be significantly different from the hypothesized parameter in order to justify the rejection of the null hypothesis. A deviation of such a magnitude or more extreme from the hypothesized mean can only occur by chance with a probability of 4.6 percent or less.

In this sense, a hypothesis-testing decision rule is simply a procedure that specifies the decision to be taken for each possible sample outcome as a choice between two possible states, in effect partitioning the sample space into two mutually exclusive and exhaustive regions, corresponding to a rejection and acceptance region. The partitioning of the sample space is accomplished by specifying the probability of making a Type I error based on the sampling distribution that results from assuming the null hypothesis is true. In this particular problem, because the question concerns mean drug dosage, the level of significance set at 4.6 percent was mandated by the dose requirements, which placed the z values at ± 2 corresponding to the upper and lower allowed dosage limits.

Therefore, to reject the null hypothesis at the 4.6 percent level of significance, the sample mean must have a value that is either below the lower critical limit 29.8 mg or above the upper critical limit of 30.2 mg. Figure 21C.3 graphically portrays the sampling distribution of the mean and the regions of acceptance and rejection of the null hypothesis, given that the null hypothesis is true. As can be seen, a two-tailed test has two regions of rejection. The z values of ± 2.0 are used to establish the critical limits because for the standard normal distribution, a proportion of 0.0456 of the area is outside these limits and located in the two tails of the distribution, which corresponds to the designated 4.6 percent level of significance. Because the normal distribution is symmetrical, the area in each tail of Graph 21C-2 is one-half of 0.0456, or 0.0228 (2.3 percent). Thus, given that the null hypothesis is true, the overall probability is 0.0456 (4.6 percent) that the mean for a random sample of $n = 100$ capsules will be either below 29.8 mg or above 30.2 mg for this example.

Furthermore, because our sample is large ($n = 100$), the sampling distribution of means is assumed to be normal. This sampling distribution, for samples of size 100 from a population, where $\mu = 30$ mg (in conformity with specifications) and $\sigma = 1$ mg, is shown in Figure 21C.3. The tail regions in this graph represent 4.6 percent of the area under the normal curve.

Referring to Table 19B.3, chapter 19B, we see that 2.3 percent (0.228 to be exact) of the area in a normal distribution lies to the right of $z = +2.0$, and correspondingly the same percentage of area lies to the left of $z = -2.0$.

Because the standard error of the mean is equal to

$$\sigma_{\overline{X}} = \frac{\sigma}{\sqrt{n}} = \frac{1}{\sqrt{100}} = 0.1 \text{ mg.}$$

The critical values beyond which we would reject H_0 is

$$\text{Critical } \overline{X} = \mu_0 \pm z\sigma_{\overline{X}} = \mu_0 \pm 2\sigma_{\overline{X}} = 30 \pm 2(.1) = 29.8 - 30.2$$

In hypothesis testing, a two-tailed test is used when we are concerned about a possible deviation in either direction from the hypothesized value of the mean. If the sample mean is used as the test statistic, two critical values of the sample mean have to be defined: one that is unusually less than the hypothesized value and one that is unusually greater than the hypothesized value. In contrast a one-tailed test is appropriate when we are concerned about possible deviations in only one direction from the hypothesized value of the mean.

In summary, upon drawing a random sample of one hundred caps from the stock and observing $\overline{X}$, the sample mean, the pharmacist should apply this decision rule:

1. If $\overline{X} < 29.8$ mg, reject H_0 (reject the stock).

2. If $\overline{X} > 30.2$ mg, reject H_0 (reject the stock).

3. If $\overline{X} \leq 30.2$ mg or $\overline{X} \geq 29.8$ mg; [$29.8 \leq \overline{X} \leq 30.2$ mg], accept H_0 (accept the stock).

Instead of establishing the critical values in terms of the sample mean (that is in terms of the original units in milligrams), we would specify the critical values in terms of z values corresponding to the $\overline{X}$ values of 30.0 ± 0.2, that is, $z = \pm 2.0$. If the z value lies to the left of the critical value of -2, H_0 is rejected; if to the right of -2, H_0 is accepted. Identically, If the z value lies to the right of the critical value of $+2$, H_0 is rejected; if to the left of $+2$, H_0 is accepted.

Table 19B.3 lists the values of z most frequently used as critical values in hypothesis testing. Note that for a two-tailed test, there are always two critical values of z. For instance, for a two-tailed test at the 5 percent level of significance, the critical values are at $z = \pm 1.96$. The $z = -1.96$ and $z = +1.96$ are at the 2.5th percentile point and 97.5th percentile point, respectively, of the standard normal z distribution. Thus, the sum of the areas in the two tails is $0.025 + 0.025 = 0.050 = 5$ percent. When the value of a sample mean is determined, it is converted into a value of z so that it can be compared with the critical value(s) of z.

In the example cited, the assigned critical value was mandated by the dose requirements which placed the z values at ± 2 corresponding to the upper and lower allowed dosage requirements. Note the z values of ± 2.0 differ slightly from the common 1.96 level. In this case, the significance level is 0.0455, which accounts for the $\alpha/2$ level of $0.0227 \cong 0.023$ in each wing.

Thus, the decision rule for this case may be formulated as follows:

| 1. If $z < -2.0$, reject H_0 (reject the stock). |
| 1. If $z > +2.0$, reject H_0 (reject the stock). |
| 2. If $z \geq -2.0$ or $z \leq +2.0$; $[-2 \leq z \leq +2]$, accept H_0 (accept the stock). |

From a practical point of view, the format expressed in the original units is certainly simpler, particularly if the procedure is bound to be repeated. A random sample is chosen, its mean is determined in actual units, and the decision is taken in accordance with the stipulated decision rule. The "z" format projects a more realistic and quantitative aspect of the relation, allowing for a more objective evaluation of the sample result.

21C.5 Control of Type II error, β

P(accepting H_0 | H_1 is true) = P(accepting false H_0) = P(type II error | H_1 is true) = β

P(rejecting H_0 | H_0 is false) = P(rejecting false H_0) = P(no error | H_0 is false = $(1 - \beta)$

Control of the β error implies the attempt to fix the probability of committing a Type II error (failing to reject a false null hypothesis) at a predetermined level associated with a given alternative hypothesis. The maneuver required in this attempt is more elaborate than the one involved in fixing the probability of committing a Type I error (rejecting a true null hypothesis). This is because, for a given test, Type I error corresponds to a unique, assigned probability value, α, whereas Type II error correspond to any one of a continuous series of probabilities denoted by β. Thus, β may assume any one of unlimited values, but whose actual current value is a function of the displacement of the true mean from the hypothesized but false mean.

Thus, before we perform a hypothesis test, we may compute many β's by postulating many values for the parameter of interest, for fixed α and n, given that the hypothesized value is false.

Suppose that H_0 is false, that is, μ_{true} is not equal to 30.0 mg. Thus, if H_0 is false, μ_{true} may assume any one value that may be greater or smaller than 30 mg. In both cases, the value of μ_{true} remains unknown.

Suppose that the true population mean is $\mu_2 = 29.7$. Then the sampling distribution under H_2 is also normal, with $\mu_2 = \mu_{\bar{x}} = \mu_{true} = 29.7$.

Having assigned a specific arbitrary value of μ_{true}, we are now in a position to calculate the magnitude of the potential β or Type II error, that is, the probability of failing to reject a false hypothesis, because the area under the distribution curve of H_2 that overlaps the acceptance region specified under the distribution of H_0 include all sample means that fail to be rejected.

The perusal of Figure 21C.3 makes it clear that the β area extends beyond the assumed critical value of the lower tail of 29.8 up to the critical value of the upper tail of 30.2.[23] Simultaneously, all values under H_2 beyond the upper critical value of 30.2 would be rejected. Needless to say that the area involved in this case is infinitesimal with no practical impact on the relevant β area.

On the practical level, when $\mu_{true} = \mu_2 = 29.7$, the probability of β is equal to $P(\overline{X} \geq 29.8)$, equivalent to the β area bounded by $\overline{X} = 29.8$ and $\overline{X} = +\infty$, which is the same as

$$
P\left(z \geq \frac{\overset{\overline{X_1}}{29.8} - \overset{\mu_1}{29.7}}{\underset{\mu_{\overline{X}}}{0.1}} \right) = p\left(z \geq \frac{0.1}{0.1} \right) = P(z \geq 1) = 1.\overset{\beta}{587}.
$$

The implication of the result is twofold: on the one hand, the probability of a sample mean that is equal or greater than the critical value of 29.8 mg ($\overline{X} \geq 29.8$) accounts for 16 percent of all possible outcomes end up in accepting the null hypothesis and thus committing a β error. Alternatively, the probability of a sample mean that is smaller than the critical value of 29.8 ($\overline{X} < 29.8$) accounts for 84 percent of all possible outcomes end up in correctly rejecting the null hypothesis with a power equivalent to $1 - \beta$.

Because $\mu_1 = \mu_{true}$ is only one of a continuum of possible sample mean values when H_0 is false, Figure 21C.4 makes it clear that the actual values of μ under the alternative hypothesis that are closer to μ_0 (μ_2 and μ_3) are associated with larger β values and correspondingly smaller $1 - \beta$.

For example, when $\mu = 30.1$ under the alternative hypothesis, β now includes 84 percent of the sample means under H_3; The power of the

---

[23]   The normal curves depicted in the chart are drawn extending 4 SE of the mean on either side of the sample mean. This pictorial liberty need not obscure the fact that the actual curves extend to $\pm\infty$.

test to correctly reject sample means of alternate distribution is now reduced to 16 percent of the total as noted from the derived areas of β and $1 - \beta$.

$$P\left(z \le \frac{\overset{\overline{X}_1}{30.2} - \overset{\mu_3}{30.1}}{\underset{\mu_{\overline{X}}}{0.1}}\right) = P\left(z \le \frac{.1}{.1}\right) = P(z \le 1) = .8\overset{\beta}{4}13$$

Possible Values of μ, When H_0 Is False	Probability of Type II Error β	Probability of Test to Detect False H_0 Power $= 1 - \beta$
$\mu_1 = 29.6$	0.0228	0.9772
$\mu_2 = 29.7$	0.1587	0.8413
$\mu_3 = 30.1$	0.8413	00.1587
$\mu_4 = 30.4$	0.0228	0.9772

Table 21C.1a. β values and their complement of $1 - \beta$ associated with the four alternate and true distribution means depicted in Figure 21C.3.

Thus, although only one value of α is associated with a given hypothesis test, there are an equivalent number of β values, one for each possible value of μ if μ_0 is not the true value of μ as hypothesized.

21C.6 One-Tailed Test

Consider now the dosage problem from a different angle forcing the pharmacist to adopt an alternative approach to the situation at hand. Given the potency of the CV drug, and complaints associated with side effects of an overdose, the pharmacist decided to test the stock solely with respect to the upper limiting dosage. Neglecting for the moment the inadequate therapeutic effect of less than optimal dosage, the test must be designed to ensure compliance with the maximum allowed dosage. With this in mind, the null hypothesis was recast to reflect the new requirement

$$H_0: \mu = \mu_0 \le 30.0$$

$$H_1: \mu \ne \mu_0 > 30.0$$

The null hypothesis, H_0, states that the capsular population mean is at most 30.0 mg. If the decision procedure leads us to reject the null hypothesis, H_0, and accept the alternative hypothesis, H_1, thereby concluding that the mean dosage exceeds the safe upper limit, we are forced to reject the whole lot.

The pharmacist is aware that any test procedure involves either a Type I or Type II errors. A Type I error will occur if the stock, whose mean capsular weight is 30.0 mg, is rejected; a Type II error will occur if the stock, whose mean capsular weight is more than 30.0 mg, is not rejected.

For the decision ruled based on the probability of Type I error, α must be fixed at a predetermined level. The significance level of 0.023, corresponding to one-tail area, was therefore maintained exclusively for the upper tail only, allowing for a risk tolerance of the order of 2.3 percent associated with the rejection of a perfectly good stock given a sample mean in excess of 30.2 mg when in fact the sample mean is a true sample derived from the upper tail of null hypothesis. Thus, the critical area above which H_0 is rejected corresponds to an upper limit of the sampling distribution marked by two standard errors of the mean,

$$\mu + 2 \cdot \sigma_{\overline{x}} = 30.0 + 2 \times 0.1 = 30.2 \text{ mg.}$$

As in the case of the two-tailed test, the decision rule was formulated to take into account the targets stipulated by the formulation of the hypothesis; thus,

If $\overline{X} > 30.2$ mg, reject H_0 (reject the stock).
If $\overline{X} \leq 30.2$ mg, accept H_0 (accept the stock).

In this case, because the assigned critical value mandated by the dose requirements which placed the z value at $+2.0$ standard errors, corresponding to the upper permitted dosage, the decision rule may be formatted as follows:

If $z > +2$ standard error, reject H_0 (reject the stock).
If $z \leq +2$ standard error, accept H_0 (accept the stock).

What is perhaps more to the point in this case, having assigned an α of 0.023, is how large is β, the probability of Type II error? In other words, how large is the probability that the pharmacist will not reject the stock, given that the sample mean is more than 30.0 mg?

Suppose that H_0 is false, that is, μ_{true} is not equal to 30 mg. Thus, if H_0 is false, μ_{true} may assume any one value that may be greater or smaller than 30 mg. In both cases, the value of μ_{true} remains unknown.

Suppose that the true population mean is $\mu_3 = 30.3$. Then the sampling distribution under H_3 is also normal, with $\mu_3 = \mu_{\overline{X}} = \mu_{true} = 30.3$.

Having assigned a specific arbitrary value to μ_{true}, we are now in a position to calculate the magnitude of the potential β or Type II error, that is, the probability of failing to reject a false hypothesis, because the area under the distribution curve of H_3 that overlaps the acceptance region specified under the distribution of H_0 includes all sample means that fail to be rejected.

The perusal of Figure 21C.4 makes it clear that the β area extends into the acceptance region behind the assumed critical value of the upper tail of 30.2. Simultaneously, all values under H_3 beyond the upper critical value of 30.2 would be rejected.

When $\mu_{true} = \mu_3 = 30.3$, the probability of β is equal to $P(\overline{X} \leq 30.2)$, equivalent to the β area bounded by $\overline{X} = 30.2$ and $\overline{X} = -\infty$, which is the same as

$$P(z \leq -1) = P(\text{accepting } H_0 | H_3 \text{ is true}) = 0.1587 = \beta \text{ error.}$$

The implication of the result is twofold: on the one hand, we have accepted 16 percent of the sampling distribution of the means labeled H_3 as legitimate samples from the assumed and hypothesized distribution, H_0, committing in the process a significant β error. On the other hand, we have correctly rejected 84 percent of the sampling distribution under H_3 as representative of a distribution of different mean.

Because $\mu_1 = \mu_{true}$ is only one of a continuum of possible sample mean values when H_0 is false, Figure 21C.4 makes it clear that the actual values of μ under the alternative hypothesis that are closer to μ_0 (μ_1 and μ_2) are associated with larger β values and correspondingly smaller $1 - \beta$.

For example, when $\mu_1 = 30.1$ under the alternative hypothesis, β now includes 84 percent of the sample means under H_1. The power of the test to correctly reject sample means of alternate distribution is now reduced to 16 percent of the total as noted from the derived areas of β and $1 - \beta$.

$$P(z \leq +1) = P(\text{accepting } H_0 | H_1 \text{ is true}) = 0.8413 = \beta \text{ error.}$$

Thus, although only one value of α is associated with a given hypothesis test, there are many values of β, one for each possible value of μ if μ_0 is not the true value of μ as hypothesized.

The appropriate test procedure is dependent on whether α or β are set at the right levels from the standpoint of the decision maker, that is, whether α and β are set at levels that are satisfactory in dealing with the restriction dictated by the problem at hand.

In setting the level, one needs to consider, the relative costs of committing either type of error.

Accordingly, if the hypothesized mean happens to be false, and the actual or true mean exceeds that of the hypothesized mean, we ought to make sure that the β error incurred is acceptable, for the given deviation from the hypothesized mean.

Here again we are faced with an unlimited number of possibilities because β can be calculated only when the true value of μ can be specified. However, the ability to calculate β for different possible values of actual and true means (μ_{true}) makes it possible to assess the magnitude of the β error for the individual values covered under the rejection range.

As noted from the previous example, the ability to perform these calculations provides the means of constructing tables or graphs from which one can determine the sample size required to keep β at a level of our own choosing.

Again faced with the unknown, we can only consider the possibilities and make our choice accordingly. In this case, however, in contrast to the previous case, the rejection region is restricted to the upper tail covering the range of possible true means extant when the assumed and hypothesized mean is false (Figure 21C.4).

A random sample drawn from the sampling distribution under H_1 yields a mean $\leq$30.2 mg with a probability of 84 percent. In effect, we have mistakenly labeled a sample that should have been rejected, being derived from a distribution of a different mean, as legitimate representative of the assumed although faulty distribution. In only 16 percent of the cases is the mean rejected as being truly inconsistent with the null.

Possible Values of μ, When H_0 Is False	Probability of Type II Error β	Probability of Test to Detect False H_0 Power $= 1 - \beta$
$\mu_1 = 30.1$	0.8413	0.1587
$\mu_2 = 30.2$	0.50	0.50
$\mu_3 = 30.3$	0.1587	0.8413
$\mu_4 = 30.4$	0.0228	0.9772

Table 21C.1b. β values and their complement of $1 - \beta$ associated with the four alternate and true distribution means depicted in Figure 21C.4.

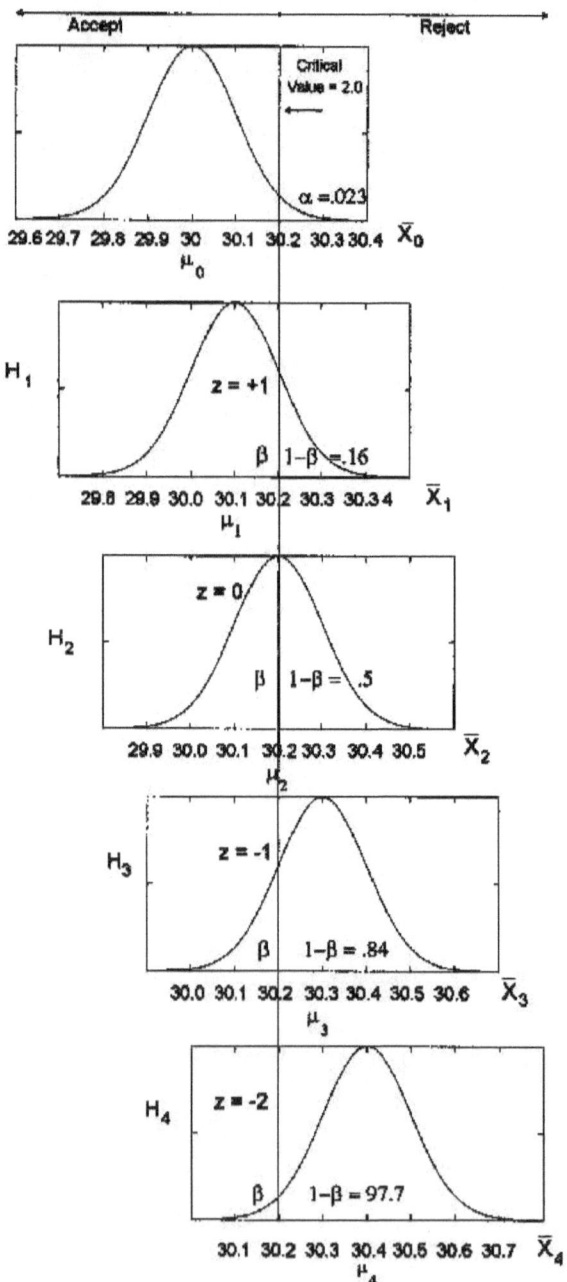

Figure 21C.4. Sampling distribution of the assumed and false hypothesis juxtaposed to the true sampling distribution of four possible population means.

A random sample drawn from the sampling distribution under H_2 is unique in that the probability of acceptance is equal to that of rejection accounting for 50 percent of the samples in each case

Under H_4, the probability of a β error is now minimal (0.023), whereas the provability of correctly rejecting a sample drawn from such a distribution is 97.7 of the total possible random sample of the size specified.

The probability of committing a β error of failing to reject a false hypothesis and its complement, the probability of correctly rejecting a false H_0, are tabulated in Table 21C.1b for the four values illustrated in Figure 21C.4.

21C.7 Operating-Characteristic Curve versus Power Curve

The β values tabled in Table 21C.1b and graphed in Figure 21C.4 are simply snapshots of the continuum of possible values assumed by the alternate hypothesis. A more realistic picture may be derived from a plot in which the acceptance probabilities are shown on the vertical axis and possible values of the alternate and true population parameters μ on the horizontal axis (Figure 21C.5a). The curve thus derived is referred to as *operating-characteristic* (OC) curve.

The $1 - \beta$ values tabled in Table 21C.1b and graphed in Figure 21C.4 may be similarly plotted (Figure 21C.5b). In this format, referred to as the *power curve,* the rejection probabilities are shown on the vertical axis, whereas the possible values of the alternate and true population parameters μ are shown on the horizontal axis.

In order to evaluate the discriminating power of a test with regard to both its possible errors, a closer look at the OC and power curves in Figures 21C.5a and 21C.5b may be rewarding.

Recall that β denotes the probability of committing a Type II error, implying the acceptance of a lot that does not meet the required dosage criteria. Specifically, β is a conditional probability based upon the assumption of a null hypothesis that is false.

$$P\left(\overline{X} < 30.0 \,|\, \mu_0\right) = P(\text{accepting } H_0 \,|\, H_0 \text{ is false}) = \beta.$$

Beta's complement $1 - \beta$ is similarly a conditional probability implying the rejection of a lot that does not meet the required dosage specification, a more realistic approach, still based on the assumption of a false null hypothesis. Thus, it shows the probability of rejecting the null hypothesis for each value for which the null hypothesis is false, which being the complement of an error is no error (Figures 21C.5a and 21C.5b).

$$P\left(\overline{X} > 30.0 \,|\, \mu_0\right) = P(\text{rejecting } H_0 \,|\, H_0 \text{ is false}) = 1 - \beta.$$

Clearly, the OC curve is simply the complement of the power curve. Furthermore, each point of either curve divides its ordinate into the same complementary values of β and $1 - \beta$.

The *power of the test*, $1 - \beta$, may be derived from the power curve for each particular value of μ satisfying the alternative hypothesis. In other words, $(1 - \beta)$ provides the relevant information by giving the probability of rejecting the false null hypothesis.

The perusal of the power curve reveals an additional feature that reveals the α value attached to the null hypothesis. In this case, the value of $\alpha = 0.023$ is shown for $\mu_0 = 30.0$, indicating the significance level of the test.

As you may recall, this is the maximum probability of erroneously rejecting the true null hypothesis H_0. In order to appreciate the significance of this statement, glance once more at the sampling distribution of associated with the null hypothesis, H_0, the first curve in Figure 21C.4.

Note that the tail area of $\alpha/2$ is marked off by the critical z value of 2, given a mean value at 30. A shift in the actual mean value to the left would shift the entire curve to the left, without affecting the critical value, which in effect would result in marking off a smaller tail area, that is, a smaller $\alpha/2$ than the original maximal area.

The same idea could be translated into the power curve, by noting that at H_{true} of 30.0, it could be seen as the minute ordinate extending 0.023 above the sampling mean axis. For values to the left of 30.0, that is, for smaller mean values of μ_0, the height of the ordinate would diminish further in conjunction with diminished marked off upper tail area of the curve.

The control of Type II error is an important feature of any particular hypothesis test. So that when the null hypothesis is false, it is helpful to know the probability that we will reject it or alternatively how frequently does the decision rule lead us to accept the null hypothesis erroneously

Legend for the Power Curve of Figure 21C.3

The heights of the ordinates to the right of $\mu_0 = 30.0$ mg give the values of $1 - \beta$, which are the probabilities of rejecting the null hypothesis when it is false. Therefore, the complementary distances from the curve to 1.00 are values of β, or probabilities of making Type II errors. Four such $1 - \beta$ values, for $\mu_1 = 30.1$, $\mu_2 = 30.2$, $\mu_3 = 30.3$, and for $\mu_4 = 30.4$ mg, are displayed in the graph. Recall that the decision rule required the rejection of H_0 if the sample mean X was greater than 30.2 mg. Thus, if the population mean is 30.2, as obtained under H_2, the probability of observing X values greater than 30.2 mg (and, therefore, of rejecting H_0) is 0.50, whereas the probability of observing X smaller than 30.2 mg (and, therefore, accepting H_0) is equally 0.50.

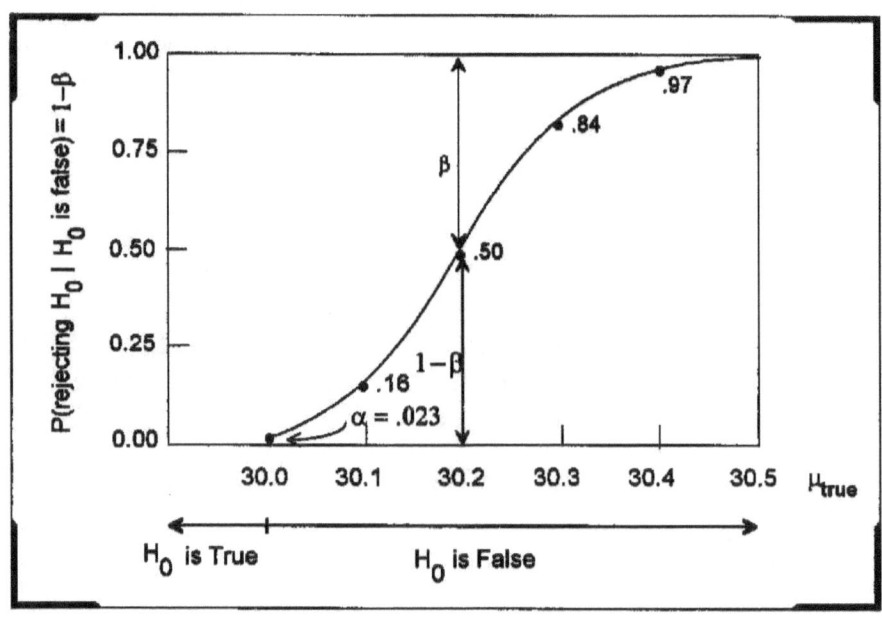

Figure 21C.5b. The Power Curve

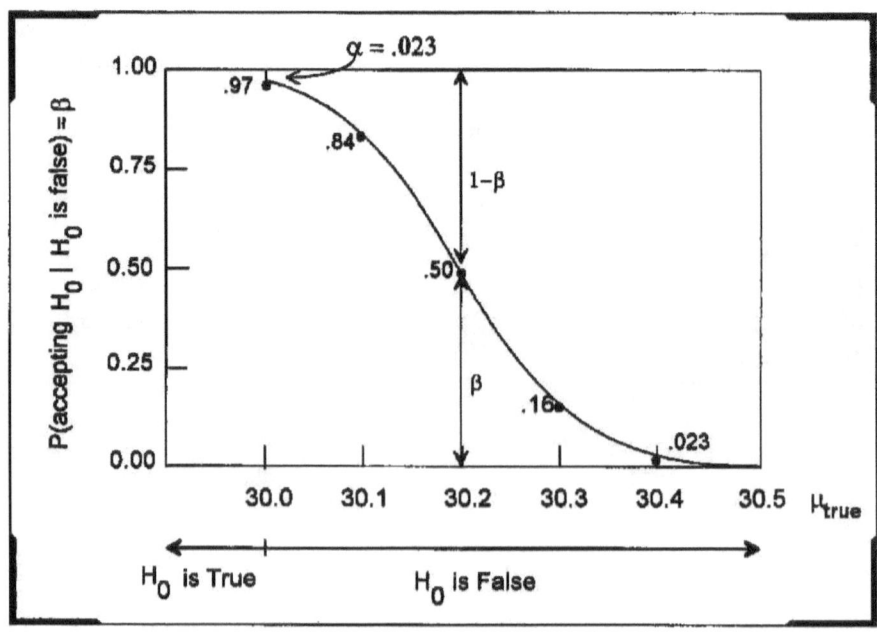

Figure 21C.5. The operating characteristic (OC) curve

21C.8 Factors Affecting Type II Error

The control of β, unlike α, is a function of several factors. Thus, in order to control β, the relation of β to each of the factors needs to be explored. The value of β, the probability of committing a Type II error, depends on three main factors

21C.8.1 Deviation of the True Mean from the Hypothesized Mean

$\uparrow$Deviation $\rightarrow$ $\downarrow$Overlap $\rightarrow$ $\downarrow\beta$
$\downarrow$Deviation $\rightarrow$ $\uparrow$Overlap $\rightarrow$ $\uparrow\beta$

The magnitude of β is inversely related to the degree of discrepancy or deviation between what is hypothesized as the mean, μ_0, although in actual fact is a false mean and the true mean, μ_1: the larger the discrepancy, the smaller the overlap, and the lower β. The extent of the deviation is beyond the control of the investigator. It is simply a fact that has to be taken into consideration and reckoned with.

If μ_1 is relatively close to the assumed but false mean μ_0, then the Type II error may be quite large. That is, if the true population mean $\mu_2 = 30.2$ mg as compared with the assumed mean of $\mu_0 = 30.0$ mg, the Type II error or β accounts for a shade short of one-half of the area (50 percent) under the distribution of the mean centered at 30.2. As noted in Figure 21C.6a, the hypothesized sampling distribution centered at the hypothesized false population mean of 30.0 mg and the true sampling distribution centered at the true population mean of 30.2 overlap to a significant degree. The critical value of 30.2 made originally with reference to the hypothesized but false distribution, to mark off the α area, is now transformed into the critical axis of the true distribution marking off the β area on the left from the $1 - \beta$ area on the right. Because sample means are to be judged by their relation to the critical value, it now becomes apparent the fully 50 percent of the random samples derived from the true distribution will fall in the β region allowing for the retention (acceptance) of the false hypothesized mean, H_0, and thus committing a Type II error.

The balance of 50 percent of the sample means would fall in the 1 − β area and would be rejected under the original mandate, which in this case would result in rejecting a false H_0 and therefore taking the right decision.

On the practical level, the pharmacist accepted a stock whose mean was 3.2, well above the desired safe upper limit with a probability of error of 50 percent. This degree of possible error is of course unacceptable under the conditions of the hypothesis.

However, if the actual or true population mean $\mu_4 = 3.4$ mg, then the Type II error is significantly reduced as noted in Figure 21C.6b. In this case, the β area accounts for a mere 2.4 percent of the sample mean, which would allow the acceptance of the false H_0 and thus committing a Type II error. On the other hand, a full 97.6 percent of the sample means would fall in the 1 − β area thus correctly rejecting the false H_0. In this case, the probability of correctly rejecting a "toxic" stock is 97.6 percent, whereas the probability of committing a Type II error by retaining H_0 and certifying the toxic stock is reduced to 2.4 percent.

As can be readily appreciated from Figures 21C.32 and 21C.3 if the hypothesis is true, the sampling distribution will center on μ_0. This is the distribution from which the region of acceptance is determined, as shown in the same Charts. Now if the hypothesis is false, the true sampling distribution of means will center on any one alternate μ rather than on μ_0 ($\mu \neq \mu_0$; $\mu = \mu_{1,2,3,4}$).

The critical decision making however is based on the significance level assigned to the hypothesized distribution. The decision maker, unaware of the prevailing situation, continues to base his decision on the sample placement with respect to the critical "axis" initially assigned to the null hypothesis.

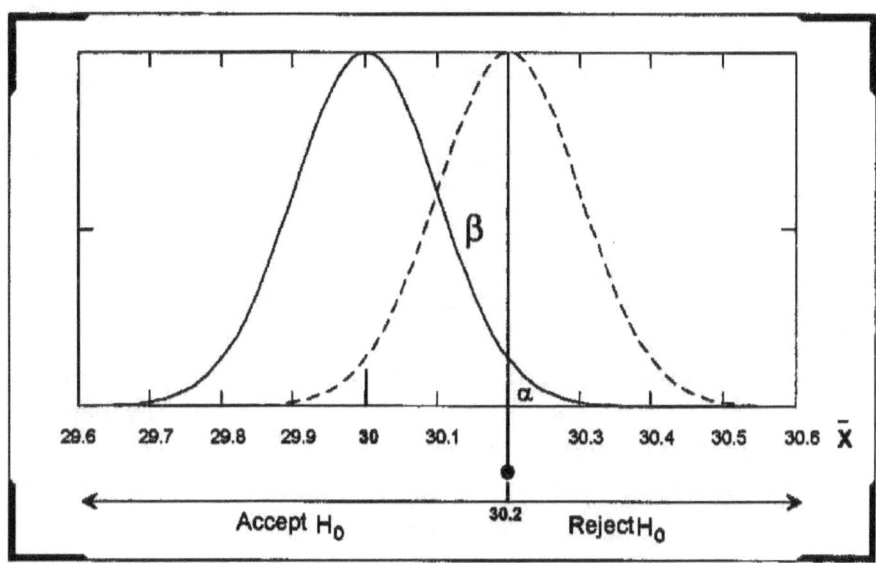

Figure 21C.6a

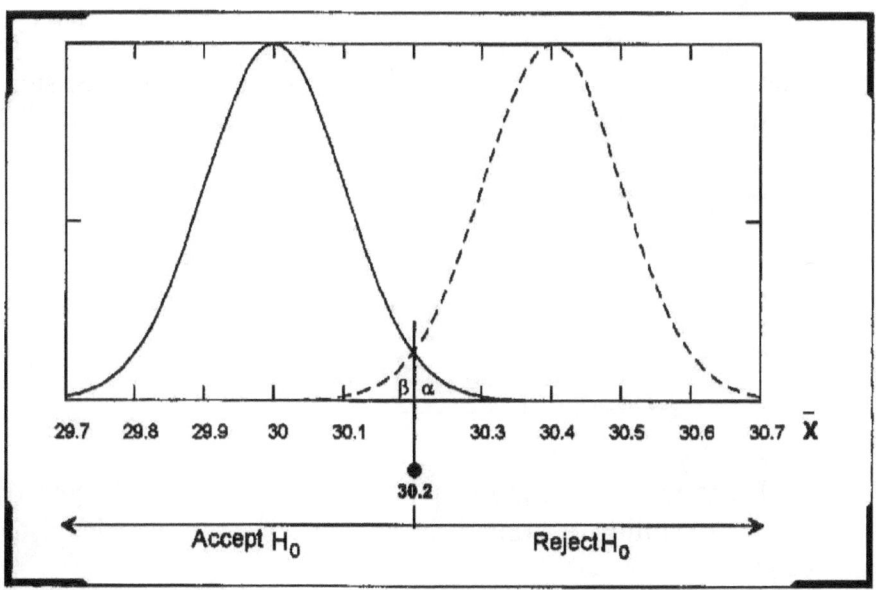

Figure 21C.6b

From Figures 21C.6a and 21C.6b, it becomes apparent that the extent of divergence or overlap of the two distributions determines the relative position of the assigned cutoff critical value with respect to the true distribution, which in turn separates the true positive (in the sense of correctly rejecting the false null hypothesis) from the false negative (in the sense of accepting a false null hypothesis).

Clearly, the probability of a Type II error is related to the extent of difference between the hypothesized but false mean and the true mean. If the two are very close, the sample means obtained from the true sampling distribution will overlap the region of acceptance to a large extent. In general, the greater the discrepancy between the alternate true μ and the hypothesized μ (μ_0), the smaller the probability of falsely accepting the hypothesis and the greater the probability of correctly rejecting the hypothesis.

Stated differently, the probability of committing Type II error could be envisaged to be related to the position of the cutoff axis bisecting the adjacent but different true distribution.

In both of the above-noted situations, the hypothesized sampling distribution remains the referent distribution on which the decision rule with a critical z of 2.0 given the assumed two-tailed test.

21C.8.2 Sample Size

$\uparrow n \rightarrow \downarrow \beta$
$\downarrow n \rightarrow \uparrow \beta$

Sample size is the most important factor in the control of Type II error. The probability of committing a Type II error is related to sample size.

Consider the test of the hypothesis related to the sampling distribution of the capsules in stock where $\mu = \mu_0 = \mu_{hypo}$.

When sample size is 100. The standard error of the mean will be

$$SE = \sigma_{\bar{x}} = \sigma / \sqrt{100} = \frac{1}{10}\sigma.$$

If sample size were 400, the standard error of the mean would be

$$SE = \sigma_{\bar{x}} = \sigma / \sqrt{400} = \frac{1}{20}\sigma.$$ Thus, quadrupling the sample size

resulted in a standard error only half as large.

In general, the larger the size of the samples, the smaller the standard deviation $(\sigma_{\bar{x}})$ of the sampling distribution of $\overline{X}$. A comparison of the two situations illustrated in Figures 21C.7a and 21C.7b shows that when sample size is larger, there is less overlap between the two distributions. Consequently, the risk is less of drawing a sample that leads to (false) acceptance of the hypothesis. Other things being equal, the larger the size of the sample, the lower is the probability of committing a Type II error. Control of sample size offers the simplest technique of controlling the risk of a Type II error without affecting other important consideration (Figures 21C.7a and 21C.7b).

The experimenter can choose the size he wants without having an adverse effect on other important considerations.

21C.8.3 Choice of Level of Significance (α)

$\uparrow\alpha \rightarrow$ $\downarrow\beta$
$\downarrow\alpha \rightarrow\uparrow\beta$

α is inversely related to β. The larger the value of α, the lower β and vice versa. Although it would be possible to alter the choice of α in order to gain a desired value for β, it is a poor idea. α ought to be decided on its own merits and other means (see points 2 and 3 above) used to control β. The inverse relationship between α and β

does remind us, however, of the danger of choosing an unnecessarily small value for α.

From Chart 21C-1 and 21C-2, the inverse relationship between a and b is best appreciated by visually moving the critical line cutting through both the hypothesized sampling distribution and the actual distributions left and right.

In general, reducing the risk of a Type I error increases the risk of committing a Type II error, which clearly demonstrates the price one pays and the associated danger one is likely to encounter in choosing an excessively small value for α.

21C.9 Simultaneous Control of Type I and Type II Errors (α and β)

What is readily apparent is that the simultaneous demand to minimize both α and β requires delicate maneuvering of the variables that will become apparent in due course

The discussion so far treated the errors α and β as separate entities. The tests were constructed with an assumed sample size, whereas the risk of Type I error was assigned by the decision procedure. Of the three factors affecting β, only two, namely, sample size and the significance level, are directly controllable. Therefore, the optimal choice for a given problem may be resolved through the analysis of the OC/power curves that may be constructed for each proposed change in the sample size and/or the significance level. In case control of Type I error was the main concern, only α was specified, which in turn determined one point on the power curve.

In order to control the levels of both Type I and Type II errors simultaneously in the same test, two specific points on the power curve need to be determined.

Consider once more the two-tailed test problem in which the stock was tested with respect to an upper limiting dosage. To this end, the probability of Type I error was fixed at an $\alpha = 0.023$ in which the pharmaceutical company ran a 0.023 percent risk of having a "good" stock with $\mu = 30.0$ mg rejected in error. The pharmacist after a second look at the power curve decided that the β error associated with the true mean of 30.3 mg was uncomfortably high at the level of 16 percent, which in the context of the problem at hand posed a substantial risk to the patients involved. In other words, because a stock whose caps have a mean weight of 30.3 mg does not meet specifications, it was decided to reduce the probability of erroneously accepting such a stock to the 5 percent level instead of the previous level of 16 percent.

From Figure 21C.4, the sampling distribution for μ_0 = 30.0 (null hypothesis; top curve), it is immediately apparent that the significance level of α = 0.023 is associated with an upper limiting mean value of 30.2 mg corresponding to a critical value of z = 2.0

From H_3, the sampling distribution mean of 30.3 is associated with a β = 0.16 for which the critical value is located at 30.2 corresponding to a z value of -1.0. Obviously the common boundary depicted in 21-10 is the one dictated by the fact that the sample size in both cases was taken at 100. How then is it possible to have these two distributions share a common border that would keep a at its original level while simultaneously reducing the b error to a tolerable 0.05 or 5 percent?

Of the three factors affecting Type II error noted previously, sample size provides the necessary solution that would simultaneously satisfy the constraints imposed on both error.

Once determined, the new sample size is used in deriving the new critical value that would simultaneously satisfy the limits imposed on both errors.

We are dealing with two different critical points. The original point lying two standard error units to the left of the of the mean μ_0 = 30.0 mg. Therefore, z_0 = 2.0. Under the alternative μ_3 = 30.3, the critical point is required to move from its original point to a point where β cuts off 5 percent of the area rather than the original 16 percent. From Table 19B.2, chapter 19B, we ascertain that 0.05 of the area in a normal sampling distribution lies to the left of a value 1.65 standard error units below the mean. Hence, z_3 = 1.65.

The following two equations need to be solved simultaneously in order to derive n, the required sample number, that would yield a common critical point that would satisfy the constraints on both α an β simultaneously:

$$\text{Critical point} = \mu_0 - z_0 \frac{\sigma}{\sqrt{n}} = 30.0 - 2 \cdot \frac{0.1}{\sqrt{n}}$$

$$\text{Critical point} = \mu_3 - z_3 \frac{\sigma}{\sqrt{n}} = 30.0 - 1.65 \cdot \frac{0.1}{\sqrt{n}}$$

Skipping over the algebraic manipulation, the necessary new sample size may be derived by simple substitution in the following final relation

$$n = \left[\frac{(z_0 + z_3)\sigma}{(\mu_0 - \mu_3)} \right]^2 = \left[\frac{(2 + 1.65) \times 1}{30.0 - 30.3} \right]^2 = \left[\frac{3.65}{-.3} \right]^2 = [12.1667]^2 = 148$$

The new sample size yields a different standard error of the mean, which is this case

$$\frac{1}{\sqrt{148}} = 0.082 = \text{Standard error of the mean for the new sample size.}$$

Substituting the new sample size, the same critical value is obtained for both $\alpha = 0.023$ and $\beta = 0.05$ that would satisfy the initial constraints imposed by the pharmacist on the tolerable errors allowed.

$$\text{Critical value} = 30.0 + 2 \cdot \left(\frac{1}{\sqrt{148}} \right) = 30.0 + 0.164 = 30.165.$$

$$\text{Critical value} = 30.3 - 1.65 \cdot \left(\frac{1}{\sqrt{148}} \right) = 30.3 - 0.136 = 30.165.$$

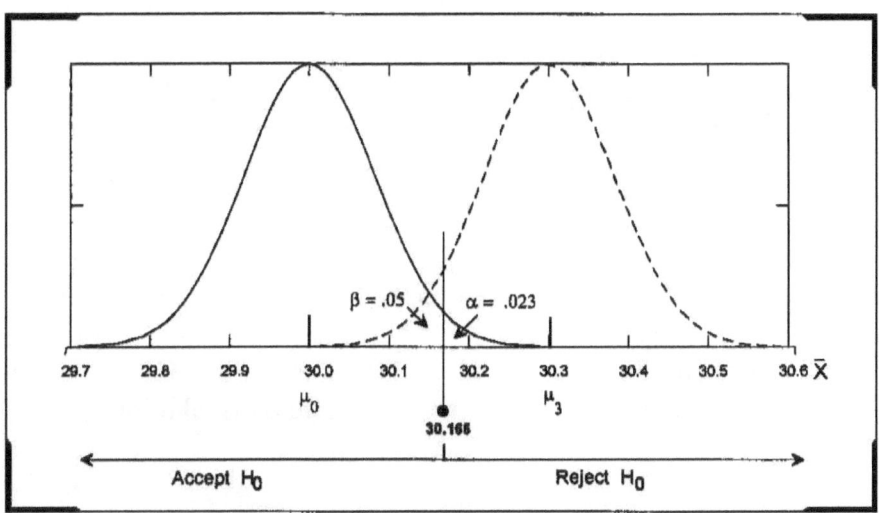

Graph 21C-5a

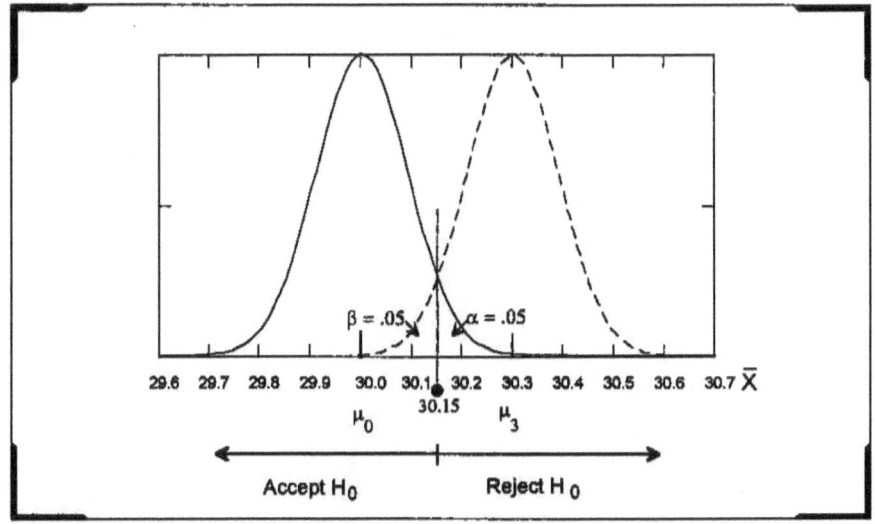

Graph 21C-5b

Note that the critical value shared by both α and β partitions the common $\overline{X}$ axis at the critical value of 1.65 to satisfy both the predetermined α and β errors (Figure 21C.5a).

For the pharmacist, the decision rule may stated in terms of the new sample size, such that

If $\overline{X} > 30.165$, reject H_0 (reject the lot).
If $\overline{X} \leq 30.165$, accept H_0 (accept the lot).

For a different error assignment, n must be reevaluated anew. So that for both α and β errors to equal 0.05 each, the derived sample size of 111 is now associated with a standard error of 0.091. The critical point in this case is set at 30.15, resulting in equivalent corresponding areas in the respective tails of the distributions.

Chapter 22

Bayes' Theorem from a Statistical Perspective
Statistical versus Bayesian Inference

22.1 Inductive versus Deductive Reasoning

As the reader may have been aware, the reasoning associated with the three main topics of this monograph, probability, Bayes' theorem, and statistical inference was based on the inductive branch of logic. A moment of reflection on the inductive process might prove rewarding. In essence, inductive reasoning's main concern is to be able to generalize from the particular to the generic, however, no matter how large the sample or the number of individual cases or items surveyed, the conclusion can never be established with absolute certainty. A single exception to the established norm renders the conclusion untenable. Of all the pink flamingoes in the world, one white flamingo is enough to refute the conclusion "all flamingos are pink." An argument is thus said to be inductive if the conclusions derived from the premises (observation, sample data) are stated with probability and not with certainty.

The deductive process, on the other hand, familiar from Euclidean geometry, culminates in a definite conclusion which must logically be true, if the given premises on which it is based are true. However, the definite conclusion so derived owes its absolute certainty to the premises that are accepted without question. Whereas certainty is sacrificed in the inductive process when based on realistic data, certainty is achieved in the deductive process when based on absolute acceptance of premises that may ultimately be refuted or redefined. The premises in this case include axioms (postulates) and arbitrarily defined terms that form the key stone of the deductive structure. Figure 22.1 illustrates their opposite modes of origin and conclusions.

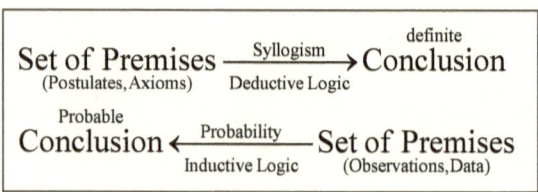

Figure 22.1

22.2 Probability versus Statistics: Deductive Inference versus Inductive Inference

Probability and its counterpart statistics are in essence two main applied forms of inductive logic. The main thrust of probability is its ability to foretell the composition of a future sample, given the parameters of the population from which it is to be derived. In probability, the contents of the urn or the black box are given, the inference in this case is to deduce the probable composition of a randomly drawn sample.

Statistics, on the other hand, is concerned with eliciting the characteristics of a population from observations made on a sample. In statistics, the contents of the black box are unknown, the inferential technique is designed to deduce the composition of the population, with a certain degree of confidence, from which the sample is purported to have been derived. In this sense, statistics deals with the relationship of sample to population as it presently exists. The polarity of the two inductive approaches is again graphically portrayed in the Figure 22.2.

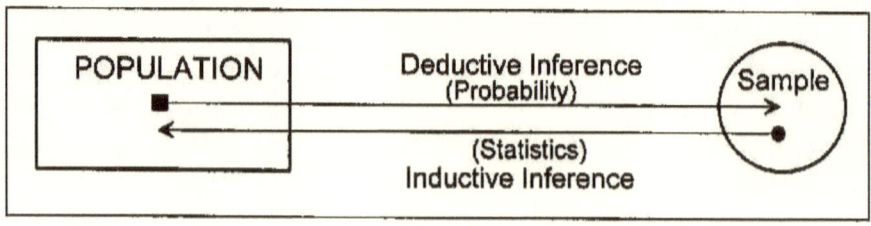

Figure 22.2

22.3 The Scientific Method: Applied Inductive Reasoning; Applied Hypothesis Testing

Hypothesis formulation and testing constitute the basic framework within which the scientific method is applied, ultimately ending in the formulation of a theory capable of binding the observed data within a simple relationship, and equally important, capable of predicting the outcome within the constraints of the initial conditions and the current available data.

In general, "scientific method" may be resolved into three interrelated steps beginning with the *Collection of Data*, followed by *Formulating the Hypothesis*, and finally by confirming it through *Hypothesis Testing*.

The first step, "data collection," refers to collecting *all* the observations relevant to the topic being studied. The important point here is that we must have *all* the evidence.

The second step of scientific methodology is "formulating the hypothesis." In doing this, two rules must be followed: (a) the hypothesis must explain all the observed data through a simple relationship and (b) the hypothesis should explain the existing observations by making the fewest assumptions.

The familiar judicial rule alluded to in the introduction of chapter 21A states that a man is to be assumed innocent until he has been proved guilty is based on the same fundamental principles underlying the process of scientific methodology. In this case, as in all scientific endeavors, it is simpler to assume the null hypothesis of innocence (not guilty) because no man can prove the absence of guilt except by the impossible task of proving innocence for every past moment of life.

Because it is true that a general negative cannot be demonstrated, we are entitled to make that general negative assumption under the rule of the simplicity of scientific hypothesis, and to demand refutation of such an assumption by specific positive proof.

Thus, by formulating the null hypothesis in terms of the general and negative assumption of innocence, we can disprove this assertion by much easier procedure of producing evidence of guilt by specific positive proof for a single act in time and place.

Similarly, a scientific theory is thus assumed to be correct until proved otherwise by finding a single exceptional case. Thus, scientific theories must be recognized as hypotheses and as such subject to refutation on the strength of specific contradictory evidence.

The third step of scientific method is testing the hypothesis. This can be done in two ways: (a) by predicting new observations, and (b) by experimentation with controls.

In a scientific experiment involving hypothesis testing, members of the experimental group are paired with member of the control group. If all other conditions are the same for both groups, then the data generated by the experimental group that is not shared by the control group, should provide the evidence in support of the alternate hypothesis.

22.4 The Reference Interval: Arbiter of the Test Result

Consider The fasting blood sugar level in normal men, 30 years or older. As noted in

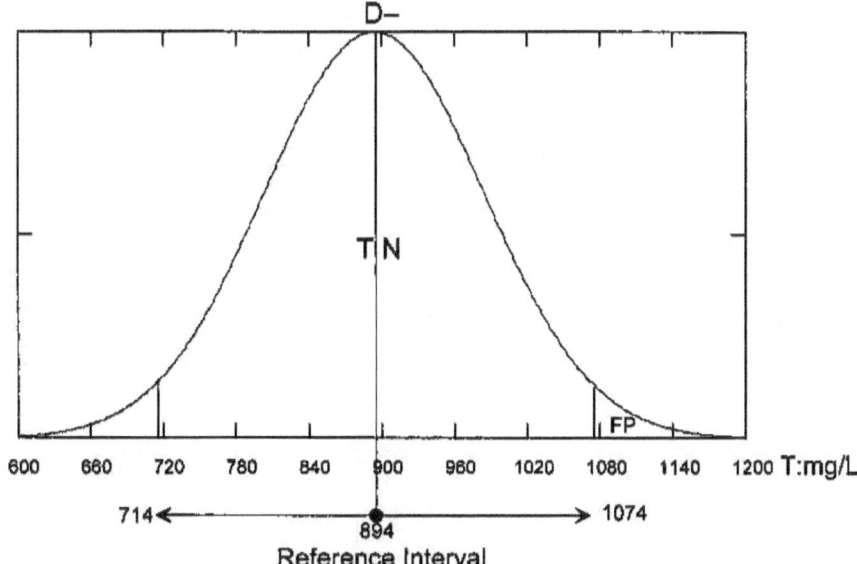

Figure 22.3 Graph of the fasting blood sugar levels obtained form 106 normal men >30 years using the hexokinase method. A mean of 894 mg/L was obtained associated with a standard deviation of 90.1. The 95 percent range is given at 714-1,074 corresponding to ± 2 standard deviations (894 − 2 × 90.1 = 713.8; 894 + 2 × 90.1 = 1,074.2) (Geigy Scientific Tables)

Figure 22.1, the normal distribution was obtained by plotting the frequency of a given value of blood sugar level on the continuous scale of mg/L. The normal curve may be considered as representative of the fasting blood glucose level in men older than 30 years. The reference range posted at 714-1,074 embracing 95 percent (95.4) of the 106 men tested was set as the norm for the nondiabetic population. This arbitrary definition of the reference range left 5 normal nondiabetic subjects outside the range either on hyperglycemic or hypoglycemic sides. Leaving for the moment the lower tail end of the curve, a normal nondiabetic subject whose fasting blood sugar level turns out to be 1,140 for example, would be classified as a potential diabetic, a false-positive result given the imposed reference range.

The normal distribution of fasting blood sugar in a sample of equal number of diabetic patients whose mean was calculated at 1,200 mg/L, superimposed on the same scale of the nondiabetic sample is shown in Figure 22.4.

The cutoff level of 1,074, the level determined for the normal sample, resulted in a crossover marked by a significant false negative equivalent to 8 percent of the area under the normal distribution of the diabetic sample ($1,074 - 1,200 \div 90.1 = -1.4z \Rightarrow 8$ percent). In contrast to the 2.5 percent false-positive area for the nondiabetic subject.

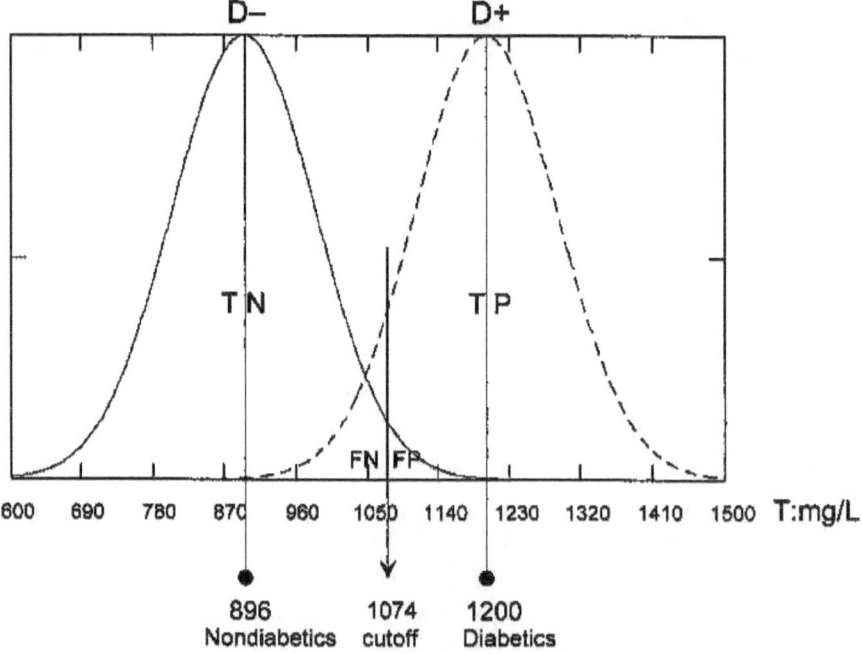

Figure 22.4 Graph of the normal distribution of fasting blood sugar in an equivalent sample of diabetic patients, whose mean was calculated at 1,200 mg/L, superimposed on the same scale of the nondiabetic sample.

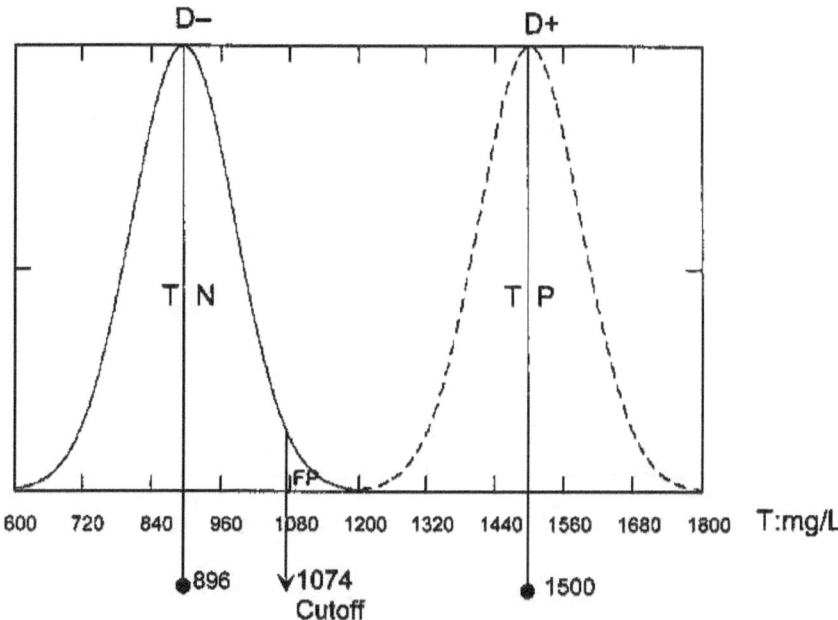

Figure 22.5 Graph of the normal distribution of fasting blood sugar in an equivalent sample of diabetic patients whose mean was calculated at 1,500 mg/L, superimposed on the same scale of the nondiabetic sample.

In this case, the crossover is practically eliminated, resulting in a clear demarcation at the 1,200 level between the diabetics and nondiabetics. Had this been the case, the reference interval could have been extended to include 99.9 percent of the subjects whose fasting blood sugar falls within ±3.37 standard deviations from the mean of 896 ($1,200 - 896 \div 90.1 = 3.37z$). Recall, however, that both the solid curve and the dashed curve extend underneath each other territory, so that the rate possibility of a false positive and false negative can never be eliminated.

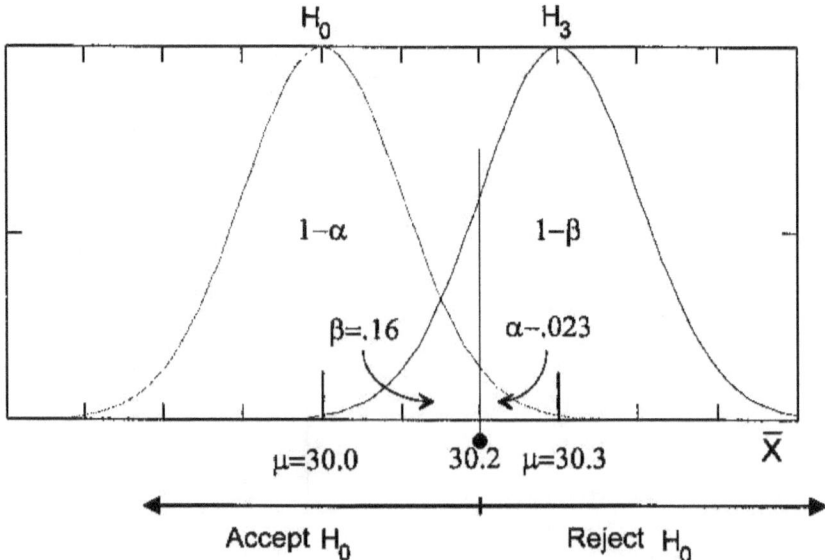

Figure 22.6 Graph of the sampling distribution of the mean of the null hypothesis centered at μ_0 of 30.0 mg juxtaposed to the sampling distribution of the alternative hypothesis H$_3$ centered on μ_3 of 30.3 mg.

Recall the sampling distribution of size n (100) drawn from the stocks of capsule by the pharmacist for validation of the accepted dosage. In contrast to the nondiabetic/diabetic curves noted earlier, whose continuous random variable was the actual level of fasting blood sugar in milligrams per liter in a given subject, the normal curves in the capsular case define the value of a given sample mean (size n) in milligrams, drawn from the population of the capsular stock. This is reflected in the labels associated with the x axis. In the diabetic case, the actual test value, T(X), constituted the random variable; whereas in the caps case, it is the sample mean value associated with a given sample size, $\overline{X}$, that constitute the random variable.

Finally, note that the partition of the sample space into four mutually exclusive and exhaustive subsets was fully explored in chapters 6, 7, and 8. Figure 22.7 parallels the definition of sensitivity and specificity (and their complements) in terms of the four conditional probabilities associated with clinically determined probability of a positive or negative test given the presence or absence of disease.

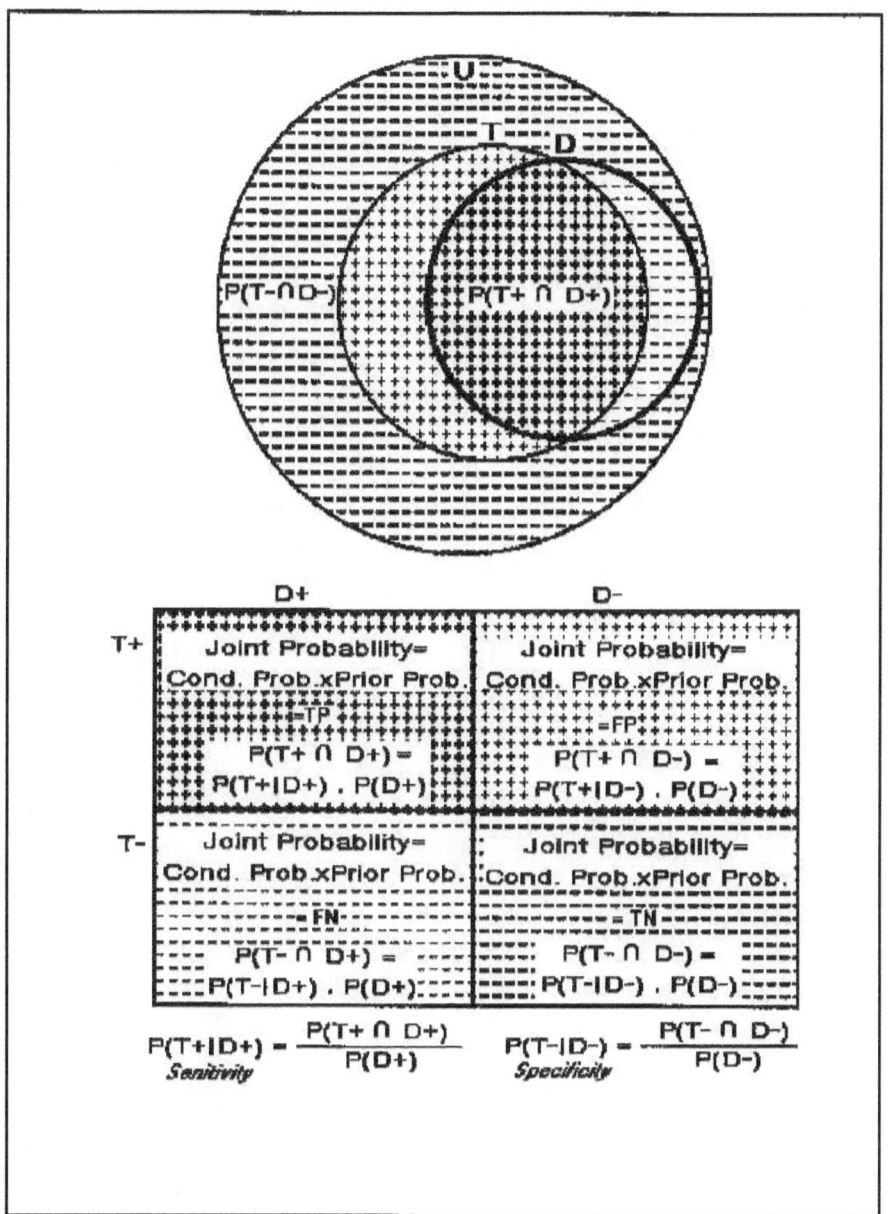

Figure 22.7 Venn diagram of the partition of the sample space into four conditional probabilities associated with clinically determined probability of a positive or negative test given the presence or absence of disease.

22.5 **Statistical versus Bayesian Inference**

The null hypothesis constitutes the classical instrument of statistical inference. Its central position requires a brief reference to its relationship to the Bayesian inference as presented in this monograph.

Bayes' theorem, as has hopefully been made clear, is essentially a technique of inductive inference in which the opinion (prior probability) held before the experiment or test is integrated into the sample evidence resulting in a modified or posterior probability. In terms of the black box, its contents in this case are presumed to be known based on an educated estimate or published data. In view of the sample at hand, a reevaluation of the actual contents is thus made possible.

In order to consolidate the inherent similarity in the variables involved in both inferential approaches Tables 22.1 and 22.2 portray the analogous and corresponding role of the variables in the two approaches.

As can be seen, the α level may be considered as the analog of the complement of specificity. However, α is arbitrarily set to reflect the tolerated error in the decision-making process. Specificity and its complement, on the other hand, are experimentally derived parameters of a given random variable or test result. The Type I error is thus analogous to the false-positive results associated with any given test.

Once α is set, β, the risk of making Type II error, may be determined from the power curve. In this sense, β is the analogous equivalent of the complement of sensitivity.

The binary table thus reflects an analogous construction in both Bayesian and statistical inference. The key element, however, is the comparison of the decision-making process in both cases.

Table 22.3 translates the variables involved in the construction of the posterior probability. At the basic level, both theories require the integration of three variables in the decision-making process.

Table 22.1

		Decision	
True State, Actual Situation — Unknown to Decision Maker		Reject H_0 — Test: T^+	Accept H_0 — Test: T^-
H_0 is false, H_1 is true $\mu_{True} > \mu_{Hypo}$ $H_1: \mu_1 > \mu_0$ Evidence in support of H_1 D^+		Correct decision Inference of difference $P(\text{Reject } H_0 \mid H_0 \text{ is false})$ $=P(\text{No error} \mid H_1 \text{ is true})$ $=1-\beta=$ Power $P(T^+ \mid D^+) \cdot P(D^+) = P(T^+ \cap D^+)$ Conditional probability (Sens) • Prior probability = Joint probability (True positive) $P(T^+ \mid D^+) =$ sensitivity	Erroneous prediction Inference of No difference $P(\text{Accept } H_0 \mid H_1 \text{ is False})$ $=P(\text{Type II error} \mid H_1 \text{ is true})$ $=\beta$ $P(T^- \mid D^+) \cdot P(D^+) = P(T^- \cap D^+)$ Conditional probability (1 − Sens) • Prior probability = Joint probability (False negative)
H_0 is True, H_1 is False D^- $\mu_{True} \leq \mu_{Hypo} \rightarrow$(upper-tailed) $H_0: \mu_1 \leq \mu_0 \rightarrow$ No evidence in support of H_1		Erroneous prediction Inference of difference $P(\text{Reject } H_0 \mid H_0 \text{ is true})$ $=P(\text{Type I error} \mid H_0 \text{ is true})$ $=\alpha$ $P(T^+ \mid D^-) \cdot P(D^-) = P(T^+ \cap D^-)$ Conditional probability (1 − Sp.) • Prior probability = Joint probability (False positive)	Correct decision Inference of no difference $P(\text{Accept } H_0 \mid H_0 \text{ is true})$ $=P(\text{No error} \mid H_0 \text{ is true})$ $=1-\alpha$ $P(T^- \mid D^-) \cdot P(D^-) = P(T^- \cap D^-)$ Conditional probability (Sp) • Prior probability = Joint probability (True negative)

Critical Value

H_b(Hypo) H_1(True) T^- T^+

H_0 is True $1-\alpha$ TN β FN α FP

H_0 is False $1-\beta$ TP

D^- H_0 D^+ H_1

True state / Actual situation	H0 : H1	Prior probability	D⁻ : D⁺
Specify / Significance level	α	Determine specificity	1 – specificity
Graph sampling / Distribution (α and β)		Graph Venn diagram: FP and FN	
Set / Critical cutoff value	$\overline{X}; z_a$	Set normal reference interval	T⁻
Specify / Alternate population mean	$\mu1$	Specify Abnormal interval mean	T⁺
Specify / Acceptable error	β	Determine sensitivity	1 – sensitivity
Determine test statistic	$\overline{X}$	Determine test result of sample	T
Action; decision	Accept H_0 / Reject H_0	Action; decision	Accept D⁻ / Reject D⁻
Outcome: error	α / β	Outcome: error	FP / FN
Outcome: correct	$1 - \alpha$ / $1 - \beta$ (Power)	Outcome: correct	TN / TP

Table 22.2

True State; Actual Situation		
D^- H_0 is true H_1 is false	D^+ H_1 is true H_0 is false	
Predictive error $P(D^- \mid T^+) = (1 - PV[+])$ $= FP / TP + FP$ Posterior probability $P(H_0$ is true $\mid$ Type I error) $\alpha / (1 - \beta) + \alpha$	Predictive accuracy $P(D^+ \mid T^+) = PV[+]$ $= TP / TP + FP$ Posterior probability $P(H_1$ is true $\mid$ No error) $1 - \beta / (1 - \beta) + \alpha$	Positive T^+ Abnormal test
Predictive accuracy $P(D^- \mid T^-) = PV[-] =$ $TN / TN + FN$ Posterior probability $=$ $P(H_0$ is true $\mid$ No error) $(1 - \alpha) / (1 - \alpha) + \beta$	Predictive error $P(D^+ \mid T^-) =$ $(1 - PV[+]) =$ $FN/TN + FN$ Posterior probability $=$ $P(H_1$ is true $\mid$ Type II error) $\beta / (1 - \alpha) + \beta$	Negative T^- Normal test

Table 22.3

True State; Actual Situation		
D⁻ H_0 is true H_1 is false	D⁺ H_1 is true H_0 is false	
Predictive error $P(D^-|T^+) = (1 - PV[+])$ $= FP / TP + FP$ Posterior probability $P(H_0$ is true | Type I error$)$ $\alpha / (1 - \beta) + \alpha$	Predictive accuracy $P(D^+|T^+) = PV[+] = TP$ $/ TP + FP$ Posterior probability $P(H_1$ is true | No error$)$ $1 - \beta / (1 - \beta) + \alpha$	Positive T⁺ Abnormal test
Predictive accuracy $P(D^-|T^-) = PV[-] = TN$ $/ TN + FN$ Posterior probability $=$ $P(H_0$ is true | No error$)$ $(1 - \alpha) / (1 - \alpha) + \beta$	Predictive error $P(D^+|T^-) = (1 - PV[-])$ $= FN / TN + FN$ Posterior probability $=$ $P(H_1$ is true | Type II error$)$ $\beta / (1 - \alpha) + \beta$	Negative T⁻ Normal test

Table 22.3(reversed)

Books on Statistics
of
Different Disciplines

Epidemiology

Friedman, G. D. *Primer of Epidemiology*. 3rd ed. McGraw-Hill, 1987.

Fletcher, R. H. *Clinical Epidemiology*: *The Essentials*. 2nd ed. Williams and Wilkins, 1988.

Sackett, D. L., R. B. Haynes, G. H. Guyatt, and P. Tugwell. *Clinical Epidemiology: A Basic Science for Clinical Medicine*. 2nd ed. Little Brown, 1991.

Wassertheil-Smoller, Sylvia. *Biostatistics and Epidemiology*. Springer-Verlag, 1990.

Biostatistics

Dawson-Saunders, Beth, and R. G. Trapp. *Basic & Clinical Biostatistics*. Appleton & Lang, 1994.

Motulsky, H. *Intuitive Biostatistics*. Oxford University, 1995.

Rosner, Bernard. *Fundamentals of Biostatistics*. Duxbury, 1990.

Clarke, G. M. *Statistics and Experimental Design*. E. Arnold, 1980.

Riegelman, Richard, and Robert P. Hirsch. *Studying a Study and Testing a Test: How to Read the Health Science Literature*. 3rd ed. Little Brown, 1996.

Hirsch, Robert P., and Richard Riegelman. *Statistical Operations: Analysis of Health Research Data.* Balckwell, 1966.

Hirsch, Robert P., and Richard Riegelman. *Statistical First Aid: Interpretation of Health Research Data.* Blackwell Scientific, 1992.

Duncan, Robert, Rebecca G. Knapp, and M. Clinton Miller III. *Introductory Biostatistics for the Health Sciences*. John Wiley, 1977.

Rees, D. G. *Essential Statistics for Medical Practice: A Case Study Approach.* Chapman & Hall, 1994.

Norman, Geoffrey R., and David L. Streiner. *PDQ Statitistics*. B. C. Decker, 1986.

Glantz, Stanton A. *Primer of Biostatistics*. 2nd ed. McGraw-Hill, 1987.

Sokal, Robert R., and F. James Rohlf. *Introduction to Biostatistics*. 2nd ed. W.H. Freeman, 1969.

Sokal, Robert R., and F. James Rohlf. *Biometry*. 2nd ed. W.H. Freeman, 1981.

Lewis, Alvin E. *Biostatistics*. Reinhold, 1966.

Everitt, Graham Dunn Brian. *Clinical Biostatistics: An Introduction to Evidence-Based Medicine* (Xerox copy). Edward Arnold, 1995.

Colton, Theodore. *Statistics in Medicine*. Little Brown, 1974.

Bailar, John C. III and Frederick Mosteller (Eds). Medical uses of statistics. *New England Journal of Medicine*, 1986

Ingelfinger, Joseph A., Frederick Mosteller, L. A. Thibodeau, and H. Ware James. *Biostatistics in Clinical Medicine*. Macmillan, 1983.

Mosteller, Frederick, Stephen W. Fienberg, and E. K. Rourke Robert. *Beginning Statistics with Data Analysis*. Addison-Wesley, 1983.

Mosteller, Frederick, E. K. Rourke Robert, George B. Thomas Jr. *Probability and Statistics*. Addison-Wesley, 1961.

Munro Barbara Hazard, Madelon A. Visintainer, and Batten Ellis. *Statistical methods for Health Care Research*. Lippincott, 1986

Dunn, Olive Jean. *Basic Statistics: A Primer for the Biomedical Sciences*. John Wiley, 1964.

Croxton, Frederick E. *Elementary Statistics with Application in Medicine and the Biological Sciences*. Dover, 1953.

Langley Russel. *Practical Statistics Simply Explained*. Dover, 1970.

Sox, Harold C. Jr., Marshal A. Blatt, C. Higgins Michael, and Keith I. Marton. *Medical Decision Making*. Butterworth-Heinemann, 1988.

Glaser, Anthony N. *High-Yield Biostatistics*. Williams & Wilkins, 1995.

Phillips, Jr. John L. *How to Think about Statistics*. Revised ed. W. H. Freeman, 1973

Phillips, John L. Jr. *Statistical Thinking*. W. H. Freeman, 1971.

Williams, Frederick. *Reasoning with Statistics.* Holt, Rinehart & Winston, 1968

Kranzler Gearald, and Janet Moursund, *Statistics for the Terrified.* 2nd ed. Prentice Hall, 1999

Bernstein, Leonard A. *Statistics for Decision: A Tool for Everybody*. Grosset and Dunlap, 1965

Bahn, Anita K. *Basic Medial Statistics*. Grune & Stratton, 1972.

Galen, Robert S., and Gambino S. Raymond. *Beyond Normality: The Predictive Value and Efficiency of Medical Diagnosis*. John Wiley, 1975

Larson, Harold J. *Statistics: An Introduction*. R. E. Krieger, 1983.

Kapadia, R., and Anderson G. *Statistics Explained: Basic Concepts and Methods*, Ellis Horwood, 1987.

Schmidt, Marty J. *Understanding and Using Statistics basic concepts*, D.C. Heath, 1975

Rowntree, Derek. *Statistics Without Tears: A Primer for Non-Mathematicians,* C. Scribner, 1981

Wulff, Henrik, R. *Rational Diagnosis and Treatment*. Blackwell, 1976

Gigerenzer, Gerd. Calculated Risk: *How to know when numbers deceive you*, Simon & Schuste, 2002

Statistics for Psychology and Behavioral Sciences

Minium, Edward W. *Statistical Reasoning in Psychology and Education.* 2nd ed. John Wiley, 1978.

Glass, Gene V., and Kenneth D. Hopkins. Statistical Methods in Education and Psychology, 2nd ed., Allyn & Bacon, 1984

McCall, Robert B. *Fundamental Statistics for Psychology.* 2nd ed. Addison-Wesley, 1983.

Keiss, Harold O. *Statistical Concepts for the Behavioral Sciences,* Allyn & Bacon, 1989.

Welkowitz, Joan, Robert B. Ewen, and Jacob Cohen. Introductory Statistics for the Behavioral Sciences. 3rd ed. Addison-Wesley, 1982.

Welkowitz, Joan, Robert B. Ewen, and Jacob Cohen. *Introductory Statistics for the Behavioral Sciences* 4th ed. Addison-Wesley, 1982

Hildebrand, David K. *Statistical Thinking for Behavioral Scientists.* Duxbery, 1986.

Clayton, Keith N. *An Introduction to Statistics for Psychology and Education.* C. E. Merrill, 1984.

Runyon, Richard P., and Audrey Haber. *Fundamentals of Behavioral Statistics.* 6th ed. Random House, 1988.

Garrett, Henry E. *Elementary Statistics,* David McKay, 1962.

Peatman, John G. *Introduction to Applied Statistics: For the Students of Psychology and the Behavioral Sciences,* Harper & Row, 1963.

Gravetter, Frederick J., and Larry B. Wallnau. *Statistics for the Behavioral Sciences,* West Pub., 1985.

Erickson, B. H., and T. A. *Nosanchuk, Understanding Data.* 2nd ed. University of Toronto, 1992

Business Statistics

Plane, Donald R., and Edward B. *Oppermann. Business and Economic Statistics*. Business Pub., 1981

Hamburg, Morris. *Statistical Analysis for Decision Making*. 3rd ed. Harcourt Brace Jovanovich, 1983.

Griffin, John I. *Statistics: Methods and Applications*. Holt, Rinehart and Winston, 1962.

Kohler, Heinz. *Statistics for Business and Economics*. 3rd ed. Harper Collins, 1994.

Brightman, Harvey, and Schneider Howard. *Statistics for Business Problem Solving*. 2nd ed. South Western Pub., 1994.

Ben-Horim, Moshe, and Haim Levy. *Statistics: Decision and Applications in Business and Economics*. 2nd ed. Random House, 1984.

Ott, Lyman, and David K. Hildebrand. *Statistical Thinking for Managers*, Duxbury, 1983.

Keller, Gerald, Brian Warrack, and Henry Bartel. *Statistics for Management and Economics: A System Approach*, 2nd ed. Wadsworth Pub., 1990

Freund, John E., Frank J. Williams, Benjamin M. Perles. *Elementary Business Statistics. The Modern Approach*. 5th ed. Prentice Hall, 1988.

Gordon, Gilbert, and Israel Pressman. *Quantitative Decision Making for Business*. Prentice-Hall, 1978.

Cook, Thomas M., and Robert A. Russel. *Introduction to Management Science*. 2nd ed. Prentice-Hall, 1981

Lapin, Lawrence L. *Statistics for Modern Business Decisions*. 3rd ed. Harcourt Brace Jovanovich, 1982.

Lapin, Lawrence L. "A Study Guide to Accompany Statistics for Modern Business Decisions," In *Introductory Statistics for Business and Economics*, eds. Thomas H. Wonnacott and Ronald J. Wonnacott. 4th ed. John Wiley, 1990

Spirer, Herbert F. *Business Statistics: A Problem Solving Approach*. R. D. Irwin, 1975.

Daniel, Wayne W., and James C. Terrell. *Business Statistics: For Management and Economics*. 6th ed. Houghton Mifflin, 1882.

Bechtold, Brigitte, and Ross Johnson. *Statistics for Business and Economics*, PWS-Kent Pub. 1989

Kazmier, Leonard J., F. Pohl Norval. *Basic Statistics for Business and Economics*. McGraw-Hill, 1984

Wallis, W. Allen, and Harry V. Roberts. *Statistics: A New Approach*. The Free Press, 1956.

Kroeber, Donald W., and Lawrence R. LaForge. *The Managers Guide to Statistics and Quantitative Methods*. McGraw-Hill, 1980.

College Statistics

Jarrell, Stephen B. *Basic Statistics*. Wm. C. Brown, 1994.

Freedman, David, Robert Pisani, and Roger Purves. *Statistics*. W. W. Norton, 1980.

Devore, Jay, and Roxy Peck. *Introductory Statistics*. West Pub., 1990.

Freund, John E. *Modern Elementary Statistics*. 7th ed. Prentice Hall, 1988.

Triola, Mario F. *Elementary Statistics*. 5th ed. Addison-Wesley, 1992.

Kohler, Heinz *Essentials of Statistics*. Scott, Forseman, 1988.

Iman, Ronald L., and W. J. Conover. *A Modern Approach to Statistics*. John Wiley, 1983.

Comrey, Andrew L, Paul Al Bott, B. Lee Howard. *Elementary Statistics: A Problem-Solving Approach*. 2nd ed. Wm. C. Brown, 1975.

Brase, Charles Henry, and Corrinne Pellillo Brase. *Understandable Statistics*. 4th ed. D. C. Heath, 1991.

Witte, Robert S. *Statistics*. 3rd ed. Holt, Rinehart and Winston, 1989.

Walpole, Ronald E. *Introduction to Statistics*. 2nd ed. Macmillan, 1974.

Harshbarger, Thad R. *Introductory Statistics: A Decision Map*. Macmillan, 1971.

Bluman, Allan G. *Elementary Statistics: A Step by Step Approach*. Wm. C. Brown, 1992.

Sincich, Terry. *Statistics by Example*. 3rd ed. Dellen Pub, 1982.

Mansfield, Edwin. *Basic Statistics with Applications*. W. W. Norton, 1086.

Huntsberger, David B. *Elements of Statistical Inference*. Allyn and Bacon, 1961.

Snedecor, George W. *Statistical Methods*. 5th ed. Iowa State College Press, 1956.

Bhattacharyya, Gouri K., and Richard A. Johnson. *Statistical Concepts and Methods*. John Wiley, 1997.

Fisher, Sir Ronald A. *Statistical Methods for Research Workers*. 13th ed. Oliver and Boyd, 1958.

Probability and Statistics

Stigler, Stephen M. *Statistics on the Table: The History of Statistical Concepts and Methods*. Harvard University, 1999.

Newmark, Joseph. *Statistics and Probability in Modern Life*. 4th ed. Saunders College Pub., 1988.

Schmitt, Samuel A. *Measuring Uncertainty: An Elementary Introduction to Bayesian Statistics*. Addison-Wesley, 1969.

Mosteller, Frederick, Robert E. K. Rourke, and George B. Thomas Jr. *Probability: A First Course*. Addison-Wesley, 1969.

Mosteller, Frederick. *Fifty Challenging Problems in Probability with Solutions*. Dover, 1965.

Adler, Henry L., and Edward B. Roessler. *Introduction to Probability and Statistics*. 4th ed. W. H. Freeman, 1972.

Dwass, Meyer. *First Steps in Probability*. McGraw-Hill, 1967.

Mendenhall, William. *Introduction to Probability and Statistics*. 5th ed. Duxbury Press, 1979.

Devore, Jay L. *Probability and Statistics for Engineers and the Sciences*. 4th ed. Duxbury, 1995.

McCord, James R. III, and Richard M. Moroney Jr. *Introduction to Probability Theory*. Macmillan, 1964.

Meyer, Paul L. *Introductory Probability and Statistical Applications*. Addison-Wesley, 1966.

Mode, Elmer B. *Elements of Probability and Statistics*. Prentice-Hall, 1966.

Goldberg, Samuel. *Probability: An Introduction*. Dover, 1960.

Freund, John E. *Introduction to Probability*. Dover, 1873.

Laplace, Marquis de. *A Philosophical Essay on Probabilities*. Dover, 1951.

Mises, Richard von. *Probability, Statistics and Truth*. Dover, 1957.

Rozanov, Y. A. *Probability Theory: A Concise Course*. Dover, 1969.

Chernoff, Herman, and Lincoln E. Moses. *Elementary Decision Theory*. Dover, 1959.

Bross, Irwin D. J. *Design for Decision: An Introduction to Statistical Decision Making*. Free Press, 1956.

Mandel, John. *The Statistical Analysis of Experimental Data*. Dover, 1964.

Adler, Irving. *Probability and Statistics for Everyman*. Signet Science Library, 1963.

Weaver, Warren. *Lady Luck: The Theory of Probability*. Anchor Books, 1963.

Baskin, John T. *Probability: A Noncalculus Introduction*. Helix Books, 1986.

Johnson, Donovan A. *Probability and Chance*. McGraw-Hill, 1963.

Wentzel, E. S. *Probability Theory: First Steps*. Mir Pub. 1977.

D'Arcy, J. A. *Chance and Choice*. Thames and Hudson, 1968.

Lowry, Richard. *The Architecture of Chance: An Introduction to the Logic and Arithmetic of Probability*. Oxford University, 1989.

Edwards, Anthony William. *Likelihood*. Johns Hopkins University Press, 1992.

Everitt, Brian S. *Chance Rules: An Informal Guide to Probability, Risk and Statistics.* Copernicus Books, 1999.

Holland, Bart K. *Probability without Equations, Concepts for Clinicians* (Xerox copy). Johns Hopkins University Press, 1998.

Holland, Bart K. *Probability without Equations: Concepts for Clinicians.* Johns Hopkins University Press, 1998.

Eigen, Manfred, and Ruthild Winkler. *Laws of the Game: How the Principles of Nature Govern Chance.* Knopf, 1981.

Goren, Charles. *Go with the Odds*: *A Guide to Successful Gambling,* Macmillan, 1969.

Orkin, Mike. *What Are the Odds: Lotteries, Blackjack, Zero-Sum Games.* B&N, 2000.

Logic

Ballard, Keith Emerson. *Copi: Introduction to Logic*. 4th ed. Macmillan, 1972.

Warring, R. H. *Logic Made Easy* (Tab book), 1985.

Kreyche, Robert J. *Logic for Undergraduates*. 3rd ed. Holt, Rinehart & Winston, 1970.

Carney, James D., and Richarad K. Scheer. *Fundamentals of Logic*. Macmillan, 1964.

Cohen, Morris R., and Ernest Nagel. *An Introduction to Logic and Scientific Method*. Harcourt Brace, 1934.

Lytel, Allan. *ABC's of Boolean Algebra*. SAMS, 1967.

Hohn, Franz E. *Applied Boolean Algebra: An Elementary Introduction*. Macmillan, 1960.

Hutchison, David, and Peter Silvester. *Computer Logic: Principles and Technology*. John Wiley, 1987.

Benrey, Ronald M. *Understanding Digital Computers*. Rider, 1964.

Polya, G. *Mathematics and Plausible Reasoning: Vol. II, Pattern of Plausible Inference*. Princeton University, 1968.